Americans
with Disabilities

Americans with Disabilities

Exploring Implications of the Law for Individuals and Institutions

Edited by
**Leslie Pickering Francis
& Anita Silvers**

Routledge
a member of the
Taylor & Francis Group

NEW YORK   LONDON

PUBLISHED IN 2000 BY

Routledge
29 West 35th Street
New York, NY 10001

Published in Great Britain by
Routledge
11 New Fetter Lane
London EC4P 4EE

Routledge is an imprint of the Taylor & Francis Group.

Library of Congress Cataloging-in-Publication Data

Americans with disabilities : exploring implications of the law for individuals and institutions / edited by Leslie Pickering Francis and Anita Silvers.
     p. cm.
    Includes bibliographical references.
    ISBN 0-415-92367-0 (hbk. : alk. paper) — ISBN 0-415-92368-9 (pbk. : alk. paper)
      1. Handicapped—Legal status, laws, etc.—United States. 2. United States. Americans with Disabilities Act of 1990. I. Francis, Leslie, 1946– II. Silvers, Anita.
KF480.A32 F73 2000
342.73'087—dc21

00-021869

This book is dedicated to the memory of
Jack Achtenberg, Greg Kavka, Jacobus tenBroek
and other early writers on the significance of
civil rights for people with disabilities. Their
pioneering scholarship enlarged our understanding
of justice and jurisprudence.

Contents

PART C Practical Applications: Work, Health, Congress and the Courts

PART C-1 Work

PART C-2 Health

PART C-3 Congress and the Courts

PART D Viewing U.S. Law from Elsewhere: Canada, the United Kingdom and Australia

Acknowledgments

Leslie Pickering Francis thanks Jay Jacobson for his helpful comments on the introduction, Cynthia Lane and Troy Booher for their help in bringing this project to fruition, and the Excellence in Research and Teaching Fund at the University of Utah College of Law for funding in partial support of this research.

Anita Silvers thanks Thomas Ehrlich for his many kindnesses, Nina Fendel for her wisdom and focus, and Dean Nancy McDermid for her generosity of spirit and her practical support. She is grateful to the late Jack Achtenberg, whose 1975 article (University of San Fernando Law Review, v.5, n.2) introduced her to the idea that people with disabilities might acquire protection against discrimination.

Both editors thank the many scholars and activists whose insights have enriched this book, and Heidi Freund for her unfailing commitment to bring liberatory scholarship to the American public.

INTRODUCTION

Achieving the Right to Live in the World
Americans with Disabilities and the Civil Rights Tradition

LESLIE FRANCIS AND ANITA SILVERS

SEEKING THE RIGHT TO BE IN THE WORLD

Writing two years after the passage of the 1964 Civil Rights Act, Jacobus tenBroek, S.J.D., Harvard; J.D., University of California, professor at the University of California, began an article for the *California Law Review* by observing: "nothing could be more essential to personality, social existence, economic opportunity—in short, to individual well-being and integration into the life of the community—than . . . the public approval, and the legal right to be abroad in the land."[1]

To be denied this right, or to experience the ire of others because one exercises it, invites the direst disadvantages segregationist policy inflicts on those whom it isolates. Accustomed himself to being denied access to the civic and commercial infrastructure because of his blindness, and often himself deprived of the right to be in the world, tenBroek was propelled throughout his career by the ambition to secure equality. His writing teems with illustrations of the growing national commitment to desegregation and equal opportunities for minorities, and the article is infused with the emancipatory optimism of the period.

Yet in 1966 Professor tenBroek himself had no legal recourse when he was precipitously and arbitrarily denied carriage on a train or plane for which he had purchased a regular ticket. Nor did he have a legal remedy when restaurants declined to serve him, or banks refused to let him deposit his money. Despite his accomplishments and inarguable competence, he expected to be held the responsible party if, in traversing the university campus, he fell into any open pit left by a repair crew or was injured in a collision with a campus vehicle. For, in virtue of his blindness, Professor tenBroek, founding president of the National Federation of the Blind and editor of *The Braille Monitor,* suffered an attenuation of the right to be in the world.

So in 1966, in the early days of an unprecedented era of liberation brought by new civil rights laws to previously marginalized groups, tenBroek probed to see what protections the law offered people who, on the basis of their disabilities, encountered inferior treatment in, and even segregation from, the civic and commercial worlds. The disabled lacked the civil rights protections afforded women and minorities by the Civil Rights Act of 1964. But beyond the lack of civil rights protection, tenBroek observed, people with disabilities lacked critical legal support in their efforts to negotiate the world. He asked:

> Does the law assure the . . . disabled, to the degree they are . . . able to take advantage of it, the right to leave their institutions, asylums, and the houses of their relatives? Once they emerge, must they remain on the front porch, or do they have

the right to be in public places . . . and to receive goods and services in . . . places of public accommodation? . . . What are the standards of care and conduct, of risk and liability, to which they are held and to which others are held in respect to them? Are the standards the same for them as for the [nondisabled]? (tenBroek, p. 842)

In the next four pages, tenBroek adduces statute after statute and case after case to learn whether the law of the time acknowledges that people with disabilities have a right to be in the world: integration is "the policy of the nation" (tenBroek, p. 847) . . . but it is widely disregarded by courts. A principal explanation is the erroneous attitudes of actors within the legal system: "jurors are almost entirely ablebodied (blind people are excluded from jury service), and the judge has sound . . . limbs, fair enough eyesight, and, according to counsel, can hear everything but a good argument." Drawing only from their own experience and ignoring the perspectives of people with disabilities, "The judge or juror . . . provide . . . a standard of reasonableness and prudence . . . including some often quite erroneous imaginings about the nature of . . . disability." (tenBroek, p. 917)

For the nondisabled are situated very differently from the disabled, tenBroek reminds us. Their "basic rights of effective public access have been long established and newly vindicated." (tenBroek, p.848) He then observes that, in sponsoring and affirming the 1964 Civil Rights Act, both President Johnson and the Supreme Court declared that denying equal access to public facilities to any group of citizens was a moral and social wrong and a burden on commerce. Although the protection the Civil Rights Act offers explicitly is against discrimination based on race, color, national origin, sex and religion, tenBroek supposes that being in the world is a human right, pertaining to all persons who are members of the community. Therefore the legal system must evolve to acknowledge the right of the disabled to access public facilities equitably. People with disabilities are human persons with community membership, he says, yet they are frequently subjected to arbitrary action and are for the most part without legal redress when turned away from trains and planes, travel, lodging, rental housing and "from bars, restaurants and places of public amusement, from banks to rent a safety deposit box, from other kinds of banks to give a pint of blood, and from gambling casinos." (tenBroek, p. 851)

Other public policy approaches to disability outside of the civil rights paradigm both predate tenBroek's powerful discussion and continue in effect today. The United States tax code contains an additional personal exemption for blindness, amounting to $850 in 1999, included on the theory that personal subsistence costs are higher for the blind.[2] Social Security provides two quite different benefit programs, both, however, rooted in the assumption that people with disabilities cannot work. Disability benefits (SSDI) replace work-based income; disabled individuals are eligible to receive disability benefits if they qualify for Social Security by having met income thresholds for forty quarters, and if they accumulated at least twenty of these quarters within the ten years before they became disabled. (These requirements are reduced proportionately for younger workers). Individuals qualify as disabled if they have a disability that is expected to last (or has lasted) at least one year, or to result in death, and that prevents them from doing any substantial gainful work. Benefits are based on a formula that reflects average earnings and age; and individuals who are receiving disability become eligible for Medicare benefits after 24 months.[3] The justification for Social Security disability benefits parallels that for retirement benefits: those who are no longer able to work should have access to income replacement as a form of insurance "earned" at least in part by their earlier participation in the workforce.

The second Social Security program, Supplemental Security Income (SSI), is an income supplement for certain low-income, categorically needy persons, including those with disabilities.[4] Unlike Social Security disability, SSI is fully need-based. To qualify, disabled individuals must fall below very strict asset ($2000 for an individual and $3000 for a couple) and income ceilings ($500 per month for an individual and $750 per month for a couple). Legal resident aliens who arrived in the United States after August, 1996, are ineligible for SSI unless they meet the requirement of forty work quarters to qualify for Social Security. SSI is a "welfare" program, justified as providing a minimal safety net for the categorically needy. As such, it has been criticized by opponents of welfare, who see it as paternalistic and encouraging of dependency; this criticism played a major role in the decision to exclude legal immigrants from SSI if they arrived in the United States after the effective date of congressional welfare reform. Whatever their plausibility against welfare programs, however, it is important to recognize that these criticisms are inappropriately directed against the income insurance or tax programs, which at least begin with the assumption that disabled people formerly or presently earn income.

As the civil rights paradigm developed, particularly after passage of the Americans with Disabilities Act (ADA), critics of these older approaches claimed that they were inconsistent with the civil rights ideal. In law, this criticism took the form of cases contending that individuals could not both claim the protection of the ADA in their struggles for equal opportunity, and at the same time seek the protection of disability benefits. However, the United States Supreme Court recently held that ADA and Social Security disability claims are not inconsistent, at least if the claimant can explain why she was both unable to work given the opportunities available to her and able to work with reasonable accommodations.[5] Nonetheless, as the discussions in this collection indicate, there remain deep tensions between the view of disability discrimination as a civil rights problem, and the view of disability discrimination as a social safety net issue.

THE CIVIL RIGHTS TRADITION: EXTENDING PROTECTION FROM NONDISABLED TO DISABLED PERSONS

Attempts to amend the 1964 Civil Rights Act to gain explicit recognition for the right of people with disabilities to be in the world began in the 1970s, but all such undertakings were defeated. The reasons were both political and conceptual, with traditional civil rights groups joining the usual opponents of government regulation to block adding disability discrimination to the list of offenses against citizens' civil rights. Representatives of the groups protected under earlier legislation feared opening it to amendments that might weaken it.[6] They also resisted increasing the numbers of groups entitled to special protection against discrimination because they did not want to compromise the interests of the originally protected groups by diffusing the focus of antidiscrimination enforcement and enlarging the number of persons eligible for compensatory programs.

Further, many people found it objectionable, and even absurd, to equate the social isolation experienced by people with disabilities with the historical exclusion of individuals on the basis of race, color, national origin, sex and religion. Representatives of groups traditionally disadvantaged on the basis of these characteristics often simply could not conceive that people with disabilities were similarly mistreated, for they supposed that people with disabilities were naturally deficient in their capability to make good use of opportunity. That is, they thought of the disabled as being naturally limited rather than as being artificially limited by arbitrary and prejudiced social practice.

To make disability a category that activates a heightened legal shield against exclusion, it was objected, would alter the very purpose of legal protection for civil rights. For doing so inevitably would transform the goal from creating opportunity for socially exploited people to providing assistance for naturally unfit people. Some even took as definitive of the disabled the selfsame attributions of incompetence they had always deemed biased when applied to women and racial minorities.

Similar reasoning brought into question Congress's authority to force compliance with measures that protect people from socially imposed disadvantage on the basis of disability. Congress can abrogate a state's Eleventh Amendment immunities only as empowered by the Fourteenth Amendment, from which issues broad power to remedy discrimination and prevent future discrimination. But when disability is defined as impairment-related dysfunction and equated with being biologically deficient, weak and incompetent, the inferior economic status and powerless political position of the preponderance of people with disabilities appear to result from their personal limitations, not from the kind of arbitrary and irrational discrimination which warrants intervention in the name of the constitutional guarantee of equal protection.

To understand disability in the former rather than the latter way suggests that the right to be in the world is an entitlement to assistance that disabled people need in order to participate in civic and commercial activity instead of a claim for eliminating arbitrary barriers to access. But the Fourteenth Amendment in no way entitles people to get help because they have corporeal or cognitive deficits. To identify disability with ill-health and deficiency undercuts the propriety of construing access for the disabled as equal protection for civil rights. Consequently, those who thought about disability in this medicalized way doubted the appropriateness of invoking Congress's Fourteenth Amendment enforcement powers to safeguard people with disabilities.

A further complication was that some of the affirmative measures required to remedy the effects of discriminatory practices were not encompassed by traditional civil rights standards. These included such concepts as the removal of barriers caused by thoughtless architectural and transportation design, and the provision of information through alternative media and adaptive modes of communication. Civil rights advocates had traditionally emphasized the similarities of excluded people to the dominant class and obscured their differences in order to highlight the arbitrariness of their exclusion. But to be integrated, people with disabilities require that their differences be acknowledged and accommodated. The difficulty was, then, how to square this need for acknowledgment with the traditional civil rights goal of equal opportunity.

So it seemed to some that, as the United States Commission on Civil Rights pronounced in 1983, "[h]andicap discrimination and, as a result, its remedies differ in important ways from other types of discrimination and their remedies."[7] From the perspective of the then-prevalent politics of homogenization, religious bigotry, racial segregation and sexism manifested themselves primarily in prohibitions against the admission of the practitioners of minority religions, people of color and women to desirable programs and positions. At the time, it was thought that simply purging practices of these prohibitions—opening the doors of schools to children of all races and the doors of workplaces to employees regardless of sex—would result in members of these groups whose achievement heretofore had been limited becoming integrated into the practices of existing institutions and thereby being launched toward success. Thus, people whose race or sex previously disadvantaged them would come to be perceived as not importantly different from the prototypically productive citizen.

But that perspective did not equally envision that boosting the warmth of the invitation to participate would successfully integrate and eventually homogenize people with disabilities. For it is one thing to effect integration simply by repealing the ordinances that require certain kinds of people to use the back door, but it might seem to be quite another when integration requires constructing ramps, instead of or in addition to stairs, up to the door. Similarly, it seems one thing to require that no one be denied full social participation because her spoken English bears the accent of a non-U.S. national origin, but quite another to require that full social participation be effected for people who cannot speak, or hear, at all. Integrating persons of the first sort appears to mean nothing more than ignoring their differences when they practice everyday speech, while integrating persons of the second sort appears to involve supplementing everyday speech by providing an interpreter who Signs.

In sum, even had it been granted that practices prohibitive to the disabled are usually arbitrary, the general thrust of remedying these exclusions was supposed to be of an order different from the remedies needed to repair or forestall discrimination against other groups. One question was whether accommodating a disability requires affirmative steps and consequently calls for public and private effort that exceeds the simple remedy of being tolerant of difference. A further issue was whether prohibiting segregation and exclusion of the disabled, who by definition are uncommonly limited in their ability to perform, would require fundamental alteration of the purpose and nature of commonplace practices. Would, for instance, nondiscrimination demand that cognitively impaired workers be employed side by side with normal ones, and would doing so devastate the efficient productivity that defines commercial aims, thus fundamentally compromising the institution of work? A remedy like this could not help but seem excessive to someone who believes that efficiency is paramount, much less to someone who believes that an individual's cognitive impairment naturally disqualifies that person from useful pursuit of opportunities for self-support and social advancement.

BUILDING LEGAL SAFEGUARDS AGAINST DISABILITY DISCRIMINATION

Of course, from the transformative standpoint brought about by the past two decades of the politics of difference, it now is clear that repairing a long history of discrimination against any group requires changes in institutions that deny recognition to people by neglecting their differences. Equality calls for adjustment to difference, not just tolerance of it. However, for the quarter-century that followed the Civil Rights Act of which Jacobus tenBroek had such high hopes, few provisions to relieve people with disabilities of their exclusion from the opportunities made available to everybody else were integrated into comprehensive legislation aimed at safeguarding them along with other minorities. (The Fair Housing Amendments Act of 1988, 102 Stat. 1619, is a notable exception.) Instead, their protections against discrimination were fashioned mainly by enacting or amending statutes pertaining solely or principally to the disabled.

Important laws of this kind include the Architectural Barriers Act of 1968, 82 Stat. 718; the Rehabilitation Act of 1973, 87 Stat. 355; the Education for All Handicapped Children Act of 1975, 89 Stat. 773; the Developmental Disabilities Assistance and Bill of Rights Act Amendments of 1975, 89 Stat. 486; the Voting Accessibility for the Elderly and Handicapped Act of 1984, 98 Stat. 1678; and the Air Carrier Access Act of 1986, 100 Stat. 1080. Section 504 of the Rehabilitation Act was considered the most far-reaching provision against discrimination. Embedded in a multipronged legislative program meant to resituate people with disabilities by facilitating their getting work, Section 504 enjoined recipients of federal funds against excluding such individuals: "No otherwise qualified handicapped individual . . . shall, solely by reason of his handicap, be excluded from the participation in, be denied the benefits of, or be subjected to discrimination under any program or activity receiving federal funds."[8]

What these laws have in common is a delineation, either implicitly—as in the Architectural Barriers Act—or explicitly—as in the Rehabilitation Act, of the minority of people they are targeted to protect. Originally, the Rehabilitation Act defined the "handicapped" people it benefited as: "Any individual who (a) has a physical or mental disability which for such individual constitutes or results in a substantial handicap to employment and (b) can reasonably be expected to benefit in terms of employability from vocational rehabilitation services."[9] In 1974, the act was amended to define a person with a disability as someone who satisfies the following disjunctive test: (a) has a physical or mental impairment, (b) has a record of such a physical or mental impairment, or (c) is regarded as having such a physical or mental impairment.[10]

A year earlier, in 1973, Sections 503 and 504 had been included in the Rehabilitation Act. Section 503, 29 U.S.C. § 793 (a), specifies that holders of federal contracts in excess of $10,000 "shall take affirmative action to employ and advance in employment qualified individuals with disabilities." Section 504, 29 U.S.C. § 794 (a), provides for "nondiscrimination under federal grants and programs." It directs that: "No otherwise qualified individual with a disability in the United States . . . shall, solely by reason of handicap, be excluded from the participation in, be denied the benefits of, or be subjected to discrimination under any program or activity receiving Federal financial assistance or under any program or activity conducted by any Executive agency."

Although these provisions were groundbreaking at the time the Rehabilitation Act incorporated them, they had much less strength and scope than the civil rights laws of the time offered women and minorities. Section 504 prohibited discrimination "solely by reason of . . . disability," which at least suggests that disability discrimination is acceptable when conjoined with other kinds of bias. In 1986, the National Council on the Handicapped observed that while public policy aimed at eliminating discrimination against other groups generally, the Rehabilitation Act attacked disability discrimination *per se* and prohibited it only "when it is found in a pristine, isolated, unadulterated form."[11]

Moreover, the means required to remedy discrimination, such as the removal of barriers and the provision of reasonable accommodations, were described only in the implementing regulations for the Rehabilitation Act[12] and thereby were subject to challenge as outside the statutory mandate. The first federal disability rights law that explicitly requires making reasonable accommodations to people's disabilities is the Fair Housing Amendments Act of 1988.[13]

As for scope, only federal contractors and other recipients of federal money were prohibited from discriminating. Further, the Rehabilitation Act does not give victims of disability discrimination a private right of action, and only very rarely did the federal agencies charged with enforcement do anything more in response to complaints than issue findings. The absence of effective enforcement and the indifference of many covered entities to compliance with the Act are evidenced by the pervasive disregard of Section 503's requirement, 29 U.S.C. § 793 (a), that employers receiving federal funds act affirmatively to employ and promote people with disabilities: almost all universities developed affirmative action plans for women and minorities, but almost none have such a plan on file for people with disabilities.

Finally, the Rehabilitation Act, in all its sections, concentrates on providing vocational rehabilitation through individualized training, rehabilitation counseling, and independent living and support services to individuals with disabilities, in order to facilitate their employment and economic self-sufficiency. Inclusion and integration into society form a secondary goal. Thus, the Rehabilitation Act's main emphasis is helping people with disabilities overcome their personal limitations, not helping society overturn the limitations biased practice imposes on the disabled.

Frustrated in respect both to drawing the disabled under the shield of the Civil Rights Act and to achieving the equivalent of civil rights protection through other kinds of laws, the disability community turned toward the idea of developing a comprehensive federal statute aimed at forbidding discrimination based on disability. In 1986, the National Council on the Handicapped, a federal agency, published *Toward Independence,* a report that recommended provisions such a law should include and gave the prospective statute a name, "The Americans with Disabilities Act."[14] Subsequently, the council drafted its own bill and had it introduced into the 100th Congress in 1988, but the Congress expired without action being taken.

On behalf of the bill, there was call for greater political visibility. Thousands of Americans with disabilities lobbied their federal representatives, and many engaged in pro-ADA civil disobedience.[15] Disability groups not normally in alliance forged a strong coalition and courted the civil rights leadership. Such organizations as the Leadership Conference on Civil Rights and the American Civil Liberties Union contributed lead personnel who worked full time on securing broad-based support to extend civil rights protection to the disabled.[16]

A revised bill was introduced in May 1989. Testimony in support of the bill played upon two main themes. One was reducing the fifty-seven-billion-dollar cost to the nation of disability benefits paid out to people who could become productive taxpayers if discrimination no longer kept them from the employment rolls.[17] This potential outcome was portended by a Harris Organization survey, which found two thirds of unemployed working age individuals with disabilities wanted to work but could not find employment.[18]

The second major theme evidenced in the testimony deplored the irrational and harmful segregation that pervaded the experience of Americans with disabilities. Examples in congressional committee reports cite an individual banned from an auction house because she used a wheelchair and was deemed disgusting to look at, children with Down syndrome denied admission to a zoo so as not to upset the chimpanzee, a woman with arthritis denied a job at a college because the trustees believed "normal students shouldn't see her," and a woman fired from a job because her son had AIDS.[19] Sharon Mistler, who helped to coordinate nationwide ADA advocacy, recalled "being refused service in restaurants and theaters because I was a fire hazard, dehydrating so that I could go to school because my chair wouldn't fit into the bathroom, being kicked off airplanes, being directly told 'We don't want you people next door or on the bus or on the street.'"[20]

After several amendments and two conferences to reconcile differences in the House and Senate versions, the House approved the final version on July 12, 1990, by a vote of 377 to 28. The Senate approved the act on the following day, by 91 to 6. On July 26th, 1990, President George Bush signed the Americans with Disabilities Act, stating that the nation was "taking a sledgehammer . . . to a wall which has, for too many generations, separated Americans with disabilities from the freedom they could glimpse, but not grasp."[21] Americans with disabilities had achieved what they hoped would prove a legal remedy against abrogation of their right to be in the world.

THE AMERICANS WITH DISABILITIES ACT

Although achieving the right to be in the world was the primary goal of advocates for disability rights, the Americans with Disabilities Act as enacted was multipurposed. Indeed, Congress enumerated nine separate findings in support of the act. Grouped thematically, the aims of the act included eliminating arbitrary prohibitions against being in the world, ending inequality of opportunity, and reducing the costs to the United States of unnecessary dependency. While not necessarily incompatible, these aims do not always point in the same direction, and the strains among them have become increasingly significant over the ten years since passage of the ADA.

More specifically, Congress, in passing the ADA, found that over 43 million Americans had at least one disability, and that the number was increasing as the population aged, 42 U.S.C. § 12101 (a) (1). In support of achieving being in the world, Congress noted the historical segregation of people with disabilities, (a) (2); the discriminatory effects of architectural, transportational and other barriers, (a) (5); the inferior educational and economic status of people with disabilities, (a) (6); and the various ways in which people with disabilities have been treated as a "discrete and insular minority," (a) (7). In support of achieving equal opportunity, Congress observed that people with disabilities have continued to experience discrimination in critical areas such as voting or employment, (a) (3); that they encounter unequal opportunities in public benefits, (a) (5); and that, unlike other victims of discrimination, they frequently have no available legal means to address such discrimination, (a) (4). Finally, Congress observed that "the continuing existence of unfair and unnecessary discrimination and prejudice . . . costs the United States billions of dollars in unnecessary expenses resulting from dependency and nonproductivity," (a) (9). The next-to-last finding summarized all three of these basic aims: "the Nation's proper goals regarding individuals with disabilities are to assure equality of opportunity, full participation, independent living, and economic self-sufficiency for such individuals. . . ." (a) (8).

Toward these ends, the ADA pursues three major strategies. Title I addresses inequality in employment, Title II, inequality in public services, and Title III, inequality in services and accommodations offered by private entities. In addition to the general statement of purpose just described, some critical further elements are common throughout all three titles. Most importantly, "disability" is defined to include "a physical or mental impairment" that substantially limits at least one "major life activit[y]," a record of having such an impairment, or being regarded as having such an impairment, 42 U.S.C. § 12102 (2). Specifically excluded from the definition of disability, however, are illegal drug use, 42 U.S.C. § 12210; homosexuality, bisexuality and tranvestism, 42 U.S.C. § 12211 (a) (b) (1); and compulsive gambling, kleptomania, or pyromania, (b) (2). Individuals are protected from retaliation and coercion for asserting their rights under the act, 42 U.S.C. § 12203. Individual choice is specifically respected; no one may be required to accept accommodations or other rights under the act, § 12201 (d), unless they choose to do so. Attorneys' fees are available for prevailing parties in proceedings under the act § 12205, and alternative dispute resolution is encouraged for resolving disputes, § 12212. Finally, the act § 12212 claims to abrogate state sovereign immunity from suits seeking any remedies available against private entities under the ADA.

Title I of the ADA, the employment discrimination title, balances equality of employment opportunity against costs of accommodation to employers in a compromise that has proved controversial, as many of the articles in this collection demonstrate. Title I applies to employers with more than 15 employees (but not the United States, Indian tribes or certain private clubs), § 12111 (5). It prohibits job discrimination against "qualified individual[s]" with disabilities, because of the disability, in terms and conditions of employment. An individual is "qualified" by virtue of his or her ability to perform "essential functions" of the job, with or without accommodation; however, the employer's judgments as to essentiality are critical, particularly if they have been incorporated in a prior written job description § 12111 (8). Prohibited "discrimination" includes practices that curtail equality of opportunity, although once again there are employer-protective limitations. Employers are required to make "reasonable accommodations" for people who can, as a result, succeed on the job; examples of such accommodations include making facilities accessible, restructuring work schedules and providing readers or interpreters, § 12111 (9). But "reasonable accommodations" do not include actions of "significant difficulty or expense," measured in terms of costs of the accommodation, financial resources of the facility at issue and financial resources of the employer as a whole, § 12111 (10). The Interpretive Guidance issued by the Equal Employment Opportunity Commission (which indicates the commission's positions but does not have the legal force of regulations) recommends that employer and employee use a problem-solving approach to work out which employment practices would afford the disabled employee opportunities to perform on the job that are equal to those of a similarly situated nondisabled employee.[22] As several of the contributions to this volume indicate, there has been ongoing tension over the meaning of reasonable accommodations. One source of the tension has been the multiple goals of the ADA itself: whether the goal of reasonable accommodation is to achieve work in the world for people with disabilities, or whether it is principally to "level the playing field" between the disabled and the nondisabled. On the former view, the ADA is an affirmative action statute, aimed to further the right to be in the world of work. On the latter view, however, the ADA is a nondiscrimination statute, simply requiring employers not to erect unjustified barriers in the path of opportunities for people with disabilities.[23] Another source of the tension has been how to balance opportunities for the employee against expenses for the employer.

Title II of the ADA prohibits discrimination in publicly provided services, activities or programs. It parallels Title I in requiring reasonable accommodations for individuals who are "qualified" to receive the public services, in the sense that they meet essential eligibility requirements, with or without reasonable accommodation, § 12131 (2). And it has generated controversies similar to those that have arisen under Title I. In addition, Title II sets out quite specific standards for public transportation, § 12141-12165, surely a critical aspect of the right to be in the world for people with disabilities.

Finally, Title III of the ADA governs public accommodations provided in the private sector. Unlike the other major sections of the ADA, Title III affords protections that are not limited to "qualified individuals." Instead, Title III, § 12182, requires nondiscrimination "in the full and equal enjoyment of the goods, services, facilities, privileges, advantages, or accommodations of any place of public accommodation." This requires the provision of goods and services in "the most integrated setting appropriate to the needs of the individual" and the opportunity to participate in mainstream activities even if separate activities are also available. It specifically prohibits the failure to remove barriers, the imposition of eligibility criteria unless "necessary for the provision" of the goods or services, and the failure to take steps to avoid excluding people with disabilities unless "taking such steps would fundamentally alter the nature" of the good or service. Title III also has specific accessibility requirements for new construction and for transportation serving the public.

Even here, however, there are noteworthy, cost-motivated exceptions that surely affect being in the world: newly constructed and altered buildings of fewer than three stories are not required to have elevators, unless they are shopping centers, shopping malls or offices of health care providers, § 12183 (b); and over-the-road (that is, long-distance) buses are not required to have accessible rest rooms if the result would be a loss in seating capacity, § 12186 (a) (2) (C). Despite these limits, Title III is the section of the ADA which affirmatively pursues the right to be in the world most directly, although as the chapter by Ruth Colker in this volume indicates, it is not immune from criticism in this regard.

THE ADA IN THE COURTS

Not surprisingly, it took nearly ten years before the United States Supreme Court attacked problems of interpretation under the ADA. In its initial decision interpreting the ADA, the Court held that nonsymptomatic HIV infection is a "disability" under the ADA because it interferes with a major life activity (reproduction), and that a dental office is a public accommodation under Title III of the ADA. The Court also concluded that a practitioner's judgment about whether treatment posed a health or safety threat was entitled to deference only if it was objectively reasonable.[24]

In five decisions in 1999, the Court addressed several contentious issues under the ADA. The import of these decisions for persons with disabilities is mixed. First, the *Cleveland* decision held that an individual's application for welfare-based disability benefits does not preclude pursuit of remedies under the Americans with Disabilities Act; if the individual can show that although she or he was denied employment, and thus could not work, she or he nonetheless remained qualified to work.[25] In an appropriate case, therefore, it is possible for an individual both to claim the need for support because she was denied the opportunity to work, and to assert that she was unfairly denied equal opportunity to exercise her capacity to work.

Second, the *Olmstead* case challenged a state's refusal to provide recommended community placements for patients with mental disabilities. The state's justification for refusing to provide the placements was financial; because of limited funding, the state contended, requiring immediate community-based placements would "fundamentally alter" the nature of state-provided services.[26] The Court of Appeals had concluded that unwarranted institutionalization was discrimination, and that in assessing the state's "fundamental alteration" defense, the trial court should weigh the costs of providing the two community-based placements at issue in the litigation against the overall state mental health budget, a comparison favorable to the plaintiffs since it was unlikely that the costs of two community-based placements would radically alter the structure of state services. In remanding to the District Court, the Supreme Court agreed that it is discrimination under Title II to fail to provide recommended community-based services, but accepted a far less stringent understanding of the fundamental alteration defense: "In evaluating a State's fundamental-alteration defense, the District Court must consider, in view of the resources available to the State, not only the cost of providing community-based care to the litigants, but also the range of services the State provides others with mental disabilities, and the State's obligation to mete out those services equitably."[27] This language in Justice Ginsburg's opinion was joined by only three other justices; Justice Stevens would have supported the Court of Appeals' position,[28] and Justice Kennedy would have given more deference to physicians and state policy-makers, including a decision not to provide community-based placements at all.[29] *Olmstead* is an important recognition that the ADA opposes the segregation of people with disabilities. On the other hand, disability rights advocates may find it a pyrrhic victory if it results in increased difficulty for plaintiffs seeking to challenge chronic under-funding of state services or if it signals that the Court is willing to take a generally broad view of the costs and hardships that limit ADA requirements. Eva Kittay's discussion, in Part A below, is powerful testimony to the importance of the support that allows people with disabilities to remain in their homes and communities rather than experiencing the segregation of institutionalization.

The other three cases decided in 1999 significantly curtailed and confused the under-standing of disability under the ADA. Unlike other civil rights statutes, the ADA requires a threshold determination that an individual is disabled before he or she can claim the act's protection. Narrowing the understanding of disability will both limit the scope of the act and could, depending on the form the narrowing takes, reconceptualize the act as being nothing more than a reduction of dependency statute for individuals whose impairments significantly compromise their competency. The three 1999 decisions point to an under-standing of disability that insists on significant personal loss of capacities—what has been called the "medical model" of disability[30]—and grants employers wide discretion in mak-ing business decisions. If interpretation of the ADA continues in this direction, it will in-creasingly function as a statute that balances limited opportunities against their perceived costs. The discussions in Part B of this volume defend different approaches to defining dis-ability, and the discussions in Part C explore whether cost-based limits are justifiable.

In *Sutton,* the principal case of the three defining disability, the plaintiffs challenged United Airlines' vision requirements for pilots (uncorrected vision of at least 20/100). The Court held that the Sutton sisters' myopia should be assessed in its corrected rather than its uncorrected state, and that they should be regarded as disabled only if, with correction, they were unable to perform a major life activity such as working. Although they could not meet United Airlines' standard for pilots despite the fact of vision that was fully correctable, the sisters could and did work as pilots for a United feeder airline, and so were not dis-abled.[31] The Court offered three reasons for this conclusion: the language of the ADA indi-cates that its focus is whether a person is presently disabled; disabilities must be evaluated on an individualized basis; and Congress's statement of purpose in the ADA did not include all of the people whose disabilities are sufficiently corrected to enable them to function effectively. Indeed, the Court said, Congress's estimate of the numbers of people with disabilities (43 million in 1990), clearly indicates that Congress did not mean to sweep the majority of Americans with corrected disabilities within the reach of the ADA.[32]

In a second decision handed down with *Sutton,* the plaintiff Hallie Kirkingburg chal-lenged a refusal by Albertson's to continue to employ him as a commercial truck driver because he had monocular vision. Albertson's decision rested on a federal safety require-ment; although waivers of the requirement became available, in fact, because of doubts about whether the regulation really was justified, Albertson's did not seek a waiver for Kirk-ingburg. Before his vision was properly assessed by Albertson's, Kirkingburg had worked for over a year without any vision-related difficulties; although he later received a federal waiver, Albertson's refused to rehire him. In rejecting Kirkingburg's challenge, the Court first commented that Kirkingburg's monocular vision should not be regarded as a disability unless it was a "substantial limitation," judged on the basis of his ability to compensate for the impairment.[33] The principal focus of *Kirkingburg,* however, was whether the plaintiff was "otherwise qualified," and the Court held that Albertson's was entitled to rely on a federal regulation in determining that he was not, without further inquiry into the reasonableness of the regulation or its application in the particular case.[34] Kirkingburg thus faced a paradox: he was not disabled because of his ability to compensate for his lost vision in one eye, but Albertson's was free to rely unquestioningly on a federal regulation that judged individuals with monocular vision to be unsafe drivers.

In the final decision, Vaughn Murphy challenged his dismissal from United Parcel Service because of hypertension that exceeded federal safety regulations for truck drivers. The Court held that whether the impairment—hypertension—substantially limited a major life activity must be determined based on the quality of the individual's life with mitigating measures taken into account. Thus Murphy could be considered disabled only if, with medication, his hypertension made him unable to continue working.[35] Unfortunately for Murphy, although his hypertension was not controlled to the level that permitted him to meet federal safety standards, it was sufficiently controlled to permit him to perform at least some jobs, and so, the Court concluded, it did not interfere with the major life activity of working.

These decisions understand disability to be a property of the individual that can be superceded by corrective treatment or mechanical devices. Their result is that individuals will find it more difficult to claim the protections of the ADA to the extent that they have overcome or corrected their disabilities, as Arlene Mayerson and Matthew Diller point out forcefully in Part B below. They may also find it more difficult to claim that the major life activity of "working" means the ability to explore a range of options, rather than merely being able to obtain any kind of employment at all. As this book goes to press, this and many other issues about the direction and impact of the ADA remain unresolved in the courts; their resolution may greatly affect the extent to which the ADA furthers the rights of people with disabilities to be in the world.

UNRESOLVED ISSUES

Despite the passage of ten years and the exponential growth of litigation, theoretical treatment of the ADA remains sparse and much more limited than that afforded other civil rights statutes. Compared with the enormous volume of literature about race and gender, little attention has been paid to the theoretical understanding of disability. Nor is there agreement about how to integrate the health-related and socially conditioned aspects of the disability experience. In general, there has been almost no progress in linking the conceptualization of disability to efforts to facilitate understanding and achieve the purposes of disability discrimination law.

Moreover, the fundamental question of what approach to justice the ADA represents—whether it should be viewed as a nondiscrimination or an affirmative action statute—left unresolved in the congressional statement of purpose has not been explored extensively. But it is critical to understanding the ultimate directions that will and should be taken with respect to the ADA as interpretation of the statute evolves. This neglected discussion is taken up in the contributions to Part A of this volume, especially in those by Patricia Illingworth and Wendy Parmet, Richard Arneson and Thomas Pogge. So is the further theoretical question of whether justice offers the best foundation for pursuing the purposes of the ADA, or whether appeals to other values—the good, the virtues, or the moral quality of social roles—are more compelling.

The initial premise of citizens with disabilities who believed disability discrimination law would secure their right to be in the world was that they are just people seeking the same opportunities others take for granted.[36] Nevertheless, the threshold issue in applying the ADA is not whether an individual is the same as other people but whether the person is disabled. Mark Kelman addresses the importance of this special assignment of disability status in the opening essay in Part B of this volume; in essays in the same section, Mary Crossley and David Wasserman both question whether disability or the stigmatization of difference is the underlying issue of justice that is most compelling. In Part A, Lawrence Becker, Eva Kittay and Alasdair MacIntyre all consider this question.

Despite the Court's 1999 decisions, there are many uncharted areas about the meaning of disability, several of which are explored in Parts B and C of this volume. The Court's apparent embrace of the understanding of disability in terms of deficiencies in the disabled person has already drawn much criticism. The essays by Ron Amundson, Mary Crossley and Anita Silvers in Part B criticize various aspects of this medicalized understanding of disability as individual impairment. Amundson addresses the assumption that biological normality can be distinguished from biological dysfunction, Crossley criticizes the coherence of the distinction employing the examples of pregnancy and obesity, and Silvers considers the complexities of employing a functional account of disability in the context of disability discrimination law. Whether the Court will continue down this path remains to be seen.

Moreover, deciding who is disabled continues to be troublesome in other respects. Imprecisions in the ADA's definition of disability, which requires that limitations be substantial and that the limited activities be major, contribute to the confusion about who is protected by the ADA. If current legal trends continue, it appears that "major life activity" will be defined in very basic terms, to include activities such as breathing, moving, thinking, working or reproducing. If a person must be substantially incapable of executing such broad activities to qualify as disabled, the class of people who are disabled will be limited to the more severely incapacitated, and the applicability of the ADA will be correspondingly limited. As Iris Marion Young points out in Part C, such narrowing has the risk that those who do not qualify for the protection of the ADA will resent those who do. At present, as Ruth Colker's empirical work demonstrates, a very high percentage of plaintiffs lose on summary judgment on issues involving the definition of disability, and it seems possible that the Court's 1999 decisions will only entrench this trend.[37]

Perhaps the problem with the 1999 cases is that they did not raise the third prong of the ADA's definition of disability: whether the individual was "regarded as" disabled. How this prong is understood will surely make a major difference to the reach of the ADA. This is the prong that brings the ADA most in line with other civil rights statutes, for in order to come within it, an individual need not prove an actual feature of him or herself but merely that a judgment made by someone else invoked the relevant category—in the case of the ADA, the category of disability. Some appellate court decisions, however, appear to be reading the definition of actual disability into the "is regarded as" prong. Courts have held, for example, that an employer must regard the individual as unable to perform a major life activity, and not just erroneously judge the individual's ability to do the job under consideration, in order to "regard" the individual as disabled.[38] On the remedy side, another critical issue for "is regarded as" plaintiffs is whether they are able to claim the advantages offered by the ADA to actually disabled plaintiffs. "Is regarded as" plaintiffs may be able to demonstrate that they are "otherwise qualified" by showing that they are able to perform essential functions of the job, rather than all of the position's functions. They also may be entitled to reasonable accommodations.[39] Linking "is regarded as" plaintiffs to "actually" disabled plaintiffs in this way seems to make particularly good sense for the case of plaintiffs who have limited impairments requiring accommodations but are erroneously viewed by their employers as completely unable to work in their current jobs. The approach has been criticized as "absurd," however, because it may entitle plaintiffs who are not actually disabled to claim protections as though they were disabled.[40] This controversy, like others about the ADA, reaches deeply to questions about the nature of justice the ADA is meant to provide.

A further "gatekeeping" issue in applying Title I of the ADA is whether the individual is "otherwise qualified." In *Kirkingburg,* the Court indicated a willingness to defer to employer judgment, at least where the employer was relying on federal safety regulations. How far this deference will extend, however, remains an open question. At least some lower court decisions have indicated a willingness to impose standards on employers. For example, plaintiffs have been required to show only that they can perform "essential functions" of the position,[41] and employers have been required to reassign employees to other available jobs that are within their capacities.[42] *Kirkingburg,* however, viewed the statutory language as quite deferential to employer judgment. How "otherwise qualified" is understood is critical to the kind of protection afforded by the ADA. If individuals must be able to fit within employer judgments, understood in a broadly deferential way, then the ADA will require limited rethinking on the part of employers about what they have traditionally expected of employees. But if employers must meet substantive standards of reasonableness in judging qualifications, they may be forced to reassess traditional patterns, to reconsider whether it is how jobs are constructed that has led to judgments that people with disabilities cannot "do the job." In Part C–1 below, Peter Blanck, Gregory Kavka, Michael Stein and Iris Marion Young take different stances in considering this issue.

If individuals are "otherwise qualified," the ADA requires "reasonable accommodations," but not if these result in "undue hardship" to the employer. Once again, the extent of deference to employer judgment is critical to the reach of the ADA. So, too, is the issue of costs; one of the standard economic objections to the ADA is the costs its critics allege it imposes on employers—an objection directly criticized by Michael Stein in his contribution to this volume. If "reasonable accommodations" require only inexpensive assistive devices, significant job restructuring will not take place. By contrast, if employers are required to rethink how jobs are organized and job responsibilities are assigned, the world may adjust far better to the differences of individuals. Thomas Pogge, writing in Part A, and Anita Silvers, in Part B, disagree about whether it is reasonable to demand the reform of common practices so as to include people with disabilities.

Both "reasonable accommodations" and "undue hardship" are highly fact-specific judgments, so it is not surprising that there is little legal theory interpreting these concepts. Some cases, however, once again suggest deference to the employer; for example, USAir was not required to rethink its decision to abandon part time positions in order to accommodate an employee whose working hours were limited by carpal tunnel syndrome.[43] Another issue here that has yet to be decided is what it means for the employer to concentrate on facility-specific costs, rather than costs for the enterprise as a whole, in arguing that costs are too great for accommodations to be required. Still a further cost-based issue will be the difference between discrimination and actuarially justified differences that are allowed for insurance benefits.

Yet another issue is the defense that making a structure, program or activity accessible will fundamentally alter its nature. In deciding whether to accept such a defense, courts have accorded great deference to the conventions of some kinds of endeavors—for instance, to universities' academic requirements—but less deference to others—for instance, to professional sports associations' rules of play. Unfortunately, there is almost no legal or philosophical theory to guide judgment about whether a change in practice, made to accommodate an individual's disability, is a fundamental or instead an inessential alteration.[44] There is also dispute about whether it is discriminatory to reduce the resources on which the disabled especially rely for support. Current calls for rationing health care and social services make this a particularly pressing problem to resolve, as many people with disabilities have special health and service needs. In Part C–2, Dan Brock and David Orentlicher take different positions on the ADA's implications for health care allocation, Joel Feinberg considers the intersection of disability and illness, and Norman Daniels explores equality of opportunity for people with mental impairments.

Many critical questions remain unanswered about the significance of the apparent trends to narrow the reach of the ADA. Does the Court's current direction undercut the premise that the disabled are just people seeking to fulfill expectations common to all citizens, such as the right to work defended by Gregory S. Kavka in Part C, or the right to health care? If protection against disability discrimination is interpreted as applying only to a narrowly defined group, are others who do not qualify more likely to resent the statute's protection of those who do? Is the statute more likely to be perceived as unfairly imposing inefficiencies on employers? More likely to impose problematic demands on the health care system? Will there be a call for prohibiting practices that aid only the disabled because these are perceived as discriminating in reverse? This prospect is not simply a legal issue, for it emerges from political concerns about acting preferentially towards minority groups. These practical and political issues are the substance of Part C of the volume.

Can action pursued under the ADA eventually eliminate the social disadvantages from which citizens with disabilities suffer today? In Part C–3, Andrew I. Batavia and Richard Scotch wrestle with this question. Harlan Hahn posits that it will be difficult to make real progress against disability discrimination until courts recognize the extent to which the disadvantageous conditions imposed on the disabled are intentional and not a by-product of benign neglect. Lennard Davis offers a similar analysis, arguing that the justice system unwarrantedly discounts the extent to which hate fuels practices that are injurious to people with disabilities. In their essays, both Ruth Colker, and Lori Andrews and Michelle Hibbert examine trends in judicial responses when people with disabilities seek compensatory relief.

A final set of unresolved problems, for the ADA as well as for other civil rights statutes, is Congress's power to authorize lawsuits that seek to remedy violations by state governments or their agencies. In *Kimel v. Florida Board of Regents*,[45] the U.S. Supreme Court held that Congress does not have the constitutional power under the 14th amendment to enforce prohibitions against age discrimination by state governments. *Kimel* gives no explicit indication of the Court's position about disability discrimination, although it cites *Cleburne*[46] for the proposition that age classifications, unlike classifications based on race or gender, should not be deemed to reflect prejudice. Federal appellate courts are divided on the parallel issue for the ADA.

Under current constitutional doctrine, Section 5 gives Congress the power to remedy violations of the Fourteenth Amendment but not to expand the Amendment's scope.[47] If differential treatment of the disabled must pass only a rational-basis test to comport with equal protection, the ADA would appear to expand the scope of the Fourteenth Amendment, or so the Eighth Circuit argued.[48] On the other hand, if the Fourteenth

Amendment prohibits invidious discrimination against the disabled, and Congress explicitly adopted the ADA to this end, then the ADA is properly regarded as a remedial statute.[49] The underlying philosophical questions here are the federal power to shape a standard of equal protection and to hold the states to it.

In the decade since the passage of the ADA, regulations to guide implementation of the law have been developed, promulgated and revised; compliance plans have been written (although some entities required to do so have no such plan on file); and cases have been tried, decided, appealed and decided even by the United States Supreme Court. Yet the extent to which the ADA and the exercise of civil rights can or should secure the well-being of people with disabilities remains unresolved. Do the disabled really benefit from a rights-based approach aimed only at removing barriers and leveling the playing field of opportunity? Or should public policy focus instead on making provisions to relieve their special needs? Or should the effort be cultivating virtuous conduct toward people with disabilities on the part of the nondisabled majority?

As the ADA reaches its tenth anniversary, we appear not much theoretically advanced beyond the Supreme Court's unsuccessful attempt to distinguish between nondiscrimination and "affirmative efforts to overcome the disabilities caused by handicaps" in *Southeastern Community College v. Davis,* a case decided over twenty years ago under Section 504 of the Rehabilitation Act.[50] In *Davis,* the Court insisted that only nondiscrimination had been authorized by Congress. Subsequently, the Court acknowledged, in a footnote to *Alexander v. Choate,*[51] the confusion this earlier language had caused. The footnote includes an attempt to distinguish between reasonable accommodation and affirmative action by characterizing the latter as substantially modifying or fundamentally altering the nature of a program.[52] Yet interpretation of the ADA remains beset by this fundamental unclarity.

From a global point of view, the ADA stands as powerful testimony to the expansiveness of civil rights law. In Part D, Jerome Bickenbach, Mairian Corker, and Melinda Jones and Lee Ann Basser Marks contrast the ADA with how disability is treated in English legal systems that lack a civil rights tradition. Their contributions offer a comparative method for weighing whether affirmative measures of support are more central than prohibitions against discrimination in remedying the disadvantages experienced by citizens with disabilities.

Despite standing as a beacon of hope for disabled people around the globe, the ADA has its critics. To them, the statute raises more questions than it answers, and invites more problems for society at large than it resolves for people with disabilities. To a large extent, failure to examine the conceptual, philosophical, political and legal foundations of the ADA invites such complaints. To advance beyond the absence of theory that has attenuated progress during the first decade of the ADA, this volume brings together leading philosophers, legal scholars and political theorists—many of whom have backgrounds in bioethics or in disability studies—to explore these critical issues. In honor of the ADA's tenth anniversary, this volume aims to provide both philosophical and legal analysis that will guide achievement not only of the right to be in the world that Jacobus tenBroek invoked over thirty years ago, but also of the broader goals of opportunity and inclusion envisioned by the civil rights movement that transformed American life in the last half of the twentieth century.

NOTES

[1]Jacobus tenBroek, "The Right to Live in the World: The Disabled in the Law of Torts," 54 Cal. L. Rev. 841 (1966).

[2]26 U.S.C. § 63(c)(3), (f). See also John K. McNulty, *Federal Income Taxation of Individuals*. St. Paul, MN.: West Publishing Group, 1999.

[3]42 U.S.C. § 423. For a useful discussion of the differences between Social Security disability and SSI, see Carolyn A. Kubitschek and Barbara Samuels, *Social Security and SSI Disability*. New York: Practising Law Institute, 1999.

[4]42 U.S.C. § 1382c. For a discussion of the impact of the 1996 welfare reforms on the elderly and disabled, see Leslie P. Francis, "Elderly Immigrants: What Should they Expect of the Social Safety Net?" 5 *The ElderLaw Journal* 229 (1997).

[5]*Cleveland v. Policy Management Systems Corp.*, 119 S. Ct. 1597 (1999).

[6]Robert L. Burgdorf, Jr., "The Americans With Disabilities Act: Analysis and Implications of a Second-Generation Civil Rights Statute," 26 *Harv. C.R.-C.L. L. Rev.* 413, 429 (1991).

[7]United States Commission on Civil Rights, "Accommodating the Spectrum of Individual Abilities," Washington, DC: 1983,149.

[8]29 U.S.C. §749 (1994).

[9]Pub. L. 93–112, § 7(6), 87 Stat. 355, 362 (1973).

[10]Rehabilitation Act Amendments of 1974, Pub. L. 93-516, 88 Stat. 1617 (1974) this volume.

[11]National Council on the Handicapped, *Toward Independence*. Washington, DC: National Council on the Handicapped 1986, A–19.

[12]29 C.F.R. part 1630 (1998).

[13]42 U.S.C. §§ 3604(f)(3)(C) and 3604(f)(3)(B)(1988).

[14]*Toward Independence*, 18–21.

[15]President's Commission on Employment of People with Disabilities, *Worklife*, Special ADA Issue vol. 3, no. 3, Fall 1990. Washington D.C., p. 2.

[16]*Worklife*, 7, 16.

[17]*Worklife*, p. 13.

[18]Lou Harris and Associates. "The ICD Survey of Disabled Americans: Bringing Disabled Americans into the Mainstream" (1986), 50.

[19]Robert L. Burgdorf, Jr., "The Americans with Disabilities Act: Analysis and Implications of a Second-Generation Civil Rights Statute," 26 *Harv. C.R.-C.L. L. Rev.* 413, 418–419 (1991).

[20]*Worklife*, 18.

[21]*Worklife*, 11.

[22]"Interpretive Guidance on Title I of the Americans with Disabilities Act, 29 C.F.R. part 1630, Appendix (1998).

[23]For an argument that the ADA is a "level the playing field" rather than an "affirmative action" statute, see Allen Dudley, "Comment: Rights to Reasonable Accommodation Under the Americans with Disabilities Act for 'Regarded as' Disabled Individuals," 7 Geo. Mason U. L. Rev. 389 (1999) (arguing that the rights of "regarded as disabled" individuals should be narrowly construed).

[24]*Bragdon v. Abbott*, 524 U.S. 624 (1998).

[25]*Cleveland v. Policy Management Systems Corp.*, 119 S. Ct. 1597 (1999).

[26]*Olmstead v. L.C.*, 1999 U.S. LEXIS 4368 (June 22, 1999).

[27]1999 U.S. LEXIS 4368, at *30.

[28]1999 U.S. LEXIS 4368, at *46 (Stevens, J., concurring in part and concurring in the judgment).

[29]1999 U.S. LEXIS 4368, at *47 (Kennedy, J., concurring in the judgment).

[30]See, e.g., Adam A. Milani, "Living in the World: A New Look at the Disabled in the Law of Torts," 48 *Cath. U. L. Rev.* 323, 329 (1999) ("the focus of the medical model is on how the individual adapts to his or her disability, not how society as a whole should deal with people with disabilities").

[31]*Sutton v. United Airlines, Inc.*, 1999 U.S. LEXIS 4371 (June 22, 1999).

[32]1999 U.S. LEXIS 4372, at *22.

[33]*Albertson's, Inc. v. Kirkingburg*, 1999 U.S. LEXIS 4369, at *18 (June 22, 1999).

[34]1999 U.S. LEXIS 4369, at *39.

[35]*Murphy v. United Parcel Service, Inc.,* 1999 U.S. LEXIS 4370 (June 22, 1999).

[36]See, e.g., Robert Burgdorf, "'Substantially Limited' Protection from Disability Discrimination: The Special Treatment Model and Misconstructions of the Definition of Disability," 42 *Vill. L. Rev.* 408–585 (1997).

[37]Ruth Colker, "The Americans with Disabilities Act: A Windfall for Defendants," 34 *Harv. C.R.-C.L. L. Rev.* 99 (1999).

[38]See, e.g., *Weber v. Strippit, Inc.,* 186 F.2d 907 (8th Cir. 1999); *Lessard v. Osram Sylvania, Inc.,* 175 F.3d 193 (1st Cir. 1999); *Standard v. A.B.E.L. Services, Inc.,* 161 F.3d 1318 (11th Cir. 1998).

[39]*Deane v. Pocono Medical Center,* 142 F.2d 138 (3d Cir. 1998) (en banc).

[40]Allen Dudley, "Comment: Rights to Reasonable Accommodation Under the Americans with Disabilities Act for 'Regarded as' Disabled Individuals," 7 *Geo. Mason L. Rev.* 389 (1999).

[41]E.g., *Deane v. Pocono Medical Center,* 142 F.3d 138 (3d Cir. 1999) (en banc).

[42]E.g., *Smith v. Midland Brake, Inc.,* 180 F.2d 1154 (10th Cir. 1999) (en banc).

[43]*Terrell v. USAir,* 132 F.3d 621 (11th Cir. 1998).

[44]See Anita Silvers and David Wasserman, "The Double Edge of Convention: Disability Rights in Sports and Education," 18 *Newsletter of the Institute for Philosophy and Public Policy,* 1 (1998).

[45]2000 U.S. LEXIS 498.

[46]*Cleburne v. Cleburne Living Center,* 473 U.S. 432 (1985).

[47]*City of Boerne v. Flores,* 521 U.S. 507 (1997).

[48]*Alsbrook v. City of Maumelle,* 184 F.3d 999 (8th Cir. 1999) (en banc).

[49]*Dare v. California,* 1999 U.S. App. LEXIS 22351 (9th Cir., Sept. 16, 1999).

[50]442 U.S. 397 (1979).

[51]469 U.S. 287 (1985).

[52]300–301, n. 20.

Foundations
Justice, Goodness and Disability Rights

Civil rights statutes may reflect a wide variety of approaches to justice and rights. Different theoretical approaches, to be sure, will recommend corresponding differences in the range of protections offered. Libertarians will be concerned to protect people from force, fraud and the unjustified deprivation of property. Those who see justice as fair equality of opportunity will aim to remove barriers that make it more difficult for some than for others to have access to major means for achieving the good life, such as education, employment or health care. Others will go further, seeking to assure that each individual is guaranteed at least a minimally decent life.

With respect to the prohibition of discrimination based on race, these theoretical differences are at play in the debates among defenders of limiting remedies to compensation for past injuries and correction of existing discrimination, who believe that the vestiges of discrimination have largely been eliminated in contemporary society; proponents of ongoing efforts to eliminate current and future discrimination; and advocates for more extensive affirmative action. In the area of disability rights, this debate has been complicated by a history of misguided paternalism. Discrimination against people with disabilities has been rationalized by false beliefs about inadequacy, incompetence and difference. The disabled have been segregated by being placed in custodial care in supposedly protective institutions. They have been excluded from public life out of unfounded fears that their attempts to participate would humiliate them, put them at risk or be uncomfortable or burdensome to nondisabled people. This history raises questions about whether a statute directed specifically to preventing discrimination against people with disabilities furthers their equality or threatens to undermine it. Should the ADA be understood as making the ordinary right of equal protection meaningful to people with disabilities? Or, should it be viewed as extending special rights they need if protection for them is to be meaningful? Which of these, or perhaps other, interpretations of the statute and its goals best furthers genuine equality?

In the first essay of this section, Wendy Parmet and Patricia Illingworth attack this concern head on. They argue that positive and negative rights cannot be distinguished, and that the Americans with Disabilities Act is properly viewed as a statute establishing positive rights. Parmet and Illingworth argue that when we see the ADA as a positive-rights statute, and disability as spread broadly throughout the community, we will fully support genuine equality for all.

Richard Arneson also criticizes the nondiscrimination approach, but from the perspective of a prioritarian theory of justice. On Arneson's welfarist, responsibility-catering prioritarianism, institutions and practices should be arranged to maximize moral value, which roughly corresponds to welfare. Adjustments should be made, however, for the responsibility or lack of responsibility which individuals bear for their circumstances. Arneson's prioritarianism would recommend significant commitments to accommodations for people with disabilities, at least when such accommodations would enhance welfare for individuals who are not otherwise responsible for their disadvantageous situations.

Also within the liberal tradition, Thomas Pogge distinguishes consequentialist and semiconsequentialist forms of liberalism. Semiconsequentialism would require removing barriers which thwart the efforts of persons with disabilities to hold jobs, but would not require affording them the means to make up for their individual disadvantages. Pogge contends that the distinction between the elimination of discrimination and the assignment of special rights to compensate for inequalities cannot be sustained in the effort to understand justice for people with disabilities.

The other three writers in Part A shift the focus from the theory of justice to the good life and the good community. All do so by questioning whether claims about rights constitute the most propitious basis for enhancing the social inclusion of people with disabilities. In Lawrence C. Becker's view, the foundational point is recognition of the fundamental good of agency. If we see the ADA in terms of this indisputable good, rather than in terms of contentions about rights, we will not be caught up in the problem of whether it is a "nondiscrimination" or an "affirmative action" statute. Instead, we will interpret the ADA as an instrument for achieving the value of agency; all individuals should be offered the support necessary to achieve at least conventional levels of agency to the extent they are able.

While Becker focuses on the good of independent individuals, Eva Kittay explores the moral value achieved by promoting interdependence and connectedness between people with and people without disabilities. Narrating what she has learned from her relationship with her profoundly disabled daughter, Kittay observes that institutional segregation sacrifices this value, impoverishing both the lives of people with disabilities and the lives of their families and communities. Thus it is broadly beneficial to interpret the ADA as requiring that people with disabilities be given the option of living in the community. By placing the Supreme Court's *Olmstead* decision within a framework derived from recent work in feminist ethics, Kittay offers an expanded foundation for understanding the purpose of the "most integrated setting" provision of the ADA.

Alasdair MacIntyre likewise both welcomes the result of *Olmstead* and criticizes the reasons given by the Court for its decision. MacIntyre is committed to a standard of care for the mentally disabled that enables them to live with as much independence in the community as they can. But he does not think the nondiscrimination norm of the ADA can yield this conclusion. What we need instead is an understanding of the "standard of care" required of the community, which can then be enforced evenhandedly by the courts. MacIntyre is not contending that the disabled are an "other" to be patronizingly tended by the abled. Rather, we are all dependent and interdependent throughout our lives, and we must recognize our mutual needs. In the end, MacIntyre suggests, even laws such as the ADA are in some sense beside the point. For it is only when we act virtuously toward each other that we will see the standard of care as a source of self-understanding important to us all, and not as an adversarial, costly drain on existing resources.

Positively Disabled
The Relationship between the Definition of Disability and Rights under the ADA

PATRICIA ILLINGWORTH AND WENDY E. PARMET

Since the enactment of the ADA in 1990, the seemingly simple question "who has a disability?" has dominated analysis and interpretations of the Act. In 1998, in *Bragdon v. Abbott*,[1] the Supreme Court faced the question in the case of HIV disease, concluding in a closely divided opinion that an individual who was infected with HIV but not overtly ill did in fact have a disability, because she had a condition which interfered with the major life activity of reproduction. More recently, the Court appeared to veer in the opposite direction, ruling in *Sutton v. United States*[2] that an individual whose impairment is controlled by medication or other mitigating measures does not have a disability within the meaning of the Act.

As a result of the *Sutton* decision, individuals with a wide array of chronic conditions, from epilepsy to diabetes, will likely be found not to have a disability. To the Supreme Court, this narrowing of the Act's coverage was necessary, despite the opposition of the Federal administrative agencies which enforce the Act,[3] because of the statute's definition of disability.

The debate about who has a statutory disability is closely connected to larger cultural and political debates about the nature and prevalence of disability.[4] Moreover, the statute's text appears to invite these queries. In contrast to other civil rights statutes, such as Title VII of the Civil Rights Act of 1964,[5] Titles I and II of the ADA generally prohibit discrimination only against an "individual with a disability," rather than anyone who is discriminated against on the basis of disability.[6] The statute thus usually requires that an individual who brings a claim show that he or she falls within the protected class, before the existence of discrimination can be considered. As a result, defendants can seek summary judgment on the question of disability and, when they succeed, forego a trial on the merits. The question of disability therefore can serve as a barrier to a plaintiff's ability to obtain relief under the statute.

The ambiguity of the statute's definition of disability is also surely to blame. The definition states that an individual with a disability is one who:

(i) has a physical or mental impairment which substantially limits one or more of such person's major life activities, (ii) has a record of such an impairment, or (iii) is regarded as having such an impairment.[7]

This language is amenable to an infinite array of interpretations. For example, the statute on its face leaves unclear the question before the Supreme Court last year: whether an impairment that can be corrected by medication is one that substantially limits one or more major life activities.[8] Also uncertain is whether the third, "regarded as," prong of the definition includes individuals who are regarded as having an impairment which is

3

substantially limiting because of the attitudes of others, or whether the prong applies only when a defendant actually believes that an individual is substantially limited in one or more major life activities due to the physical impact of the impairment.[9]

Other textual ambiguities can be demonstrated, but they alone cannot fully explain why the determination of disability in the context of the ADA is so controversial. After all, the ADA is not the only statute with textual uncertainties. Yet the ADA's definition of disability has been subject to unusually intense debate and litigation. And, to a degree never anticipated by the statute's drafters, the definition has served to defeat ADA claims.[10] The reason why this has occurred, we believe, stems in part from a deeper and ultimately misguided concern about the nature of the rights that the Act creates. In effect, the disability question acts as a proxy for debates about the nature of rights under the ADA and how widely available they should be.

To pursue these arguments, we begin with a brief discussion about the nature of legal rights. In so doing, we contrast positive rights and positive freedoms with negative rights and negative freedoms, and we explore the criticism that has often greeted the recognition of positive rights. Despite that criticism, we argue that in important respects all rights are positive. We then turn to the ADA itself, and consider the type of rights it promises, and why those rights do not fall neatly into any simple dichotomy of positive and negative rights. We then explain why the novelty and complexity of ADA rights has led many courts to seek a narrow and limited definition of disability. In conclusion, we argue that this response is ill advised, and that the type of rights provided by the ADA require a broad and generous interpretation of disability. In other words, we suggest that the gate should be kept open.

I

To begin, let us consider the nature of rights. In general, to have a right is to have a claim on someone or some institution. Rights are not gifts, to be given or not. They are a demand that must be met. Thus, as Henry Shue points out, rights are closely connected to human dignity.[11]

Rights can be classified in a number of ways: moral and legal, and positive and negative. We consider each of these in turn. Moral rights, such as various rights to liberty (e.g., Locke's life, liberty and property) and what have come to be called "natural rights" generate ethical claims and corresponding obligations by others. For example, when people claim that there is a universal right to health care, they seek to impose upon others the duty to provide health care. But moral rights are not enforceable by legal mechanisms. Jeremy Bentham therefore dismissed one species of them, natural rights, as "nonsense on stilts."[12] Moral rights are not, however, completely impotent in social debate. Certainly they can influence the public discourse over legal rights.

The legal theorist Wesley Newcomb Hohfeld developed an important analytic framework for understanding legal rights.[13] Hohfeldian legal rights create a legal claim to protection against interference by others or permission to forego providing assistance to others.[14] A legal right in this sense generates a corresponding legal duty in someone else. And it is the job of the state to enforce these legal rights.

There are many legal rights. There are rights to sue and rights to contract. There are rights to criticize the government and rights to not be denied a job due to one's race. These rights have some bite to them because they have the force of the state behind them. But this neutral description of Hohfeldian rights is silent about the highly politicized quality rights have taken on.

Rights also serve to protect freedom. Isaiah Berlin put it nicely when he said that rights have to do with the "frontiers of freedom which nobody should be permitted to cross."[15] As protectors of freedom, rights occur against a particular concept of liberty. Isaiah Berlin drew a distinction between negative and positive liberty. Negative liberty refers to a sphere in which an individual cannot be interfered with by others, including government.[16] Recall John Stuart Mill's famous harm principle. Roughly, the only time the state is justified in interfering with a person's freedom of action is when the action harms another person.[17] Thus the harm principle reflects a concern with negative liberty. By limiting state action to those instances when actions harm other people, the harm principle limits state intrusion on individual liberty as much as possible.

Underlying this view of freedom and the significance placed on it is a seventeenth century view of human nature that C. B. Macpherson called "possessive individualism."[18] For Hobbes, the essence of human freedom is: "freedom from dependence on the wills of others."[19] The individual is a: "proprietor of his own person and capacities, owing nothing to society for them."[20] This view, which is reflected in contemporary forms of libertarianism including law and economics,[21] envisions society as a series of voluntary relations among proprietors.[22] To further freedom in this sense, the less government the better.

But as Isaiah Berlin pointed out, negative liberty does not exhaust the concept of freedom. There is also positive freedom. According to Berlin, "the positive sense of the word 'liberty' derives from the wish on the part of the individual to be his own master."[23] Liberty in this sense has to do with the desires people have to be in control of their own lives, to have self-determination over their actions. But self-determination in this sense should not be equated with simply being let alone. Instead, it has to do with having some understanding of one's desires and motives and having some control over how they influence one's actions. Others have referred to freedom in this sense as "autonomy."[24]

Corresponding to these different concepts of "freedom" are different views of what rights should look like. If freedom is envisioned as negative liberty, rights protect that liberty in so far as they too are negative. Negative rights protect people from interference from others and from state intrusion. Rights such as the right to free speech are characterized as negative because they impose on the state a duty to refrain from interfering with an individual's speech. In contrast, positive rights are connected to positive freedom. Positive rights, such as the rights to education and health care, consist in the state having a duty to provide the right's holder with something. If people have a right to education, then the state has actually to provide them with schools, teachers, books, pencils, and so on. Positive rights are also called entitlements or subsidies, and they are often associated with welfare politics. Individuals, however, may also have a claim for positive rights from other individuals, as a child has a right to care and support from parents. Although Holmes and Sunstein argue that it is confusing to identify positive liberty with positive rights, there is certainly a connection between paradigmatic positive rights and how we conceive of positive liberty.[25] For example, education and health care are paradigmatic of positive rights because they are tools for self-development.

When freedom is understood as negative, serving the interests of possessive individualism, it may be seen as inconsistent with recognizing positive rights. Since possessive individualism privileges the individual's independence from others, including the government, it is skeptical of positive rights that by definition necessarily require interaction and interdependence between the individual and others. Once individuals receive positive rights and thereby are given something, they become dependent in a way that is disfavored by those who view liberty through the lens of negative freedom.

Arguably, providing people with only negative rights is not enough to ensure that they will be their own masters, that is, truly autonomous. For some people, autonomy might well require more than simply being left alone. Many if not all individuals require the help of the government (or others) to become their own masters. Put differently, C. B. Macpherson points out that if we recognize only negative rights "to naturally unequal individuals, we are in fact denying equal freedom and humanity to all but the stronger and more skillful."[26]

Ultimately, the distinction between negative and positive rights may be spurious. Holmes and Sunstein, building upon the insights of the legal realists,[27] argue that all rights are in part positive. "To the extent that rights enforcement depends upon judicial vigilance, rights cost, at a minimum, whatever it costs to recruit, train, supply, pay and (in turn) monitor the judicial custodians of our basic rights."[28]

Holmes and Sunstein do a good job of outlining some of the costs associated with the state protection of so-called negative rights. To begin, they point out that when a person has a negative right, she can seek relief from a judge in the event of its violation. Rights will be respected and corresponding duties met only if the state and its various enforcement mechanisms are viewed by the community as possessing relevant authority.[29] This involves costs. Courts are one important way that remedies are provided to people who have had their rights violated. But they are an expensive publicly financed mechanism that needs to be made available at all times.[30] Judges must be paid, courts housed, purchased and maintained, records kept and research done. Moreover, in order to protect yet other rights, such as the Fourth Amendment's negative right against unreasonable searches and seizures, state mechanisms must themselves be monitored, an effort which requires further public financing.[31]

There are other publicly funded mechanisms for protecting rights. For example in 1996, the Consumer Products Safety Commission spent $41 million in protecting consumers against hazardous products.[32] In the same year, the Occupational Safety and Health Administration (OSHA) spent $306 million ensuring that employers met their duties to provide safe workplaces to their employees.[33] Despite these costs, the rights protected by these agencies are typically framed as negative rights: the right to be free from hazardous products and places.

Traditionally, rights to equal opportunity have been conceptualized as negative rights because they limit the way in which others may treat the rights-bearer, without obligating others to bestow any resources or benefits upon the rights-bearer. Hence equal opportunity to higher education implies that admissions offices not artificially limit opportunities for admission (on racial grounds, for example). It does not require a school to alter its standards or provide a student with financial aid in order that he or she can actually attend and succeed at the school.

Just as apparently negative rights are not wholly negative, rights to equal opportunity, upon close examination, are also more complex. Alan Goldman claims that: "opportunities are equal in some specified or understood sense when persons face roughly the same obstacle or obstacles of roughly the same difficulty of some specified or understood sort."[34] Goldman believes that equal opportunity is necessary for fairness reasons, in order for people to deserve the positions they have.[35] He reasons that people deserve the fruit of their labor only if the competition has been fair. Thus corrections need to be made for arbitrary differences among people that might impair their ability to compete. Consequently, access to employment qualifications should be equal. To achieve such equality of opportunity with respect to qualifications, society must correct for social and natural qualifications, because both are potentially undeserved. Goldman argues that society accepts that people deserve what they make for themselves.[36] But when society is responsible for establishing obstacles to people's well-being, then the burden is on society to remove these obstacles. Nothing in this explanation of equal opportunity restricts society to using only negative rights to correct for arbitrary advantages. Indeed, this view implies that positive rights or entitlements may be necessary to ensure that equal opportunity is realized.

A fair competition guarantees that people deserve their benefits and thus should enjoy them. Presumably, this guarantee will be at least as valuable to those who have an abundance as to those who do not. This point is not to be minimized because it shows that the entitlements of equal opportunity may most clearly benefit those in the worst-off positions, but insofar as they justify the distribution, they also benefit the best-off. Holmes and Sunstein make a related point about the mutually beneficial nature of rights when they explain that rights, even private rights, are publicly funded and supported because they are "social bargains generating mutual benefits and providing the terms for social cooperation."[37]

Despite the arguments suggesting that the demands of equal opportunity cannot be realized on a strict negative-rights model, laws designed to guarantee equal opportunities have traditionally been conceptualized as protecting negative liberties, or, in common parlance, guaranteeing equal opportunity.[38] Thus Title VII of the Civil Rights Act of 1964,[39] the cornerstone of American civil rights laws, prohibits employers from disadvantaging individuals due to their race or gender. The act, however, does not require employers to take affirmative steps to alter the underlying conditions that may make women or minorities appear less qualified.[40] For example, Title VII does not require that an employer provide paid maternity leave, even though the lack of such leave may harm female employees. Instead, Title VII requires only that if the employer provides paid sick leave, it may not be denied to new mothers.[41]

The practice of affirmative action, of course, challenges the idea that civil rights laws are purely negative. Affirmative action changes the status quo in fulfillment of Goldman's understanding that when individuals are differentially situated due to arbitrary factors, equal opportunity requires that adjustments be made in order to equalize qualifications. Yet the controversy over affirmative action and the fact that courts see it as antithetical to rather than necessary for equal opportunity illustrate the preference granted to negative rights.[42] In a regime of negative rights, the claim that affirmative action is appropriate to redress past discrimination against groups that have historically suffered from systematic discrimination will be limited by the demands that such remedies be closely tailored to specific instances of past discrimination.[43] In the absence of a close connection to a breach of negative liberty, affirmative action is seen as a demand for problematic positive rights, which may appear especially troubling when the rights are aimed against other individuals instead of the state. Given the belief that such positive entitlements infringe upon the rights of others, our legal and political systems seek to keep such rights limited.

For whatever historical and cultural reasons, freedom in the United States has been largely (if mistakenly) understood as negative freedom. Recognition of positive rights has been reluctant. Where they are forthrightly recognized, such rights have either come under attack (as in the case of welfare rights or affirmative action), or have been distributed parsimoniously.

II

The genius of the ADA is that it forthrightly melds positive and negative rights, creating a civil rights statute that goes beyond the simplistic equal-opportunity-as-negative-rights model represented by Title VII. Unfortunately, given the powerful grip of possessive individualism and its preference for negative rights, the novelty of the ADA's blend of rights creates confusion, particularly with respect to the key question of to whom the statute applies. As noted above, most civil rights laws have been envisioned as declarations of negative liberty. To that extent, courts have seldom displayed great concern over whether a plaintiff should be entitled to a statute's benefits. No one, after all, should be denied a right to "equal opportunity."

As a result, although Title VII was enacted to provide protections to racial minorities and women, it has consistently been held to provide identical rights to men and European-Americans.[44] Indeed, the critical inquiry in Title VII cases is never the parties' membership in the protected class,[45] but the question of whether the defendant was motivated by a forbidden ground (race or sex).

Disability law has traditionally departed from this convention because laws concerning disability have usually taken the form of positive entitlements. Assuming that disability constituted an incapacity or inability to be self-sufficient in a world of negative liberty, American law has historically endorsed the differential treatment of individuals with disabilities. Usually that differential treatment meant lesser or harsher treatment. Thus laws have supported the segregation, disenfranchisement and even confinement of individuals with disabilities.[46]

More recently, the differential treatment of individuals with disabilities has taken the form of positive entitlements to benefits or services that are designed to assist individuals with disabilities who are presumed unable to be self-sufficient.[47] Vocational training, income replacement and even special educational programs were enacted throughout this century to provide individuals with disabilities with positive rights not otherwise available to the general population.[48]

Political acceptance of these positive rights for individuals with disability rights has been largely dependent upon first accepting a narrow understanding of disability. Thus, because these positive rights are seen as paternalistic, exceptional and corrosive of negative freedoms, they have been politically sustainable only because they were made available to discrete groups of individuals who could not otherwise be self-sufficient in a regime of negative rights.[49]

The tight correlation between positive rights and narrow definitions of disability is evident from recent attempts to limit the definition of disability in public income replacement programs. As Matthew Diller has shown, both the Social Security Disability Insurance (SSDI) and Social Security Income (SSI) programs have historically been privileged, as compared to other public assistance programs, because of their close association with a medical model of disability.[50] In other words, these rights were widely accepted as long as individuals with disabilities were perceived of as ill, not at fault and incapable of independence. In 1990 those assumptions were threatened when the Supreme Court, in *Sullivan v. Zebley*,[51] interpreted the Social Security Act in such a way as to expand greatly the number of children eligible for benefits. An intense political debate ensued. Testifying before the Senate Finance Committee in 1995, Carolyn Weaver, Director of Social Security and Pension Studies at the American Enterprise Institute, traced the "rapid growth" of children enrolled in SSI to the *Zebley* case and questioned whether the children receiving benefits are "seriously disabled" and whether, in any event, they should receive payments. Perhaps to emphasize the point that those who received payments after *Zebley* were not "truly deserving," of the positive rights SSI gave them, Weaver pointed out that two thirds of the growth in the system went to children with "behavioral problems."[52] She also noted reports suggesting that children were being "coached" to misbehave, in other words, that an expansion of the definition of disability in light of *Zebley* had enabled those who do not deserve the positive entitlements of SSI to obtain them.

Responding to such concerns, Congress amended SSI by narrowing the definition of eligibility to ensure that children with "less serious" conditions were no longer considered disabled.[53] Thus, because it served as a gatekeeper into a program of positive rights, the definition of disability in SSI was narrowed so that a program designed as an exception to the dominant model of negative rights did not become commonly available.

III

The dispute over the ADA's definition of disability reflects the close and problematic relationship between constructions of disability and the nature of disability rights. To the extent that the ADA is thought to follow in the footsteps of prior civil rights laws and enforce negative liberties, a broad construction of disability is widely accepted as appropriate, for the rights protected are deemed universal. If, in contrast, the ADA is seen as an extension of earlier entitlement programs for individuals with disabilities, a broad definition of disability appears problematic, for it threatens to make positive rights commonplace. The problem for those construing the definition of disability, of course, is that the ADA is the heir to both traditions.[54] It is both a civil rights statute and a grant of special treatment. As such, neither a narrow nor a universal construction of its definition quite makes sense.

The hybrid nature of the ADA is apparent throughout the statute. Like other civil rights statutes, the ADA broadly prohibits discrimination on the basis of disability. However, in contrast to Title VII, the ADA does not stop with a guarantee of equal opportunity understood within a negative-rights framework. The ADA does not simply say that individuals with mobility impairments have the same rights as others to climb the stairs. Instead, in a variety of ways, the ADA follows Goldman's insights about equal opportunity by requiring employers (and others) to accommodate the needs of individuals with disabilities and reorder the social world to take into account the interests and needs of such individuals. Thus the ADA gives individuals with disabilities the positive right to demand changes (and contributions) from others, including private actors, to enable individuals with disabilities to become self-sufficient and participate more fully in public life.

This complex fusion of positive and negative rights can be seen by reviewing briefly the ADA's employment provisions. Title I of the act prohibits discrimination and appears to foster the negative goal of allowing individuals with disabilities to compete in the workplace. Unlike SSI or other more clearly paternalistic statutes, Title I provides no entitlement of either cash or a job. It only ensures that "qualified" individuals with disabilities may work free from discrimination.[55] In this sense, the ADA promises only equal opportunity as a negative right. It does not create a positive entitlement.

On the other hand, Title I is not your typical employment discrimination statute. While it applies only to individuals who are "qualified," it also requires employers to adjust their workplaces so that individuals with disabilities are more likely to be "qualified." Under Title I, a qualified individual with a disability is not an individual with a disability who meets the employer's stated job qualifications. Rather, a qualified individual with a disability is one who is able to meet the "essential functions" of the job "with or without reasonable modifications."[56] Moreover, the act requires employers to use "qualification standards, employment tests or other selection criteria" in such a manner as not to screen out or tend to screen out individuals with a disability unless the standard or test can be shown to be "job-related for the position in question and is consistent with business necessity."[57] Although individuals with disabilities are not given an entitlement to a job, they are given the right to demand "reasonable accommodations" and to prohibit employers from imposing job qualifications that disadvantage individuals with disabilities unless they are actually necessary to ensure that hired employees can do the job.

Advocates for the ADA such as Anita Silvers[58] have argued that these provisions do not demand positive rights and that the ADA contrasts sharply with prior paternalistic legislation for individuals with disabilities because of the lack of enfeebling entitlements. In some ways, this is true. The ADA provides neither cash assistance nor fundamental modifications of the workplace. Individuals with disabilities are given no assurance that they will be given a job or that all of the their needs will be met. In this sense, the ADA contrasts radically with more clearly positive entitlement programs such as SSI.

Moreover, modifications demanded by the ADA can also be fashioned into the negative-rights model by describing them as mere recompense for past discrimination. Workplaces, as well other social institutions, have traditionally been designed without the needs or interests of individuals with disabilities in mind. If that neglect is described as discriminatory, as it surely is, then the modifications demanded by the ADA are merely remedies for past wrongs rather than prospective positive entitlements.

But while there is significant validity to such arguments, they fail to recognize the extent to which the ADA actually moves beyond the simple protection of negative rights. These arguments deny the degree to which the ADA makes demands upon individual employers and public accommodations far above any which can be characterized as purely retributive justice. An ADA claim does not require a plaintiff to demonstrate the defendant's *mens rea* (or intent to discriminate). Nor are the benefits of the ADA limited to the victims of past discrimination. All individuals with disabilities, after all, benefit from the prospective design changes demanded by the statute. Ramps and elevators (unlike affirmative action) are not to be limited to a class of past victims. Moreover, the argument that the ADA compensates for past neglect cannot fully explain why the ADA requires modifications that result from benign neglect with respect to disability while employers remain free to benignly neglect a whole host of other needs of employees (such as the needs of employees with small children or long commutes). The ADA, after all, does not simply require that the employers treat individuals the same as (which can mean as badly as) other employees. Instead, the ADA requires that some affirmative steps, reasonable modifications, be made to ensure that the particular impediments faced by individuals with disabilities are overcome. Thus the ADA requires more than the cessation of invidious intent to individuals. The statute requires the positive consideration of those in the protected class.

Moreover, the attempt to disclaim the ADA's positive entitlements may have unfortunate consequences for those who are most in need of the act's positive features.[59] Some individuals with disabilities require certain modifications and supports that are more costly or burdensome than others. If the ADA is characterized as first and foremost a right to "simple equality," then the claims of those individuals whose needs are greater are easily dismissed as outside of the scope of the statute.[60] In addition, by focusing so much attention and hope on the ADA as the guarantor of self-sufficiency, the needs and aspirations of those for whom self-sufficiency is a quixotic goal are ignored—and the benefits the community can obtain when positive rights lead to greater participation in the marketplace and civil society are lost. Self-sufficiency is perhaps not the only goal nor the highest goal of the act.

More important, the attempt to deny the extent to which the ADA imposes positive obligations wholeheartedly accepts possessive individualism's critique of positive rights and assumes that the other widely accepted rights are in fact truly negative. However, as Sunstein and Holmes have shown, any attempt to defend legal rights as truly negative is doomed to failure. Despite their appearances, traditional nondiscrimination rights are positive because the claimant can call upon the resources of the state to limit the ability of the employer to deny the individual employment based upon the whims or bigotries of the employer. While this "entitlement" is both less costly and less overtly paternalistic than a welfare-state program, it nevertheless shares more "positive" characteristics with such programs than is commonly recognized. It is because of those "positive" characteristics that opponents of antidiscrimination laws are able, sometimes successfully, to claim that such laws create "special preferences."[61] Rather than question the appropriateness of such laws because of their positive-rights characteristics, should we not acknowledge the universality of dependence and dispel the myth that freedom ever consists in total independence from one another?

IV

We have argued thus far that the ADA combines grants of negative liberty with entitlements to positive rights. In effect, the ADA draws upon the traditions of both civil rights laws as well as disability entitlement programs to create a complex, "second-generation"[62] statute that aims to achieve the negative liberty of self-sufficiency while fostering the positive right to accommodation.

Both elements are reflected in the genesis of the statute's definition of disability. The ADA's definition derives from 1974 amendments to the Rehabilitation Act.[63] When it was first enacted, the Rehabilitation Act provided federal financial support for a variety of vocational training programs for individuals with handicaps. In effect, the statute provided positive rights to training programs that were intended to help those who could not work without the special training provided by the statute.

Because the original Rehabilitation Act had this limited goal and provided rights to programs that were not intended to be available to everyone in the population, the statute used a relatively narrow definition of handicap. Since the statute created "special" rights, it required strict eligibility criteria. Thus the definition of disability served as an eligibility criterion in the original Rehabilitation Act, limiting the availability of the programs to those who would not be employed without the benefits of the program.

In 1973 the Rehabilitation Act was amended to include an antidiscrimination provision. With surprisingly little debate, Congress added language to the Rehabilitation Act that prohibited all recipients of federal financial assistance from discriminating against "otherwise qualified" individuals with a handicap "solely by reason of . . . handicap."[64] This was not a right to a particular benefit program, designed for those who could not work without the program. It was instead a "right" meant to be more widely available to all individuals with a handicap, whether or not they could benefit from the vocational programs financed by the Rehabilitation Act.

As the nature of the right provided by the Rehabilitation Act changed, the earlier, narrow definition of handicap made little sense. A definition that applied only to those who could work only with training was inappropriate for a statute that now attempted to prohibit discrimination against those who could work without training. In other words, the original entitlement statute required a definition of disability that was narrow and applied only to those who otherwise could not work. The new antidiscrimination provision which was aimed at ensuring the right to work and study for those who could work and study required a far broader, less exceptional definition of disability.

Recognizing this incongruity, Congress amended the Rehabilitation Act in 1974 to include a new definition of disability that would apply solely to the act's nondiscrimination provisions. The new definition stated that: an individual with a disability was:

> Any individual who (i) has a physical or mental impairment which substantially limits one or more of such person's major life activities, (ii) has a record of such an impairment, or (iii) is regarded as having such an impairment.[65]

The ADA incorporated this definition almost verbatim.

Interestingly, there was little debate or confusion about the definition prior to the enactment of the ADA. For the most part, courts construing the Rehabilitation Act simply assumed that individuals who claimed to have a handicap within the meaning of the statute did indeed have one. Conditions such as diabetes and depression were simply assumed by the courts to constitute handicaps.[66] And in the only Supreme Court case to discuss the definition of disability, *School Board v. Arlene,* the Court construed the definition broadly, finding that the Rehabilitation Act's definition could apply to a nontraditional disability such as a contagious disease. [67]

With the enactment of the ADA, however, matters changed. The reach of the antidiscrimination mandate first crafted in the Rehabilitation Act was greatly expanded so that more of the private sector was now obligated to respect the disability rights granted. With this expansion of the rights' reach, the definition of disability that previously had presented a relatively low hurdle for plaintiffs began to appear insurmountable. Case after case began to question whether an individual who brought a claim under the ADA was "truly disabled."[68] More often than not, plaintiffs who were found to meet the statutory definition were also found to be too limited to be qualified to work. Plaintiffs, in effect, were caught in a bind between the competing conceptions of rights that the ADA tried to integrate. If plaintiffs presented with common or mild impairments, they were found not to be exceptional enough to warrant the grant of a positive right. Thus during oral argument in the *Murphy* case, Justice Breyer asked: "Is it then necessary to say that everyone who uses false teeth or glasses is disabled, or is there a way of drawing a line?"[69] His point was clear. In our individualistic world, less than perfect physical characteristics should not entitle us to claims from others; otherwise, we could all make such claims. Only those who are significantly "impaired," and unable to compete in our individualistic market, should be entitled to and deserving of positive rights.

On the other hand, because the ADA also protects negative rights, which do not undermine the individualism of our market economy, those who are so impaired that they require major modifications or assistance in order to achieve their aims also generally find no solace in the act. Thus employees who are frequently absent from work due to severe and chronic health problems have almost always lost their ADA claim, on the theory that they are not qualified to work because attendance is invariably an essential function of the job.[70] While such employees might be deserving of a positive entitlement in order to refrain from working, the negative-rights aspect of the ADA is insufficient to serve their purposes.

In short, while the definition of the ADA was designed to meet the statute's hybrid goals, the danger now is that it will meet neither. Because of our national predisposition toward negative rights, the positive rights in the statute have led courts and critics to insist that the definition of disability be read narrowly to preclude any possibility of universal positive rights. Yet because the statute predicates all of its positive rights in the context of a negative antidiscrimination statute, those individuals who are most likely to be found deserving of positive rights are the least likely to benefit from the ADA. The result is that an act both bold in its promise and creative in its design has been less than earth-shattering in its impact.

Ironically, many disability advocates do not disagree with the courts' parsimonious constructions of disability. They also believe that the positive benefits promised by the ADA are highly problematic and must be granted sparingly. These advocates believe that positive rights should not ordinarily be given, and that when they are, stigma will inevitably follow. On this view, the definition of disability must be kept narrow so that the rights bestowed by the ADA do not undermine the ability of the statute to realize significant change for those who do fall (most centrally) within its purview. Such a view unnecessarily and erroneously accepts the supremacy of liberty understood in negative terms.

While the ADA interweaves positive and negative rights in a more complex and explicit manner than earlier civil rights laws, this is not unique—it is only more overt. As we noted above, no legal rights are totally negative. All civil rights laws entail enforcement costs and all bestow positive benefits to the intended recipients. For example, laws against sex discrimination in the workplace are enforced through the not-inexpensive efforts of the EEOC and state employment agencies. More fundamentally, the realization of equal gender opportunity in the workplace has led to an accommodation or alteration of workplace norms so that sexual harassment—once a widely accepted form of workplace behavior—is no longer legal. In essence, Title VII has provided women with a positive right to a less offensive workplace. Thus, if the presence of positive rights entails stigma and necessitates the narrowing of the protected classification, then each gender, as well as every racial group, should face an analysis similar to that which has been granted to the question of disability.

However, even if we posit that the ADA combines elements of positive and negative rights to a greater degree than other civil rights laws and thus carries with it the risk of greater stigma and hence backlash stemming from its association with positive rights, a narrowing of the definition of disability is not necessarily the correct response. This argument accepts that positive rights should remain the exception, assuming the validity of a possessive individualism whereby individual self-sufficiency is both the norm and the ideal. But if the debates about the definition of disability and the fears of opening the floodgate reveal anything, it is that physical and mental impairments are extraordinarily commonplace and that few if any of us can truly sustain independence. And even if we could, why would we want to? In their understandable rejection of forced dependency, disability advocates may be too quick to accept that the highest freedom is freedom from others. In so doing, they may neglect the interests of those individuals with disabilities who cannot prosper in a regime of negative freedom as well as making it unnecessarily difficult for those who can get by only by superhuman feats. More generally, critics of dependency

overlook the opportunity the ADA provides to educate the public about both the prevalence of disability and the human dignity and worth of everyone with disabilities, even
those who cannot be self-sufficient. Such critics forego the opportunity to revitalize the
dialogue around the conceptions of freedom and social responsibility.

These arguments, however, will not satisfy those who believe that the definition of disability should be read narrowly because the ADA's positive rights are inherently inefficient
and therefore should be provided only to those with exceptional need.[71] These critics point
to the ADA's positive elements, such as the requirement that employers provide reasonable
accommodations, and worry that if the definition is read broadly the demands upon businesses will be infinite, undermining American productivity and competitiveness.

Given the dismal rate of success enjoyed by ADA plaintiffs, these cries seem misplaced.[72] Moreover, they falsely assume that just because the ADA provides for some elements of positive rights, it creates unfettered entitlements. In fact, all of the positive rights
created by the ADA are substantially curtailed to ensure that the costs upon defendants are
modest at most.[73] Thus, as we noted above, the ADA's employment provisions apply only
to individuals who are qualified for the job,[74] and reasonable accommodations need not be
offered if they impose an undue burden on the employer.[75] For the most part, courts have
been extremely sympathetic to defendants who raise such issues.

Moreover, the fact that the ADA mandates positive benefits in certain cases does not
mean that all individuals who are found to be within the protected class are given a carte-
blanche right to such benefits. Implicit in the ADA is the idea that accommodations need
to be provided only when necessary.[76] Individuals with impairments that are controllable
and do not otherwise interfere in their ability to work (such as those with correctable vision
impairments or asymptomatic HIV disease) should receive nothing from the ADA other
than the negative right not to be the subject of invidious discrimination. In such cases, it
makes sense to say to that the individual has a disability and is protected by the statute not
because she requires accommodations, but because she can compete in the workplace if
only permitted to do so. To deny that she has a disability for fear of supposedly inefficient
positive rights is to risk the inefficiency of losing her productivity in the workforce and rel-
egating her to the fully positive-rights regime established by our welfare and disability
insurance laws.

In effect, as Justice Stevens recognized in his dissent in *Sutton,* the Court's narrowing of
the definition of disability undermines the ability of the Act to protect negative rights, for
the Court has, in essence, decreed that individuals with correctable impairments, who are
fully capable of working efficiently, even without accommodation, can be denied the right
to do so simply on the basis of the myths and stereotypes that our culture harbors about
physical and mental impairments.[77] Thus fearing the statute's bestowal of positive rights,
the Supreme Court has impaired the act's ability to preserve negative liberty.

In conclusion, the fact that the ADA combines elements of positive and negative rights
should not be cause for unduly narrowing the definition of disability. In crafting a complex, "second-generation" civil rights statute, the drafters of the ADA sought to enact a
vision of equal opportunity in which the norms of justice ensure that equality is more than
a hollow promise to some and a confirmation of the status quo to others. To realize this
vision, the definition of disability can be read neither narrowly nor defensively. Instead, it
must be read broadly and contextually to ensure that all individuals who face impairments
are assured the right to be self-sufficient when they can be, and to be accommodated when
they need to be.

ACKNOWLEDGMENTS

We wish to thank Maryam Koupaie and Bronwyn Page for valuable research assistance and Steve Nathanson for insightful dialogue.

NOTES

[1]118 S. Ct. 2196 (1998).

[2]*Sutton v. United Airlines,* 119 S. Ct. 2139 (1999); *Albertson's, Inc. v. Kirkingburg,* 119 S. Ct. 2162 (1999); *Murphy v. United Parcel Service, Inc.,* 119 S. Ct. 2133 (1999).

[3]Wendy E. Parmet, "Plain Meaning and Mitigating Measures: Judicial Interpretations of the Meaning of Disability," forthcoming in *Berkeley J. Employment Lab. L.*

[4]42 U.S.C. § 2000e.

[5]42 U.S.C. § 2000e.

[6]42 U.S.C. § 12112 (a); 42 U.S.C. § 12132.

[7]29 U.S.C. § 706(B).

[8]This issue was before the Supreme Court this term in the cases of *Sutton v. United Air Lines,* 119 S. Ct. 2139 (1999); and *Murphy v. United Parcel Service,* 119 S. Ct. 2133 (1999).

[9]*Ellison v. Software Spectrum, Inc.,* 85 F.3d 187 (5th Cir. 1996).

[10]Steven S. Locke, "The Incredible Shrinking Protected Class: Redefining the Scope of Disability Under the Americans with Disabilities Act," 68 *Colum. L. Rev.* 107 (1997).

[11]Henry Shue, *Basic Rights: Subsistence, Affluence and U.S. Foreign Policy,* 2nd ed. New Jersey: Princeton University Press, 1996, 14.

[12]Jeffrie G. Murphy and Jules Coleman, *Philosophy of Law: An Introduction to Jurisprudence.* San Francisco: Westview Press, 1990, 14.

[13]Wesley Newcomb Hohfeld, "Some Fundamental Legal Conceptions as Applied in Judicial Reasoning," in *Fundamental Legal Conceptions as Applied in Judicial Reasoning.* New Haven, CT: Yale University Press, 1923, 23–64.

[14]Cf. Matthew H. Kramer, "Rights Without Trimmings," in *A Debate Over Rights,* eds. Matthew Kramer, N. E. Simmonds and Hillel Steiner. Oxford, UK: Clarendon Press, 1998, 8.

[15]Isaiah Berlin, "Two Concepts of Liberty," in *Liberalism and its Critics,* ed. Michael Sandel. New York: New York University Press, 1984, 28.

[16]Ibid., 16.

[17]John Stuart Mill, *On Liberty, in Three Essays,* introduction by Richard Wollheim. Oxford, UK: Oxford University Press, 1975, 93.

[18]C.B. Macpherson, *The Political Theory of Possessive Individualism.* Oxford, UK: Oxford University Press, 1962, 3.

[19]Ibid., 3.

[20]Ibid., 3.

[21]Richard Epstein, *Forbidden Grounds.* Cambridge, MA: Harvard University Press, 1992, 481-494.

[22]Macpherson, *Political Theory,* 264.

[23]Berlin, *Liberalism and its Critics,* 22.

[24]Gerald Dworkin, *The Theory and Practice of Autonomy.* Cambridge, UK: Cambridge University Press, 1988, 13.

[25]Stephen Holmes and Cass R. Sunstein, *The Cost of Rights.* New York: W.W. Norton and Company, 1999, 239.

[26]C. B. Macpherson, *The Real World of Democracy,* for the Canadian Broadcasting Corporation. Toronto: The Hunter Rose Company, 1965, 61.

[27]Robert L. Hale, "Coercion and Distribution in a Supposedly Non-Coercive State," 38 *Political Science Quarterly* 470 (1923).

[28]Holmes and Sunstein, *The Cost of Rights,* 45.

[29]Ibid., 46.

[30]Ibid., 46.

[31]Ibid., 80.

[32]Ibid., 46.

[33]Ibid., 46–47.

[34]Alan H. Goldman, "The Justice of Equal Opportunity," in *Equal Opportunity,* eds. Ellen Frankel Paul, Fred D. Miller Jr., Jeffrey Paul and John Ahrens. Oxford, UK: Basil Blackwell, Inc., 1987, 88.

[35]Ibid., 98.

[36]Ibid., 100.

[37]Holmes and Sunstein, *The Cost of Rights,* 217.

[38]Pamela S. Karlan and George Rutherglen, "Disabilities, Discrimination and Reasonable Accommodation," 46 *Duke L. J.* 9 (1996).

[39]42 U.S.C. § 2000e.

[40]Karlan and Rutherglen, *Duke L. J.,* 9.

[41]42 U.S.C. § 2000e (k).

[42]*City of Richmond v. J.A. Croson, Co.,* 488 U.S. 469 (1989).

[43]Ibid.

[44]*Newport News Shipbuilding & DryDock Co. v. EEOC,* 462 U.S. 669 (1983).

[45]*Oncale v. Sundowner Offshore Services, Inc.,* 523 U.S. 75 (1998).

[46]Marcia Pearce Burgdorf and Robert Burgdorf, Jr., "A History of Unequal Treatment: The Qualifications of Handicapped Persons as a 'Suspect Class' Under the Equal Protection Clause," *Santa Clara L. R.* 15:861–91 (1975).

[47]Jonathan C. Drimmer, "Cripples, Overcomers, and Civil Rights: Tracing the Evolution of Federal Legislation and Social Policy for People with Disabilities," *UCLA L. R.* 40: 1359–70 (1993).

[48]Ibid., 1341.

[49]Ruth Colker, "Hypercapitalism, Affirmative Protections for People with Disabilities, Illness and Parenting Responsibilities Under United States Law," *Yale J. L. & Feminism* 9: 222 (1977).

[50]Matthew Diller, "Entitlement and Exclusion: The Role of Disability in the Social Welfare System," 44 *UCLA L. R.* 361 (1996).

[51]493 U.S. 521 (1990).

[52]Testimony of Carolyn L. Weaver, Senate Committee on Finance, March 27, 1995.

[53]Andrew Schepard, "Defending the Most Vulnerable: Children's Rights to SSI," *N.Y. L. J.,* March 24, 1998. This definition was revisited in further amendments in 1997. See P.L. 105–33.

[54]Robert Burgdorf, Jr., "The Americans with Disabilities Act: Analysis and Implications of a Second Generation Civil Rights Statute," 26 *Har. C. R.-C. L. L. R.* 413 (1991).

[55]42 U.S.C. § 12111.

[56]42 U.S.C. § 12111(8).

[57]42 U.S.C. § 12112(b)(7).

[58]Anita Silvers, "Formal Justice," in *Disability, Difference, Discrimination,* eds. Anita Silvers, David Wasserman and Mary B. Mahowald. New York: Rowman & Littlefield Publishers, Inc., 1998, 138–39.

[59]David Wasserman, "Distributive Justice," in *Disability, Difference, Discrimination,* eds. Anita Silvers, David Wasserman and Mary B. Mahowald. New York: Rowman & Littlefield Publishers, Inc., 1998, 179–177.

[60]Such individuals are found not to be "qualified" within the meaning of the statute. 42 U.S.C. § 12111(8).

[61]*Romer v. Evans,* 517 U.S. 620 (1996).

[62]Burgdorf, op. cit., 413.

[63]Pub. L. 93–516, § 111, 88 Stat. 1617, 1619 (1974), codified at 29 U.S.C. 706(8)(B).

[64]29 U.S.C. § 794. The Rehabilitation Act originally used the term "handicap." This was altered with the enactment of the ADA.

[65]29 U.S.C. § 706(B).

[66]A good example is *Davis v. Meese,* 692 F. Supp. 505 (E.D. Pa. 1988). That case concerned an individual with insulin-dependent diabetes who wished to be an FBI special agent. In considering the application of the Rehabilitation Act, the court, with almost no analysis, asserted that insulin-dependent diabetes is "clearly" a handicap within the meaning of the Rehabilitation Act. Ibid., at 516.

[67]480 U.S. 273 (1987).

[68]Wendy E. Parmet, "Plain Meaning and Mitigating Measures: Judicial Interpretations of the Meaning of Disability," forthcoming in *Berkeley J. Employment L. L.*

⁶⁹Linda Greenhouse, "Justices Wrestling with the Definition of Disability: Is it Glasses? False Teeth?" *New York Times,* 28 April 1999, sec. A, p. 26.

⁷⁰E.g., *Tyndall v. National Education Ctrs.,* 31 F.3d 209 (4th Cir. 1994).

⁷¹Epstein, *Forbidden Grounds,* 481–494.

⁷²Colker, *Yale J. L. & Feminism,* 213.

⁷³Peter David Blanck, *The Americans with Disabilities Act and the Emerging Workforce: Employment of People with Mental Retardation.* Washington DC: The American Association of Mental Retardation, 1998, 148.

⁷⁴42 U.S.C. § 12112.

⁷⁵42 U.S.C. § 12112.

⁷⁶Wendy E. Parmet, Mark A. Gottlieb and Richard A. Daynard, "Accommodating Vulnerability to Environmental Tobacco Smoke: A Prism for Understanding the ADA," *J. L. & Health* 12 (1997–1998):1, 20.

⁷⁷*Sutton,* 1999. 119 S. Ct. at 2157–58.

Disability, Discrimination and Priority

RICHARD J. ARNESON

Is having a disability more like being a member of a racially stigmatized group or like lacking a talent? Both analogies might be apt. The Americans with Disabilities Act stresses the former analogy. The framing thought is that people with disabilities are objects of prejudice and prejudiced behaviors that wrongfully exclude them from participation in important social practices such as the labor market. Think, for example, of a blind person whose job applications are always automatically rejected because she is blind and without any consideration of her aptitude for this or that specific job. Such a person suffers wrongful discrimination and is denied equality of opportunity.

A further thought along the same line is that a long-standing pattern of discrimination can alter the shape of institutions and practices, so that even if individuals now are chosen for jobs strictly on the basis of their likely productivity, current productivity may reflect past discriminatory practices, so equality of opportunity properly understood can be violated even if no employers are currently acting from prejudice. An example would be a factory in which for many years only men have been hired for skilled jobs, and the workplace is designed for their convenience with bathrooms regularly spaced. Now women are hired and retained for skilled jobs along with men according to productivity, but women systematically produce less than men because at the skilled work site bathrooms for women are few and far between. In this example, an investment in bathrooms would create a level playing field for men and women to compete on fair terms.

This case and others we might invent suggest the need to analyze the ideals of nondiscrimination and equality of opportunity. Another type of case would feature identical output productivity on the part of blacks and whites, but labor by whites would be preferred by an unprejudiced, rationally profit-maximizing employer who sells his product to prejudiced consumers who are unwilling to buy products that have been built by the labor of blacks if the blacks are employed in skilled jobs. (We suppose that consumers can readily obtain information about what sort of workers are employed in what sort of jobs that produce the products they are reviewing for possible purchase.) In this setting, a rational business decision by the employer would produce a workforce that is segregated by race, with only whites performing all skilled jobs. Yet in some clear sense, blacks and whites in this example do not enjoy equal employment opportunities.

This essay distinguishes some possible ideals of equality of opportunity construed as a nondiscrimination norm. Stated baldly, my conclusion is that any and all versions of such norms are at best incomplete accounts of the substance of social justice and at worst flawed by making a moral fetish of talent and by falsely supposing that a perfect meritocracy in which all with the same ambition and talent have the same expectation of lifetime rewards would be a just society. What we owe to one another by way of social justice requirements goes beyond meritocratic nondiscrimination. In my judgment the provisions of the ADA cannot be fully justified by appeal to even the most plausible versions of the nondiscrimination ideal.[1] That suggests not a criticism of the ADA but rather the imperative of exploring what, beyond nondiscrimination, we owe to one another. I sketch a prioritarian response to this question and describe how this approach handles difficult issues of disability and justice. Once we are liberated from thinking of the problem of disability exclusively within the antidiscrimination framework, the way is open to consider other types of appropriate remedies for the condition of the disabled as viewed from the standpoint of social justice.

NONDISCRIMINATION AND EQUALITY OF OPPORTUNITY

Equality of opportunity is a powerfully resonant norm in contemporary societies with histories of racial exclusion and pervasive discrimination against women. This section surveys several candidate conceptions of equality of opportunity. To limit the discussion, I focus on equality of opportunity as it might be interpreted to apply to the labor market and more broadly the economic marketplace.

Contract at Will

Perhaps the simplest equal-opportunity ideal is absence of government constraint (such as legal enforcement of Jim Crow segregation or apartheid) in the relationship between employers and employees. An employer may hire as she pleases and a potential employee is free to accept or reject any offer, and once an employment relationship is established, either party may terminate the relationship at will. Each individual under this regime has equal opportunity to initiate any offer of employment or service and to accept or reject any offer that is tendered. During the specified duration of a contract, one is bound to carry out the agreed terms, but if the contract is breached, specific performance may not be demanded as reparation for breach, but only compensation for the money's-worth of the breached terms to the party who is damaged.[2]

Under contract at will, all employers might refuse, on any ground whatsoever, to hire women, blacks or deaf or blind people for any skilled job. This policy could represent nothing more than a collective whim or deep-seated prejudice on the part of employers against women, blacks, the deaf or the blind. Hence many people will find this interpretation of equal opportunity to be too weak.

Careers Open to Talent

On this construal, equal opportunity obtains when jobs are open to all applicants, applicants are judged solely on their qualifications for the post, and the most qualified applicant is offered it. Each of the phrases in this formulation requires interpretation. In the succeeding paragraphs I offer construals of some of these elusive phrases.

Jobs are open to all. A firm might find it cheaper to advertise only by word of mouth if this minimal advertising will elicit sufficient applicants. Or a firm might choose to advertise more or less widely, balancing the cost of advertising against the likely expected improvement in the pool of applicants from further advertising. For similar reasons, a firm might accept applications for a post only from firm members. An additional consideration might operate in this case: a ready internal ladder of advancement might be an inducement provided by a firm to attract more qualified individuals to entry-level positions and to help retain current firm members. In deciding what constitutes a reasonably open search for a particular firm seeking to fill a particular job, we might be most concerned when scant advertising disproportionately prevents members of groups who have been victims of past discrimination from applying.

Applicants are judged solely on their qualifications for the post. Several complexities enter once one recognizes that qualifications are not transparent either to the hiring firm or to the individual applicant. The firm chooses applicants on the basis of data it gathers that it deems to be predictive of job performance.

Since gathering information about candidates is not costless, a firm might find it profit-maximizing to hire the first applicant found to satisfy some threshold set of qualifications rather than carefully to investigate who is most qualified. For similar reasons, a firm might find that its profit-maximizing search procedure uses very rough but readily observable indicators to screen out from further consideration applicants who are marked as likely to possess traits that will impede job performance. Hence one gets statistical discrimination, which might involve excluding all black applicants (statistically more prone to absenteeism in this industry than applicants of other races), all women applicants (more likely than men to become pregnant and suspend their careers for childbearing and child rearing) and all blind applicants (more prone to on-the-job accidents that are costly for employers). Such statistical discrimination might be efficient from the standpoint of the firm (profit-maximizing), or inefficient.[3] But from the perspective of the black who never misses work, the woman who has resolute career aspirations and abhors the thought of having children, and the blind person with a spotless safety record, statistical discrimination means "I never had a chance." Such procedures may well prevent the most qualified from being hired, but of course any selection based on probabilistic indicators may do this.

Mark Kelman presses this difficulty. Suppose the employer uses a test to screen applicants that weakly but fairly predicts good work performance. The test is a weak predictor in that some of those who fail the test would succeed on the job and some who pass the test would not succeed on the job. The test is fair with respect to a group whom we fear might be victims of hiring discrimination, say, those with disabilities. (For simplicity, suppose the disabled are all deaf.) The test is fair in the sense that it predicts whether deaf applicants would succeed at the job as accurately as it predicts whether nondeaf applicants would succeed on the job. Suppose the employer hires all who pass the test and some smaller percentage of those who fail. The deaf, let us suppose, have higher fail rates on the test, so fewer of them are hired. But Kelman notes that it turns out to be a robust result under these assumptions that, of the group that does poorly on the test, fewer of those who would succeed will be hired than will be hired from the remainder group that does better on the test. If our view of equal opportunity as careers open to talents is that individuals who are equally able to succeed on the job have the same chance of being hired, then: "for almost all values of pass and accuracy rates, a test that predicts equally well for [two groups] will become less fair as the relative pass rates on the test diverge and as validities decline."[4] It does not follow that to implement equality of opportunity we should ban or discourage the use of such tests. That depends on what the feasible alternatives are. Perhaps the lesson is that the ideal of careers open to talents, in its most plausible construal, is not fully satisfiable in actual circumstances.

The notion of being judged on one's qualifications can take what might be called perfectionist and nonperfectionist forms. Suppose carpenters are being hired to put up shoddy, cheap houses favored by consumers. Being a consummately skilled carpenter may mean one is overqualified for this job; the firm suspects the master craftsman may resist doing the job the way the firm wants it done. From the firm's standpoint, the ideally qualified are the moderately skilled, but one might hold that only tests of meritorious and skilled carpentering are relevant to one's qualifications; there is an objective ideal of good carpentering, and those who most approximate this ideal are most qualified, profits be damned. A similar case would arise if a mathematician were deemed overqualified and denied employment as a clerk on the ground that she would likely get bored and quit after a brief tenure on the job. For these sorts of cases I shall stipulate that the appropriate sense of "most qualified" is the nonperfectionist sense, so that the most qualified applicant is the one reasonably best deemed to match the traits that in context are most conducive to the appropriately weighted fulfillment of the firm's legally permissible objectives. For private firms, this will be the set of traits most conducive to the firm's profitability. If one takes the other tack, one is in effect opting for some version of a substantive meritocratic ideal. The idea is that those who are truly qualified can be identified as such by discerning their intrinsic traits, and independently of relations among those traits and contingent circumstances such as market demand. Taking this line, one incurs the obligation to explain what this intrinsic notion of qualification is and why it gives rise to moral entitlements. I doubt that this obligation can be fulfilled.

Another complication in the idea of being judged solely on one's merits arises if one considers age discrimination. Consider a society that has a legally mandatory retirement age or that legally allows firms to set a mandatory retirement age or to take age into account in assessing applicants. Such practices might seem straightforwardly to violate the ideal of careers open to talents. They allow that the less-qualified younger applicant is selected for the post over the more-qualified older applicant.

Age and the mental and physical deterioration that eventually accompanies old age might be regarded as a disability to which all people are prone. But since everyone who does not die young becomes old, age discrimination can be compatible with equality of opportunity construed as careers open to talents over one's lifetime even though it is not compatible with equality of opportunity at a particular time. The ideal of careers open to talents could be perfectly satisfied for all prime-age adults of eighteen to sixty. School-age youth and those over the age of sixty are permitted to work only under constraints. If we abstract for the moment from the phenomena of childhood death and early adulthood death, then in a society that satisfies careers open to talents to this extent, everyone enjoys equal opportunity construed as careers open to talents over the life cycle. Since everyone is young once and becomes old eventually, if premature death does not intervene, all individuals can enjoy the same equality of opportunity over the life cycle in a society that limits access to jobs for aged persons. (Moreover, those who die prior to old age and hence never face the permitted or enforced discrimination against the aged are not thereby advantaged compared to those who do live to old age.)[5]

Fair Equality of Opportunity

Careers open to talents require only that those who are equally qualified have the same prospects of success in competitions for jobs. Conceptions of fair equality of opportunity add the further requirement that individuals must have a fair opportunity to become qualified. The idea that justice requires that society make available schooling to all children via a public school system or some other means goes beyond the ideal of careers open to talents and embraces some ideal of fair equality of opportunity.

If we accept that some obligation falls on us to provide opportunities for all individuals to develop their native talent potential so as to become qualified according to their capacities, the question immediately arises of how far this obligation extends. John Rawls presses the idea of fair equality to its limit in his formulation, which holds that fair equality of opportunity among persons obtains when any persons who have the same native talent and the same ambition will have the same prospects for success in competitions for positions that confer advantages.[6] This is, if you will, the ideal of a classless society in the sense that no advantages accrue to individuals in virtue of their initial placement in the social order. Whether one is born into a rich or poor family, on the right side or the wrong side of the tracks, of parents who are well educated or the reverse—none of these social factors nor any others affect one's competitive prospects compared to those other individuals face. Nothing but one's native talent endowment and ambition determine one's competitive prospects. This means that if especially well-off or socially influential parents follow their natural instincts to give their own children a competitive advantage by their educational and child rearing practices, social intervention such as special educational programs for the underprivileged occurs, so that in the end the effect of social factors in boosting one individual's prospects above another's is entirely eliminated. Since we do not know how to carry out such interventions, fair equality of opportunity might better be regarded as an aspiration postulated by justice rather than as a strict justice requirement.

Two aspects of the fair-equality norm call for comment.

First, the idea of having the same native talent as another is unclear. Consider a simple example. Suppose we could install just one of two educational programs in a two-person society consisting of Smith and Jones. One provides more intensive education, the other a more relaxed schooling. Under the intensive regime, Jones ends up with higher earnings prospects, and under the relaxed regime, Smith ends up with higher earnings prospects. Which to choose? Fair equality does not say. Or taken strictly, with the construal that the capacity to respond to schooling is a talent, fair equality requires only that persons with identical dispositions to develop exactly the same talent in response to any schooling and socialization regime qualify as having the same talent, and the proposal is silent about choices that would produce different results for individuals with different talents in this strict sense. Since in practice we only discover what talents people have by subjecting them to one or another schooling regime, fair equality, which had looked severely strict, now looks to be quite lax and undemanding. What we need to add to fair equality is some sensible continuity requirement, so that if two individuals' capacities to develop talent through schooling are "close," the developed talents they acquire should not be "too dissimilar."

A second comment is that fair equality will not rule out what will intuitively strike us as discriminatory outcomes unless its ambition component is qualified. Suppose that fair equality of opportunity obtains perfectly in a society, and it turns out that no one with a disability obtains any desirable employment. This is so because those deemed to have disabilities are trained to have low ambition, so it never occurs that a disabled person with the same native talent for a desirable type of employment as a nondisabled person develops the same ambition to achieve it. Hence fair equality of opportunity in its Rawlsian formulation is satisfied even though disabled and nondisabled persons who have the same native talent for a type of desirable employment do not have the same prospects of obtaining it. To solve this problem we would need to clarify the idea of ambition by specifying that if two people have the same native talent, but one ends up with lesser prospects for success in competitions for positions of advantage because her ambition has been reduced by prejudiced or discriminatory socialization, then fair equality of opportunity is violated.

THE NONDISCRIMINATION NORM: NOT SUFFICIENT

If equality of opportunity is inflated to appear the whole of justice, what one reaches is the view that provided equality of opportunity is sustained, any distribution of resources and life prospects thrown up by a competitive market economy in which individual property rights are firmly accepted is just. The ideal of justice becomes the market economy with careers open to talents. This amounts to justice as meritocracy.[7]

Equality of opportunity in all of the guises considered so far places no constraints on the processes that determine how jobs are defined and individuated. If I am found unqualified for a post, I might truly observe that if the job were reconfigured, or if the work setting in which the job is set were reorganized in a certain way, then I would no longer be unqualified. The fact that I am unqualified is due to the fact that my traits do not match those required for the job, and one could get a match either by changing my traits to fit the job or changing the job description to fit my traits. Obviously some complaints of this sort that one might voice do not rise to the level of registering a *prima facie* claim of injustice. Lacking hand-to-eye coordination, I can imagine a large reconstruction of the surgeon's or baseball pitcher's trade such that I could qualify, but that is neither here nor there. But some complaints of this sort do seem to raise issues of social justice.

Catharine MacKinnon has posed an interesting challenge to the ideal of equality of opportunity (regarded as sufficient for social justice). Suppose that men and women compete on absolutely fair terms for jobs that are designed by men for men. For example, male owners over the years might structure the workplace so that employees need to display aggression and competitiveness, qualities men tend to have, rather than cooperativeness and solidarity, qualities women more often display. Fair selection processes then select men rather than women as best qualified for these male-oriented workplaces. In this hypothetical case, men are more qualified than women according to the standards of qualification that are set by powerful men and reflect male proclivities. In this scenario the steady fulfillment of equal opportunity norms could coexist with continued exclusion of women from the most desirable jobs. MacKinnon suggests that actual labor markets might well function much as in the hypothetical example. As she puts it, the entire structure of contemporary economic life is "a giant affirmative action plan for white males."[8] In a possible retelling of this story, job applicants marked with conventional disabilities are excluded from desirable employment in procedurally fair competitions for work roles that are substantively biased against the interests of the disabled.

Many people have regarded it as unexceptionable that individuals confined to wheelchairs have typically experienced severe lack of access to social functions entry to which is gained via steps and stairs. But the lack of access the wheelchair-bound suffer in these circumstances is not the result only of their physical impairment but of that coupled with the design of buildings, a social construction that we could alter. In many cases of this sort, natural misfortunes do not by themselves limit the opportunities and effective liberties of various categories of disabled persons. The combination of natural misfortune plus human doings and allowings produces the limitation of opportunity we observe. Roadways and streets are designed to be safe given a certain level of manual dexterity and quickness of vision and bodily response that most people can achieve easily provided they take due care. But for some people, driving cars and walking through urban streets as currently designed require more skill than they can muster. However, we could have designed streets and walkways and cars differently so that they would be useable by (many of) the persons currently excluded. Bit by bit, through a host of design and engineering decisions along with choices of laws and social norms, we create a social environment that forms a scheme of cooperation from which some, labeled the disabled, are excluded. In a clear sense we create the categories of able and disabled individuals by patterns of individual and collective decision-making.

No version of equality of opportunity canvassed to this point, not even the most stringent and far-reaching, addresses the issue just posed, which has been called the problem of inclusion.[9] Nor should it. The problem of inclusion is an aspect of the general problem of distributive justice, the theory of what we owe to each other and what properly belongs to whom. The moral principles of nondiscrimination and equality of opportunity, no matter how you stretch them, are not suited to address this range of problems. It is not plausible to make a norm against discrimination do all the work of distributive justice.

To see this plainly, consider that a severely disabled person might be treated entirely fairly according to the norms against discrimination and for equality of opportunity, yet face miserable life prospects. Suppose Arneson is legless, blind and deaf. He does not suffer employment discrimination; in fact we might suppose he secures an unskilled job, the best job he is qualified to hold. He has little native talent, and the society is organized so that a suitably revised version of fair equality of opportunity is satisfied as it applies to his case. He faces the same prospects of success in competition for advantageous positions as anyone else with the same native talent and the same ambition he has. Moreover, his ambition levels are not stunted by prejudice or discriminatory socialization; he has always been encouraged to be all the best he can be. If one compares his lot with that of other persons whose native talent levels are roughly comparable to his, one sees that their prospects are roughly comparable to his—there are no glaring discrepancies. His problem is not that he faces any sort of discrimination but rather that his talents are meager. In assessing his talents, a sensible talent measure will include among his talents the important negative talents that render him disabled. Though fairly treated, we stipulate, by norms that aspire to make the society a perfect meritocracy, he still ends up with a very low quality of life. In rating his quality of life, we do not worry that he cannot afford baubles and trivial but fashionably chic goods. His quality of life is poor in terms of opportunities for genuinely important human goods. The question arises whether social justice requires us to do something for Arneson or whether his plight is a "don't care" from the standpoint of enlightened social justice. Equality of opportunity either does not address this question, or if viewed as addressing it, gives an implausible answer.

The Americans with Disabilities Act requires more of employers than that they do not discriminate against the handicapped. It requires that if one can do a job if one's handicap is given a reasonable accommodation by the employer, and if one would be best qualified among the applicants if that reasonable accommodation was made, one must be hired for the job. In a similar way, if one is currently employed at a job, and acquires a disability, but one could continue to perform the job competently if the employer made a reasonable accommodation in response to one's disability, the employer must do so. Examples of reasonable accommodation would be adjustments in break times, hours, or equipment. The relevant point for our purposes is that a required reasonable accommodation for a disabled applicant might render it the case that the disabled most qualified applicant is not the applicant whom it would be profit-maximizing for the employer to hire. The employer might make higher profits if she hired another applicant for whom no costly reasonable accommodation would have to be made.

It has been suggested, not altogether implausibly, that the "reasonable accommodation" rule is a form of compensation to the disabled that roughly offsets the impact of past discriminatory practice on their employment prospects. There would be a rough analogy here to one sort of rationale for affirmative action programs for blacks and other underrepresented minority groups and women. But the justification of reasonable accommodation for the disabled as a form of compensation for past discrimination comes to an end when past discrimination is compensated for or so far past that current disabled persons cannot plausibly be regarded as its victims. In these circumstances, no plausible form of antidiscrimination norm will justify the special treatment of the disabled mandated by the "reasonable treatment" provisions of current law. To my mind, these provisions might well still be intuitively justified. Thus we must search further to find a justification for help for the disabled beyond what antidiscrimination norms can plausibly warrant.

PRIORITARIANISM

The starting point for my reflections on distributive justice is the common thought that life is a jumble of chosen and unchosen lotteries. The latter are perhaps especially disquieting. Good and bad fortune falls on individuals randomly in ways that are entirely beyond their power to control, but which fundamentally determine their life prospects. By good luck, some start adult life prosperous, healthy, handsome, charming and talented, while others face miserable prospects. Many principles of distributive justice hold that the lucky ought to compensate the unlucky in ways that tend to equalize the life prospects that attach to individuals through processes that are beyond their individual power to control. The advocates of principles in this broad class have been called "luck egalitarians." The version of luck egalitarianism that I find most plausible is welfarist, responsibility-catering and prioritarian.

A *responsibility-catering* conception holds that the moral value of obtaining benefits and avoiding losses for individuals varies according to the degree of responsibility they bear for their current condition. The less one is responsible for one's condition, if it is bad, the greater the moral value, other things being equal, of improving one's condition or preventing further losses, and the more one is responsible for one's condition, if it is good, the greater the moral disvalue, other things being equal, of allowing it to deteriorate or failing to improve it. One is more responsible for one's condition, if it is bad, the more it is the case that over the course of one's life one has behaved either culpably imprudently or virtuously imprudently or deliberately undertaken courses of action with known risks, whether prudently or imprudently.

This may sound convoluted, but the idea is simple. What we owe to one another depends in part on what each of us does for herself, given the available opportunities. If my condition is bad, but the background includes the fact that I deliberately undertook a gamble and lost, or culpably behaved without care for my well-being, or virtuously sacrificed my interests for what reasonably seemed a worthy cause in a manner that was morally optional, then in any of these cases, the moral urgency of alleviating my plight lessens. (And a similar point holds if my condition is comparatively good.)

An account of responsibility includes a specification of what is expected of people and a specification of the extent to which it is reasonable to shift costs or allow costs to lie where they fall when people fail to do what is expected of them. A "soft" response to the latter issue strikes me as morally best. According to such a soft view, one should not be held responsible for what lies beyond one's power to control and, within the region of the controllable, one should be held less responsible for making and implementing an unreasonable choice, the more difficult and painful it would be for one to make and implement that difficult choice. (Suppose that making a prudent and reasonable choice requires solving a mathematical problem which is easy for you and extremely difficult for me. It would be morally unreasonable to hold me as responsible as you for making the wrong choice if we both make the wrong choice. Also, it would be morally reasonable to give me more credit if we both make the right choice.) Adjusting the moral value and disvalue of achieving gains and imposing losses on an individual depending on the extent of her responsibility for her present condition, we should, when prudence is the relevant norm that sets what we expect people to do, calculate someone's degree of responsibility depending on how far she deviates above or below the level of prudent conduct that it would be morally reasonable to expect of her (given her circumstances that fix the difficulty and cost for her of making and implementing prudent choices).

A *welfarist* conception is one that holds that the appropriate distributive-justice standard for measuring the initial opportunities that an individual faces is the well-being or welfare that those opportunities enable her to attain. The notion of welfare in play here is objective, in the sense that something can be good for a person in itself (not as a means to some further end) independently of the person's own subjective opinion about the value of that good and independently of her own attitudes toward it.

A *prioritarian* distributive justice principle holds that we should act and arrange institutions and practices so that moral value, which is a function of well-being, is maximized. According to the prioritarian, the moral value of achieving a small gain or avoiding a small loss in well-being for a person is greater, the larger the amount of well-being gained or conserved, and greater, the lower the person's level of expected lifetime well-being prior to receipt of this benefit.

Responsibility-catering prioritarianism (RCP) treats personal traits that are deemed disabilities (that befall an individual prior to the onset of adult status) just as it treats native personal abilities. Both are included in the comprehensive set of circumstances that determine one's lifetime expectation of welfare at a given moment of one's life. Distributive justice calls on us to reconfigure these circumstances by distribution of resources or in other ways to achieve what the theory of justice counts as a fair distribution. This means that if two individuals face identical circumstances, except that one is armless and the other has two functioning arms, then a distribution of resources that fails to compensate the one for armlessness will likely not be fair, because with the same external resources, the person with arms will have a far higher expectation of well-being.

I say "will likely not be fair" advisedly. According to prioritarianism, what we owe each other depends on two factors: (1) how badly off or well-off you would be in the absence of further receipt of benefits; and (2) the extent to which your well-being prospects would improve if further benefits were bestowed on you. Suppose that I am unlucky in my personal endowments. I am schizophrenic and also have borderline/narcissistic personality disorder. It may unfortunately be the case that I am an extremely poor transformer of resources into a good life. You could give me a lot of money and I would fritter it away. You could impose strict paternalistic rules designed for my benefit, or alter the social environment in other ways, but I would chafe at the paternalistic rules and find ways to subvert the good intentions of the socially altered environment. What society owes me by way of distributive justice is responsive both to the extent of my bad luck and the extent to which I can benefit from compensation. Moreover, the decision as to what should be done for me will be comparative. The issue is: (1) how badly off I am, by comparison with the well-being expectation levels of others who might be helped or might be called on to assist me; and (2) how much I can benefit from measures that might be taken to aid me, by comparison with the extent to which others can benefit if the compensatory measures are instead directed toward the improvement of their quality of life. Justice involves calculation of costs and benefits and trade-off rules to determine the moral value of the policies we might choose.

Why accept prioritarianism? Consider again the morality-of-inclusion problem. One way or another, individuals or society regulating the choices of individuals must make many decisions that will establish entry requirements for roles that involve being a productive contributor to cooperative schemes. The ensemble of these role requirements determines the terms of cooperation in these schemes to which any individual has access. The threshold requirements for being a useful contributor might be set higher or lower by establishing the scheme in one way or another. Within a broad range, setting the requirements lower is better for those who just barely pass the entry requirements at each lowered threshold but worse for those who could participate in a more restricted scheme and would be better off in it because it would be more productive per capita.

In the face of this problem, it is implausible to insist that cooperative terms must be set so that no one is excluded. Lowering the bar to productive contribution so that severely mentally retarded or severely mentally ill individuals can be full productive members might reduce the net benefits of cooperation almost to nothing. If this problem is regarded from a consequentialist standpoint, the argument for prioritarianism is that it lies between two unacceptable extremes. At one end, one might insist on the priority of inclusion no matter what. This would be tantamount to a maximin consequentialist approach: arrange institutions and practices and choose actions and policies so that the benefit level of the worst-off individual is as high as it can be made. But here, as elsewhere, maximin is an implausibly stringent priority rule. It insists that any gain, however tiny, that can be obtained for the worst-off should be chosen at the cost of any loss in benefits, however great, for no matter how many better-off people stand to lose.

At the other extreme, one might adopt the neutral-counting rule of aggregative utilitarianism. This tells us to arrange institutions and practices and choose actions and policies so that the sum of benefits over the long run is maximized. The straight maximization rule of utilitarianism tells us to accept severe losses for already badly off individuals if that loss will purchase a marginally higher sum of offsetting benefits for those who are already very well-off. Many find this sort of implication unacceptable, and reject utilitarianism on this basis. One might say that any consequentialist position that cares about how benefits are distributed across persons as well as the total amount of benefits that are produced will reject utilitarianism. The positions that lie between straight summation of benefits all involve tilting in favor of the worse-off, but to an extent less stringent than strict lexical priority. In this range lies the family of positions included within prioritarianism. Since weighting rules that are very close to either the extreme of maximin or the extreme of straight maximize-the-sum-of-benefits will attract objections very close to the criticisms that adhere to the two extremes, I suppose that the versions of prioritarianism that are most defensible and that yield most acceptable implications in practical decision problems will lie toward the middle of the range between these extremes. But I have no precise weighting rule to propose.

THE MORAL STATUS OF DISABILITY

The ADA does not analyze the idea of a disability, which is simply identified with a "physical or mental impairment that substantially limits one or more of the major life activities" of the one who has it. It is useful to distinguish a physical impairment, a chronic or permanent condition of an individual's body that impedes normal physical and mental functioning, from a disability, a physical impairment that leads to a significant diminution of opportunity to function in some valuable way. Nearsightedness is a physical impairment but it does not qualify as a disability on this definition when it is easily correctable and actually corrected by eyeglasses, laser surgery or some other treatment. A physical impairment that affects only an individual's ability to do higher mathematics is not a disability in a hunter-gatherer culture in which no one, impaired or not, would have the opportunity to do higher mathematics. A disability so construed is an uncorrected mismatch between the individual and her environment. What is a disability in one environment is not a disability in another.

Why should disability trigger a requirement of "reasonable accommodation," which, as we have seen, goes beyond anything that could be fit under the protection of a nondiscrimination norm? Suppose a wealthy, talented, charming, legless person is competing for employment with people who are nondisabled but generally lacking in desirable endowments; by any reasonable standard the legless person is better off, all things considered, in the sense that he has higher well-being prospects. Granting that it would be wrong for the employer to pick another less qualified applicant over the legless person on the ground that he has a primitive revulsion against working next to someone with a physical handicap, we might wonder why the law should require the employer to hire the legless person if he is less qualified than the other applicants. Here "less qualified" is meant in the straightforward sense that the net value to the firm of hiring the disabled person is less than the net value added that would accrue to the firm from hiring one of the nondisabled. One must add the proviso that the difference in net value added does not arise via causal processes that are tainted by prejudice (as would be the case if the job involved building widgets, and customers are unwilling to purchase widgets produced by skilled labor of disabled persons). With these stipulations in place, it turns out that the law is intervening in the market to produce a better outcome for an already better-off person at the expense of those who are worse-off. Why do this? What warrants a policy that implies such a result?

One aspect of the matter seems not to touch any issue of principle. Any legal rule will be coarse-grained and will eschew fine-grained distinctions that are difficult to administer. It is better that differential legal treatment of persons should be based on readily observable features of persons that are difficult to fake. It is better that rules should be simple rather than complex, other things being equal. Hence any redistributive policy that aims to help the truly needy and deserving will be framed in terms of easy-to-administer proxies for the subtle matters we should care about. Hence just pointing out that a government policy or legal rule does not perfectly track what we should be caring about is not yet any sort of objection to it. Such an observation rises to the level of an objection only if one can propose an alternative policy that would yield better results overall in the long run from the standpoint of the values we should care about. So perhaps the class of people who are missing one or more legs is a class of people who, on the whole and on the average, are disadvantaged in well-being prospects, all things considered, and that trying to define the class more narrowly would not be worthwhile in the terms of a cost-benefit analysis done in terms of the relevant moral values.

From a prioritarian standpoint, we might raise two kinds of concerns about any given classification scheme in a redistributive policy. One concern is whether we might alter the classification scheme to take account, of course in a rough-grained way, of people's differential responsibility for their unfortunate condition. Here are four persons lacking a leg: one lost a leg while attempting a murder, a second became legless in the course of exemplary battlefield conduct during a war, a third lost a leg while drunk and skiing, and a fourth has a congenital condition. Is there a feasible, administrable, legal classfication scheme that channels redistributive transfers toward the more deserving? If so, prioritarianism will prefer this policy, other things being equal.

A second concern is that according to prioritarianism, the obligation to aid the disadvantaged is in principle an obligation only to aid those who are disadvantaged, all things considered. So in principle we should be on the lookout for social policies that separate the people with a particular disability who are, all things considered, disadvantaged in well-being prospects from those with the same disability who are not disadvantaged in this way. Return now to the example of the very well-off disabled person competing for employment with the generally luckless nondisabled. One might limit the reasonable accommodation requirement to competitions for unskilled and semiskilled employment on the theory that persons lacking a leg who are competing for very lucrative and desirable types of employment are less likely to be truly disadvantaged than those who aspire to simple employment at low pay.

In this connection one should consider the overall consequences of alternative policies that dictate helping or refraining from helping some category of the disabled. For example, a problematic feature of the ADA is that it places the social burden of helping potentially employable disabled persons on the particular employers to whom they apply for jobs and on the customers of their employers, insofar as the employers can pass along the imposed costs of accommodating disability in the form of prices. One can easily cook up examples in which this feature of the act produces ethically suspect results. Imagine a segment of an industry that serves the very poor, for example, producers of cheap plain-quality bread. Suppose that these producers are large firms, which can afford rather high costs when extending accommodations to the disabled to the upper limit of reasonableness. Suppose further that highly desirable jobs at these firms are especially attractive to disabled persons who have lucrative marketable skills and many employment opportunities. If cheap bread has no good substitutes, then the costs of reasonable accommodation of the disabled are for the most part passed along to consumers. In this case the very poor, who are disproportionately among the worse-off members of the population, would be required by the act to subsidize disabled bakers who are disproportionately among the better-off members of the population. Prioritarianism condemns this outcome.

Of course, it is an open question to what extent the hypothetical example just described points to an empirically significant problem for the actual operation of the ADA. After all, it would be a mistake to suppose that being better-off in terms of income and wealth and even employability is closely correlated with being better-off in welfare prospects, the sense of "better-off" to which the prioritarian principle is responsive. The problem that the ADA arbitrarily assigns the costs of subsidizing the disabled is perhaps more likely to be genuine. In principle, prioritarianism would likely favor subsidies to the disabled, varying with the severity of the disability, paid from general tax revenues gathered by progressive taxation.

According to responsibility-catering prioritarianism, there is reason to favor aid to the disabled. The reason is the same as the reason that those born to favorable circumstances should be made to give up resources to better the lot of those born to unfavorable circumstances. Those who are better-off in welfare prospects, especially when this comes about through no merit of their own, should help those who are worse-off in welfare prospects, especially those whose poor prospects have come about through no fault or choice of their own. Prioritarianism offers qualified endorsement of the ADA. It is an instrument—probably not the best available instrument—for providing significant assistance to a group of people who tend to be worse-off than others in welfare prospects. The attitudes toward the ADA that prioritarianism recommends strike me as sensible attitudes, and the fact that prioritarianism generates good-sense recommendations for this difficult problem for theories of justice speaks in its favor.

OBJECTIONS AGAINST THE PRIORITARIAN JUSTICE RESPONSE TO DISABILITY

The responsibility-catering prioritarian approach to the problem of what constitutes fair treatment of the disabled can invite the objection that it is overly solicitous of the disabled as well as the objection that it is not solicitous enough. Consider the former worry first. We then consider the objection that prioritarianism responds to what it takes to be well-being deficits in a way that is unfair to persons.

Prioritarianism is too solicitous. If we claim that what distributive justice requires depends on the well-being that individuals can expect under given arrangements, it is sometimes supposed that distributive justice will end up dictating that virtually all available resources should go to those with the lowest welfare prospects, even if they can hardly be helped by further provision of aid. After all, after helping them some, they will still be worst-off, hence entitled to ever more help. In this way the hopelessly worst-off would become a basin attracting all resources. (Of course we should not crudely identify the class of the disabled with the class of the worst-off, but it is plausible to think that severely disabled individuals will be frequently among those worst-off in overall well-being.)

It should be evident that a prioritarian approach to justice is not vulnerable to this objection. The moral value of obtaining a benefit for an individual, we recall, depends on the size of the benefit that can be obtained as well as the welfare expectation of the potential beneficiary. Prioritarianism, given plausible weights attached to the various factors that compose it, will not generate the result that justice demands that better-off people should make huge sacrifices in well-being to obtain negligible increases in the well-being of every worst-off. Prioritarianism is not the same as the excessively rigid maximin.

Prioritarianism is insufficiently solicitous. The prioritarian welfarist approach can also invite the objection that it does not ask us to do enough for the disabled. To illustrate the problem, consider an example first posed by G. A. Cohen.[10] Think of Tiny Tim, the crippled boy in Charles Dickens's story *A Christmas Carol.* Though crippled, Tim is extremely cheerful, so one might suppose that overall he has high welfare. So a theory of distributive justice that scans society for individuals with low welfare expectation and directs resources and other forms of aid to them will miss Tim or, rather, will regard him as fortunate (high in welfare), not unfortunate. But most of us would think that a decent society will provide Tiny Tim a wheelchair or some other aid that will improve his mobility capability. If welfarist justice does not support that result, it stands condemned.

In response, we should first of all be careful not to confound subjective feelings of happiness or subjective preference satisfaction with true welfare. It may well be the case that a sensible objective measure of well-being, presented with Tim's comprehensive circumstances, would judge that he has a low well-being expectation despite his jaunty cheerfulness. The conviction that Tim merits aid on a basis of distributive justice may well stem from convictions about true welfare. I would, however, not shrink from the possibility that someone like Tim might be very badly off along one dimension of welfare such as mobility, but very well endowed along other important dimensions, so that overall Tim is well-off, one of the lucky ones, despite his physical impairment. That surely is possible, and not an embarrassment to a welfarist theory.

But another confusion may enter into our reaction to the case. We need to distinguish different levels of abstraction in the theory of justice. It might, for all that I have said, turn out that at the level of social policy, distributive justice in its practical mode will call for compensation for observable physical impairment but pay no heed to more elusive psychological traits such as cheerfulness, which are less easy to observe and perhaps more easily faked by persons wishing to manipulate the distributive justice agency unfairly. (The issue is not whether Tim's external demeanor appears cheerful, but whether his internal mood is happy or morose, and this may be hard to discern.) Moreover, if Tim is genuinely cheerful in a way that boosts his welfare score, this cheerfulness may reflect arduous virtuous effort on his part, rather than being part of his overall initial endowment of traits and circumstances. If feasible distributive justice agencies cannot reliably distinguish the case of a Tim who is cheerful through his own efforts from the case of a Tim who is naturally cheerful, that is another reason not to let individual cheerfulness directly control what one owes to society and is owed from it according to distributive justice at the social policy level. In short, it seems to me that prioritarianism provides appropriate guidance in thinking of fair social policy responses to Tim's plight.

Prioritarianism might be thought to recommend an inherently inadequate response to the problem of inclusion and exclusion. The costs and benefits of altering the social environment so that various classes of disabled persons can become full participants in the scheme of social cooperation might be such that prioritarianism would recommend setting the social environment so that some are excluded. How can this be moral? Surely morality must require arranging institutions and pactices so that all who can be made full participants are accorded that status.

I do not believe that the requirement of inclusion can be plausibly regarded as a trumping value in social policy. It is not entirely clear in this context what it is to be included as a full participant in social cooperation, but suppose that a particular society is arranged so that some people with severe and intractable cognitive disabilities and mental illness have no opportunities to secure employment, become heads of families, or vote and participate in other standard duties of citizens such as jury duty. Suppose we agree that whatever social inclusion involves, in this example these people fail to gain this valued status. This need not be wrong. The costs of inclusion might be too great for other members of society in the long run. To insist on inclusion being a trumping value, whatever the cost in well-being for everybody else, is tantamount to adopting a maximin principle that holds that society must be arranged so that the least well-off in well-being is made as well-off as possible. Here, as elsewhere, maximin gives too extreme a priority to the interests of the very worst-off.

Prioritarianism wrongfully insults people and fails to respect their dignity. Some philosophers see at the root of the conception of distributive justice that I endorse an insidious devaluation of the lives of the disabled and a tilt toward failing to treat them in ways that respect their equal dignity as persons. The problem as they see it starts with the basic assumption that social justice consists in identifying unfortunate people with bad life prospects, who need help, along with lucky people with good life prospects, who are tagged with the obligation to help. Anita Silvers expresses this suspicion when she writes that for people with disabilities, "justice must offer, first, the visibility of full participatory citizenship, not a spotlight that targets them as needing more than others do."[11]

Two aspects of this objection may be distinguished. One is that the focus on identifying fortunate and unfortunate individuals deflects attention from the more fundamental justice concern of identifying unfair practices and institutions, especially deeply embedded ones. This train of thought leads Silvers to welcome the ADA on the ground that it enacts "a conceptual shift in the meaning of 'disability.' Rather than defining 'disability' as a disadvantageous physical or mental deficit of persons, it codifies the understanding of 'disability' as a defective state of society which disadvantages those persons."[12]

A second aspect of the objection is the idea that a conception of justice that demarcates classes of advantaged and disadvantaged citizens inevitably insults the worth and dignity of those it singles out as needing help. Illustrating this idea, Elizabeth Anderson has imagined an "egalitarian" dystopia in which the Distributive Justice Equality Agency sends compensation checks to those identified as disadvantaged along with explanatory letters such as: "To the disabled: Your defective native endowments or current disabilities, alas, make your life less worth living than the lives of normal people. To compensate for this misfortune, we, the able ones, will give you extra resources."[13]

Responsibility-catering prioritarianism is alleged to make matters even worse. Besides demeaning those singled out for aid by declaring their lives absent aid to be defective, responsibility-catering prioritarianism, in attempting to distinguish responsible and irresponsible agents, involves those charged with implementing the principle in making morally offensive and inappropriate judgments about the merits of individuals' private choices about how to lead their own lives.

These are significant concerns intelligently expressed. But prioritarianism in my view is already an adequate response to them.

First, prioritarianism does not take existing social conditions as fixed and immutable. The status quo is privileged only in that it exists. What is just, according to prioritarianism, depends on how we can achieve the best long-run state of affairs that maximizes moral value from here—from our current starting point. Prioritarianism might, in given circumstances, require money payments as compensation to individuals, or it may be that the efficient way to make progress toward justice is to alter social arrangements in some small-scale or large-scale way. Distributive justice might require changes in the laws, transformation of the economy, the dissolution of sovereign nations in favor of a world government, or whatever. Prioritarianism does not make the mistake of assigning a normatively privileged status to the social status quo.

Second, consider the claim that any implementation of responsibility-catering prioritarianism inherently imposes morally wrongful insult and stigma. The problem of insult is significant. Since individuals do in fact tend to identify their worth with their personal endowments, which have fallen on them through processes of inheritance that are entirely beyond their power to control and for which they can claim no credit, social policies that involve public assignment of compensation on the basis of a public assessment of one's comprehensive circumstances and personal traits can be stigmatizing and insulting to the extent that they become counterproductive. However, this point can lead us astray. Being judged and graded and measured according to the quality of one's traits as perceived by others is a routine and everyday occurrence in social relations, whether in the job market, the marriage market, the dating scene, family life, spheres of voluntary association, spheres of friendship, professional associations and so on. Would public-sphere official judgments on these sensitive matters be more hurtful and debilitating than the private-sphere judgments that we cope with every day?

Perhaps so. To the extent this is so, prioritarian justice will seek to tailor social policies that mitigate the harm that is thereby done. For example, paternalistic policies might perhaps better be made in a coarse-grained way that does not institute different rules for those judged to be good choosers and bad choosers, because the cost of stigma involved in being a bad chooser may outweigh the benefits of having separate policies catering to distinct types of people. But this depends on calculation. In some cases, all things considered, a social policy that imposes some stigma and insult may be best overall, because these costs are outweighed by offsetting benefits as measured by prioritarian justice standards.

The same point holds for responsibility catering. If it is possible to establish a workable policy that discriminates between the more and the less responsible, this may make the less responsible feel bad, but if the policy satisfies responsibility-catering prioritarianism, then it would not be possible to alleviate these bad feelings except by sacrificing well-being for others that has greater moral value by RCP calculation.

The point of justice, I would say, is not to avoid stigma and insult at all cost, but rather to promote people's well-being while giving greater weight to well-being gains for the badly off and those picked out by a reasonable responsibility standard as more deserving of aid.

NOTES

[1]For a challenging argument for a position directly counter to mine, see Anita Silvers, "Formal Justice," in Anita Silvers, David Wasserman, and Mary Mahowald, *Disability, Difference, Discrimination: Perspectives on Justice in Bioethics and Public Policy.* Lanham and Boulder, CO: Rowman & Littlefield, 1998, 13–145.

[2]One might also interpret contract at will asymmetrically, so that during the term of a labor contract the employer cannot fire the employee except as specified in the terms of the contract and can be compelled by law to rehire if he breaches the contract by terminating employment. But on the side of the employee, a voluntary quit that breaches the terms of the contract can only trigger legally compelled payment of monetary compensation for damages, not legally compelled resubmission to employment according to the terms of the contract.

[3]If the market is perfectly competitive, there are no nonfiscal externalities, and other standard conditions obtain, then the outcome in which statistical discrimination occurs will be efficient in the sense of Pareto-optimal.

[4]Mark Kelman, "Concepts of Discrimination in 'General Ability' Job Testing," *Harv. L. Rev.* 104:1175–1247, 1226 (1991). See also, Mark Kelman, "Does Disability Status Matter?" this volume.

[5]Notice that a teenager who is denied employment opportunities on the ground that it is a more urgent matter to ensure employment opportunities for adults and who dies at an early age does suffer disadvantage, perhaps unfair disadvantage, via this form of age discrimination. This teenager marked for early death does not benefit from the discrimination in favor of prime-age adults. One might consider the case of a teenager who has a known uncorrectable propensity to contract an ailment that might result in his early death and who suffers age discrimination. This case looks morally problematic in a way that uniform discrimination against the old, applying equally to all who live to old age, does not.

[6]John Rawls, *A Theory of Justice.* Cambridge, MA: Harvard University Press, 1971.

[7]This section considers whether or not an antidiscrimination norm is sufficient for social justice, and answers in the negative. A further question arises: Is satisfaction of the antidiscrimination norm as standardly conceived in contemporary society necessary for social justice? Is the idea of a just society that tolerates discrimination a contradiction in terms? For arguments for negative answers to these questions, see my "Against Rawlsian Equality of Opportunity," *Philosophical Studies* 93:77 (1999).

[8]Catharine MacKinnon, *Feminism Unmodified.* Cambridge, MA: Harvard University Press, 1987.

[9]By Allen Buchanan in "Choosing Who Will Be Disabled: Genetic Intervention and the Morality of Inclusion," *Social Philosophy and Policy* 13 (1996).

[10]See G. A. Cohen, "On the Currency of Egalitarian Justice," *Ethics* 99:904 (1989).

[11]Silvers, "Formal Justice," p. 145.

[12]Anita Silvers, "(In)Equality, (Ab)normality, and the 'Americans with Disabilities Act,'" *Journal of Medicine and Philosophy* 21:209 (1996).

[13]Elizabeth S. Anderson, "What Is the Point of Equality?" *Ethics* 109:287 (1999). For a response, see my "Luck Egalitarianism and Prioritarianism," *Ethics* 110 (January 2000).

Justice for People with Disabilities
The Semiconsequentialist Approach

The dominant school of political philosophy in the Anglo-American world, egalitarian liberalism, has spawned two fundamentally different views of social justice. The first view conceives injustice in terms of *unchosen inequalities* and as inhering, first and foremost, in a social state. On its simple, strictly egalitarian version, a social state is unjust insofar as persons in it are rendered worse off than others by factors beyond their control. This version, duly specified, defines an ideal social state in which no person is worse-off than others except only as a consequence of (free and informed) choices this person has made. Many humanly controllable factors influence the extent to which a given social state fulfills this ideal; and these factors, on the basis of their impact on the justice of this social state, can then receive a derivative assessment as more or less just. Social institutions—and then, presumably, also our more informal social practices, conventions, ethos, culture and personal conduct—should, as far as feasible, promote equality of opportunities, or a solely choice-sensitive overall distribution of quality of life.[1]

The second view conceives injustice as *denial of equal (or evenhanded) treatment*, as manifested in the formulation or administration of coercively imposed social rules.[2] On the simple, strictly egalitarian version of this view, a social order is then unjust insofar as it treats some of its participants worse than others.[3] Here equal treatment means that each participant receives equivalent helps and hindrances, or benefits and burdens. Such equal treatment is not, then, equality-promoting treatment. Personal (for example, genetically based) differences among persons—however unchosen—are not seen as a collective responsibility and are not required (by this view of social justice) to be corrected or compensated at public expense.

There are more loosely egalitarian versions of both of these views—notably versions that have recently come to be known as prioritarian.[4] On such versions, the ideal may involve departures from strict equality, provided these departures raise the lowest position relative to what it would be with strict equality. Thus a prioritarian version of the first view would permit persons to be rendered worse off than others by factors beyond their control, but only insofar as this affords them superior opportunities relative to the strictly egalitarian baseline. And a prioritarian version of the second view would permit some participants to receive less-than-equivalent packages of benefits and burdens, but only insofar as these packages are superior to the (mutually equivalent) packages all participants would receive with strict equality.

Both these views (in their prioritarian versions) can appeal to John Rawls, the patron saint of anglophone egalitarian liberalism.[5] Adherents of the first view can invoke the original position with its veil of ignorance, consequent to which, Rawls holds, the criterion of social justice is chosen pursuant to the maximin rule.[6] They can argue that parties in the original position should be presumed to know that citizens' quality of life depends not only on social benefits and burdens, but also on their personal constitution or natural endowments.[7] If the parties know this, and if they choose rationally pursuant to the maximin rule, they will seek to raise the floor of quality of life by aiming for a social order under which no one must cope with *both*: poor natural endowments *and* a paltry bundle of social benefits and burdens. Reasoning in this way, the parties would then select a criterion of justice that favors basic structures under which the social and natural distributions are negatively correlated, so that those with an unfavorable personal constitution tend to have greater social advantages.[8]

The second view can point to the fact that the criterion of social justice Rawls has actually proposed, his two principles of justice, does not favor such a negative correlation. Rather, it assesses each social order exclusively on the basis of the distribution of *social* primary goods it produces: "a hypothetical initial arrangement in which all the social primary goods are equally distributed . . . provides a benchmark for judging improvements" (*TJ* 62). Rawls's two principles of justice disregard all information about the distribution of natural primary goods, such as "health and vigor, intelligence and imagination" (*TJ* 62): "The natural distribution is neither just nor unjust" (*TJ* 102).

My discussion and extension of Rawls's theory, which treated the two competing views under the more general labels of "full consequentialism" and "semiconsequentialism" respectively, sought to resolve the tension in favor of the second view.[9] I have later come to the conclusion that such a reconciliation is not workable—that there is no plausible way of deriving a semiconsequentialist criterion of social justice from the prudential perspective of prospective citizens (as modelled in a hypothetical contract of the sort Rawls imagines).[10] Rawls is, then, as I now see it, deeply divided against himself. And so is egalitarian liberalism: into a fully consequentialist—or, as I would now prefer to say, "purely recipient-oriented"—variant and one that (for lack of a better name) I will continue to call semiconsequentialist.

Both views face a severe challenge in the question of how a just society should respond to its members' diseases and disabilities. Here the two variants of egalitarian liberalism clash most forcefully. One side seems committed to the indefinite expansion of our health care system by devoting it to neutralizing (through medical research, treatment, alleviation and compensation) all handicaps, disabilities and other health problems from which persons may suffer through no fault of their own. The other side seems committed to the callous judgment that we, as a society, need do no more for those who have diseases or disabilities through no fault of ours than we need do for any healthy citizens.

It is not surprising, then, that concern for people with disabilities and support for the first view often go together. Thus it is argued that, because a just society is one in which unchosen inequalities are rectified, people with disabilities ought to be entitled, at public expense, to all the "services needed to maintain, restore, or compensate for normal species-typical functioning."[11] And it is also argued, in the opposite direction, that the first variant of egalitarian liberalism must be superior because justice as the second variant conceives it would require only modest, ungenerous, stinting and highly contingent provisions for people with disabilities.[12]

A prominent exception to this pattern is Anita Silvers, who is a strong advocate for people with disabilities and nevertheless defends a version of the second view, which she believes to be the philosophical position that informs the 1990 Americans with Disabilities Act.[13] In doing so, she reproduces some of the usual arguments against conceiving social justice as requiring compensation for the disabled. Thus she makes the point of principle that no good reason has been advanced why nondisabled persons should have a duty of justice (rather than reasons of charity or beneficence) to make transfers to the disabled, when the former are not responsible for the prevailing discrepancy in endowments and also have not discriminated against or taken advantage of the latter.[14] And she makes the pragmatic points that: (a) viewing people with disabilities as entitled to compensatory transfers grounded in their special needs is associated with the medical model of disability on which people with disabilities are viewed as defective, needy, dependent, weak, incompetent and fit to be pitied;[15] (b) there is no nonarbitrary or uncontroversial way of determining, in the face of persons claiming to be impaired or handicapped, who really is owed compensation, and how much;[16] and (c) recognition of a legal right to compensation encourages people to claim all sorts of handicaps and impairments, which in turn leads to excessive growth in the scope and cost of compensatory programs as well as to fierce struggles among different claimant groups over a pool of compensation funds which, in the end, can only grow so much (Silvers 25, 29, 98, 119, 140).

To appreciate the full force of these last two pragmatic arguments, one should bear in mind that people with disabilities are not the only ones who can claim native disadvantage. The quality of human lives may be considerably reduced by a whole host of unchosen personal features that, though not considered severe enough to qualify for the title of a disability, can be the source of considerable distress and disadvantage. Examples are (the milder cases of) bad memory, excessive self-consciousness, various anxieties and phobias, weight problems, sexual dysfunctions, infertility, premature hair loss, ugliness, shortness, addictive personality, melancholy short of depression, concentration difficulties short of attention deficit disorder and so on.[17] The attempt to maintain an institutional scheme that appropriately compensates for all such handicaps could easily be highly divisive, producing endless battles among claimant groups over the proper allocation of compensation funds.

Silvers also adduces a second group of arguments, which are based more directly on the interests of people with disabilities. The mere fact that a person has a disability can ground a right to compensation only if having this disability is bad for that person, only if, other things being equal, lives with this disability are less rewarding or less worthwhile than lives without it. Silvers, however, rejects as largely false and highly pernicious the belief that people with a disability are, by this fact alone, worse off than others. This belief is pernicious because it attributes the hardships people with disabilities currently encounter to fate or misfortune and thereby diverts attention from the important role that social factors—discrimination and exclusion—play in the production of these hardships. Only after discrimination and exclusion will have been overcome will it be possible to make an accurate assessment of whether there are any disabled persons whose lives are less worthwhile as a consequence merely of their disability.[18]

The belief that the lives of people with disabilities are less worthwhile is also pernicious in another way: by suggesting that we have reason to want the number of such lives to be reduced through eugenic measures. Silvers deplores this suggestion in several contexts. Thus she holds that couples with disabilities should not be discouraged from having children who are likely to share their disability (Silvers 94) and that such couples should not be denied genetic counseling on how to improve their chances of conceiving a child who will share their disability (Silvers 77, where her example is deafness). And she restates with approval Jenny Morris's view that even severely disabled (quadriplegic) persons should be no more (or less) entitled to choose death than unhappy but healthy adults.[19]

Silvers sets forth, then, the vision of a just society that treats disabilities on the social rather than on the medical model, that is, treats disability as on a par with race, gender and sexual orientation. Justice requires the eradication of all social barriers excluding people with disabilities and of all discrimination against them in the public sphere. Once this will have been fully achieved, a just society owes no special services, benefits or advantages to people with disabilities—just as such a society owes no special services, benefits or advantages to women, to gays and lesbians, or to persons of color.

Having briefly sketched the main thrust of Silvers's position, let us now examine how well her treatment of the topic of disabilities in the context of the second, semiconsequentialist variant of egalitarian liberalism can withstand attacks in behalf of the first, fully consequentialist variant. The central idea of such attacks is nicely illustrated in a story Silvers tells about her two dogs, a Great Dane and a little dachshund (Silvers 127). The point of this story is that equal, or fair, treatment of the two dogs requires that both be given their food at a location that is equally accessible to each. The dogs would be treated unequally, Silvers writes, if their food were placed on top of the kitchen counter, where the Great Dane but not the dachshund can reach it. In response to this little story, Wasserman maintains that it would be equally unfair to give each dog the same amount of food: "If the dog-sitter fails to treat the two dogs equally when she sets the dachshund's food at the Great Dane's height, she also fails to treat them equally when she gives the Great Dane a dachshund-size portion" (Wasserman 269). But this is not a winning argument. It would indeed be wrong to starve the Great Dane by feeding it dachshund-size portions. But the wrongness of such conduct does not diminish when the dachshund is taken out of the picture entirely. The Great Dane's entitlement to adequate food would thus seem to be based not on a right to fair or equal treatment *vis-à-vis* the dachshund, but on the special obligations that come with pet ownership. Since Wasserman does not attribute to nondisabled citizens analogous special obligations toward their disabled compatriots, his extension of Silvers's story does not damage her case.

Let us translate the story into the context it was meant to illuminate. Providing clerical employment at a location that can be reached only by stairs is unfair to wheelchair-bound applicants, Silvers maintains, and a just society would be one in which employment opportunities are equally accessible to all those capable of doing the job. Would it be equally unfair for an employer to offer equal pay for equal work to wheelchair-bound and nondisabled clerical workers? Wasserman suggests that this would be unfair in light of the greater needs of wheelchair-bound persons who, through no fault of theirs, face additional expenses associated with their disability. But this is just what Silvers denies, holding that a just society need not force its nondisabled citizens to help their disabled compatriots cope with the special challenges that the latter face through no fault of the former. The question is still open.

To make progress, a more detailed reconstruction of Silvers's position is needed. We might begin by distinguishing three kinds of harm that a person might suffer on account of a disability. There are, first, immediate harms, such as pain or the frustration resulting from the inability to perform certain mental operations or physical activities. There are, second, harms caused by the disability in conjunction with features of the natural environment. Allergies are an example: harm materializes only when the allergenic substance (e.g., pollen, peanuts) is present in the environment of the person with the allergy. There are, third, harms caused by the disability in conjunction with features of the social (and perhaps also the natural) environment.[20]

Silvers holds that it is not unjust to deny any and all compensatory help for harms of the first two kinds, however undeserved they may be and however untraceable to choices by those who are suffering these harms. Thus, according to her, justice does not require that people with disabilities receive subsidies at public expense toward the purchase of (insurance for) any corrective equipment—such as hearing aids, eyeglasses, canes for the blind, crutches, wheelchairs and so forth.[21] Holding this view leaves Silvers free to acknowledge that there are other kinds of moral reasons to help: that offering such help would, for instance, be kind or generous (cf Silvers 31). But the issue here before us concerns our responsibilities under the title of justice—and these responsibilities, Silvers claims, extend only to harms of the third kind.

I will probe Silvers's position by asking whether the key distinction, whose moral significance she asserts, can be drawn precisely enough, and whether justice demands either less or more than she contends.

I

Silvers uses as a paradigm example of a harm of the third kind the lack of access that walking-impaired persons suffer due to the fact that many public locations are accessible only by steps or stairs. In order to classify this lack as a harm (and also in order to assess how great a harm this is), we need to identify some baseline (or "no-harm") environment. We can then say of particular people with disabilities that they are harmed by a social environment if and insofar as they are worse off in it than they would be in the baseline environment. How, then, is the relevant baseline environment to be identified in a plausible way?

Silvers answers this question through a thought experiment which she calls "historical counterfactualizing" (Silvers 129–131): we are to imagine how the members of our society would have shaped their social environment (for the sake of their own productivity and convenience), if the large majority of them had been disabled. People with disabilities here and now have a right in justice to the hypothetical social environment imagined through the thought experiment, and they are harmed if and insofar as they are worse off in the existing social environment than they would be in the one imagined through the thought experiment, which Silvers imagines as "an environment fully suited to them" (Silvers 133).

There are several main issues that need clarification here. To begin with, it is unclear how the great diversity of disabilities is to be incorporated into Silvers's test. Are we to conduct separate thought experiments for each kind of disability or a single thought experiment for all kinds? And if the latter, are we to imagine that most citizens have all disabilities or that most citizens have some disability or other? The first of these options (separate thought experiments) makes little sense because it would lead to conflicting justice claims in the real world: it is evident that a population of mostly deaf persons would not shape their social environment as a population of mostly blind persons would. The second option also makes little sense, because a society in which most citizens have *all* disabilities is so remote. It is quite unclear how such a society and its majority of very severely disabled members would reproduce themselves over time and what technologies they would have developed. The third option seems to be the most promising: we can imagine existing disabilities to be more frequent than they are among us, so that no persons, or only a few, are nondisabled.

But how frequent would each kind of disability be in this imagined world? It may be tempting to respond that all disabilities should be imagined to occur at exactly the same frequency (much higher than in the actual world), so as to preclude advantaging or disadvantaging any disability group on the basis of their larger or smaller imagined size. But this proposal runs into the fatal question of how disabilities are to be individuated in a nonarbitrary way: Are all those with cognitive impairments to be considered to constitute one disability group, or several? Are persons struck with some combination of impairments

(Down syndrome and blindness; deafness and quadriplegia) to be viewed as a separate disability group or as the intersection of several such groups?[22]

The only promising alternative response I can see would propose that the thought experiment should increase the frequency of each disability proportionately (multiplying the existing percentage in each disability category by some uniform factor n). But this proposal runs into three difficulties:

(1) The thought experiment would once again be sensitive to how the relevant categories of disabilities are defined. To illustrate: Assume that in the actual population 2 percent are blind and 3 percent are deaf, and assume also that these disabilities are not correlated, so that 0.06 percent are both blind and deaf (1.94 percent blind only, 2.94 percent deaf only, 94.06 percent neither). Now there are two ways of specifying Silvers's thought experiment based on a factor of n equals 10. On the one hand, one could imagine that 20 percent would be blind and 30 percent deaf and, since there would again be no correlation among these two disabilities, 6 percent would be both blind and deaf (14 percent would be blind only, 24 percent would be deaf only and 56 percent would be neither). On this specification, however, the number of those who are both blind and deaf has increased a hundredfold rather than merely tenfold. To fix this, one might consider being both blind and deaf a separate disability, so that in the imagined world of the thought experiment, 0.6 percent would be blind and deaf, 19.4 percent would be blind only, 29.4 percent would be deaf only and 50.6 percent would be neither. On this construal, however, one is introducing a (negative) correlation between blindness and deafness, which (by assumption) does not exist in the actual world.

(2) Basing the thought experiment on existing frequencies of the various categories of disability may not square with a central moral intuition Silvers is apparently seeking to communicate through her thought experiment—the intuition, namely, that the valid justice claims that persons with a specific disability have on their society are independent of the frequency of this disability. If the extent to which our common social environment should be shaped so as to accommodate people with disabilities is (as Silvers's thought experiment suggests) independent of how numerous this group is relative to that of the nondisabled, then the fair way of balancing the interests of different disability groups in shaping this common social environment should also be independent of how numerous these various disability groups are—or so it would seem. A uniform factor n, however, preserves the numerical strength of the various disability groups. Very small disability groups would still be small in the parallel world, because the existing frequency of disabilities places tight limits on how large a factor n can be chosen: if, as matters stand, 20 percent of the population have one disability, then n must be below 5. And if n is below 5, then the smallest disability groups would, even after multiplication by n, still be quite small, too small perhaps to make much of a difference to what our social environment would be like. For these small disability groups, the thought experiment would, then, yield weaker justice demands than, I presume, Silvers would want to endorse.

Lest these queries seem overly pedantic, let me make clear why Silvers's thought experiment needs the kind of precision I ask for. Clearly, the shaping of our common social environment has a differential impact on different groups.[23] We can see this most clearly by considering how alternative feasible social environments should be ranked, taking account of how the various features of each such environment as well as the cost of maintaining it would affect people's discretionary income. The outcome of this exercise would be highly sensitive to the standpoint from which these alternatives are assessed. This standpoint might be characterized through the standard interests of the nondisabled, of the blind, of the deaf, of the walking-impaired, of persons with Down syndrome or of any of an indefinite number of other groups. In many, many ways, what is better for some is worse for others. And if Silvers's thought experiment is to provide any guidance for how the many diverse standard interests of all these different groups are to be balanced against one another, then it must be clear how strongly these various standard interests would be represented in the hypothetical parallel world she is asking us to imagine.[24]

Even if a more precise specification of Silvers's thought experiment were offered, with clear-cut instructions about how frequent the various disabilities should be imagined to be among the people in the parallel world, it is still doubtful whether the thought experiment would yield determinate results. One problem here is the general uncertainty surrounding historical counterfactuals. Ask yourself how the last thirty years would have gone had Lyndon B. Johnson not decided to quit the 1968 presidential election. Who would have won the election? What would have happened in Vietnam? Would Deng and his reformers have won in China? Would Gorbachev have come to power? Would the Soviet Union still be in business? Would nuclear war have broken out? If no one really knows even the rough probabilities with respect to such a relatively minor divergence from the actual history, then how are we supposed to have determinate knowledge about the social arrangements that would have resulted from the political struggles among the very differently composed population Silvers imagines?

Further difficulties arise from the fact that Silvers specifically asks us to speculate about alternative technologies and infrastructures: these are highly path-dependent and also highly sensitive to research and development efforts. In the parallel world, where most people are disabled, many fabulous technologies would probably have been developed. Some of these we cannot even imagine. In reflecting on these matters, Silvers seems hopelessly unimaginative, asserting, for instance, that the parallel world would be dominated by two-door cars, which make it much easier to stow a wheelchair behind the front seat (Silvers 63). But who says that the population of that world would have developed cars at all, let alone have spent untold trillions of dollars as well as enormous amounts of human ingenuity to build and maintain them, together with the paved roads they require? With lots of blind people in the population, and lots with other disabilities that prevent them from driving a car safely, it is quite possible that they would have developed a highly automated public transportation system capable of smoothly conveying millions of persons and shipments simultaneously to their intended destinations, with very little effort on the part of persons in transit. In any case, we simply do not know how that population would have shaped their transportation infrastructure and their world more generally, and we therefore cannot judge our world by reference to that parallel world Silvers invokes.[25]

Let me make the same point once more in a way that sticks as closely as possible to Silvers's paradigm ramps-versus-stairs example. Is it true that, if a much larger proportion of citizens were walking-impaired, public spaces would feature ramps instead of steps and stairs? Probably so. But perhaps not. Recently a wheelchair has been developed that allows its occupant to surmount minor obstacles and, in particular, steps and stairs. It is quite likely that something of this kind would have been developed much earlier in the parallel world, so that in it the choice between ramps and stairs might have become a matter of indifference to the walking-impaired.[26] Assuming this to be so, and taking our moral cues from the parallel world as Silvers suggests, we are then compelled to conclude that perhaps the walking-impaired in our world have a right in justice *not* to a social environment in which steps and stairs are replaced by ramps, but rather to a social environment that includes the opportunity to buy advanced wheelchairs (or superadvanced personal transportation devices) at whatever prices would prevail if their disability were much more fre-quent than it is.

II

The issues just pondered bring us to our second question: whether the thought experiment can have the moral significance Silvers attaches to it—can help us correctly identify what justice demands. Our discussion has suggested two weak spots. First, Silvers's appeals to the thought experiment attach great moral importance to the distinction between two differ-ent kinds of variables through which the situation of people with disabilities may be greatly improved: the maintenance of a social environment "fully suited to them," on the one hand, and the provision of special services, benefits and advantages, on the other. Silvers holds that people with disabilities have a right in justice to the former, even if quite expen-sive, but none to the latter, even if quite cheap. Second, Silvers's appeals to the thought experiment assume that the number of people with disabilities has no moral significance: as a matter of justice, society owes people with disabilities the social environment that would exist if they were quite numerous, irrespective of how numerous they actually are.

II.1

Silvers may seem to be drawn to her view by associating it with the idea of negative rights and duties as these are often thought of in the world of anglophone legal and philosophical theory. A conduct or policy choice that *unduly harms* some persons is thought to violate a (negative) right of these persons and thus to breach a (negative) duty of justice—even if the harm is slight, the number of persons affected by it is small, and the opportunity costs of not imposing the harm are great.[27] Even if millions of dollars could be saved by falsely con-victing a few persons of minor misdemeanors, it would still be an injustice. By contrast, a conduct or policy choice that *fails to help* people is not thought of as an injustice—even when such help would quite substantially reduce the great suffering of very many persons at low cost.

Tying Silvers's position to these Anglo-American moral intuitions about positive and negative agency has some plausibility in the context of her paradigm ramps-versus-stairs example, in which it may make sense to view the building of steps and stairs as the active imposition of impediments to freedom and thus as the violation of a negative duty of jus-tice (while the denial of wheelchairs is merely a failure to help and thus, at most, a lack of charity).[28] As one goes beyond Silvers's paradigm example, however, it becomes clear that this hypothesis cannot explain her position—that what she demands by way of a social environment fully suited to persons with disabilities asks much more of a society's citizens and government than that they cease to harm such persons unduly. Thus consider another example she briefly discusses: access to communication for the deaf. Silvers reports that under older legislation (the Individuals with Disabilities Education Act, or IDEA): "sign language interpreters are mandated as a service to those deaf youngsters who cannot other-wise perform adequately in school but are not a right of those whose academic perfor-mance is at least average despite their having only the partial access to information that lipreading can achieve" (Silvers 134). By providing a targeted benefit to those most in need on account of their handicap, this legislation is informed by the medical model of disabil-ity, which Silvers rejects. "But under the ADA, sign language interpreters are considered a necessity for all deaf youngsters who can benefit from them, regardless of how well these students perform in the absence of signing. The assumption is that those who perform well without interpreters nevertheless deserve the same opportunity to excel, by having the same full access to information that their hearing peers enjoy" (Silvers 134). This more recent legislation is informed by the social model of disability, which Silvers endorses, inasmuch as it seeks to provide no special benefit to anyone but merely aims to give all students equal access to the society's educational facilities.

According to Silvers, the ADA's requirement of sign language interpreters achieves this goal only imperfectly and should be regarded as: "a makeshift remedy required to adapt to a discriminatory practice that cannot easily be reformed" (Silvers 258). This discriminatory practice is communication by sound only: "conveying information through speech rather than pictures is a convention that excludes people who are deaf. Reforming the practice to make it nondiscriminatory requires all conversationalists to add signing to their speech, a formidable demand on hearing individuals that is partially and temporarily relieved by the use of sign language interpreters" (Silvers 258). In a similar vein, one could argue that the written language we use, as well as the existing car-centered transportation network, discriminate against the blind. If all writing were done in Braille, texts would be equally accessible to the blind and to the seeing. And if we had a highly automated public transportation system, travel would be as easy for the blind as for the seeing.

These further examples bring out clearly what the ramps-versus-stairs example may conceal: that accommodation can have considerable social costs.[29] Such costs highlight the two weak spots I have diagnosed: Does it really make sense to insist on the moral significance of Silvers's distinction between the maintenance of a social environment fully suited to persons with disabilities and the provision to them of special services, benefits and advantages? And does it really make sense to say that justice requires the addition of signing to speech—insofar as this can be accomplished without undue burdens (*cf* note 29)—regardless of how many persons are disadvantaged when we fail to make this addition?[30]

However one may answer these questions, the specific efforts Silvers demands toward giving people with disabilities full access to all communications and to a transportation system fully suited to them do not seem to be justifiable by a negative right or duty. It is hard to see how our *failure* to build a highly automated public transportation system, say, could be viewed as *restricting* the liberty of people with disabilities and thus as violating a negative duty of justice toward them. And it is also hard to see how our *failure* to add sign language to our oral communications (and our failure to choose Braille for our written ones and for the Internet) could be viewed as unduly *harming* those who then cannot understand us. After all, others have no right that we direct communication at them at all, let alone that we do so in a language they can understand; we are well within our rights when we remain silent or communicate selectively. Or so it is generally thought.

The challenge that Silvers's position, understood as invoking negative rights, faces here can be further illuminated by three additional arguments. First, by communicating in some particular language, conversationalists and authors could be said to discriminate against those who lack mastery of this language. Do the excluded, then, have a right in justice to have such communications translated into a language they can understand—or a right in justice that there should be as much communication available in their language as is available in any other? Most would find such a demand patently absurd. So, I assume, would Silvers. But how can she differentiate from it the demand she makes in behalf of people with disabilities? She could point out, quite correctly, that her demand is different in that native speakers of Estonian or Icelandic have the capacity to learn other languages (e.g., English), in which much more communication is available, whereas the blind cannot learn to read and the deaf cannot learn to process speech. But this truth is irrelevant to the issue at hand, irrelevant to the question of whether those excluded have been harmed unduly, have suffered the violation of a negative right. To see this, consider a more familiar parallel case: whether my refusal to give you food harms you unduly (violates a negative right of yours) does not depend at all on whether you have other ways of getting food. Rather, it depends on whether you are entitled to receive food from me—because you own it, for example, or because I have made a contract or promise to give it to you.

Second, one might say that people with disabilities are unduly harmed by the way in which the large majority of the nondisabled have been shaping the common social environment for their own convenience. But this explication of Silvers's position, too, has absurd offshoots. Our common social environment is shaped to the detriment of many small groups whose members might then equally well complain of injustice. Our country is saturated with cars, roads and pollution, with advertisements and pop music, golf courses and shopping malls. Some of us would greatly prefer to live with much less (or nothing) of all that and to have more unspoiled nature and high culture, and less noise and smog. But the decisions that the majority are making, individually or through the political process, frustrate these preferences. Moreover, the prices of many goods and services depend on the market demand exercised by others, which may raise some prices through competition among buyers, and lower others through competition among sellers or through economies of scale. Again some may suffer by having to pay more for what they need or want or by receiving less for what they have to sell—even while others thrive thanks to having skills that are in high demand or tastes for things few covet. And again those who suffer may invoke historical counterfactualizing *à la* Silvers: "Justice requires that our common social environment be shaped as it would be if our love for unspoiled nature and our distaste for cars were more widespread." Or: "Justice requires that our common social environment be shaped as it would be if we Amish were in the majority." If such claims are absurd, why is not the claim Silvers makes in behalf of people with disabilities absurd as well?[31]

Third, one might think that Silvers's position, understood as invoking negative rights, makes sense at least for those parts of the environment that are maintained by the government at public expense. People with disabilities are harmed unduly when they are required to contribute through their taxes to public facilities and services that are, for them, unusable. But conceding this point shows much less than Silvers wants to show. The requirement "to add signing to their speech" would then apply not to "all conversationalists" but only to public employees while on duty. It would apply, for instance, to teachers in state schools, but not to those in private colleges and universities. Analogously, only government-run trains and buses would have to be accessible to the walking-impaired. And perhaps not even them. For the government might have the option to finance such services through an "exchange branch," as proposed by Knut Wicksell. Here the government acts merely as a catalyst in order to solve a collective-action problem. It does so by distributing the entire cost of a public good or service in such a way that every contributor derives a net benefit.[32] In this scenario, the fact that some public good or service maintained by the government is unusable for certain people with disabilities does not then constitute an injustice (conceived as a violation of a negative right), because the same people are also exempt from contributing to the maintenance of the public good or service in question.

I conclude that the demands Silvers makes in behalf of people with disabilities cannot be justified by appeal to negative rights and duties. And I doubt that Silvers herself in the end believes otherwise.[33] But if this first candidate rationale for Silvers's position does not work out, what then *is* the justification for the demands she formulates and, in particular, of the moral significance she attaches to the distinction between the maintenance of a social environment fully suited to people with disabilities and the provision of special services, benefits and advantages?

II.2

Let us consider a second rationale that may better explain and justify Silvers's position—the idea that justice requires a society's government and public space to be as far as possible equally supportive of and hospitable to all citizens of this society, whatever their worldview, lifestyle, sexual orientation, ethnicity, native language, skin color, gender or disabilities (or lack thereof). Silvers's commitment to the second (semiconsequentialist) variant of egalitarian liberalism, "equally supportive and hospitable" does not mean that society must be so organized that persons across these various groups are roughly equally well-off, but rather that society must be so organized as to generate roughly equal—or at least roughly equivalent—helps and hindrances, benefits and burdens, to persons across the various groups.[34]

This idea is sometimes expressed by saying that justice requires a society's social order and its government to be *neutral* in regard to the dimensions in which the members of this society are diverse. This expression is, however, problematic in various ways. In respect to some of the distinctions among citizens, a society can come quite close to achieving neutrality—at least this seems in principle possible with regard to skin color which, in an ideal society, would matter no more than hair color or eye color matter in ours. Neutrality can be achieved only rather imperfectly with regard to religion and gender: the choice of facially neutral rules governing the tax treatment of religious donations is likely to affect different religious communities differentially; and the choice of rules governing abortion and divorce will certainly have a differential impact on women and men. In respect to these differences, the best one may hope for is a rough balance. This is even more clearly true in regard to the various cultural groups, as Will Kymlicka reminds us:

> Many liberals say that just as the state should not recognize, endorse, or support any particular church, so it should not recognize, endorse, or support any particular cultural group or identity. . . . But the analogy does not work. It is quite possible for a state not to have an established church. But the state cannot help but give at least partial establishment to a culture when it decides which language is to be used in public schooling, or in the provision of state services. The state can (and should) replace religious oaths in courts with secular oaths, but it cannot replace the use of English in courts with no language.[35]

An analogous point holds for our topic, too, as we saw when we discussed policy decisions in regard to infrastructure: decisions with regard to a society's transportation and communications technologies and networks are bound to affect different disability groups and the nondisabled differentially.

If there is no "disability-neutral" way of organizing our society, how are we to estimate whether some particular organization is fair among disability groups and the nondisabled? A plausible rough answer might be: a fair social order is one that distributes benefits and burdens in such a way that the net benefit of social interaction is roughly equal across the various groups. For this answer to be meaningful, we need some baseline relative to which the net benefits derived by the various groups are to be measured. This baseline could be defined by reference to some state of nature (a state without government) or by reference to some minimal ("nightwatchman") state, which merely aims to ensure that its members are secure from attack by one another.

It may seem that if this is what justice requires, it requires very little for people with disabilities. This would be so because such persons would, in the baseline state, tend to have far worse life prospects than nondisabled persons. An equal-net-benefit requirement would not mitigate this discrepancy in any way. And a social order under which people with disabilities are far worse off than the nondisabled would then be perfectly just, provided only that the discrepancy between each disability group and the nondisabled is no greater than it would be in the baseline state. Justice so understood—presumably easily satisfied already by the status quo—would give no support to the more ambitious demands Silvers makes in behalf of people with disabilities.

It would nevertheless be a mistake to dismiss the second candidate rationale for Silvers's position quite so quickly. There are at least two reasons for believing that the reasoning of the preceding paragraph is too rash. First, this reasoning simply assumes that there are no social causes that contribute to the occurrence of disabilities. But this is patently false. Many persons become disabled through their participation in an ongoing society—for instance, through accidents or crimes, through any of a very large number of human-made poisons (alcohol and other drugs, asbestos, pesticides, etc.) and radiation, or through infectious diseases. And even when disabilities are caused exclusively by defects in their original genetic code, these defects may in turn have social causes—radiation, pollution, medications, practices of inbreeding or drug consumption, and so forth.[36] So one cannot simply say with respect to particular persons with disabilities that *they* would be very much worse off than ourselves even if social institutions were far more minimal or nonexistent. Yes, walking-impaired persons would presumably be very much worse off than the nondisabled in a state of nature. But this fact is of no relevance in our debate with a person who would not be walking-impaired but for having been rear-ended on the New Jersey turnpike. Insofar as disabilities are themselves counted as among the (benefits and) burdens of social interaction, quite ambitious demands in behalf of people with disabilities could be justified as requirements of justice. These demands would resemble those arising from the first (fully consequentialist) variant of egalitarian liberalism. But they would be justified and viewed quite differently—not as special benefits due to those with special needs, but as compensation due to those who suffer harms or wrongs engendered by a social life that brings great benefits to most.

Second, this reasoning also assumes too quickly that the comparison should be made in terms of *overall* net benefit, in which all benefits and burdens are aggregated into a single magnitude. There may be reason to keep various categories of benefits and burdens separate in our thinking about social justice.[37] This is especially true, perhaps, for the benefits and burdens of citizenship: it is widely viewed as unjust for adult persons to be denied the right to vote, no matter how privileged these persons may be in other respects; and it is also widely believed to be unjust that some persons should be able to buy their way out of jury duty or military service. If justice does not allow the benefits and burdens of citizenship to be offset against benefits and burdens in other spheres, then it requires *equal* citizenship, namely an equal net benefit in terms of citizenship relative to a baseline of equality (e.g., a state of nature in which there is no such thing as citizenship for anyone). And it may then be possible to support the demands Silvers makes in behalf of people with disabilities from the right in justice these people have, along with everyone else, to equal citizenship. This right entitles everyone to a real opportunity to participate fully in the political and civic institutions of the society and, more broadly, in its public life: culture, education, employment, travel, shopping and so on. I do not know whether Silvers would be interested in developing such an argument.[38] The ADA, in any case, does include language that could be interpreted in this direction. In its Section 2, Findings and Purposes, the Congress declares that: "(7) individuals with disabilities . . . have been . . . subjected to a history of purposeful unequal treatment, and relegated to a position of political powerlessness in our society; . . . (8) the Nation's proper goals regarding individuals with disabilities are to assure equality of opportunity, full participation, independent living, and economic self-sufficiency for such individuals."[39]

I conclude that if the argument I have just sketched (from a requirement of equal benefits and burdens to a requirement of equal citizenship) can be satisfactorily filled in, then the second rationale presents a genuinely promising way of supporting Silvers's position.

II.3

More prominent in the same Section 2 of the ADA is yet a third rationale—one that Silver also repeatedly invokes in her essay[40]—the idea that people with disabilities have in the past been subjected to discrimination based on prejudice and that justice requires the eradication of such discrimination. In this vein, the Congress also finds that:

> (7) individuals with disabilities are a discrete and insular minority who have been . . . subjected to a history of purposeful unequal treatment . . . based on characteristics that are beyond the control of such individuals and resulting from stereotypic assumptions not truly indicative of the individual ability of such individuals to participate in, and contribute to, society; . . . (9) the continuing existence of unfair and unnecessary discrimination and prejudice denies people with disabilities the opportunity to compete on an equal basis and to pursue those opportunities for which our free society is justifiably famous, and costs the United States billions of dollars in unnecessary expenses resulting from dependency and nonproductivity.

While the second rationale tends to liken disability groups to cultural (ethnic, religious, linguistic and lifestyle) groups, which are entitled to evenhanded treatment by the rules and government of a society, the third rationale tends to liken them to groups identified by skin color, gender or sexual orientation, which have suffered discrimination based on irrational prejudice and stigmatization.[41]

There is no question that people with disabilities have suffered and are still suffering discrimination, especially in the area of employment. Often such discrimination is irrational, such as when hiring decisions are made in ignorance of the fact that a disabled applicant could do the job quite well so long as minor, inexpensive accommodations are made. Such accommodations might consist of one or more of the following: allowing disabled employees to do the job somewhat differently (e.g., seated rather than standing), giving them special consideration in the allocation of assignments, providing them with somewhat different equipment (e.g., a TTY/TDD line rather than a telephone), providing them with additional equipment (e.g., a face mask for removing allergens), or changing the workplace setting (e.g., adding a filtration device to the air conditioning system). In many cases, such discrimination is "rational" in the sense that the hiring agent correctly perceives that the people on whom the success of her organization depends are prejudiced against persons with certain disabilities. As some clientele may dislike being visited by a black saleswoman or being served by a gay waiter, so they may also dislike being visited by a wheelchair-bound salesman or being served by a waitress with Down syndrome (cf Silvers 112–113).

But the fact that justice permits, even requires, the eradication of all such discrimination based on prejudice cannot support most of the demands Silvers makes in behalf of people with disabilities. Even in a society without any such prejudices, employers may prefer to hire nondisabled people over equally qualified ones with disabilities. They may want to save the expense of making special accommodations, for example, or they may correctly assume that people with certain disabilities have on average higher absentee rates than nondisabled persons or cannot work as fast as nondisabled persons during hours of peak demand. Even in a society without prejudices, the nondisabled would be unwilling to add signing to their speech, let alone to legislate a requirement to this effect. The benefit to them of developing this capacity simply seems not worth the effort, just as learning Estonian seems not worth the effort to most non-Estonians. Even in a society without prejudices, the nondisabled may build stairs and narrow bathrooms in their residences and prefer to use computer software with mouse-click icons (Microsoft Windows over DOS; *cf* Silvers 107–109). To be sure, prejudice may in fact contribute to such choices. But an unexceptional (though not therefore unexceptionable) concern with one's own goals and projects is alone quite sufficient to explain them. Thus, if justice requires us to choose differently, as Silvers asserts, then justice must require more than the eradication of prejudice.

III

I have looked at three candidate rationales for the position Silvers advances in sympathy with the ADA: negative rights, evenhanded treatment, and nondiscrimination. None of these rationales seems to me to support the full range of the demands Silvers makes in behalf of people with disabilities, though an extension of the second rationale (equal citizenship) may be within striking distance of supporting many of them. My discussion is evidently too brief and preliminary to allow any definitive conclusions. In particular, it is quite possible that a more convincing justification of Silvers's position can be constructed by combining some of these (and perhaps other) rationales.

It seems more doubtful, however, whether any specification of Silvers's semiconsequentialist position can yield plausible conclusions about those with the most severe disabilities, who could not meet their own needs in *any* feasible environment. It is hard to see how Silvers can avoid the unpalatable conclusion that, once our practices and environment will have been fully reformed, justice gives us no further responsibilities toward such people.

I realize that the set of people who cannot meet their own needs in any environment may not be large. For the relevant question here is not whether a person can do without the help of other people. Stephen Hawking needs a lot of help from others, but this is true of most non-disabled people as well. I meet most of my needs through purchases out of my income, and so does Stephen Hawking, who can easily meet his own needs even in the existing environment. In a fair environment many disabled persons who are unemployed and excluded from various social amenities today could similarly meet their own needs with some accommodations from employers.

And yet, even if we grant that the reforms required by justice would enable all physically and many mentally disabled persons to meet their own needs in the relevant sense, we would still face a residual group of persons with severe mental disabilities who cannot be productively employed in any feasible environment, however hospitable. While Silvers, in developing her view, has focused mainly on physical disabilities, such as blindness and walking impairments, she has not exempted such mental disabilities from its scope. This raises the question whether her semiconsequentialist view is plausible when extended to the severely mentally disabled.

The existence of such persons puts pressure on Silvers's social model of disability, or so it seems to me. One difficulty here is that of providing and justifying a list of practices and environmental features that are unfair to the mentally disabled. This list is needed to specify both our goal of removing unfairness and our compensatory responsibilities while unfairness persists. Another difficulty is that of supporting the view that, once our environment will have been made fully fair to people with severe mental disabilities, justice will require no support for them from the rest of us. If collective support through the state is discretionary, the immediate relatives of people with severe mental disabilities may end up bearing much of the cost of caring for them, exposing such families to serious financial hardship and its effects.

Maintaining a strictly semiconsequentialist approach, Silvers could say that, even if *justice* does not require financial support for households with a severely disabled member, such support instantiates other virtues which we ought to exercise, either individually or collectively, without legal constraint. Even with an environment and practices that are perfectly fair, it is good to help people meet special expenses they incur through no fault of their own. Silvers could add that any moral benefit of requiring such subsidies as a matter of justice would be outweighed by the moral cost of reverting to the medical model of disability, which she sees as associated with the idea that certain kinds of people are inferior and their existence undesirable.

But must the medical model really carry such associations? Can we not *affirm* that certain persons, irrespective of any social factors, have defects that make them needy and dependent and yet *deny* that their lives are any less worthwhile than ours? This friendlier medical model of disability seems to me to be strongly supported by Eva Kittay's paper in this volume—not for all people with disabilities, to be sure, but for some and the severely mentally disabled in particular.[42] Rather than throw out the medical model of disability altogether, perhaps we should try to cleanse it of the traditional associations with inferiority and pity and then apply it to, in particular, people with severe mental disabilities.

This proposal still faces the important procreative issues Silvers raises. Is it unjust to discourage mentally disabled couples from having children likely to share their disability (*cf* Silvers 94)? And is it unjust to deny genetic counseling to such couples who want to improve their chances of conceiving a severely mentally disabled child (*cf* Silvers 77)? On the friendlier medical model we might say that such practices are not unjust. They do not reflect the belief that the lives of severely mentally disabled persons are less worthwhile, but rather the belief that such lives are more expensive. A decent society, if reasonably affluent, must stand ready to share such expenses, but it may then also take steps to limit their rate of incidence.

Perhaps because she finds this conclusion hard to accept, Silvers seems drawn toward relaxing her semiconsequentialist approach by holding that justice requires state financial support—not to people with severe mental disabilities themselves, but to their families who take care of them. These family members are entitled to support because they would otherwise be less included in the community than others who have no severely mentally disabled person to take care of. I have seen only a brief version of this view, so cannot comment on it in detail. But, in general terms, it seems to me to sit on a slippery slope inclined toward a fully consequentialist approach, which recognizes no morally significant distinction between social factors that exclude persons from common activities and personal factors that limit their opportunities to involve themselves. If justice requires us to help pay for a caretaker for a severely mentally disabled child in order to enable her parents fully to participate in the social life of our society, then why does not justice also require us to help pay for equipment necessary for the full participation of people with physical disabilities? And if society ought to help pay for wheelchairs and hearing aids, then why must we not also help pay for measures designed to promote the social inclusion of shy, ugly, awkward and stammering people?

Perhaps we ought to do just that. But Silvers's view thus far has been the opposite: That I need a wheelchair is no fault of yours, and justice does not require you, society, to help pay for my wheelchair in order to facilitate my inclusion. What justice does require, however, is that our common practices and environment be shaped so that people in wheelchairs are not excluded or discriminated against. My question is then: If this is the right view about facilitative equipment, why isn't it also the right view about caretaking services for a severely mentally disabled family member?

I realize that I have raised more questions that I have been able to answer and I can only hope that this essay will nevertheless be of some use in clarifying our views about these urgent and difficult moral issues. Let me add in conclusion that I have looked at the arguments here discussed solely as arguments. But arguments may entail more than merely conclusions—they may have psychological and political effects. Silvers is aware of this point when she stresses that the ADA brings an important practical benefit by drawing on the social rather than the medical model of disability: the ADA fosters respect for (and thereby enhances the self-respect of) people with disabilities by presenting itself as "protecting them against external obstructions of their physical and social access rather than from their internal flaws and failings" (Silvers 120).[43] I take no position here on the extent to which arguments we make in a public setting may or should be adjusted toward such objectives. I merely point out that I have not tried to look beyond the soundness of the arguments.

ACKNOWLEDGMENTS

This essay has greatly benefited from the very helpful comments I have received from Ling Tong, Sophia Wong and especially Anita Silvers. Many thanks.

NOTES

[1]The view described comprises a large number of more specific conceptions of justice, which differ in various dimensions—and notably in regard to how quality of life, or human flourishing, should be specified for purposes of an account of social justice. Among the main champions of this view are Richard Arneson, G. A. Cohen, Will Kymlicka, and Amartya Sen. The most elaborate defense of conceiving justice as, first and foremost, a property of distributions is provided in G. A. Cohen: "Where the Action Is: On the Site of Distributive Justice" in *Philosophy and Public Affairs* 26 (1997), 3–30.

[2] Such pervasive social rules, which organize the collective life of a social system (e.g., a society) are often referred to as social institutions or, collectively as a social order or "basic structure" (Rawls). We can ignore the fine distinctions one might draw among these various expressions, since we are here concerned with the core idea that is shared by one division of liberal-egalitarian conceptions of social justice (and distinguishes these from the liberal-egalitarian conceptions of social justice in the other division).

[3]The adjectives "equal" and "worse" can, of course, be specified in various ways. Consider a tax system that applies to persons whose gross incomes are diverse. Here one might argue that equal treatment requires equal taxes, or equal tax rates, or progressive tax rates. Again, I bypass such issues in order to focus on the core idea.

[4]This adjective was first introduced in a still-unpublished work by Derek Parfit, or so I believe.

[5]Cf. John Rawls, *A Theory of Justice*, Cambridge, MA: Harvard University Press, 1971/1999; and John Rawls, *Political Liberalism*. New York: Columbia University Press, 1993/1996. I will refer to these works as *TJ* and *PL*, respectively.

[6]The veil of ignorance is explained in *TJ* §24, the maximin rule in *TJ* §26. Someone using the maximin rule of decision-making strives to maximize her minimum payoff. In the case at hand, prospective participants using the maximin rule rank candidate criteria of justice by the worst life prospects that might be generated by a social order informed by this criterion. Thus the parties in the original position choose that criterion of social justice which secures them the highest minimum life prospects.

[7]My use of the expression "quality of life" is a simplification. Rawls stipulates that the parties in the original position seek to optimize the fulfillment of three higher-order interests of the prospective citizens they represent (cf. *PL* 75: "the parties have only the three higher-order interests to guide their deliberations"). These are the interests (1) to develop and exercise a sense of justice, which involves a sincere allegiance to some conception of justice (whose content remains unspecified so as not to prejudge the parties' decision); (2) to develop and exercise the capacity to form, to pursue, and rationally to revise a conception of the good; and (3) to protect and advance one's particular conception of the good (*PL* 74). Adherents of the first view can argue that it would be clear to the parties in the original position that citizens' capacity to fulfill their three higher-order interests, and the third of these in particular, depends not only on social benefits and burdens but also on their personal constitution or natural endowments.

[8]This reasoning models, *within* Rawls's theory, the argument Sen has given to the effect that a criterion of social justice should be formulated in terms of capabilities rather than social primary goods. See Amartya K. Sen "Equality of What," in his *Choice, Welfare and Measurement.* Cambridge, UK: Cambridge University Press, 1982, 353–369, esp. 366; and *Inequality Reexamined.* Cambridge, MA: Harvard University Press, 1992, esp. 79–87.

[9]*Realizing Rawls,* Ithaca: Cornell University Press, 1989. I will refer to this book as *RR.* According to the definition I proposed there, a semiconsequentialist conception of justice holds, while a fully consequentialist (or purely recipient-oriented) conception of justice denies, that "any benefits and burdens an institutional scheme brings about are always more important that any goods and ills it merely lets happen (so that the latter can figure at most as a tiebreaker in the assessment of institutions)" (*RR* 45). Against "deontological" conceptions of justice, both kinds of consequentialist view deny that "within the domain of what an institutional scheme brings about, benefits and burdens it establishes have, sometimes at least, more weight than equivalent benefits and burdens it foreseeably engenders" (*RR* 45, cf. *RR* 46–47).

[10]"Three Problems with Contractarian-Consequentialist Ways of Assessing Social Institutions" in *Social Philosophy and Policy* 12: 241–266 (June 1995).

[11]Norman Daniels, *Just Health Care.* Cambridge, UK: Cambridge University Press, 1985, 79.

[12]See David Wasserman, "Distributive Justice" and "Response—Wasserman on Silvers and Mahowald," both in Anita Silvers, David Wasserman and Mary Mahowald, eds., *Disability, Difference, Discrimination.* Lanham: Rowman & Littlefield, 1998, 147–207 and 267–283. He applies these four characterizations to the demand for fair equality of access to health protection, which I had formulated in *RR* (Wasserman 163, 165, 205). I leave aside his characterization of my position as inflexible (Wasserman 165), because it rests on his mistaken assumption that I define health protection as "resources for restoring or maintaining health" (Wasserman 159; cf. *RR* 185).

[13]Anita Silvers, "Formal Justice" and "Response—Silvers on Wasserman and Mahowald," both in Anita Silvers, David Wasserman and Mary Mahowald eds., *Disability, Difference, Discrimination.* Lanham: Rowman & Littlefield, 1998, 13–145 and 253–266.

[14]"It is not at all clear why we should be required to compensate for disadvantages that are not the result of one group's having enjoyed privilege to the detriment of another" (Silvers 254). For such "natural" disadvantages justice requires no compensation, according to Silvers—though justice does require rectification of *social* disadvantages, as when people with disabilities are being discriminated against or treated worse in other ways.

[15]Silvers 97–98. Silvers does not oppose such transfers but, rather, accepts elsewhere "the goodness of acting charitably to the disabled" (Silvers 31) as well as the "intuition that the resources of society should be tapped to obtain a wheelchair for a citizen who cannot walk" (Silvers 30). In that context she insists, however, that justice permits but does not require such compensatory transfers: "there are circumstances in which allocating an unusually large amount of resources to those who are more than usually disadvantaged is neither to privilege them nor to be unfair to everyone else. However, we should not conflate the permissibility of an unequally large allocation with the obligation to allocate greater than usual amounts of resources" (Silvers 30–31). Her view is, then, that conceiving such transfers as charity (and

permitted by justice) can—whereas conceiving them as fulfilling obligations and entitlements of justice cannot—avoid the offensive perception of people with disabilities as needy, dependent, weak, incompetent and fit to be pitied. This view contains an empirical-psychological assertion, which reverses the way the contrast between the attitudes associated with justice and charity is usually presented in the rights literature. It would be interesting, then, to learn more about Silvers's grounds for this reversal.

[16]"Nor is it clear how we are to rank competing claims for restoration from nature's harms" (Silvers 254, cf. 31).

[17]Some theorists would also include here genetically based or involuntarily acquired "expensive tastes"; see, for example, Richard Arneson: "Liberalism, Distributive Subjectivism, and Equal Opportunity for Welfare," *Philosophy and Public Affairs* 19 (Spring 1990):158–194.

[18]Silvers 133. The fact that a disability, by itself, prevents a person from engaging in some potentially worthwhile activities does not show that her life is worse. All persons must do without many activities that greatly enrich the lives of others, if only because life is too short to engage in all such activities (cf. Silvers 91).

[19]Silvers 41, citing Jenny Morris: "Tyrannies of Perfection" in *The New Internationalist* July 1, 1992.

[20]I use the expression "social environment" rather than Silvers's "artificial environment" in this context, because the former expression better brings out that she has in mind here also, I believe, harms resulting directly from our social practices and conventions, and not only harms produced indirectly through the ways in which we shape our physical habitat and produce and consume goods and services. The attitudes persons display through their conduct can be quite as excluding and devastating as physical and legal barriers. I should add that any attempt to make this tripartite distinction operational would run into very great difficulties. I will come back to this point below.

[21]"Although public transportation systems must be made accessible, the disabled are owed only that level of mobility enjoyed (or deplored) by public transportation users, not the higher level achieved by private automobile users, despite the fact that many people with disabilities cannot drive and thus do not have mobility equivalent to nondisabled car owners" (Silvers 124).

[22]The proposal faces an additional problem in that it may lead to implausible conclusions in the case of extremely rare disabilities: incorporating into our social environment some costly feature that significantly enhances the productivity of persons with a certain disability may seem prohibitively expensive when this disability affects only 20 persons, even while the same accommodation would seem quite reasonable if the disability in question affected 20 percent of the population. I will come back to this point in the next section, which discusses the moral plausibility of Silvers's position.

[23]Silvers downplays the importance of this fact by avoiding examples in which one group's gain is another group's loss. Her paradigm examples are the choice between competing software designs and the architectural choice between ramps and stairs. She suggests that with both of these choices one option is Pareto-superior to the other: Software not requiring a mouse would be just as good for the seeing and better for the blind, and ramps are better than stairs for the walking-impaired while being otherwise equivalent in financial cost and aesthetic value. Even if a Pareto-efficient option is indeed available in these two cases, this is certainly not the case with most of the choices we face concerning our social environment.

It should also be noted that, even in her two paradigm examples, Silvers's preferred option is Pareto-superior only if one follows her in disregarding the cost of rectifying unjust prior choices, i.e., the cost of replacing Windows software and the cost of replacing stairs by ramps and elevators. Ignoring such transition costs seems plausible insofar as they can be imposed on those who had made the unjust prior choices. But in the actual world, much of the transition costs will have to be borne by persons who neither have contributed to nor (by Silvers's own assumption) now benefit from the prevailing exclusive software or architecture. When this is so, two demands of justice are in tension, and some further argument is then needed to show why the claim of people with disabilities—to be able, without assistance, to use standard computer software and to reach all public spaces—should prevail.

[24]This thought shows, incidentally, that one important advantage Silvers claims for her position may be illusory. She criticizes those who hold that justice to people with disabilities demands a pool of resources for corrective equipment and compensation on the ground that such a pool tends to "place the interests of individuals with disabilities in competition with one another for access to whatever resources nondisabled people are willing to allocate to the disabled" (Silvers 25). But her own position that justice to people with disabilities demands a social environment fully suited to them hardly engenders the

harmony of interests among people with disabilities that Silvers advertises. To the contrary, it, too, engenders competition with regard to how scarce resources should be deployed and, in some cases, even straight conflicts (which would persist even if resources were unlimited). A simple example of conflict would be that the addition of auditory information for the blind (e.g., beeps synchronized to traffic lights) would go against the interests of those who are hypersensitive to noise.

[25]One may well doubt that, even if we did have the requisite knowledge about that parallel world, people with disabilities here and now have a right in justice to have the existing transportation infrastructure replaced by whatever alternative system the people of the parallel world would have constructed. I will come back to this point below.

[26]To be sure, the (Johnson and Johnson) advanced wheelchair soon to go into production is quite expensive and inconvenient. But the hypothesis is that the people of the parallel world would have developed a way of mass-producing, relatively cheaply, much more sophisticated personal transportation devices that would greatly enhance their occupants' mobility even out in nature, allowing them to venture far beyond paved trails and roads. If this is what they would have done, which seems quite conceivable, ramps would have become obsolete in their world.

[27]These duties are called "negative" because they do not require us to do anything in particular but, rather, require us to refrain from performing certain actions. Of course, making this distinction precise is anything but easy. Much depends on how acts are individuated. The duty of keeping a contract or promise, for instance, may often seem to require the promisor to perform some specific action. It is nevertheless generally viewed as a negative duty, on the ground that it requires us to refrain from the complex act of promising-and-not-doing-what-one-has-promised. For a sustained discussion of this negative/positive distinction, see Jonathan Bennett, *The Act Itself.* Oxford: Oxford University Press, 1995.

[28]There are also brief allusions to this negative-duty theme in Section 2 ("Findings and Purposes") of the ADA, as reference is made to "(5) . . . the discriminatory effects of architectural, transportation, and communication barriers, overprotective rules and policies" and it is acknowledged that "(7) individuals with disabilities are a discrete and insular minority who have been faced with restrictions and limitations."

[29]These costs are, in the first instance, reductions in productivity and pleasure arising from conversationalists spending time on learning sign language rather than on learning or doing other things. In response to a draft of the present essay, Anita Silvers has commented that these costs could be quite small, if sign were taught in schools as part of the curriculum. She also writes that, where transition costs are large (adding signing might well be a "formidable demand" on current adults), they constitute "undue burdens" recognized as grounds for an exemption under the ADA. Insofar as conversationalists' failure to add signing to their speech is excused by undue burdens such addition would impose on them, Silvers considers them to be engaged in a practice that, though discriminatory, is not unjust. On Silvers's view, justice would then seem to require the gradual addition of signing to speech (and the transition to writing in Braille?) through curricular reforms rather than adult retraining.

[30]To sharpen the challenges posed by these questions, imagine something that at this stage of computerized technology is hardly far-fetched: a handheld device that converts spoken into printed words and vice versa. A sophisticated such device is a full functional equivalent for the deaf of everyone adding signing to their speech. Could it really be that even a very small minority of deaf persons have a justice claim to the universal use of sign language even while they would have no claim to help in purchasing those overall less costly translation devices?

[31]Again, it is true that persons generally have a choice about being Amish or nature lovers, and no choice about being disabled. And again this difference is, for reasons given in the preceding paragraph, irrelevant to the question whether the groups in question suffer negative-right violations.

[32]See Knut Wicksell, "A New Principle of Just Taxation," in R. A. Musgrave and A. T. Peacock, eds., *Classics in the Theory of Public Finance.* London: Macmillan, 1958. Cf. Rawls, *TJ* 282–283.

[33]There are a few places where she invokes the idea, most notably when she writes that "absence of access to public transportation limits impaired people's freedom" and that "failure to provide instrumentally effective accommodation illegitimately impinges on the negative freedom of" people with disabilities (Silvers 127). My sense is that just as we nondisabled folk are often far too oblivious of the standpoints of people with disabilities, Silvers may sometimes be too focused on her own case of a walking impairment. In regard to this case, the invocation of a right to negative freedom is at its most plau-

sible: a curb may impede a wheelchair-bound person's freedom of movement just as a wall may restrict that of a nondisabled one. The more distant cases are from such locomotion impairments—other physical disabilities, sensory impairments and finally mental disabilities—the less mindful Silvers tends to be of them, and the less well the demand for a social environment fully suited to people with such disabilities would seem to fit under the negative rights/freedom banner. Let me add that Silvers's tendency is quite understandable, given that one way in which people with physical disabilities are routinely mistreated in our society is by dealing with them (or preferably with any nondisabled person accompanying them) as if they were mentally disabled.

[34]As I have stated at the beginning of this essay, both views permit persons to be worse off as a consequence of choices they have made. My formulation in the text assumes that the effects of such choices roughly balance out across groups. It also gives the strictly egalitarian (rather than the prioritarian) version of each view.

[35]Will Kymlicka, *Multicultural Citizenship: A Liberal Theory of Minority Rights*. Oxford: Oxford University Press, 1995, 111.

[36]Cf. Silvers 54.

[37]For a sustained development of this idea, see Michael Walzer, *Spheres of Justice*. New York: Basic Books, 1983.

[38]She writes that one reason for the measures she demands in behalf of people with disabilities is that of "eliciting their contributions through full and meaningful citizenship" (Silvers 143). "For them, justice must offer, first, the visibility of full participatory citizenship" (Silvers 145).

[39]See also the U.S. Supreme Court decision in *Olmstead* (98–536, 1999).

[40]Cf. Silvers 52, 84, 95, 112–117.

[41]For a good recent discussion of this approach, see Andrew Koppelman, *Antidiscrimination Law and Social Equality*. New Haven: Yale University Press, 1996.

[42]In response to some formulations in the ADA, Kittay points out that "independent living and 'productivity' or economic self-sufficiency cannot be goals for all disabled persons, no matter how one wants to stretch these terms, most especially perhaps with very severely mentally disabled persons" ("At Home with My Daughter," in Leslie Francis and Anita Silvers, eds.: *Americans with Disabilities: Exploring Implications of the Law for Individuals and Institutions*. New York: Routledge, 2000, 73.

[43]The expression "flaws and failings" seems a little unfair to the medical model, which is associated with the goal of eliminating or mitigating disabilities. This goal need not imply that persons are somehow responsible for their disabilities or worse on account of them. No such implication is attached to the goal of curing a person's infection, straightening his teeth or thinning his blood. In my view, the medical and social models are both one-sided. The hardships people with disabilities bear in our society arise from the conjunction of their own condition and social circumstances. While we surely can, and should, reduce these hardships by altering the social environment in various ways, we cannot realistically hope solely through such alterations to erase all of these hardships completely.

The Good of Agency

LAWRENCE C. BECKER

APPRECIATION

The Americans with Disabilities Act has been an extraordinary success in many respects. Predecessor statutes from the early 1970s, such as the Rehabilitation Act of 1973, were important in upgrading vocational training and in making crucial opportunities for independent living available for people with severe disabilities, but the ADA has much wider application for education, employment, public accommodations and travel. Moreover, while the predecessor statutes helped sustain a useful level of activism among the disabled and their advocates, and that, combined with other liberalizing social forces, raised the consciousness of some people in government agencies, private business, education and medicine, those earlier statutes were also widely ignored. People who worked on committees to evaluate access issues in the seventies and eighties were often dismayed by the results. Reports were written; recommendations were made; a few recommended changes were made; the reports were filed, and eventually lost.[1]

By comparison, the ADA has typically been taken seriously by people who control serious money. In responding to this statute, people in both the public and private sectors have opened up a remarkable range of education, work, housing, travel and entertainment opportunities—at least for paraplegics, amputees, the deaf, the blind and the mobility impaired. Admittedly, much of this was already well under way, often as an unexpected by-product of other changes, such as the dramatic increase in nonbusiness air travel brought about by that other ADA, the Airline Deregulation Act.[2] Moreover, the record has been disturbingly mixed with regard to mental illness, mental retardation, certain lethal and infectious diseases, and a whole array of rather low-profile issues. Nothing goes perfectly.

And of course the ADA is as much an *effect* of social changes (reaching back at least to the end of World War I) as it is a cause of such changes. In the United States, there has been a fairly steady expansion of opportunity for the disabled throughout the last half of the twentieth century. The ADA marks a sharp broadening of all of this, perhaps a change in velocity, and certainly a change in the legal cover given to the claims of the disabled. But it does not mark a change in general direction.

DISMAY

That said, we need to face an exasperating fact. Now that we have begun in earnest to funnel disability rights through legal channels, we have produced a huge body of legal briefs, judicial opinions, political speech, activist manifestos and philosophical argument—a body of work that, among other things, amounts to a baroque elaboration of standard legal and philosophical theories of rights and distributive justice. Disability rights often seem to follow (or fail to follow) from such theories in the form of "me too" claims, added as afterthoughts to our concerns about equal opportunity, discrimination and affirmative action for women and minorities. The result is confusion—or so it seems to me.

I shall argue here that disability rights are not "me too" matters. They are implicit in long-held, fundamental commitments about the value of human life and agency. The history of rehabilitation and vocational training makes it plain that we have not always needed legal sanctions to bring that to our attention. In my view, much of the current discussion that should be premised upon a simple, satisfying, philosophically sound consequence of liberal-democratic ideals has been corrupted by adversarial debate. Perhaps this is inevitable, given the way we organize efforts to achieve significant social change. Perhaps it is even good. Nevertheless.

AGENDA: GAINING SOME ALTITUDE

What follows is an attempt to make a fresh start. The idea is to offer a compact restatement of what I take to be the simplest, most politically plausible way to justify the sorts of social subsidies invoked by the ADA, as well as to generate defensible decisions about the details of their implementation. This restatement will take the form of a consistency argument, proceeding from premises that are no longer seriously debated in Western liberal democracies. It would be tiresome, in this context, to go all the way down to philosophical foundations on these things—to rehearse once again why we protect human life, liberty, property and the pursuit of happiness with an assortment of moral and legal rights understood as human rights. Most of the disagreements people in liberal democracies have with each other about such rights—the extent of them; the enforcement of them—will turn out not to matter in the argument I will outline.

The point of making this fresh start is simply to get some distance on the current debates. The ancient stoics used to recommend as a remedy for perplexity that people fasten their attention repeatedly on pithy, memorable maxims—or at worst, nutshell versions of knockdown arguments—designed to bring into sharp relief the ultimate values at stake. The purpose of this was to gain the altitude necessary to get an uncluttered, reassuring overview of one's ultimate destination.[3] Such an overview in the disability case reveals that the only plausible destination for dealing with it has almost nothing directly to do with justice, rights, caring, benevolence, dependence or independence, *except as those things are means to an end*. It has almost everything to do with the good of human agency.

ARGUMENT: PUTTING AGENTS FIRST

Here is the maxim: if you are going to save the life, save the Agent in it first. The nutshell consistency argument for that maxim is this: (1) being an active, effective human agent is overwhelmingly more valuable than merely being a human who is alive, or conscious or capable of agency; (2) if we are ever committed to saving and sustaining *mere* human life, consciousness or capacity, even though doing so is expensive and inconvenient, then it is inconsistent with the values involved (not to mention cruel and wasteful) not to have a superordinate, prior commitment to saving and sustaining that human being as an active, effective agent; (3) we are often committed to saving and sustaining human lives in expensive and inconvenient circumstances; (4) we ought not to be inconsistent, cruel or wasteful; (5) therefore, in every case where we are committed to saving or sustaining the life, consciousness or agency potential of a given human being, we ought to commit ourselves first to saving or sustaining the active, effective agency of that human being, even when doing so is expensive and inconvenient.

All the rest is elaboration, and there need not be much of that.

The Superordinate Value of Active, Effective, Rational Agency (Agency, Agent, etc.)

Let us confine our attention to human beings, and think of the class of active, effective, rational human agents as including everyone who is (while awake) persistently, consciously goal-directed, who represents and deliberates about achieving such goals in a language, remembers prior activities, makes choices and takes action to accomplish goals, is typically effective in making at least local changes in the world as a result of those actions, and is (with the help of others and circumstance) sometimes successful in achieving those goals.

This notion of an Agent covers a very wide range of human beings, beginning with young children. The reference to rationality is meant to be minimal, referring only to the use of language to represent goals, to deliberate about means to those ends, and to make choices about achieving them. The range of goals is left undefined, so as to include at one extreme people who have grandiose ambitions for a wide variety of projects and at the other extreme people whose goals are mostly defensive—aimed at carving out a tranquil, unambitious existence. The category includes the moral philosopher's paradigm of independent, fully autonomous people, but also includes people who absorb their values and goals unreflectively from outside sources and who quite effectively subordinate their own agency to the control of others. Similarly, the notion of effectiveness here is much broader than the notion of success in accomplishing one's goals. It would be odd to call an agent effective if she *never* accomplished anything she set out to do, but equally odd to call her ineffective simply because she was often defeated by circumstance and sometimes defeated by lack of ability.

Contrast the notion of an Agent with that of its polar opposite among the living: someone in a persistent vegetative state. Next consider, for the sake of argumentative convenience, two intermediate points: one at which there is the ability to formulate projects but not to act on them, and the other at which there is mere sentience—consciousness without even the capacity to formulate and deliberate about projects. We now have before us four types of human existence: (a) active, effective rational Agents; (b) activity-disabled Agents—that is, rational Agents who have projects but wholly lack the ability to act on them; (c) agency-disabled human beings who are sentient but who lack the capacity for any form of rational agency; (d) human beings in a persistent vegetative state—alive as a biological organisms but irreversibly lacking all awareness of it, let alone self-awareness and conscious, goal-directed activity.

I take it there is no serious question about what the ordinal values are here, in the sense of what human beings generally prefer for themselves as well as for those they care about. It is a>b<>c<>d. The preference for Agency dominates all the others, and the relations among those others varies with the circumstances and personalities of the valuers. Moreover, I take it that the preference for Agency is a very strong one. The only evidence I have for this is in the conversational atmosphere—in what is regarded as uncontroversial, commonsense speech about the various possibilities. It would be gratifying to have empirical confirmation of this, but if any direct, systematic evidence exists, pro or con, I am not aware of it.

(If some vagrant philosophical reflex requires that more be said, this parenthesis will have to suffice. We regularly wish for the temporary oblivion of dreamless sleep (d), both for ourselves and for those whose welfare we care about, and we certainly wish for such oblivion during major surgery. We may wish for respite from our restless agency from time to time, and take refuge in an aimless form of tranquil self-awareness (b) or even in mere pleasant sensation (c), whether induced by meditation or medication. But I take it that such desires do not disturb the ordinal structure a>b<>c<>d, because they are part of a deliberate project of implementing and ultimately enhancing Agency, to which we expect to return. Temporarily disabled agent activity may dominate temporarily disabled agency (b>c), especially if we expect the return from it to Agency to be easier or more certain. For the same reason both disabled activity and disabled agency usually dominate a persistent vegetative state (b<>c>d) because, by definition, d virtually always precludes return to Agency. But when the return to Agency is blocked from all these states, the preference order changes. Or so it seems to me. This is so because, without the possibility of return, both (b) and (c) define forms of the "locked-in" syndrome characteristic of some horrific neurological injuries and the last stages of degenerative diseases such as amyotrophic lateral sclerosis (ALS). Faced with the certainty of becoming locked in, it is difficult to believe that one would not prefer death—or possibly, out of fear or hope, a persistent vegetative state. Since there is generally a very strong preference for active, effective, rational agency over either death or a persistent vegetative state, it follows that there is an even stronger preference for such Agency over being locked into either disabled activity or disabled agency.

(It is of course true that certain more or less self-sustaining forms of mental illness and chemical dependency persistently reduce Agency to one of the other states in a way that raises difficult questions about what the agents' preferences "really" are. On the one hand, people in such straits are typically in great distress and struggle against their situation in periods when they are Agents. On the other hand, in some attenuated sense they repeatedly choose to reduce their Agency rather than to enhance it. Further, certain Eastern religious practices are incautiously proffered—at least by some Western enthusiasts—as projects that change the a>b<>c<>d preference order in the sense that they value Agency only for its usefulness in securing ever more extensive forms of, say, tranquil sentience. I say the proffer is incautious because it is typically coupled with great concern about how such tranquility is to be achieved. We are expected to achieve it as the result of Agency rather than, for example, by the deliberate introduction of disease or neurological injury.)

A Commitment to Life Entails a Superordinate Commitment to Agency

I made the preceding section as long as it is mainly out of mild embarrassment at how quickly the rest of what I want to say follows from it. Given our strong preference for active, effective agency in ourselves and other human beings, this maxim follows directly:

> *If* we are going to go to great lengths to create and save human lives, *then* it is inconsistent (not to mention cruel and stupid) to aim merely for the life alone, absent whatever potential for Agency there is in it, rather than aiming to save the Agency in it. No matter how much some of us insist that human beings who are in a persistent vegetative state must be protected and cared for, or even that human lives without any form of agency at all are in some sense as precious as those with it, deliberate attempts to put people into such states or to keep them there when they could become Agents, are out of the question, not to mention criminal.

So to subsidize childbearing but neglect child welfare and early education is inconsistent. And indeed we are not inconsistent in this way. To subsidize rescue and neglect the rehabilitation necessary to raise mere life into Agency is inconsistent, and we recognize this also. There are huge social subsidies for child welfare, education and rehabilitation. Moreover, these subsidies for agency are superordinate in the sense that they are required of us all in a way that reproduction and rescue are not. We do not force people to have children, but if they do, we bring them (and ourselves) under stringent requirements with respect to the welfare and education of those children. We do not force communities to have rescue squads, or hospitals to have emergency rooms and acute care units, or doctors to begin treatment whenever an emergency presents itself. But if rescue attempts begin, we put the rescuers (and ourselves) under stringent requirements to strive to save the Agent, not merely the life. If we fail to save the Agent in the life, we may (or may not) require that mere life be preserved. But aiming for mere life rather than Agency, or failing to invest as much in saving the Agency as in saving the life and therefore failing to save the Agency, would be inconsistent. That much, as pilots say of some skies, is severe clear.[4]

Consequences for Disability Issues

The problems addressed by the ADA and its predecessor statutes concern the large area between a conventional baseline of full-fledged Agency and fully disabled agent-activity or less. At or below fully disabled activity there are of course significant ethical issues to consider—issues about palliation, custodial care, assisted suicide and various forms of euthanasia. But they are not pertinent to what may reasonably be called disability issues. Here we are concerned with the extent to which we ought to offer socially subsidized opportunities for people to achieve full-fledged Agency, as well as with defining the range of people to whom we should offer such opportunities and how we should fund those opportunities.

The obvious inference from the consistency argument is that we should subsidize Agency at a level of effort and expense at least comparable to our investment in saving and sustaining human life itself. Anything less is inconsistent with the values that underwrite our commitment to protecting human life. Moreover, it follows that these subsidies should be available to anyone to whom life-saving and life-sustenance subsidies are available. It matters not at all whether one's Agency has been limited by disease or by injury, by a psychologically damaging childhood or by poor nutrition, by genetic predisposition or by social or economic constraints.[5] If we are going to save the life when it is threatened, we must if possible save the Agent in it first.

That leaves two issues: how to fund these opportunities, and the level of active Agency they should aim to make available. Take funding first. Nothing at all appears to follow directly from this high-altitude consistency argument about the details of funding. And this is as it should be. The method of funding is troublesome for many reasons (e.g., efficiency, fairness, unintended consequences, political theory), but not with respect to whether the funds ought to be socially guaranteed, given a prior social commitment to saving and sustaining human lives. Once the underlying social guarantee is secured, how we work out the details does not amount to a special disability issue. The ADA's mandates for funding arrangements are remarkable, but assuming we can guarantee equally effective outcomes in other ways, there is no special reason in terms of disability issues to insist, for example, that the "reasonable accommodations" must be paid for by each employer in turn, as a worker changes jobs, rather than through some form of portable social insurance that the disabled worker carries from job to job. For complicated reasons, we follow the employer-pays pattern for some things (including some very expensive things such as start-up costs for scientists' research laboratories in universities), and we follow the social insurance pattern for other things. Similarly, assuming equal trickle-down burdens that are not self-defeating, it does not matter whether access to government offices, transportation, public accommodations, shopping and entertainment are funded through broad-based taxes or through the budgets of individual agencies and businesses who pass on the cost to their whole customer base.

The level of Agency that should be guaranteed, however, is always a disability issue. And the target given by the argument here is clear enough: the target is to offer all individuals the support necessary for them to achieve a conventional level of Agency. The argument assumes that efforts to reach this target would not be forced on the disabled except under the general conditions that justify paternalistic interventions. (We do, of course, make early education compulsory for everyone, with or without disabilities, for paternalistic as well as political reasons.) And it is important to be clear that the argument does not assume that reaching the target is tantamount to erasing all the socially controllable burdens of a disability or to providing the opportunity for disabled people to satisfy their every desire—or even their heart's desire—with respect to education, work, civic life, entertainment, travel and play. Time and circumstance limit options for us all. The peculiarities of our bodies and personalities do the same. We do not judge ourselves to be less than Agents just because our options are limited in a frustrating way—or limited relative to more fortunate people.

Hence, if all we can say of a given physical or mental disability is merely that it limits our options, or limits them in relation to what others have, that should not trigger a social subsidy for improvement unless mere quirks of time or circumstance, physique or personality also do it. (This is a consistency argument.) So when do such quirks trigger socially guaranteed support? The Rehabilitation Act and the ADA say that the trigger point is the limitation of a "major life activity,"[6] but defining that has proved to be difficult.[7] The sort of argument I am making here suggests that we back up a step and get an overview of the possibilities.

In order to do that, I suggest we speak first about activities that are "natural and necessary" for developing and sustaining Agency. They certainly deserve the label "major life activities," and the warrant is clear for saying that limitations on them ultimately push us below the conventional baseline for full-fledged, active, effective, rational Agency.

The notion of a necessary activity is fairly straightforward. Some activities are necessary for sustaining life itself—namely, securing basic goods and carrying out basic life-sustaining projects with the available resources. These certainly count as major life activities if anything does. Some of these activities (breathing, for example) we expect healthy people to be able to accomplish effectively on their own, and count them as less than effective agents if they cannot do so (given the availability of air, in the case of breathing). Other necessary activities, such as securing food, clothing and shelter, we now organize through a complex division of labor. As a consequence, we do not typically count people as less than effective agents if they cannot directly produce their own food, make their own clothing or build their own houses. Rather, we think their Agency is compromised if they cannot secure such basic goods *either* on their own *or* through participating in the division-of-labor system, given the availability of work in it. Compromised Agency with respect to necessary activities—whether due to accident, injury or social circumstance—should trigger a helpful social response comparable to that we make for saving and sustaining life itself. It is a simple matter of consistency.

The extension of this argument beyond the class of necessary activities is not always a straightforward matter, but is unavoidable because it is patently obvious that dramatic limitations of Agency are possible in ways that have nothing to do with strictly basic or necessary goods. Legs are not strictly necessary for farming; one can work around the loss of them, especially with our technology. But it would be preposterous to insist that, because legs are not strictly necessary, losing them does not cripple one's Agency. The question is how to extend the argument while keeping it within plausible limits.

Perhaps we can best minimize the difficulties of this in the following way. First, we should stay focused on the aim of describing, in a commonsense way, what counts as less than active, effective, rational Agency itself. The simple inability to get what one wants in a given case, even if one wants it desperately, does not rise to this level. Second, we should limit our attention to activities that are not only characteristic of *all* active, effective human Agents but are, when frustrated, especially potent in diminishing the human being's Agency quite generally, not just in a particular case or range of cases. Doing those two things will restrict discussion to matters that are clearly "major life activities," limitations on which we have reason to believe would threaten Agency itself.

No doubt any list we make along these lines will reflect some transient cultural preoccupations which, from the vantage point of succeeding generations, will seem anything but "natural." But this simply presents us with another version of the familiar epistemological problem of identifying and coping with persistent biases and doing the same with the all but invisible distortions introduced by the forms and filters overlaid on experience generally. That problem is unavoidable in every context.

In the present context this epistemological problem does not seem overwhelming. Think of activities that are strongly and persistently "called for" in the normal course of events by the impulses of a healthy human physiology and psychology operating in a reasonably hospitable environment. (We have plenty of history and anthropology to correct hasty, culture-bound generalizations about this.) Examples include unconstrained body movement, variety in one's activities, self-expression and communication, reciprocal social relationships, achievements through work, the satisfaction of sexual impulses, and play. Such impulses are persistent and strong throughout the lives of all humans who are Agents, though of course these impulses vary in form, frequency and amplitude with age, attention, nutrition and various socially constructed circumstances.

Moreover, it does not seem especially daunting to decide, in terms of the available anthropological, historical, medical and psychological evidence, which of these persistently impelled activities meet our second condition—namely, that their persistent and thorough frustration, *in a healthy human physiology and psychology*, tends to degrade the capacity for Agency itself. Voluntary abstention from sex, for example, does not necessarily do this, but living in an isolation cell from the age of two to twenty almost certainly does. If we can decide, then, which of these impulses are "natural" in the requisite sense, we will have a commonsense way of excluding any extension of the argument to the occasional or partial frustrations typical of human life generally or to the frustrations of impulses that are themselves already pathological.[8]

A persistent incapacity to engage in natural and necessary activities drops us below the conventional baseline of what counts as full-fledged, active, effective, rational agency. Whether that incapacity is the result of disease, injury, time, circumstance or the peculiarities of our physiology or psychology, the social protections surrounding Agency should thus be triggered, given that we are committed to saving and sustaining human lives generally.

A Rich Set of Opportunities Is Saved by the Scale, Complexity and Velocity of Modern Life

How many opportunities must we provide for each person who needs social support? How many specially equipped schools, job sites with automatic doors, television programs with closed captioning? It is hard to think that much in the way of variety is strictly natural or necessary for Agency, given the range of human lives (some of them very cramped and oppressive) we see around us—lives lived by people who are clearly active, effective, rational Agents. Suppose we make sure that the blind can make a living making brooms, and that paraplegics can make a living as telemarketers. Is that enough social support to meet the test of consistency? As a purely theoretical possibility, yes. But the yes is irrelevant as a practical matter for us. As a practical matter, the answer is no.

The theoretical yes must be given because the consistency argument does not require that the same range of opportunities be available for everyone. It is not an equality argument, and it is not about human capabilities of all sorts—for example, reproductive ones, athletic ones, artistic ones and so forth. It is thus not a version of Sen's equal-capabilities argument.[9] But as a practical matter, given the way we have organized ourselves in complex, large-scale societies, any level of social support that meets the consistency test will provide a great deal of opportunity—and variety of opportunity—to any disabled person who can develop or be restored into active, effective, rational Agency.

To see why this is so, begin by considering why the equal-capability approach may not be especially well suited for discussions of disability, even when it is filtered (as it is for Sen) through a sophisticated Aristotelian account of the capabilities required for human virtue and flourishing. In the first place, for the seriously disabled (those who have disabilities that are more than transient inconveniences), it is futile to press for the creation or restoration of equality with the nondisabled because it is futile to think that one can restore the capability that has been lost, or replace it with something equivalent. Artificial limbs and money are welcome gestures, but not an adequate substitute for the limbs lost. Moreover, focusing on the full range of human capabilities involved in full-fledged Aristotelian flourishing invites us to think that we must address disabilities as a matter of justice whenever they are serious losses of capacities, even though the losses have not noticeably compromised Agency, and even though the people thus disabled can themselves redirect their energies and activities into a form of life that (in other circumstances) we find not only acceptable but good.

For example, suppose there are some Aristotelian virtues that are inaccessible to people who do not have children—certain forms of unconditional love and self-sacrifice, for example. If so, childlessness is incompatible with an Aristotelian ideal. Yet when people choose not to have children, perhaps as a consequence of a religious vocation or the demands of another sort of career, Aristotelians as well as the rest of us are accustomed to regarding this loss of virtue as compatible with a socially acceptable good life, though perhaps not an ideal one. If that is so, then when childlessness is the result of sterility rather than chastity or contraception, and when acceptably good alternative forms of life are successfully adopted by those who are sterile, it is hard to see why we should insist on the existence of a social obligation to address it further (unless we are perfectionists in social policy as well as moral theory, or unless the incidence of sterility threatens social welfare).

That said, the focus here on the good of Agency is obviously very closely allied to the concerns of equal-capabilities theorists, because both accounts focus on what appears to be the central, indispensable element of specifically human flourishing. The Agency account is, however, more Stoic than Aristotelian in its insistence that full-fledged Agency is a sufficient locus of concern, and then only with respect to natural and necessary activities. Stoics notoriously deny that a variety of opportunities is necessary for a good life. So if the argument here is in the Stoic tradition, it is no surprise that it does not *directly*, as matter of theory, generate a social obligation to provide variety for the disabled. Yet it is not hard to see how, *in practice here and now*, the consistency argument will support extensive social obligations that yield such variety.

Consider work, which is certainly something natural to Agency and is often necessary to it. And take the worst case by confining the argument to paid employment and then supposing, with the Stoics, that it is not necessary to have any variety at all in the available jobs in order to develop or sustain Agency. Does this, as a practical matter, doom the disabled to one option each? It does not, given the way we have organized ourselves with respect to the division of labor, the location of workplaces and the productivity demands on workers. Making sure that everyone who needs it gets assistance in developing and sustaining a conventional baseline level of Agency is a large-scale undertaking. This is required by the consistency argument to be comparable to the social investment we make in saving and sustaining lives. There is simply no way to do this effectively and efficiently without making schools, public places and work environments generally available to very large classes of people with disabilities. Very many people are mobility impaired; or are vision- or hearing-impaired; or are unable to do strenuous physical labor; or are unable to do strenuous intellectual labor.[10] It is much easier and more efficient to arrange access across the board for a wide variety of common disabilities than to arrange exactly one adequate opportunity for each disabled person. Variety is saved by circumstance, if nothing else.

Vulnerability to Circumstance

It is clear that the consistency argument here is only as strong as the initial commitment to saving and sustaining life. Absent that initial commitment, the argument justifies nothing about social obligations to the disabled. Given a weak initial commitment, the argument justifies only a correspondingly weak obligation to the disabled. To anyone who is a foundationalist about ethics, this is an unsatisfactory situation. To anyone who is an advocate for disability rights, it may seem to make disability rights disturbingly conventional and vulnerable to the vagaries of time and place. What if social circumstances change? What about obligations to the disabled in cultures where there is little or no social investment in saving or sustaining life? Surely we need to put the rights of the disabled on firmer footing than this consistency argument provides.

Of course we do, and I think the consistency argument calls our attention to the firmest footing imaginable on disability issues: the good of Agency. It is a footing right at the foundation of Stoic and Kantian ethical theory and versions of social-contract theory derived from them. It is similarly at the bottom of eudaimonistic versions of libertarianism and, perhaps, Aristotelian versions as well—at least as agency is central to the sort of human flourishing at stake in the "capabilities" arguments mentioned above. It is embedded, at least in a derivative way, in other plausible moral theories as well, such as in the concern for human autonomy one finds in Mill's version of utilitarianism. So if we need arguments for the good of Agency that go all the way down to the ground, we can get plenty of them. Moreover, as a practical matter, it seems unlikely that Western liberal democracies are going to give up their social commitments to protecting human lives, so this consistency argument is as secure as those social systems. It is true that the argument cannot be exported to systems that lack the requisite social commitments, but paying attention to the good of Agency provides a powerful philosophical focus that can help create such social commitments.

That said, I know of no way to put reasonable social commitments to the disabled on the sort of *a priori* footing that might make them invulnerable to changes in social circumstances. Make the commitment to life as stringent as you like, and you still have to face the possibility of not being able to save everyone—of sometimes having to choose between people. In the cold moral arithmetic of desperate times, burdens of all sorts, including burdensome human beings, must sometimes be left behind. That is a hard doctrine, but it is difficult to see how to avoid it, short of adopting the implausible injunction that no one should ever be saved unless all can be saved—or, which comes to the same thing, insisting that we make the choices by lottery regardless of whether the result saves anyone. The argument here has the reassuring consequence that if we devote any time at all to saving and sustaining lives, we must save the Agency first. Once that is done, it is hard to see why we disabled people should not take our chances along with everyone else.

NOTES

[1]It is useful to compare the opening sections of the Rehabilitation Act of 1973, 29 U.S.C. § 701, with the Americans with Disabilities Act of 1990, 42 USC § 12101. In the Rehabilitation Act, under the heading "Purpose" we have this:

> The purposes of this chapter are (1) to empower individuals with disabilities to maximize employment, economic self-sufficiency, independence, and inclusion and integration into society, through (A) comprehensive and coordinated state-of-the-art programs of vocational rehabilitation; (B) independent living centers and services; (C) research; (D) training; (E) demonstration projects; and (F) the guarantee of equal opportunity; and (2) to ensure that the Federal Government plays a leadership role in promoting the employment of individuals with disabilities, especially individuals with severe disabilities, and in assisting States and providers of services in fulfilling the aspirations of such individuals with disabilities for meaningful and gainful employment and independent living.

In the ADA, the "Purpose" is described this way:

> It is the purpose of this Act (1) to provide a clear and comprehensive national mandate for the elimination of discrimination against individuals with disabilities; (2) to provide clear, strong, consistent, enforceable standards addressing discrimination against individuals with disabilities; (3) to ensure that the Federal Government plays a central role in enforcing the standards established in this Act on behalf of individuals with disabilities; and (4) to invoke the sweep of congressional authority, including the power to enforce the fourteenth amendment and to regulate commerce, in order to address the major areas of discrimination faced day-to-day by people with disabilities.

[2]Airline Deregulation Act, 92 Stat. 1705 (1978).

[3]Pierre Hadot, *Philosophy as a Way of Life: Spiritual Exercises from Socrates to Foucault, 1987*, translated by Michael Chase, edited by Arnold I. Davidson. Oxford: Blackwell Publishers, 1995, 84–86.

[4]My thanks for this image, as well as many others, to the splendid general aviation memoir by Mariana Gosnell, *Zero 3 Bravo*. New York: Knopf, 1993.

[5]Cf. Richard Arneson, "Disability, Discrimination and Priority," this volume.

[6]From the ADA, 42 U.S.C. § 12102:

> The term disability means, with respect to an individual : (A) a physical or mental impairment that substantially limits one or more of the major life activities of such individual; (B) a record of such an impairment; or (C) being regarded as having such an impairment.

[7]Duncan C. Kinder (dckinder@ovnet.com), *Americans with Disabilities Act Document Center*, Great Lakes Disability and Business Technical Assistance Center, the ADA-OHIO Steering Committee and Duncan C. Kinder, available at http://janweb.icdi.wvu.edu/kinder/.

[8]It may be that defeating (rather than transforming) an anorexic's desire for skeletal thinness will in fact defeat her capacity for Agency. This is a good reason for insisting on treatment rather than mere control of such impulses. But as long as anorexia is defined as pathological, the anorexic's efforts to achieve skeletal thinness will not count as a "natural" major life activity understood along the lines proposed here.

[9]See Amartya Sen, *Inequality Examined*. Cambridge, MA: Harvard University Press, 1992, esp. chaps. 1–5; and Martha Nussbaum and Amartya Sen, eds., *The Quality of Life*. Oxford, UK: Clarendon Press, 1993, esp. Part I. My thanks to Anita Silvers for prompting me to include these comparative remarks.

[10]From the ADA, 42 U.S.C. § 12101: "The Congress finds that . . . some 43,000,000 Americans have one or more physical or mental disabilities, and this number is increasing as the population as a whole is growing older. . . ."

At Home with My Daughter

EVA FEDER KITTAY

> [I]n a society which defines and confines all meaning and worth in terms of production, profit and pervasive greed, intellectually disabled people will likely be exploited.
>
> —*Trent 1994, 277*

> [T]he loathing and disgust which people have at the sight of an idiot, is a feeling which, though having some foundation in human nature, is not necessarily attached to it in any virtuous degree, but is owing in great measure to a false delicacy, and . . . a certain want of comprehensiveness of thinking and feeling.
>
> —*William Wordsworth (responding to criticisms to his poem* The Idiot Boy)

SETTING THE STAGE FOR *OLMSTEAD v. L. C. AND E. W.*

At Home with Sesha

It's Sunday morning in my kitchen. Sesha, my daughter, is enjoying a breakfast of oatmeal and whole-grain toast covered with jam. Sesha, my beautiful love, who is nearly thirty years old (but looks like she's fourteen) is profoundly retarded. She sits in her modified Quickie wheelchair, which serves as her own throne. It supports her, secures her and transports her more effectively and for longer stretches of time and space than can her none-too-steady legs. Sesha speaks only with her wonderfully expressive eyes. She understands some of what we say to her—and maybe a great deal more than we fathom—but not enough to be safe when not securely seated in her chair. When she's well and enjoying her food, mealtimes are a pleasurable time. She insists on music while she dines—preferring her headphones and cassette player to the radio, where announcers are wont to interrupt the steady flow of music. These interruptions occasion one of the few times Sesha resorts to her voice, and she registers her protest until they stop their useless speech.

This morning, Sesha's caretaker has prepared small pieces of the toast and jam for finger-feeding—Sesha cannot use a spoon, fork or knife effectively. She holds a piece of the toast and jam in her hand, and her mouth is a lovely raspberry red. I sneak up behind her and kiss the still-pristine cheek. Sesha, as always, is delighted to see me. Anxious to give me one of her distinctive kisses, she tries to grab my hair to pull me to her mouth. Yet at the same time my kisses tickle her and make her giggle too hard to concentrate on dropping the jam-covered toast before going after my hair. I negotiate, as best I can, the sticky toast, the hair-pulling and the raspberry-jam-covered mouth. In this charming dance, Sesha and I experience some of our most joyful moments—laughing, ducking, grabbing, kissing. It is a pleasure I would have been denied if Sesha were not at home with us.

64

Sesha is so much a part of our home, a part of our life, that over the now nearly thirty years of her life, we have not been able seriously to consider placing her in residential care—although, given Sesha's profound retardation, she would most likely be a candidate for care not in a community setting. Although we do not think of Sesha's disability as a "blessing," we are among the most fortunate families in this world. Our financial resources have made available the possibility of hiring truly remarkable people who have helped us with Sesha's daily care.[1] These resources, together with good health insurance and legal mandates for her education, have allowed us to provide for her medical and habilitation needs, to make home modifications that would facilitate her care at home, and to integrate her special needs into our lives. As a result, we have been able to keep Sesha with us, but also to have a life not that different from the life we would have chosen for ourselves had Sesha not had such serious disabilities. The beneficiary of keeping Sesha at home has been not only Sesha. We, her family, those who come to our home, meet her, and experience her as part of our daily life, as well as those persons in the community who have been in touch with her, all have learned something important about the variety of human possibility and about the best of human love.

Olmstead v. L. C. and E. W.

The morning's pleasures are mixed with thoughts concerning the *Olmstead* decision, and the histories of institutionalizing the mentally retarded. In *Olmstead v. L. C. and E. W.,* the Supreme Court affirmed that the Americans with Disabilities Act mandates that people with mental disabilities are to be provided services in the least restrictive setting possible. The precious moments Sesha and I have shared in our kitchen provide a point of fixity for a consideration of debates about institutionalization versus community care, as well as the concerns of well-being and justice that they entail.

L. C., Lois Curtis, and E. W., Elaine Wilson, are women who were diagnosed with both mental retardation and mental illness. Both had lived at times in Georgia's psychiatric hospitals and at times in inadequate and even abusive community settings. Lois Curtis had been treated in the psychiatric hospital with medications and discharged without attention paid to her retardation. She had been discharged no less than 18 times, sometimes to her mother, who could not handle the situation, and sometimes to personal care homes. At her last stay, the psychiatric hospital and lawyers who had been retained on her behalf worked out an agreement not to discharge her until a plan had been put in place for appropriate community placement.

Elaine Wilson's story is depressingly similar. Due to meningitis, Elaine Wilson was mildly retarded and brain-damaged. She was homeless for more than twenty years after being discharged from a mental retardation facility. She was taken to Georgia's Regional Hospital over thirty times and successively released to various personal care homes, some of which were abusive. She sometimes ended up on the street. When her mother secured Legal Aid, the attorney halted discharge plans until community placement with appropriates services was provided.[2]

Lois Curtis and Elaine Wilson both had progressed to the point where the state professionals recommended community placement, and both had very much desired such placement. They were appropriately placed by order of a lower Georgia Court decision. In *Olmstead,* the Supreme Court upheld the lower court decision, thereby also affirming the ADA provision that disabled persons and their families can receive support services in the setting they determine most appropriate (but with important qualifications discussed below).[3] The *Olmstead* case has been hailed as a victory for those who advocate for community placement and deinstitutionalization. Yet it is as much a case about *receiving needed services in an appropriate environment* as it is about deinstitutionalization and community care *per se*. It is arguable that Lois Curtis and Elaine Wilson suffered as much from being moved into the community without appropriate care as they did from inappropriate institutionalization.

The Supreme Court decision was, however, qualified in some important ways: first that the least restrictive setting possible is determined by State health professionals; second that being placed in a less restrictive setting is not opposed by the disabled person herself; third that providing the service to this individual in a prompt fashion will not involve the person skipping ahead on a waiting list that moves at a reasonable pace; and last that providing service in the least restrictive setting to this disabled individual will not be so costly that it impedes a state's ability to provide a wide array of possible treatment settings appropriate to the variety of disabilities of its citizens.

A Brief History

Olmstead v. L. C. and E. W. marks an important milestone in a process that began over a quarter of a center ago. The televised exposés of the Willowbrook State School and Letchworth Village by Geraldo Rivera in 1972 awoke the nation to the fact that a great harm was being inflicted on the most vulnerable amongst us. In a relatively short time, large state institutions for retarded persons began to be dismantled, and the effort to reintegrate institutionalized persons into the community commenced. There was a call and a concerted effort to provide much smaller, community-based settings for those whose families did not want or could not continue to keep their developmentally disabled family members at home. In time, localities, to varying degrees, provided some supports to enable families to keep their disabled family member at home or close to home.

The state school institution for the mentally retarded began in the United States with a promise and a vision: educating and preparing the "feeble-minded" for "productive work." Prior to the mid-1800s, those believed to be chronically incapable of achieving the means to be self-supporting were accommodated by their families or consigned to almshouses. The progressive conception of care and education that led to the first "idiot asylums" quickly fell victim to forces that shape what Erving Goffman (1961) called "total institutions," to vicissitudes of attitudes toward the cognitively disabled, and to the opportunism, greed, and cupidity of officials and politicians.[4] The condition of the large public facility for retarded persons was, for most of its history, sad and often horrid. However, the particular conditions of the institutions at the time of the Willowbrook exposés reflected an especially unfortunate sequence of events: a rapid growth during the post–World War II years, followed by serious cutbacks over a decade later. An obsessive concern with normalcy and with the concept of the "normal" family, born in the aftermath of two world wars and a depression, bloated the state institutions in the 1950s. In the early 1960s, under the Kennedy administration, federal expenditures allowed for the building of more facilities. The expansions in facilities, fed by increasing numbers of parents who looked to house their children in them, increased the demand on state funds for maintaining the new institutions. However, in the late 1960s, cutbacks in state funding, begun under Ronald Reagan's governorship in California, propelled already squalid and uncaring institutions into cruel and truly horrific ones.[5]

Sesha was born in 1969. At the time we first suspected a problem, Sesha was four months old. At six months we were rather brutally informed that our daughter was severely to profoundly retarded. It was not until she was about one and a half years of age that we were certain that this prognosis was correct. Physicians and well-meaning relatives, subtly and not so subtly, indicated to us that placing Sesha in an institution would be the best course for her and for us. By this time—but already at birth—she was our beloved child. Parting with a baby we loved as much as any parent has loved a child was not something we could consider. Living in New York City and being *au courant* in public affairs, her father and I were surely aware of the exposés that preceded Willowbrook. In our conscious thoughts, we did not entertain the possibility of placing our own daughter in such horrid circumstances, but it is likely that the threat these presented shaped our views and contributed to our intransigence.

A study of parents conducted at about the same time our daughter was born indicated that most parents then had the same aversion to the idea of institutionalization. The urgings usually came from others. Jerry Jacobs, who conducted the study, remarked on the benevolent views of many of the parents he interviewed towards infanticide. Noting that the parents in his study were not unique, he quoted examples of parents from another study. One such parent stated: "I never really planned to kill my child, but I have thought of how much easier it would be if he died; my religion is the only thing that keeps me from killing my child" (Jacobs 1969, 89). Tellingly, Jacob wrote: "A key factor in the benevolent view that parents of retarded children took toward infanticide revolved around the prospect of their ultimately having to institutionalize their child." (Jacobs 1969, 89). The dominant stories that Jacob recounts involve parents wrestling with the idea that the time will come when they learn that their child will not develop sufficiently to become a productive member of society. It is either at this point or at a time when the child becomes too much for the parents to handle that they envision having to institutionalize their child. Recalling the exposés that preceded Rivera's, such as Robert Kennedy's 1965 assault on Rome and Willowbrook State Schools and *Look* magazine's graphic and brutal photographic essay "Christmas in Purgatory," may be sufficient to explain why loving parents would rather contemplate the death of their child than his or her institutionalization.

Yet at the same time, the advice to send a retarded child away, to institutionalize the individual who could never become a productive member of society, who would always be a "burden" to that family, was repeated again and again to parents with children who had Down syndrome and to parents of children who, whether they had a "normal" appearance or not, were labeled retarded. Today, such advice might not be offered as freely.

The exposés of the Willowbrook School and Letchworth Village forced a crucial reassessment of institutionalization *per se*. It was not simply the appalling conditions of institutions that were a problem, a problem that many previously believed was fixable by increased funding, better staffing, and improved training of staff; the very fact of "the institution" was seen to be the problem—*segregating* this population of children and adult citizens was itself suspect. Not until 1990, however, was the segregation *per se* legally prohibited in the form of the Americans with Disabilities Act. And not until *Olmstead* was the principle affirmed by interpreting the ADA to require that Lois Curtis and Elaine Wilson receive the services they need in the least restrictive settings possible.

That the situation for retarded individuals is generally far better than it was in the 1950s through early 1970s is hard to deny. Early intervention programs are available; foster care is encouraged and facilitated; schools, even local schools, are supposed to accommodate the needs of the cognitively disabled. And if placement is suggested, as it may be for a severely retarded child such as Sesha, it is likely to be placement in a private institution,[6] not necessarily small and homelike, but not the chamber of horrors that Willowbrook or Letchworth had become. In cases where parents decide that they are not prepared to care for a disabled child, foster care or adoption, rather than institutionalization, is usually proffered, although disabled infants and children are less likely to find adoptive homes than the able-bodied. However, the availability of services varies widely from state to state, and the heavy dependence on state-funded rather than federally funded programs hampers efforts to realize Federal legislative actions such as the ADA. Moreover many retarded persons are still in large institutions (though not as massive or decrepit as Willowbrook); many community-based services are inappropriate or inadequate; family support is far too meager and tends to be means-tested, providing relief only for families who are below a certain income;[7] and, as one researcher states: "when programs are limited in scope and size, returning a person with disabilities to the community may be a euphemism for returning the child to the mother" and that "little exists to support mothers in their work" (Nemzoff 1992, 20).

The Value of Community and Sesha's Value to Community

As a baby, Sesha was easy to love and easy to care for, and under no circumstance would we consider entrusting her care to strangers, much less condemning her to an anonymous institution. While we were told of the severity of her disability early on, we could not then, given the absence of any etiology, know how completely accurate the prognosis would prove. Nor could we know that nearly thirty years later Sesha would remain in our care at home. The journey has not been one of unadulterated joy, nor one of unmitigated hardship. The decision to keep Sesha at home is always up for reconsideration. Michael Bérubé writes, in *Life as We Know It,* that he and his wife always fear their son, who has Down syndrome, will die before they do *and* that they will die before he does. Like so many other parents of severely developmentally disabled children, we, too, tremble at the thought of such a vulnerable person in this harsh world without loving and devoted parents to see her through. And we, again like so many others, do not wish to burden our other children with the sort of home care we have provided for the disabled child. So the time of Sesha's placement in some facility other than her home is an immanent likelihood. What we wish for her is to find a place where she can continue to experience the sharing of love with those who see the person she is—beyond the twists of her body, the lazy eye that gets too easily distracted, the withdrawn look which one who doesn't know her, or doesn't care, mistakes for vacuity. Sesha is just the sort of person, you see, who a state official might determine would not benefit from a community placement. She will never become "independent." She will never become a "productive member of society." She will never contribute to her own support, much less become self-supporting. Sesha will be a "burden" on any economic order. But Sesha's being in the world is an inestimable contribution—even in the face of all the care and resources she requires. She is a most gentle tutor. She instructs us in the beauty of life itself. Her right to be in the world is not the bread she earns but the joy she brings. Her right to be in the world is not earned by her rationality but by her example that reason is not what defines what is human. Shut off from the community, her lessons fall on sleeping pupils.

Yet Sesha is not fully integrated into "the community" because she doesn't do things other young people her age do. Sesha truly could not take advantage of integrated classrooms, since her skills fall so far short of anything done in schoolrooms occupied by other children. She has always gone to a special school and nowadays attends a special day treatment program.

When Sesha was very young, I would take her everywhere—to school, to the park, shopping, to restaurants, to museums. When Sesha got older, she would be accompanied as often by her caretaker as by me or her father. But she would regularly go to a neighborhood playground. With care and solicitude, her caretaker coaxed children to speak and play with Sesha. I do not doubt that the exposure was puzzling for these children, yet they came to know someone quite unlike themselves, but one who was treated with love and concern. Here Sesha, with her caretaker's help, opened these children's perceptions to a new and important awareness.

Today we do not take Sesha out much in public places. Doing many activities with her in public areas is physically demanding. Shopping is too difficult for us and inundates her with too much stimulation for her to handle comfortably—she "spaces out." Mostly, we shuttle her in her specially equipped van between home and day treatment program, home and physician, home and pool or therapist. We still take Sesha for walks, to see a ballet or hear music (for music is her world, and she is enraptured when she gets to hear live music). People sometimes approach us and want to make contact. Each nonroutine activity, however, involves many difficulties. Each exposure brings looks and makes us see Sesha as others see her. But when she communicates her delight, or grabs me or her father or her caretaker and embraces us, kissing and hugging and showing her love without inhibitions, even the cold stares of strangers melt into warm smiles. Here is Sesha as we cherish her, and, not uncommonly, even strangers come to glimpse a special quality. What we learn in Sesha is that our humanity sits at our very core—that it is not vested in this skill or that, that a skill less does not mean less a human being, worthy of less care and dignity. Maybe there is no more important lesson for us to learn.

THINKING THROUGH *OLMSTEAD*

Olmstead v. L. C. and E. W. affirms a number of propositions with which we can readily agree:

- That services should be provided in the least restrictive setting that is appropriate for a given mentally disabled individual;
- That segregation is itself a form of discrimination;
- That placement to a less restrictive setting should not go against the wishes of the person affected.

But it also contains a number of points about which I have concerns. In particular, I am concerned about the limitation that maintains that such services need not be supplied if doing so would strain the state's budget for disability. I would like to take these up in turn.

Least Restrictive Setting

Reading *Olmstead* in light of my family's experiences and the history of the institutionalization of the retarded, assenting to the first proposition, "that services should be provided in the least restrictive setting," is easy. Institutions are undesirable. Large state facilities, those that remain, may not be the infernos they were in the 1960s and early seventies, but neither had they always been as squalid as they had by then become. We have seen that they are vulnerable to economic pressures that may increase the numbers of institutions and the number of residents occupying them while depleting resources available for their staffing and maintenance—even more so when these institutions become places in which society discharges an obligation to a population about which it knows little and cares even less.

Erving Goffman delineated the features of the sorts of residential facilities that were "total institutions." In his influential book, *Asylums,* Goffman drew from a range of facilities: those purporting to help their residents and those meant to punish or destroy their inmates. The need to house and control large numbers of inmates with a small number of people to oversee them and the need to place large numbers of persons into a restricted locale result in the loss of privacy, the subjection to a total authority, abuses from inmates and authorities alike, and an estrangement from self. Goffman showed that the nature and requirements of such institutions, regardless of their particular purpose, set in motion processes by which confined individuals lost their former identities and their connections to those who were closest and were constitutive of that identity. The case he so convincingly constructed portrayed the dehumanization of these institutions as an inevitable outcome of their structural features, even where the original intent of the institution was benign.

Segregation Is Discrimination

Judge Thomas, who dissented from the majority opinion, argued that segregating a population with a specific problem precisely to provide them with services and treatment *for the very same problem* was not discrimination. In this view he diverges from an important tradition that has argued that segregation *per se* is discrimination. The histories of civil rights and antidiscrimination laws have provided ample basis for arguing that segregation is a form of discrimination.[8] Thomas's argument is plausible for situations in which providing treatment can only be accomplished by confining individuals—that is, when the needed services are exceedingly rare, costly, and so filled with hazards and difficulties that they demand highly specialized personnel. But the personal care and the therapies that mentally disabled persons normally require are not services of this sort. They are normally possible in less restrictive settings, assuming a community commitment to make them available.

The effects of segregation are felt not only by those who are confined, but also by those from whom the targeted population is segregated. The fear and stigma of those who are "different" is reinforced. In turn, the targeted population becomes increasingly subject to discrimination. In the case of the disabled, "the different forms that human life and human ability can take," as one disability rights activist put it,[9] are often unfamiliar, frightening and threatening. The more disabled persons are sequestered away from the able-bodied, the more they can only be perceived as Other. As Other, persons with disabilities are excluded from the sympathies and concerns of the able-bodied. The less they enter into the configuration of equals that constitute the associations from which societies are formed, the more they are excluded from the privileges of rights-bearing citizens. Integration into the community not only is the right of disabled people as citizens but is often seen as the condition of the possibility of their citizenship.

Complications and Qualifications

Yet the two propositions to which I urged our assent—that institutions are bad, and that segregation is discrimination—are not as unproblematic as the above considerations suggest. Not all institutions in which people come together to live and lead their lives follow the dismal script that Goffman, no doubt accurately, ascribes to most. That is, there are institutions that are "total institutions," dehumanizing their inhabitants, and then there are those that have the prerequisites for becoming "total institutions" but nonetheless do not. The residential college campus comes to mind. Here, too, peers are herded promiscuously together, divorced from their previous home life. There are many 18- to 21-year-olds under the supervision of a few older teachers, administrators and dorm supervisors. They sleep, eat, work and play mostly (if not all) within the one facility, a facility frequently closed off from the rest of the world with gates (especially at night), walls or other barriers.

But few liberal arts colleges today have the regimentation, the manipulation, the stripping of self, the rituals of contamination that characterize the institutions described by Goffman.

The campus model is self-consciously adopted by one institution I recently visited. Located in a spacious, villagelike setting in upstate New York, consisting of cottages housing six to eight residents in rooms that residents and their families decorate and personalize, staffed with therapists galore and a truly caring staff who seem genuinely to enjoy their charges, incorporating a farm complete with farm animals, vegetable gardens and flower gardens, equipped with a swimming pool, a nice café with good food, a science lab, computers, a bed-and-breakfast where the family can come and stay to visit their child, and having policies that encourage the child to return home on weekends and holidays as the family desires, this institution (which houses mentally retarded and multiply disabled individuals ranging in age from 5 to 86) is the antithesis of the ones Goffman portrays. Yet it, too, is an all-encompassing setting in which residence, education, work, associations all take place in one locale under one administration and which effectively "segregates" a population. Although there is no barbed wire or high walls that separate this facility from the outside world, it is a "village" or "campus" unto itself.

Residents of this institution are not integrated into their own communities in a daily fashion. Nonetheless, this is a place that is situated in a community and attempts to involve the community. It has created a cooperative store selling farm products, so that those in the adjacent community can partake of the products produced on its site.

What are we to say of sizable institutions of this sort? What are we to say of its cloistered situation? Is this the pernicious segregation that amounts to discrimination? Would it not stretch the concept of "community care" to say that the cooperative arrangement with some members of the community integrates the residents into the community? Are all institutions bad? Is all segregation discrimination? Isn't an institution of this sort far preferable to a community setting that is completely inappropriate, such as a homeless shelter "in the community" or the "personal care home" in which Elaine Wilson was held down by one provider who "tried to pray the demons out of her" (see Bazelon Center for Mental Health Law 1999)? Or the group homes owned by uncaring and irresponsible persons who build group homes, hire incompetent staff, provide little care, poor services and hazardous conditions, but profit handsomely from public funds, supervised by unscrupulous bureaucrats? In these community-based group homes, the residents are scarcely better off than in the state institutions of the late 1960s.[10]

Might not a well-run institution with a devoted administrative staff that guarantees a uniform level of good-quality care be preferable even to a small group home in which the quality of care can be more directly subject to the vicissitudes of personnel (whose turnover rates are high) and inadequate supervision? Isn't a larger institution such as the one portrayed above, with a track record of good-quality care, an entire staff of well-trained personnel, and a committed board of directors, more of a comfort to parents of at least more severely impaired persons than the intimate setting of a group home that depends on just a few people for its continued existence and integrity? Even persons who are mildly retarded are so vulnerable to abusive behavior that placing them in the hands of unscrupulous or underpaid, undercommitted and unsupervised personal care providers can result in serious abuse.

Arguably, for someone who is very severely impaired or who requires many different services, a larger facility, one that contains most of what the person requires, that could keep a very vulnerable person more protected, and that would facilitate her movement from one activity to another, would be preferable to a setting that was more obviously community-based but involved a greater fragmentation of services and more exposure to abuse.

These, I submit, are difficult and uncomfortable questions that force us to resist simple pieties about what is good and bad with respect to caring for the needs of those with significant mental and cognitive impairments. The willingness to devote adequate material resources to the facilities, willingness properly to pay and train the staff devoted to caring for and providing services for those with disabilities, and willingness to devote energy and thought to how best to serve vulnerable persons, their families and their communities are ultimately as important as the frequent mantras (still much needed) that "institutions are bad" and "segregation is discrimination."

I have indicated that sometimes a less integrated setting may be preferable to a setting that is more community-based. A homeless shelter, which was at one point contemplated for one of the *Olmstead* plaintiffs, may be located within the community but it is hardly appropriate for a person with cognitive and other mental disabilities. (It is, one should argue, inappropriate for those without impairments as well, although it is the vulnerability resulting from the mental disability that makes such placement especially cruel.) Voice of the Retarded, an advocacy group of parents of retarded persons, has urged that while community placement is frequently preferable to institutionalization, the vulnerability of some persons with mental incapacities is such that most community settings are not sufficiently protective. They argued for, and applauded *Olmstead* for, insisting that placement to a less restrictive setting should not go against the wishes of the person affected. In the cases of L. C. and E. W., the individuals involved were capable of indicating their wishes. They very much wished to be able to receive the services they required in appropriate community-based residences. Some persons with severe mental impairments are not able to voice preferences—and arguably, those who may need more protective settings may be those least able to object to being thrown into a situation of "independent living," one for which they may be ill equipped. In any such decisions, families and whatever other persons are intimately concerned with the person's well-being, not only professionals, have to be in a position to decide on the appropriate setting.

Questions of who is to decide, and the idea that this is a decision to be made—that the decision may not be the same for all—may not be to the taste of some advocates for the full integration of persons with disabilities into the community. The disability community has insisted that often a disability need not be an obstacle, need not become a handicapping condition. It has been called to our attention that a society lacking a commitment to the well-being of all its citizens, those with disabilities as well as those without, maintains its life form and builds its structures in ways that exclude persons with disabilities. It thereby exacerbates many handicaps produced by the impairment and sometimes creates handicaps where none need exist (without steps, for instance, persons in wheelchairs would not be denied access to places reachable only by steps).

Still, what sometimes goes unquestioned is the goal toward which we aim when we insist on access and the value of integration for persons with disabilities. "Independence" and "productivity," for example, are often stressed and are often proffered as economic incentives, as the payback for building ramps and including Braille signs. Even the mentally retarded can be employed and can be productive rather than being only burdens on the community. Living in the community and integrated into the community, the disabled—and even the mentally disabled—can be part of the reciprocal social cooperation, the sharing of benefits and burdens. Locked away in an institution, segregated, people with disabilities become a drain on resources. Society pays for its prejudice in cash.[11]

Yet independent living and "productivity" or economic self-sufficiency[12] cannot be goals for all disabled persons, no matter how one wants to stretch these terms, most especially perhaps for very severely mentally disabled persons. For my daughter, no accommodations can secure her "independence." Doubtless, a very ingenious person could find a way to make whatever skills she has into some "productive" activity—but it would be productive perhaps for us, not for her. It would add little to her life. If integration into the community would not further these goals, why is it a matter of significance? Is it always desirable? What are the goals for persons impaired so severely that independence and productivity in any real sense are not within their grasp, how is the setting in which they are placed to figure in these goals and what obligations do we, as a society, have to fully dependent persons who will never be productive?

Let us first consider what goals we have in raising and educating any child. My aims in caring for our daughter are oddly similar to the goals I have with my fully able son—to help him become a happy thriving person whom I can love and who can love in return. In the case of my son, that telos has a subordinate aim of bringing forth a person who can appreciate moments of both independence and dependence, who can appreciate the importance of our interdependence. With my son I also hope to promote his ability to make use of his talents to add value to our world.

In the case of my daughter, her dependence is most prominent, but nonetheless, I depend on her as well—on her welcome when I return home and when I awake in the morning, on her laughter to remind me of sunshine when I'm overburdened with commitments and sadness, on her love when I feel alone. It's perhaps self-delusional to say that I am as dependent on her as she is on me, but perhaps not. Others could take care of her and even love her—in fact, I *must* think that she will continue to thrive with or without me. But without her, I would wither. So I have spawned in her a person who is not only dependent but interdependent—even if she can never be *in*dependent. Nor can she be productive (unless what she feeds all those who get to know her, her own special brand of *soul food*—food for the soul—counts as productivity). On any official count of burdens and benefits, Sesha is only a burden. Well, why, then, should Sesha be integrated into the community, except perhaps that it can lower the cost of her care? And in that case, why should she have any other option? Perhaps what her case really tells us is, first, that it is not productivity and independence that matter, but the full flourishing of each member of the community, and, second, that a fully flourishing life involves family, community, and the interdependence of those with whom we share family and community.

I've suggested that Sesha might be thought to be one of those individuals who cannot take advantage of integration into the community—that she requires a "more protective setting." Sesha has clearly benefited from being a part of our home. The appropriateness of community placement cannot be held hostage to a notion that a disabled person can become "productive" or live "independently" if "suitably assisted."

Yet phrases such as a "setting least restrictive of a person's freedom" "integration into the community" "a family or home-like setting" "protective environment" take on strange affinities and oppositions when one considers the full range and the varied forms disabilities take. The paternalism of "a protective environment" that may be irksome to a person with blindness who is in all other respects fully able to participate in employment and community life stands in contrast to the goal of integration into the community. Such integration is achieved in an independent home for adults and a family for a child, settings that would be properly characterized as the "least restrictive." For someone like my daughter, however, a protective environment is more crucial than many other considerations.

The most protective, in her case, is the family setting, as long as we remain the family and have the resources to care for her at home. One has to wonder how many more families would be able and willing to have the setting be their own home if a truly full array of supportive services were to be made available not only to the individual for medical treatment and habilitation but to the family to continue keeping their child (even when an adult) at home.[13]

The next best may not be a "familylike" setting. Instead it may be an institution—but only if it is one like the idyllic place described above. Of course, such facilities are not common, nor are they cheap. The claim made in the Brief for the Amici Curiae American Association on Mental Retardation that "Although needs may differ from one individual to another, the core concept of establishing a home in a neighborhood where residents can live what society perceives as a 'normal' everyday life, has proved successful time and again" may sound like a clarion call we should all rush to, but we have to think carefully about what norms of "normal" we want to subscribe to. Where the norm is "independent living" rather than a caring environment wherein individuals thrive, we have to be cautious that the prejudices which drove the mentally disabled out of the community do not resurface as neglectful "dumping" of people into the streets, homeless shelters or small residences that are poorly staffed and supervised, because such dumping is cost-effective—a danger realized in the lives of Lois Curtis and Elaine Wilson and who knows how many others. *Olmstead* can help protect against this for others in the position of these two women only if there is as much emphasis placed on the reading of *Olmstead* on the provision of adequate and appropriate services as there is on the setting in which the services are to be provided. The purpose of bringing people back into the community and of assisting families who want to keep their mentally disabled children and relatives in the community must be to connect and reconnect, to provide the bonds that assure that people will be valued with or without impairments, and to do what is needed to allow them to flourish.

As I have tried to indicate in the example Sesha sets for us, when one is allowed to flourish, no degree of impairment is so great that that person cannot contribute to the well-being of those around her—just by being in the world.

Limitations of *Olmstead*

Considerations such as these bring up some of the more problematic propositions affirmed in *Olmstead*—in particular, that providing needed services in the least restrictive setting possible cannot be made where the state's budget for disability would be strained if placement were made. This is puzzling. Are we being told that justice here demands that members of a group, in this case the disabled, have recourse to complaint only if some are treated badly, not if all are treated equally badly? Consider the following: a state determines to spend a paltry amount on its disabled population, just enough to provide for a few community-based services of a relatively poor quality. These same services are also provided in the state institutions. It turns out that if all the persons housed in segregated facilities who health officials agree would benefit from community placement were to be so placed and receive these services in the community, the state would have to shut down its institutional facilities. In that case, either those who would have to remain in the institution would have no place to go, or those who are thought appropriate for community placement would be denied such placement. But to alter the situation by placing all those who could benefit from community placement, such as it is, would worsen the situation of those for whom institutionalization is deemed appropriate. Under the current arrangements, no one is treated particularly well, since the facilities, whether in the community or in the institution, are of poor quality. And one of the two groups, those who should be in the community or those who should not, suffers as a result of the low level of expenditure. In that scenario, under the Court's interpretation of the ADA in *Olmstead,* the state is obliged to do nothing at all. But then the spirit of the ADA is violated. What a sad and bizarre state of affairs this is. Without material resources to back it, the ADA, as interpreted by the *Olmstead* decision, provides purely formal rights, not realizable substantive ones.

Beyond *Olmstead*

The decision not to institutionalize Sesha had to do with the financial resources we had at our disposal. These enabled us to care for Sesha at home and carry on lives not that different from the lives we might have carried on had we not had a disabled child or even a child as severely disabled as Sesha. That choice is available to very few. Yet were policies in place that took seriously the notion of providing services in the community or in the least restrictive setting possible, these policies and funding would be directed toward enabling and supporting those families who do choose to keep their disabled child at home, even past the period of childhood when appropriate.

Done well, when this sort of care does not mean "dumping" the full responsibility and burden on the mother and whatever family she has to call upon, it is often—but not always—the best outcome. That is, were we to have a full array of flexible supports for home care, the option I and my family have exercised would be available as a choice to many families.

It may well be that the arguments that need to be made in support of the full flourishing for all persons, disabled or not, cannot in the end rest on policies that view each person as isolated and independent of all others. The disservice that is done to the individual who ought to be treated in the community and who fails to be able to receive treatment in the least restrictive environment is a disservice not to this individual alone. The disservice is also to the parents, family and others who have a stake in the individual's happiness. Desirable as the campuslike institution/village described above is, her father and I remain reluctant even to consider it as a possible residence for Sesha—at least while we are able to keep her at home. So it is not just the awful, Goffmanesque, total institutions we fear. We fear the separation from her—losing her as a resident in our family home.

To illustrate how this consideration may be used to enlarge the thinking in *Olmstead,* consider the case that my daughter would only be granted services in an institution outside her community. The services she requires are directly related to just those incapacities that make it necessary for her to be institutionalized. While it may be possible to provide those services in the community, were all who were eligible to receive these services in the community to receive them in the community, the state institution would have to close for lack of funds. In this case, how do I claim discrimination against my daughter? Who would count as the favored class in comparison to which limiting my daughter's access to treatment to the institution constitutes discrimination? If, however, the impact on the family is considered, it is perhaps clearer that the hardships of her confinement are spread more widely—that all in her family suffer as a family. Our loss is in our ability to maintain the close family bonds with our child that another family, whose child can receive services in the community, can maintain without jeopardizing the provision of needed services. Additional costs to the state are weighed against some fundamental rights and interests of people to maintain familial relationships—relationships of care and concern to those closest to them. The segregation of disabled family members, then, may be discriminatory to her and her family insofar as it forces a separation in order to receive needed services when other families are not so impacted by a family member's need for important social, medical or habilitative services.[14]

The point concerning family integrity is perhaps best made in the case of a minor child—that is, the situation most comparable to families who do not have a person with significant disabilities. The mentally disabled person who reaches adulthood, however, occupies a peculiar position: chronologically adult, but mentally incapable of negotiating the adult world.

Sesha is, after all, a young woman of thirty. Other young women of similar age are, today at least, long gone from parental protection. And here is the rub. Most parenting involves nurturing one's young bird until it has learned to fly on its own—and then one watches with bittersweet pleasure as it tries out its wings and flies from the nest. But this bird cannot fly now and never will. Why remove her from the nest? The closer to the source of those for whom this individual's welfare is of utmost concern, the better. The bird who cannot fly is best-off close to the nest—if not in the nest. I do not believe this is infantilizing the developmentally disabled but recognizing a vulnerability that is quite unlike any other except that of a child. Mental disability spans a range from childlike incapacity to a less-than-full-adult-capacity, and it involves a vulnerability proportional to the incapacity.

The challenge is to give adequate recognition to the developmentally disabled individual's vulnerability and the protective and nurturing environment of an accepting and loving home situation (if such there is), without exploiting the resources and labor of the mother. The other challenge is to offer alternatives to those without the familial caring environment that can mimic that invested protectiveness, a protectiveness that is so crucial.

The exploitation of the intellectually disabled that Trent notes in the opening quotation of this chapter can take place in various settings. The ultimate challenge is to see in the lives of the intellectually disabled values that can speak out against the meaning of life and worth of people that is confined to "production, profit and pervasive greed." The challenge is to value their lives, to understand that their dependence is a dependency which we all share as we live together, that the contribution they make, however unrelated to production and profit, is the contribution of the bonding that relations of dependency form. Understanding that these connections are what give life its value is ultimately the best defense we have against conditions that foster the likelihood that "intellectually disabled people will . . . be exploited."

Olmstead moves us in the right direction. Its insistence on the provision of services in settings that foster the possibility of mentally disabled persons remaining connected to family and community helps to bring us closer to an ideal in which meaning and worth move beyond the values which exclude the lives of Lois and Elaine and Sesha. But it still leaves much undone. It still fails to ensure that material resources will be extended to provide adequately for the needs of the mentally disabled.

Olmstead, Dependency and Justice

To what extent, however, can we justify the expenditure of resources that are required to provide for persons as disabled as the mentally and cognitively impaired to flourish, especially in cases where they will never be fully independent or productive? Do we, as a society, have obligations to individuals who are entirely dependent, who cannot enter into a reciprocity of social cooperation, sharing both the burdens and the benefits of such cooperative arrangements? Anita Silvers (1998) has argued that what we owe to disabled persons is equality of opportunity and the elimination of discrimination. We are moreover obligated to devote resources to altering the social environment so as to realize equality of opportunity and to eliminate the barriers that are discriminatory to those with physical and mental disabilities. On this view, the *Olmstead* case appropriately has been argued on the basis of antidiscrimination law, where segregation is itself viewed as discrimination. But, she insists, we are not obligated to devote resources that will *equalize* the condition of those with disabilities, where the benchmark of equality is one of either resources, capabilities or welfare. On this view, *Olmstead* should not be seen as making a claim to equalize those with mental disabilities and those without such disabilities. Expenditures of resources are required by justice if they remove discriminatory behavior.[15] So that if nondisabled persons receive whatever services they require in their community when it is feasible, then disabled persons, even when their disability is mental, should receive services in the community whenever delivering those services in the community is feasible. The case is nicely illustrated in the case of education. Able-bodied children receive educational services in their communities, therefore disabled children should receive educational services in their community. This would be nondiscriminatory behavior that does not exclude one part of the population. If providing this education for disabled children in their community were to be more costly than providing it in segregated settings, the expense would be justified by virtue of the correctness of not engaging in discrimination against the disabled children.

Yet I argued above that providing services to severely mentally disabled persons in the community may, at times, be less preferable, from the perspective of providing *adequate services,* to being placed in a more segregated, but better staffed, better equipped and probably more costly setting. From the perspective of nondiscrimination, it does not seem that these expenditures can be justified.

We could, like Norman Daniels (1988), view access to health care as a matter of equality of opportunity—the opportunity to be restored to health—and view disability as a form of ill health, so that educational, habilitation and therapeutic services are seen as efforts to restore disabled persons to a nondisabled state (defined physically or functionally). Then we could argue that the disabled person should have the same opportunity to achieve health, which in the case of disability means restoration to a nondisabled state (defined physically or functionally). But when Silvers argues against the claim of equalization, I imagine this is precisely the argument she opposes. Restoring a disabled person to a non-disabled state—or rather attempting to do so—may be a Sisyphean effort consuming enormous resources. In the case of severe cognitive disablities, it is not clear that any expenditure of resources could achieve the task.

What if we understand equality of opportunity in its more conventional ways, as the opportunity that is opened when barriers are removed and access is facilitated (in the case of disability by eliminating prejudice and discriminatory practices in the workplace and other public spaces and suitably modifying the environment)? Then the aim is to remove obstacles that prevent disadvantaged persons from achieving as much as they are inherently capable of. This equality of opportunity is envisioned as allowing all who have the talent and interest to thrive in the competitive arena of production. Such a "leveling of the playing field" is scarcely of much help for my daughter or others like her. She couldn't survive, much less thrive on such purely formal justice. According to such a conception of justice, there is no justification for spending more for those who would thrive in a better but more segregated setting.

Behind much antidiscrimination and equality of opportunity law stands the figure of the individual who, if only freed from oppressive restrictions, can be independent, self-sufficient, and a contributing member of society. The theories of justice that justify them count contributions largely in terms of productivity. But all such theories must count the contributions of Sesha and those sharing her disabilities as outside the scheme of cooperation.

In *Love's Labor,* I argue against an understanding of society as first and foremost an association of equals—independent equals engaged in reciprocal interactions. Instead, I argue, social organization must be recognized to begin with the fact of human dependency. Because humans cannot fully be independent, because we are all dependent at some point in our lives, and most will have periods of dependency later in our lives, we require social organization and community to sustain us through these periods of dependency. If social organization—its origins and rationales—is about cooperative arrangements among independent equals, it is as much, if not more, about the need to care for dependents. I take this to mean that a theory of justice that addresses social arrangements must recognize the obligation to dependents and those who care for them.

Although those who are dependent in the way Sesha and many cognitively impaired persons are cannot reciprocate, they have as much right to the resources as able and productive persons have. For the point of society is not only to protect and enable our labors when we are fully functioning and independent, but also to offer the means to nurture and protect us in our vulnerable dependency and to provide those of us who care for dependents the means and resources to accomplish our task. I venture that those most vulnerable are justified in having *first* call to resources. They are least able to go out and get what they need or to demand a share in the benefits of social cooperation. They depend on others' moral sensibility. But if we did not need one another, depend on, that is "hang on," one another, then what could make society hang together? Without vulnerability and dependency, it isn't clear that there would be much social cooperation from which to benefit. We do not need to justify devoting resources even to the most dependent persons (by claiming, for example, to equalize them, however we construe that), for providing for dependents is in large measure the point and purpose of social organization. *Olmstead* is a case to be celebrated. Yet in relying on an antidiscrimination argument, it still fails to center the care of vulnerable persons.

Sesha and other mentally disabled persons, including those far less disabled than she is, remind us of our own vulnerability to being or becoming dependent. The more we stress the importance of independence, the more threatening and fearsome is that reminder of dependency. But we can utilize this reminder to recognize that each of us has periods of dependency in which we need to be cared for and during which we are vulnerable to need, exploitation and abuse. Then we will not allow ourselves to be lured into the fantasy that our lives are at all moments under our own control. We will allow ourselves to recognize that we are at all times dependent to some degree and sometimes, dependent to the full degree. Only then can we begin to build better social structures and protections for those times when we may be vulnerable.

To gather the political will to make rights granted by the ADA meaningful and so set policies that enable families and communities to care properly for the mentally disabled, we need to place these policies in a larger agenda of making society responsive to dependencies of all sorts. In that wider context, disabilities are not be singled out as dependencies that need to be supported. The ADA received strong support because it included a wide range of disabling conditions—wide enough that a significant portion of the citizenry could recognize its applicability or potential pertinence to their own lives. The agenda should be still wider. The dependency of disability needs to be joined to the dependency of infancy and early childhood and to a healthy but frail old age. Strategically we can say that the broader the base, the less is the danger of backlash and resistance. But beyond strategy, we can say that if we can allow ourselves to learn from those who are most dependent about the frailties that come with being human dependent animals (see MacIntyre 1999), we can reappropriate our own resources and priorities so that meeting needs and granting rights are aligned in a just, caring and effective manner.

REFERENCES

ADAPT. "ADAPT Press Release: ADA Victory in the Supreme Court." 22 June 1999. <nlaspina@ix. netcom.com>.

Bazelon Center for Mental Health Law (leec@bazelon.org). *Who are L.C. and E.W.?* 1999. Available at http://www.bazelon.org/lcandew.html.

Boo, K. "Invisible Lives: Troubled System for the Retarded." *Washington Post,* December 5, 1999, 3, Section A1.

Bulmer, M. *The Social Basis of Community Care.* London: Allen and Unwin, 1987.

Daniels, N. *Am I My Parents' Keeper? An Essay on Justice between the Younger and the Older.* New York: Oxford University Press, 1988.

Ferguson, P. M. *Abandoned to Their Fate: Social Policy and Practices toward Severely Retarded People in America.* Philadelphia: Temple University Press, 1994.

Goffman, I. *Asylums.* Chicago: Aldine Publishing, 1961.

Jacobs, A. "Pennsylvania Couple Accused of Abandoning Disabled Son." *The New York Times,* 29 December 1999, national page.

Jacobs, J. *The Search for Help: A Study of the Retarded Child in the Community.* Washington, DC: University Press of America, 1969/1982.

Kittay, Eva Feder. *Love's Labor: Essays on Women, Equality and Dependency.* New York and London: Routledge, 1999.

Landsman, G. H. "Reconstructing Motherhood in the Age of the 'Perfect' Babies: Mothers of Infants and Toddlers with Disabilities." *Signs,* 24 (1998): 69–99.

MacIntyre, A. *Dependent Rational Animals.* Chicago: Open Court, 1999.

Manning, A. "Quietly Overwhelmed." *USA Today,* January 17, 2000.

Nemzoff, R. E. "Changing Perceptions of Mothers of Children with Developmental Disabilities 1960–1992: A Critical Review." Working Paper. Working Paper Series. Center on Research on Women: Wellesley College, 1992.

Silvers, A., Wasserman, D., and Mahowald, M. B. *Disability, Difference, Discrimination.* Lanham, MD: Rowman & Littlefield, 1998.

tenBroek, J. "The Right to Live in the World: The Disabled in the Law of Torts." *California Law Review* 54 (1966): 841.

Trent, J. W. J. *The Invention of the Feeble Mind.* Berkeley, CA: University of California Press, 1994.

NOTES

[1] I speak at some length about the person who has been Sesha's primary caretaker, Peggy, who has cared for Sesha from the age of four and still continues to care for her, in Kittay 1999.

[2] Bazelon Center for Mental Retardation 1999.

[3] See the statement of ADAPT <nlaspina@ix.netcom.com>, "ADAPT Press Release: ADA Victory in the Supreme Court," 22 June 1999.

[4] See Ferguson (1994) for an account of the asylums and for a nuanced account of the "progressivism" of the early founders of the asylums for "idiots."

[5] In the above account, I follow Trent (1994).

[6] Where at least some of the funds would come from public financing.

[7] In fact, not only do poor families find it impossible to meet the needs of their severely disabled children, middle-class, and even wealthy families find themselves overwhelmed with medical and caretaking

responsibilities. Finding qualified help is both difficult and so expensive it can exhaust the resources of well-off parents as well. The tragic consequences of parents who, in spite of a generous income, are no longer able to cope is exemplified in the account of the Kelsos. The father is a chemical company chief executive and the mother is a well-known advocate for children with disabilities. In December 1999, they abandoned their 10-year-old son in the emergency room of a hospital. (See Jacobs, Andrew. "Pennsylvania Couple Accused of Abandoning Disabled Son." *The New York Times,* December 29, 1999, National Page). A subsequent newspaper article put the Kelso case into the context of the many families raising children with serious medical, physical, and mental difficulties who face the strains of caring for their specially vulnerable and dependent children with so little social support. (See Manning, Anita. "Quietly Overwhelmed." *USA Today,* January 17, 2000, cover story.)

[8]In their Amici Curiae Brief, the ACLU and Georgia's ACLU cite *Brown vs. Board of Education,* 347 U.S. 483, 494 (1954) in maintaining that racial segregation "is inherently because of its damaging effects on the excluded individuals . . . [sending] a message of racial inferiority and [perpetuating] stereotypes with their resulting stigma." Similarly, citing the Supreme Court's decision in *United States v. Virginia,* 518 U.S. 515, 534 (1996): "[Gender] classifications may not be used, as they once were, . . . to create or perpetuate the legal social and economic inferiority of women," the briefs point to the condemnation of exclusionary practices in the case of gender. The ADA was enacted "against the backdrop of our nation's other civil rights laws and with the express purpose of providing disabled individuals with equivalent protection. . . ."

[9]Marsha Sexton, personal communication.

[10]See the devastating account of the condition of group homes in Washington, D.C., exposed in a searing article by Katherine Boo in the *Washington Post,* "Invisible Lives: Troubled System for the Retarded," December 5, 1999, 3, Section A1.

[11]The Brief for the Amici Curiae American Association on Mental Retardation notes that in the Georgia Regional Hospital in Atlanta, the state psychiatric hospital where both L. C. and E. W. were housed: "The per diem, per capita cost of institutional care at the special unit for persons with mental retardation . . . was $283 in fiscal year 1996 for an annual cost of $103,295." The contrast with the Georgia Medicaid waiver program is striking, with per diem costs for community care per person ranging from $118 to $124, for an annual total cost of $43,070 to $45,260. One can probably assume that the residents were not engaged in income-generating employment.

[12]The Americans for Disabilities Act, for example, has as one of its findings the following: "the Nation's proper goals regarding individuals with disabilities are to assure equality of opportunity, full participation, independent living, and economic self-sufficiency for such individuals; . . ." (ADA, S.933, Sect. 2.a.8).

[13]Once again, states and localities differ in how much they will provide to make necessary alterations in the home, to provide sufficient home aids, to provide respite care, to help with the purchase of appliances that make home care feasible, etc.

[14]This is an argument which is due in large measure to Anita Silvers's prompting.

[15]Silvers (1998) decries "the needlessly debilitating proliferation of neediness" (p. 145), as a basis for, or result of, arguing for provisions for and environmental modifications to accommodate those who are disabled. She does remark, "Nothing I have argued here precludes supporting a distributive scheme to benefit profoundly impaired people" (p. 144), and she supports programs that "assume the extraordinary costs of caring for profoundly impaired people." Yet, she maintains, if these are requirements of justice, they are so only for the dependency workers who care for profoundly impaired individuals, not for the disabled themselves. I am arguing that justice demands such distributive schemes for *both* dependency worker and dependent.

The Need for a Standard of Care

ALASDAIR MACINTYRE

Lois Curtis and Elaine Wilson, both suffering from mental retardation and also in the past afflicted by bouts of mental illness, now live, the one in a three-person group home, the other in her own apartment, in a way that enables them both to receive the mental health services that they need and also to live in a way that fosters their independence and that they themselves have chosen. Had it not been for the Supreme Court's *Olmstead* decision that denied to the State of Georgia the right to make its mental health services available to them only if they submitted to conditions of institutionalized isolation, this happy outcome would not have occurred. Moreover, it is a consequence of that decision that it is significantly more difficult for Georgia and other state authorities to deny to others in similar conditions similar opportunities. For these reasons, and because there seems to have been in the law of the United States no alternative remedy available to Ms. Curtis and Ms. Wilson, we should welcome almost, but not quite unqualifiedly, the conclusions arrived at by the majority of Justices.

The qualifications that I have in mind are three. The first has to do with the legal grounds for the *Olmstead* decision. The majority of the justices treated the wrong done to Ms. Curtis and Ms. Wilson as a case of discrimination. In so doing they relied for the most part on wording used in Title II of the Americans with Disabilities Act. Against this position Justice Thomas, joined by Justices Rehnquist and Scalia, argued, in my view compellingly, that the majority had had to extend the concept of discrimination illegitimately in order to find grounds for their decision. "Until today," declared Justice Thomas, "this Court has never endorsed an interpretation of the term 'discrimination' that encompassed disparate treatment among members of the same protected class. Discrimination, as typically understood, requires a showing that a claimant received differential treatment *vis-à-vis* members of a different group on the basis of a statutorily described characteristic." And Justice Thomas went on to argue that this not only conforms to dictionary definitions of discrimination, but is in keeping with Title VII of the Civil Rights Act and subsequent Supreme Court decisions. Justice Thomas conceded to some degree that the use of the words 'discrimination' and 'segregation' by Congress in the Americans with Disabilities Act had already involved an extension in the meaning and use of those expressions. But he took the implications of that extension to be too unclear to provide a warrant for the reasoning of the majority. And he concluded: "At bottom, the type of claim approved of by the majority does not concern a prohibition against certain conduct (the traditional understanding of *discrimination*), but rather imposition of a standard of care." Justice Thomas found no existing legal justification for the imposition of a standard of care, and about this, too, I take him to have been right. But it is at this point that he and I sharply disagree. For I take it that what is badly needed by our society is precisely the formulation, the acceptance and the imposition of a standard of care. And if the law does not justify the imposition, where necessary, of such a standard, then this is a grave defect in the law. And the law should be amended.

What I am suggesting, but here will not argue, is that the extension of the notion of discrimination in an *ad hoc* way in the majority's reasoning marks a new stage in the attempt to justify substantive moral and/or legal conclusions by appeal to a concept of equal, nondiscriminatory treatment which by itself is far too thin to justify what it is employed to justify. It is not of course that equal treatment is unimportant, but rather that what is at stake in treating members of this or that particular class equally or unequally is always determined by some relevant standard that prescribes for some area of life how members of that class are to be treated. Once we have, for example, a standard of care governing how we act towards the mentally retarded and the mentally ill, then it is indeed important that that standard is applied in a nondiscriminatory way. But no prohibition of discriminatory conduct will itself yield a standard of care.

That the majority failed to recognize this becomes all the more important when we consider another aspect of their decision. Justice Ginsburg, writing for the majority, took care to assert that "The State's responsibility, once it provides community-based treatment to qualified persons with disabilities, is not boundless," and she endorsed the reasonable-modifications regulation that "allows States to resist modifications that entail 'a fundamental alteration' of the States' services and programs," repudiating the construal of this regulation by the Court of Appeals as permitting a cost-based defense "only in the most limited of circumstances." The majority's opinion therefore leaves intact the view that, at any given time, limits are set to what a state authority can be required to do for the mentally retarded or the mentally ill by the scale and the organization of the existing services provided by that state. But this is to get matters morally back to front.

We should not begin by asking what resources we now provide for the care of the mentally retarded and the mentally ill and then allow the present scale and organization of those resources to set limits to the care that we provide in particular cases. We need instead to begin from a justified standard of care, so that we can ask how, in the light of that standard, our overall resources ought to be allocated. Our budget-making should be informed by our standards and not vice versa. Of course it would be imprudent and therefore quite wrong for a society to risk the danger of bankruptcy by unwise and excessive allocations for this or any other purpose. But the way to avoid that risk without surrendering to the often mean-spirited allocations of the status quo is for the members of a society to think through together how their shared resources ought to be allocated in the light of their various responsibilities. And some of those responsibilities cannot be defined without a standard of care.

Consider now a third qualification to our welcome of the majority's decision. Justice Ginsburg remarked that: "the State generally may rely on the reasonable assessments of its own professionals in determining whether an individual 'meets the essential eligibility requirements' for habilitation in a continunity-based program." The judgments of the relevant professionals with respect to Ms. Curtis and Ms. Wilson were indeed both humane and informed by an adequate knowledge of mental retardation and mental illness. But it is important that judgments based on professional expertise cannot be a substitute for and must in fact, wherever appropriate, be governed by a standard of care that is the standard of the society and not just of the professionals. Professional judgment should not be treated as overriding in this or any other sphere and when and if professional judgment is at odds with the appropriate standard of care, it should be set aside. Professionally trained experts, whether mental health workers, or physicians, or lawyers or whatever, ought to be treated as the servants of plain persons and the instruments of the shared purposes of the community of plain persons. And the standard of care that should inform those purposes and govern the judgments and actions of experts is a standard that has to be formulated by and upheld by that entire community.

So far I have explained why appeal to a standard of care is important, but I have said little or nothing about what it is. And the best way in which we can approach that question is by asking: What is defective, what is lacking in someone who fails to care? Caring has two dimensions: we care for some particular individual or individuals who stands in some relationship to us and we care for them in respect of some more or less urgent need. So there are two corresponding ways in which we may fail. We may fail because in our care we do not address them as the individuals that they are or as those who are related to us in the way that they are; and we may fail because we do not address what they genuinely need. In our caring for others in their time of need and disability, we are generally and characteristically those who have been cared for by others in our own times of need and disability. We who, as small children or when ill or injured, have been cared for uncalculatingly by others, now find ourselves called upon to care for others, even if generally not the same others. We discover that we belong to a network of givers and receivers within which we are measured by not only our justice but also our generosity, and not only our justice and generosity, but also our courage in risk-taking and our temperateness in respect of our own wants and needs.

Some of those for whom we are called upon to care are those to whom we have particular responsibilities: our aging parents, our sick children, our injured coworkers or friends. But it is of crucial importance that most often we are able to care for those in serious need only by receiving help from individuals or groups who would otherwise be strangers. The network of giving and receiving relationships necessarily extends beyond family and immediate local community, so that we find ourselves called upon to give to strangers, just as they are called upon to give to us, and this in proportion to whatever need it is that has to be addressed. For we may fail in respect of care not only by not providing it for those others to whom justice and generosity require us to give, but by not addressing the real needs and the real extent of the needs of those others.

What is the reality of those needs? Often, in the first instance, we have to provide for those who are afflicted in some urgent way care or healing that they cannot provide for themselves. But in so doing, we make them dependent on us. And when others have become dependent on us, we do what is best for them by enabling them, as far as possible and as soon as possible, to become once again independent. So, too, where the needs of others have to be defined by us, as is often the case with the mentally retarded and the mentally ill, we do what is best for them by assisting them, as far as possible, to become able to define their own needs and to choose how those needs are to be met. That the limits of possibility here are sometimes very, very narrow does not diminish the importance of bearing these facts in mind. Indeed, to keep them constantly in mind is necessary if we are not to forget that to care for others is to will what is best for them, not what seems most convenient for us. And we will be the less likely to forget this if we recognize that it is only through willing that our common life should be informed by regard for this kind of care that we are able to will what is genuinely best for ourselves. Why?

This is for two different but mutually reinforcing reasons. The first has to do with the nature of the virtues. It is common to classify some virtues as other-regarding, for example, justice and generosity, and other virtues as self-regarding, for example, temperateness. But while this contrast is undeniably useful for some purposes, attention to it may obscure the extent to which and the ways in which the practice of the so-called other-regarding virtues is important for our own good, just as the practice of the so-called self-regarding virtues is important for the good of others. And this is because, as Marx rightly insisted, the self is not one thing and its social relationships another. It is true that no one is reducible to his or her social relationships. But they are in key part constitutive of what we are, and the good of each individual is not the good of that individual in isolation from others, but the good of that individual in her or his relationships to others. When such virtues as those of justice and generosity inform our relationships to others, certain possibilities are opened up for us that are otherwise denied to us. What are they?

Among them is the possibility of engaging in those types of conversation and those types of practice through which we and others may be mutually instructed about what our common good is. It is only insofar as we are disposed to give others a just hearing, to be generous in our interpretation of what they say, to be temperate in the expression of our own views, to take risks in exposing such views to refutation, and to be imaginatively sympathetic in our appreciation of opposing standpoints that we are able to participate constructively in such conversations and such practices. The corresponding vices of an adversarial attitude, the vices of insisting on an unjustly large share of the conversation, of advancing ungenerous interpretations of opposing contentions, of intemperateness in our rhetorical and argumentative modes, and generally of a lack of openness to alien standpoints preclude such conversations and such practice. So, in general, it is only insofar as we will that others should identify and achieve their own good, what is best for them, that we are likely to be able to identify and to achieve what is best for us. That this is so has special relevance to thinking about disability.

We are all of us too apt to think of the disabled as a special, especially unfortunate class of human beings, and we are most of us too apt to think of that class as one to which we do not belong, so that it is for us to decide what attitude to take up to *them. They* are available as objects of *our* benevolence, as recipients of *our* giving. But to think in this way is to ignore central features of all our lives. For, as I have already noted, we are all disabled for extended periods of those lives: as infants and small children, when old and when ill or injured, physically or mentally. And we are always vulnerable to further disability. Just because we are thus vulnerable, we are often actually and always potentially dependent on others for care. The networks of giving and receiving in which we participate can be sustained only by a shared recognition of each other's needs and a shared allegiance to a standard of care. And what a standard of care measures is not only the quality and quantity of the care afforded to those who are disabled relative to their needs, but also the success or failure in the exercise of the virtues by the members of the society to which these particular disabled belong.[1]

What an adequate standard of care for those who are disabled therefore prescribes is what the virtues require, and to spell out the details of such a standard would involve a virtue-by-virtue account. But at once it will be said that such an account could not supply what is needed, and that, indeed, any attempt to understand a standard of care in terms of the requirements of the virtues is badly misconceived. For the notion of a standard of care is the notion of a standard imposed by law. This is, after all, how Justice Thomas introduced the notion, and my own argument has from the outset presupposed that a standard of care would be a legally enforceable standard. The virtues, however, so the objection will run, are not a proper subject matter for legal prescription. It is not possible to make human beings virtuous by enacting and enforcing laws, and if what we want is to ensure conformity to a standard of care, our questions should be concerned with the content of the required laws and the means for inducing compliance, rather than with the virtues.

This sharp contrast between the way in which laws function and the part played by the virtues is central to much contemporary thinking about both. But it obscures an important difference between a legal system that is in good order and one that is not. When a legal system is in good order, the laws are generally obeyed, not just because they are the laws as enacted by sovereign authority and have the backing of the coercive resources of state power, but because they are recognized to be laws obedience to which is, in general, conducive to the achievement of the human good, in that they are laws that foster and encourage the exercise of the virtues. And they can be so recognized only within a society in which the virtues are cultivated and exercised by those who, in one way or another, set the standards for the rest of the population. Where the virtues do not inform the judgments and actions of a given society to a significant degree, the relationship between conformity to the laws and the achievement of the common good and of individual goods will not be adequately acknowledged. And where that relationship is not adequately acknowledged, laws will often be observed from fear of the consequences of doing otherwise, sometimes grudgingly and always in a way that has regard to the letter rather than to the spirit of the laws. Whether or not the legal system is in good order will therefore make an important difference to how laws that prescribe a standard of care for the disabled are obeyed and enforced. I do not want to suggest that legal prescriptions and legal enforcements are unnecessary or unimportant. But a standard of care that is acknowledged only as a legal standard will always be inadequate. Virtues without a corresponding set of laws are certainly insufficient, but so are laws without virtues.

We can bring this out further by returning to the question: What is defective in someone who fails to become what the virtues require in respect of upholding an adequate standard of care? They will, among other things, even if they are generally benevolent, tend to see the cause of the disabled as something competing with other causes for our interest and concern, a cause admirable enough, to be sure, but one that will and should be of interest to some and not to others. They will not take the possibility of their or their children pursuing a career as a provider of care for the disabled as having any great claim upon them or theirs and they will not understand the importance of raising the wages paid to and enhancing the status and prestige enjoyed by those who give their lives to such caregiving. Moreover they will not recognize what important indicators these are of the moral well-being or otherwise of their society. And one dire long-term consequence of this may be— in some countries, at least, this is already threatening—that even the most admirable and generous legal provision for the care of the disabled may be nullified by a lack of recruits to those services whose members provide everyday care for the mentally retarded and the mentally ill, for small children who cannot be adequately cared for in their own homes, especially those children living in poverty, and for the old and indigent.

It is characteristically in societies in which the nature and place of the virtues is no longer adequately acknowledged, except by moral eccentrics, that duty and obligation acquire a new centrality. When our natural inclinations are no longer transformed and redirected by our dispositions, we look for a motive for right action that will be independent of those inclinations, and we sometimes find it in a sense of duty, in a regard for what moral precepts require of us, independently of any conception of our directedness towards the human good. And in such societies, the giving of care to those in need will be apt to become a matter of duty and obligation. But while we all of us certainly do have duties to and obligations in respect of some of those who are presently disabled, it matters that duty and obligation cannot of themselves ever furnish systematically and in the long run the kind of motivation that has to inform our care. And this is because we need, in order to become the type of human being who is sufficiently motivated, to have had our inclinations transformed and redirected through the work of the imagination. No account of the place of the virtues in our lives is complete without some acknowledgment of the importance of the moral education of the imagination, and this has a peculiar relevance to our thinking about disability.

What do I mean by this? I am not speaking here of developing a capacity for imaginative empathy with those who are presently disabled, important in certain circumstances as this may be. I am speaking rather of the imagination as a source of self-knowledge, of the development of a capacity for viewing ourselves and our attitudes in a different light. An author who enlarges our imagination in a relevant way is Andre Dubus, the Massachusetts short-story writer and essayist who died earlier this year. In 1986 he lost one leg and the use of the other in an accident, thereafter spent his days in a wheelchair, and engaged constructively with his despair. Out of that despair came new thoughts expressed in the essays in *Meditations from a Movable Chair.*[2] About his legs he wrote: "I do not remember ever feeling grateful for mine," although running had been a central part of his life, and his new inability to run was one cause contributing to his despair. It is perhaps impossible to feel grateful for one's legs until and unless one has learned how to imagine oneself—oneself and not anyone else—without them and therefore come to know what cannot otherwise be known, what difference it makes to have legs—or arms or whatever. Without an imagination for bodily loss, one cannot feel genuinely grateful for bodily wholeness. And without the sense that such gratitude affords of what it is that one has, one cannot feel adequately vulnerable in respect of its future loss or share the vulnerability of others. And without adequate feelings for our own vulnerability, we are morally diminished.

So how we stand in relation to the plight of the presently disabled turns out to be a measure of ourselves and of our own moral education or miseducation. The verdict that we pass on the issues as stake in such cases as that of *Olmstead v. L. C.* is always also a verdict on us.

NOTES

[1]For an extended statement of this point of view, see my *Dependent Rational Animals.* Chicago: Open Court, 1999.

[2]New York: Vintage Books, 1999.

Definitions
Who Is Disabled? Who Is Protected?

The ADA is a unique civil rights statute because it requires proof of disability before its protections can be claimed. Unlike other civil rights statutes, it does not prohibit discrimination based on invidious attitudes about qualities such as race, religion, sex or age. Instead, it prohibits discrimination against a particular set of people, those with disabilities, as discrimination has come to be understood in the statute and in case law under it. The definition of disability thus serves a "gatekeeping" function in ADA jurisprudence: only the "disabled" can claim the statute's protection. Wendy Parmet and Patricia Illingworth argued in Part A that this feature of the ADA is tied to the understanding that in some sense it protects positive rights. The more the ADA protects, its critics assert, the more important it becomes to limit the class of the protected.

This part of the volume takes up questions about who is disabled, both as a philosophical issue and as a matter of understanding the ADA. A common theme in all of the writings is whether disability is a feature of the individual—a biological or medical personal limitation—or a feature of society—a social limitation imposed on people in virtue of their physical or mental differences.

Mark Kelman begins this section with an iconoclastic question: Should disability status matter at all to the interpretation of the ADA? His question is prompted by puzzling anomalies in the *Bragdon* Court's analysis of whether Ms. Abbott's disability entitled her to nondiscrimination in receiving dental care. Her entitlement turned on whether her HIV status substantially limited her major life activity of reproduction, hardly an activity of relevance to whether she should receive care for her teeth. The special focus on disability status, it might seem, just confuses the issue. Kelman explores whether this is so with respect to the ADA's protection from differential treatment and its requirement of reasonable accommodations. He asks whether it is disability status or stigmatizing treatment that matters in delineating discrimination.

Ron Amundson takes up the supposed ontological status of the group "people with disabilities." The direction of the law, at least from the Rehabilitation Act to the ADA, has been the gradual recognition that disability is a socially constructed category. That said, we must also acknowledge that conditions such as blindness are biological facts about people. The recognition that biological differences and socially created handicaps are separate phenomena, and that the goal of the ADA is eliminating the latter, is central to interpreting and defending the ADA, Amundson contends. Amundson locates much criticism of the ADA in unjustified adherence to functional determinism and argues that the Supreme Court mistakenly interprets disability as functional abnormality.

Mary Crossley's discussion focuses on the idea of "impairment" in the ADA definition of disability. "Impairment" is typically taken to mean "abnormal function," but Crossley, like Amundson, questions the coherence of this identification. She explores groups of cases about two kinds of individuals—pregnant women and obese people—who experience discrimination based on bodily difference but frequently do not succeed in their claims to the protection of the ADA. Categorizing these groups in medical or functional terms is deeply problematic, Crossley contends, for it ignores such people's lived experience of being discriminated against because their physical differences are held in cultural disregard.

The 1999 decisions of the United States Supreme Court narrowed the understanding of disability by requiring that the limitation imposed by any correctable impairment be assessed in its corrected state. In a forceful critique, Arlene Mayerson and Matthew Diller challenge these decisions. To dismiss disability because its limiting effects have been mitigated penalizes those who take steps to overcome their disabilities and risks making the situation worse for those whose conditions can be remedied only incompletely by medication or prosthesis but not completely cured.

Anita Silvers begins her contribution by noting the fundamental ambiguity of the ADA: Is it, like other civil rights statutes, designed to dismantle barriers that have prevented people with disabilities from full expression of their capacities? Or does it adopt an entirely new strategy in this area, offering a helping hand to those whose natural deficiencies unfairly provide them with a lesser start in life? Silvers does not locate discrimination in stigmatizing treatment only, but in the thoughtless and exclusionary design of certain human practices. Grounding the understanding of disability in this view, Silvers makes the case that the ADA does not depart from the traditional civil rights strategy of presuming the competence rather than the dysfunction of members of protected classes.

Finally, David Wasserman breaks new ground by urging reform of the ADA. The Supreme Court's 1999 decisions limit the protections of the act to those who have major impairments remaining after correction and those who are regarded in this way. According to Wasserman, the goal of the ADA is to protect people from stigmatizing misperceptions about their physical or mental differences, and such stigmatization need not rest on impairment. The idea that the ADA should be a statute for only the "truly handicapped," as it were, assumes the medicalized model of handicap, much criticized in this volume. Instead, the overall goal should be to eliminate discrimination based on differences that are stigmatized, such as obesity or ugliness.

The selections in this part thus are uniformly critical of current ADA jurisprudence. The Supreme Court's mandate that "disability" must be assessed with reference to the correction or correctability of underlying impairments is misguided because it invokes a biological model of disability. But "disability" is not of a natural kind, to be identified with physical or mental dysfunction. Instead, it is a constructed category, to be understood in terms of social and political responses to difference.

Thus far, authors in this section agree. But they do not so clearly agree on the consequences of this understanding of disability, especially in respect to its implications for policy. The question remains as to whether disability discrimination law should adhere closely to the strategies of the earlier civil rights statutes, or whether the situations of disabled people are so significantly different from those of other minorities as to call for an altered approach. Part C of this volume will explore how the understanding of disability both shapes and is shaped by employment policy, the distribution of health care, and the possibilities of the political and judicial processes.

Does Disability Status Matter?

INTRODUCTION

In *Bragdon v. Abbott*[1] the defendant, a dentist, refused to fill the cavity of the plaintiff, who was HIV-positive, outside a hospital setting. The defendant argued not only that he was justified in demanding that the patient be treated in a hospital because he would otherwise be at undue risk of contracting a life-threatening disease, but that he was entitled to refuse to treat her whether he was justified in his (highly atypical) medical judgments or not, because she was not a member of the class protected by the ADA. His argument, in essence, was that because she could be described as asymptomatic (in the sense that unlike a full-blown AIDS patient, she was not, by her own description, especially sick on a day-to-day basis) she could not conceivably be considered disabled; asymptomatic and "disabled" are, the defendant argued, virtually antonyms.

The arguments made by both the majority and the dissenters on this issue have a decidedly otherworldly quality to them. On the one hand, it is clear that the dentist, Dr. Bragdon, would have refused to treat a full-blown AIDS patient for precisely the same reason that he refused to treat Ms. Abbott. It is difficult to imagine why he should be entitled to refuse treatment to Ms. Abbott because he erroneously fears that treating her risks infection if he would not be permitted to refuse treatment to someone whose disease had progressed further based on the same irrational fear. On the other hand, the patient's argument—that she is entitled to the protection of the ADA because even asymptomatic HIV infection interferes with reproduction, a major life activity—seems grossly beside the point as well. Just as it appears peculiar to argue that the dentist could be compelled to fill the cavity of someone with symptomatic AIDS but not someone whose symptoms were less visible or manifest, it appears equally troubling to believe that a hypothetical postmenopausal Ms. Abbott, whose HIV infection unquestionably has no bearing on reproduction, would be any less entitled to protection against discrimination than the actual plaintiff is afforded.

Perhaps the Court's problem is not really one of *conceptual* confusion. Instead, the case is arguably driven by some combination of legal formalism and institutional competence concerns. The argument from formalism is straightforward. There are a host of reasons for courts to be bound by clear language directives (whether legislative language or the language of judicial precedents). Legal regulatory regimes often state substantive policies in terms of rules (or proxies)—readily discovered, verbally unambiguous features of factual situations—rather than standards—restatements of the purposes that we hope to achieve by regulating an area of social life. (Thus we tell the voting registrar to allow those who are 18 or older to vote, not to try to ascertain which voting applicants are "politically mature," in order to, for instance, reduce official discretion or administrative and litigation costs. Chronological age is merely an easily identified, linguistically unambiguous proxy for political maturity, but one can readily defend the use of such an easily administered proxy.) The argument for institutional competence is equally familiar: legislatures are the (sole) democratically legitimated source of policy judgments, and courts should simply do their best to implement the legislative scheme.

The ADA formally protects those with (actual or perceived) disabilities and defines a disability as a "physical or mental impairment that substantially limits one or more of the major life activities of [such] individual [who complains that she is the victim of discrimination]." Given what the Court (mysteriously) saw as this plain, transparent statutory language, it might appear that the Court has no choice but to ascertain, first whether the plaintiff has a physical impairment[2] and, second, that the impairment substantially interferes with a major life activity.[3] A number of the amici chose to emphasize the degree to which asymptomatic HIV infection interfered with innumerable daily activities. (Of course, this argument is politically ambiguous for disability rights advocates and AIDS activists who may well want to emphasize the degree to which people who are HIV-positive have no real problems working.) But the patient's lawyers chose instead to rely on the fact that the infection interfered with an "activity" (reproduction) that *is* "major" in the sense that it is frequently of great emotional and social significance in an individual's life plan. They did so despite the fact that reproduction can readily be differentiated from the specifically statutorily enumerated activities. It is neither a single, discrete "activity" (like walking or hearing), an activity that is repeated on a daily basis such that the inability to perform it would be manifest pretty much continuously, nor an activity thought to have largely instrumental value in meeting a range of economic production or consumption goals.

It is certainly possible, though—and analytically helpful—to imagine what it would be like to clear away all the formal and institutional underbrush here and ask whether Ms. Abbott's claim *should* turn, in any way, on ascertaining whether those with asymptomatic HIV infections are disabled. Do those with disabilities have some trait as individuals that differentiates them from those who are not disabled, that makes them candidates for legal protection not afforded those lacking the trait? Alternatively, or additionally, are they are members of some social group that is rightly afforded protection that others lack?

To put the point more broadly: What would it be like to have "disability law" that made no reference at all to whether the plaintiff is disabled? Why do, or should, we care about whether a plaintiff possesses some preliminary status trait before we decide that she is afforded protections parallel to those offered by the ADA? To answer that question, of course, it seems we must first do what legal realists conventionally taught us to do in thinking about legal "rights": view "rights" as simple instantiations of the remedies a "rights-bearer" is entitled to.[4]

REMEDIES AND DISABILITY STATUS

There are essentially two remedies the ADA contemplates granting those whose "rights" under the statute are violated: first, protection against "simple discrimination" (differential treatment despite equality along "relevant" dimensions), and second, "reasonable accommodation" (of relevant difference). Obviously, it is possible to imagine that people are unequal in ways some would deem relevant and others would not; thus the right to be free from simple discrimination requires some consensus on what traits potential defendants can deem relevant. The right to demand reasonable accommodation likewise is undefined till we've decided which distinctions should be accommodated.

These remedies have relatively precise conventional meanings, though—defined in relationship to conventional understandings of the workings of a market economy. A person suffers from simple discrimination insofar as an employer (in the employment discrimination context traditionally regulated by Title VII of the 1964 Civil Rights Act) or a public accommodation owner (in the public accommodation context traditionally regulated by Title II of the same act) fails to treat him "impersonally." Insofar as the employer or owner cares about the person's status or traits that are irrelevant to such person's economic function, he or she is breaching the duty to avoid simple discrimination. A public accommodation owner discriminates in this way if he or she does not treat a potential customer as a source of net proceeds (money he or she will receive to provide a service net of the costs of service provision); an employer discriminates insofar as he or she treats the employee or job applicant as anything but embodied net marginal product (the value of the increase in goods or services the firm will produce if the employee is added to the firm, net of the added costs that the firm will incur if she or he is employed by the firm.)

A customer or employee is entitled by the ADA to reasonable accommodation in the sense that the public accommodation owner or employer must treat the customer or worker in terms of his or her gross, not net, value added to the firm. This obligation to ignore the input costs associated with serving the customer or employing the worker or applicant holds only so long as the cost of these atypical inputs is not unduly high (reasonable in that sense) and the added inputs would not benefit other customers or potential employees nearly as much as they would benefit the plaintiff.

Thus, in the public accommodations context, the simple antidiscrimination principle would preclude the dentist from refusing to treat a hearing-impaired patient, even though his inability to communicate with the patient affected neither the price the patient would pay nor the cost of serving him. The accommodation principle would require that the dentist take steps to be able to communicate with the hearing-impaired patient if necessary to provide her with the same quality care he gives other patients, without charging the patient the incremental costs of treating her.[5] This is true even though a simple, nondiscriminating, impersonal, capitalist calculator would refuse to treat a patient who is atypically costly to serve unless permitted to charge more for the services.[6]

In the employment context, the conventional antidiscrimination norm forbids an employer from refusing to hire a blind lawyer who can do the same legal work as a sighted one. The accommodation principle demands that the employer not reduce the blind lawyer's pay if he requires a "reasonably" costly reader to generate the same work that sighted lawyers do without an aide.[7] What is critical to note is that these two distinct antidiscrimination principles need not, at first blush, make any reference to group membership status. An individual could be deemed the victim of simple discrimination if he were not treated exclusively as the source of net receipts (in the public accommodation context) or net marginal product (in the labor market context). Any individual could be said to be entitled to accommodations (costly inputs) that permit him or her to generate as much output as similarly rewarded workers (in the labor market context) or to receive the same quality services for the same price as others (in the public accommodation context), so long as these inputs are not unduly expensive and would not be valued by other workers and customers as much as she valued them.

This is especially obvious in relationship to simple discrimination. Individuals *qua* individuals might be entitled to "market-rational" treatment. In this sense, the antidiscrimination norm is simply coextensive with a norm requiring such treatment. We know that an African-American has been the victim of discrimination before we need consider his or her race; we know it because he or she, as an individual, did not get something he or she deserved.

In this view, social groups are relevant for only limited purposes, each of which could best be described as *administrative*. First, because we know that outcomes for individuals have a good deal of randomness to them, we believe we are able to discern irrational treatment by those accused of treating individuals irrationally only if we look at groups *for proof purposes*. We care about the treatment of black job applicants or workers as a group in this view largely because we will not be able to ascertain in most cases whether an individual black applicant was treated unfairly. This observation was most dramatically apparent in looking at earnings equations and trying to ascertain whether we are observing trait-based discrimination. We know that no individual's pay can be predicted very exactly on the basis of standard productivity traits (schooling, experience etc.). But we expect "randomness" to average out when there are large numbers of observations. If it does not, it is a result of unwarranted discrimination, not error or luck. Groups are created in this view as statistician's artifacts to measure the existence of discrimination against individuals with a commonality that makes us believe they will be victims of discrimination atypically often. We may suspect that those with decision-making power might exhibit animus or aversion towards those possessing the trait, or suspect that they are likely to misconceive the true virtues of those possessing the trait, as a result of false stereotyping. But the group need not have any self-conscious identity—whether as a social group into which one feels "thrown" or as a voluntarily created political association.[8] There are clearly such aggregates where we do not surmise it is even worth investigating the possibility that the group is subjected to simple discrimination: the group of those born on Wednesday constitute such an aggregation.[9]

Second, if we decide that individuals have affirmative entitlements to impersonal rational treatment, we may still believe that we will use state power to protect only members of historically subordinated social groups. We may believe that not because the entitlement is breached any less when someone who lacks that status suffers irrational treatment but because we believe that members of socially advantaged groups are unlikely to face such treatment *persistently* across a variety of settings. A straight, white, able-bodied male may, in this view, be the victim of irrational treatment by a particular employer or public accommodations owner (whom he reminds of a loathed stepfather, for instance). We expect, though, that such idiosyncratic irrationality will have few consequences, given the presence of other employers and sellers. We may reasonably believe that prejudice against African-Americans (or those with disabilities, or gays and lesbians) is widespread among those with social power. Stereotypes are both socially created and social-norm-enforced. On the other hand, the hypothetical white male applicant or customer is unlikely to run into many people whom he reminds of a hated stepfather. Both the African-American and the white are victims of discrimination, so defined, but only the one is likely to be corrected by market competition rather than state action.[10]

The idea that we focus on group membership for wholly administrative reasons appears to me incomplete even when we are talking only about simple discrimination. Part of what is wrongful about this sort of conventional discrimination is plainly that it precludes an individual from receiving some good or service she both desires and deserves; in that sense, the antidiscrimination norm vindicates legitimate material expectations that have been frustrated. And part of what the norm vindicates is a desire to be treated fairly. In this sense, what we seek to protect is not so much the interest in getting the *thing* one wants but the interest in being treated appropriately.

It seems, though, that the norm is significantly designed to protect as well against the stigma imposed on subordinated group members, and is therefore not purely individualistic as a matter of theory as well as administrative practice. In this regard, we care less that a person is denied a job he's entitled to because he reminds the employer of a hated step-father, not only because the applicant is likely to find a job elsewhere. The decision not to hire in such a case does not confirm traditional status-based hierarchies, express the social power of one group over another, or demean the victim. It is far more plainly the case from the "victim's" vantage point that he or she is dealing with a stupid jerk with some social power. It is far less plausible that he or she would believe he or she is dealing with someone whose judgment has the weight of tradition, someone who makes the sort of covert social claims for the validity of negative views that keep groups "in their place."

It is similarly possible, though considerably less conventional, to state demands for accommodation without regard to group membership. Any employee might be entitled to be treated precisely as well as those with the same gross output potential are treated, without regard to the fact that the input costs needed to generate that output differ. This formulation of the "right to accommodation" is most straightforward when the worker demands that the employer expend funds out of pocket to support his work (supplying him with more expensive capital equipment or costly aids).[11] The gross output/net output distinction is more awkwardly applied to situations in which the accommodation the employee requests is one which allows him or her to generate less output over the course of her employment, though he or she still generates as much output per unit of time. (If, for instance, an employee suffering from depression or chronic fatigue syndrome requires time off, so that his or her gross output is lower over the course of a year than his or her coworkers' but is the same per hour, this is a demand for an accommodation in this sense.)[12]

In either case, though, it is not obvious why it matters whether the employee is a member of a social group, or more particularly whether we think of her as disabled. So long as employees sought only costly physical help (aides and equipment), it was seemingly inevitably the case that only those who could be described as disabled would seek accommodation. Neither an expensive Braille printer nor a reader is of any use to the sighted; special keyboards are of no use to those without repetitive stress disorders (or at least the risk of developing them). But the question of whether or not one is disabled need not be answered prior to the question of whether one would in fact be helped by the desired accommodation. The inability to produce as much without the atypical inputs, despite the ability to do so with the aid, defined the person as disabled. We needed no separate inquiry into group status.[13]

If, though, those seeking accommodations ask not just for simple physical aids but, for instance, for less demanding schedules, there are many individuals who might claim that they (a) are as productive (per hour) as fellow employees, and (b) "need" time away from work more than their fellow workers. Those with atypical caretaking responsibilities (e.g., parents with small kids, adults with sick relatives) do not really purport to be members of a social group (and are certainly not "disabled"). Nonetheless, they might also claim that they should be treated in terms of their gross productivity, without penalizing them for generating higher input costs by demanding flextime or time off.

Naturally, it is not easy to distinguish "needs" from "wants." The claim that a worker needs accommodation is thus not readily adjudicated. For a purely hedonic utilitarian, a need appears to be nothing more than an especially intense want. For such utilitarians, a plaintiff seeking time off to play golf has a weaker claim than one who seeks time off to care for a sick child only insofar as they believe he values golf less than the competing claimant values caring for his child. Antidiscrimination law is clearly animated in part, though, by the idea that claims for social inclusion have priority over mere hedonic desires: what historically subordinated people justly seek redress for is their exclusion from participation in valued social spheres. Thus we should not evaluate the demand for a less onerous schedule as a simple claim to a state-mandated in-kind subsidy, to be allocated to whatever party values it most. Instead, the party must claim that he or she "needs" the accommodation, in the sense that but for the accommodation, he or she simply will not (and should not be expected to) participate in ordinary social life.

At this point, though, the question of group membership again becomes salient. Does antidiscrimination law simply remind us how significant social inclusion is for all individuals, or does it tell us that social inclusion is especially significant only to those who are members of groups that have been relegated to outsider status? Do we have a universalized principle that we give high priority to each individual's capacity to enter the range of social spheres—in which case it does not matter whether we think of those with caretaking duties as a social group or not? Or do we have a special interest in integrating members of groups—like those with disabilities—who share a history of having been excluded from relevant spheres?

We might differentiate the claims made by those with disabilities from the claims made by others seeking less rigid schedules. Those with disabilities alone might claim that they would simply not produce as much per hour if forced to work the more typical schedule, while those with caretaking responsibilities must claim, instead, that their losses outside the workplace are atypically high if they work a typical schedule. It is not lucid to me, though, that those without disabilities could not also claim that their productivity at work would be compromised if forced to work full-time.[14] More important, it is not clear that their moral claim is especially compromised if they seek accommodation to avoid especially large losses outside the workplace rather than productivity losses at work. Moreover, the accommodation one would expect most asymptomatic HIV-positive plaintiffs to seek in the employment setting if they required accommodation at all—time off to follow medication regimens and to monitor health status—is designed essentially to preclude atypical out-of-work losses.

It is also possible to see the demand for accommodation as the demand for resource redistribution. In essence, an entity subject to a demand for accommodation is asked to pay an implicit "regulatory tax" which is then "implicitly spent" on a program that provides certain benefits, in-kind rather than in-cash, to those benefitted by the accommodation.[15] Redistributive programs may legitimately be focused on needy individuals, without regard to group identity, for a host of familiar reasons (e.g., conventional utilitarians believe that the marginal utility of income declines so that such redistribution increases aggregate utility). They may also be directed at improving the status of certain groups. (Even methodological individualists, who believe that only the welfare and rights of individuals count, may be group-sensitive in formulating a distribution policy.) If a particular redistributive program is justified by virtue of its favorable impact on a group, then parties obviously ought not to benefit from the program unless their participation will in fact aid the group. In this regard, if the ADA is intended to redistribute income in-kind to those with disabilities in some substantial part to aid the group of those with disabilities, then group identity and membership clearly count.

HOW AND WHY DOES DISABILITY STATUS COUNT?

Assume first that the ADA is designed only to eliminate what I have labeled simple discrimination. Group status matters in such a case, I argued, largely for administrative reasons if we ignore, for the moment, the possibility that we use state power to counter such discrimination only when it imposes stigmatic injury on its victims.

If the disputed practice is one whose legitimacy cannot be ascertained in individual cases, but only by examining a pattern of cases, we need to investigate those statistical aggregates where we suspect either animus or stereotyping are widespread. In *Bragdon v. Abbott* itself, though, the dentist's conduct either is or is not "market-rational" in relationship to the particular plaintiff. The refusal to treat any party because of false beliefs about the risks of treating her could readily be interrogated (and banned) without any regard to the group status of the plaintiff.

There will be innumerable cases, though, in which the practices of an employer or public accommodation owner cannot be evaluated unless we see how he has treated a group of similarly situated plaintiffs. Most notably, refusals to hire individuals or pay and promotion decisions are often hard to evaluate looked at one at a time. We would certainly be right to suspect that the core groups Congress has protected through civil rights legislation (women, members of ethnic minorities, those with conventionally defined disabilities) as well as some it clearly has not (gays and lesbians) and others whose legal status is uncertain (people conventionally judged unattractive or overweight) are subject to aversive prejudice and stereotyping. It would thus surely be worth investigating whether members of such groups are treated irrationally. But we need no strong independent theory of groups to do the work here. If a plaintiff's lawyer can convince a fact finder that his clients are treated irrationally by demonstrating that there is a statistical aggregate of people receiving poor treatment that is more plausibly explained by their identity than by random chance, his clients should prevail. "Groups" are relevant in the very thin sense that membership in a socially cognizable "victim group" connotes that atypically bad outcomes are more plausibly attributed to social process than lottery luck.

If instead we look to the state to correct simple discrimination only when we believe the market fails to do so spontaneously, group membership may be more important. Markets presumably fail to eliminate irrational treatment where irrationalities are widespread rather than idiosyncratic. Irrationalities are widespread in relationship to traits possessed by groups, not isolated individuals. Even in the *Bragdon* context, one might believe that the market protects victims of idiosyncratic beliefs that particular patients are dangerous to treat, but does not protect those with socially stigmatized diseases. Thus, given this view, what the Court should ask is whether those who are HIV-positive, like others who are unambiguously deemed disabled, are likely to confront repeatedly the same sort of ignorant stereotypes or aversive prejudice from market actors other than the particular defendant. They are disabled, in the relevant sense, if likely to suffer such repeated prejudice.[16]

We are arguably especially prone to protect people from market-irrational treatment when and only when their failure to receive it does more than defeat legitimate expectations to receive particular economic benefits or legitimate expectations to receive fair treatment. Arguably, we invoke antidiscrimination law only for those who legitimately experience such treatment as stigmatizing. In this regard, group membership is vital. Stigmatic injuries are almost invariably injuries imposed on individuals by virtue of their group-based identity, insults to collectives with which the plaintiff associates him- or herself. There is fairly sharp political disagreement over whether parties experience significant stigmatic injury unless their group status is subordinate, but there is considerably less controversy over the significance of group identity.[17] Again, if this account is correct, a court assessing whether HIV-positive persons are "disabled" should ask itself whether they share with others conventionally dubbed disabled a vulnerability to stigmatic injury when excluded or mistreated. In this view we protect only those with a justified sense that they have sustained a wound to the identity they derive through mutual recognition of significant social commonalities. (I should note that I am quite wary of limiting antidiscrimination protection to those who can claim stigmatic injury, believing that such a restriction unduly encourages people to identify themselves in increasingly rigid group categories.)

If we protect persons who make legitimate claims to accommodation, we should decide whether claims made by members of acknowledged groups to atypical inputs are more compelling than other similar claims. "Disability law" could readily dispense with the disability category and focus explicitly on the reasonableness of the accommodation demand. To do so, we would need to address genuinely difficult questions that have been thus far evaded. Should a worker be penalized (at all) for requiring more expensive capital inputs to produce a certain amount just as she would be penalized for producing less? Should the reasonableness of an accommodation turn on the resources available to the entity that deals with the party seeking an accommodation, or should we judge more directly whether the cost of the accommodation is justified by the benefits? Does a worker "need" an accommodation solely because such an accommodation permits her to increase her output at work, or should she be granted one only if the failure to do so would (realistically) preclude her from working?

If, though, we need to decide, as in *Bragdon,* whether HIV-positive status "is" a disability, given that only those with disabilities are entitled to accommodation, we must simply decide whether the accommodations HIV-positive persons will seek closely resemble those demanded by those more unambiguously disabled. It seems to me difficult to imagine why any legislator would find demands for work-schedule reductions (or breaks to take medication) any less compelling for an HIV-positive plaintiff than one with diabetes or a cancer patient who needs to leave work to get chemotherapy. If we have decided that the demands to care for one's own body must be accommodated, even if we are less certain that demands to care for others (or to pursue other extra-work goals) need be, then HIV-positive plaintiffs are making the sorts of demands we have decided should be accommodated.

Finally, to the degree that we see accommodation orders as implicit taxes redistributed in kind to those benefited by the orders, we need to decide how compelling claims of groups to redistributive largesse really are, compared to more individualistic claims of need. An analogy might well help. We might choose to allocate medical research funds so as to maximize the number of life-years saved,[18] without regard to the group identity of those who would be saved. If an incremental dollar spent on research on *X* would forestall more premature death than a dollar spent on *Y,* we must spend the dollar on *X.* Such a metric is individualistic and need-based. There is a feature individuals have in common without regard to group identity (aversion to death), and we allocate resources so as to minimize this (universally) negative experience.

We might, though, believe that spending to avert deaths with meaning to cognizable social groups has a weight that averting other (group-random) deaths does not. If, in this view, spending to cure or prevent AIDS does not *simply* save lives but serves also to undo some degree of conventionally expressed disapproval of gays, it may take (at least some) priority. If research on breast, rather than prostate, cancer symbolizes a commitment to the social importance of (historically marginalized) women, it might be justified even if less effective in saving lives.[19]

It may well be the case that individuals' welfare is as significantly affected by the sense that they belong to a group held in reasonable social esteem as it is by access to more conventional material goods. To the degree this is so, group-sensitive distributive policies are not just acceptable but appropriate in situations in which the distribution of goods signifies esteem. Such a distributive metric may be especially apt when we are distributing not cash or cash equivalents (where individual need may be far more significant) but (in kind) opportunities to participate in publicly validated spheres. To the extent that we believe that we can use a regulatory tax to force social inclusion (at work, in public accommodations) that would not occur spontaneously in the market, it seems there are some good reasons to undo social exclusion associated with group membership (e.g., gender, disability status), rather than individual traits (poverty that precludes one from paying for the accommodation, lack of skills that preclude one from getting a desired job).[20]

If "disability law" is designed to elevate the material claims to costly social inclusion of those who reasonably identify with a social group that reasonably feels demeaned by its widespread exclusion, then accommodation requests by those with disabilities do have a certain priority. Whether a particular person or persons with a particular trait (such as HIV-positive status), is "disabled" in this sense turns on whether inclusion diminishes the sense that others "in the group" have that their group is unjustly marginalized and mistreated. There appears to be nothing physical or medical that helps us to recognize who is an insider and who an outsider in this sense. Whether (many? all?) people using wheelchairs (reasonably) "identify" with the exclusion that will befall those suffering from depression or dyslexia or asymptomatic HIV-positive status unless they are accommodated is an historically contingent, empirical question. Whether rights ought to turn on whether groups develop this sort of interdependency (to put a positive spin on it) or be linked sensitively to wounds (to give it a more negative spin) is surely open to question, too.

ACKNOWLEDGMENTS

Research was supported by the Stanford Legal Research Fund, made possible by a bequest from Ira S. Lillick and by gifts from other friends of Stanford Law School.

NOTES

[1] *Bragdon v. Abbott,* 524 U.S. 624 (1998).

[2] Both sides in the *Bragdon* case conceded that those who were HIV-positive had such an impairment because their immune response system was compromised.

[3] As a formal matter, questions arose as well in the case as to the relevance of extratextual indices of legislative intention. There is little doubt, looking at typical extratextual sources (committee reports, prior uncontested interpretations of parallel statutes by judicial bodies and administrative agencies) that Congress intended to protect all those who were HIV-positive. The dissent was forced to rely, therefore, on the perfectly credible view that courts should never look outside the four corners of the statute in interpreting the statute, at least so long as the statute's meaning is otherwise discernible.

[4] Thus, in this realist tradition, to say that one "owns" one's genetic material is meaningless. One must specify what "ownership" means in terms of discrete legal powers. Can one (merely) refuse to give it away, or is one permitted to contract to sell it, or can one recover damages if it is used by others (but not sell it)? Does it matter whether the user profits from it or not?

[5] For instance, if the dentist had to hire someone to sign-translate his questions and to translate the patient's replies into oral language, he would not be permitted to charge the patient the interpreter's fees.

[6] The court will order the accommodation only if it is reasonable. It must be reasonable first in the sense that it is not unduly costly. Under current law, we evaluate whether the accommodation is too costly in part by reference to the capacity of the particular service provider or employer to afford the accommodation, rather than inquiring whether, in some more general sense, we believe the benefits of the accommodation outweigh the social resource costs of providing it. I believe that procedure is indefensible, but it is surely current practice. We would also ask whether it is a "reasonable accommodation"

or an "unreasonable" demand for improvement in service. If the person with a disability is seeking some change in the service structure (or some "aid" at work) which makes the product he is receiving (at ordinary market prices) more desirable for typical customers (or amplifies any worker's product), the change he is seeking is not an "accommodation" to which the ADA entitles him.

[7]In *Bragdon* itself, the dentist claims that he would not serve the client unless the patient paid the bulk of the cost of what the dentist saw as a necessary accommodation, performing the procedure in the hospital. Now the plaintiff claims that no accommodation is needed, and that the refusal to treat her in his office is itself simple discrimination (and would be stigmatizing even if she were not asked to pay for the hospital treatment). The dentist claims, though, that the refusal to treat her at ordinary prices in an ordinary setting stems from the ways in which she is distinct in relevant ways from his other patients: he says that she is riskier to treat. In a sense, the plaintiff is complaining that the dentist has engaged in simple discrimination (falsely claiming that she cannot be treated in the conventional office setting). If this claim were rejected, though, I imagine that the patient would then complain that if she indeed requires accommodation (i.e. she is riskier to treat), she cannot be charged for the cost of providing these accommodations, both because they are not unduly costly and because they do not represent improvements in service that nondisabled customers would seek, but distinctions in service necessitated by her disability.

[8]Thus we can ascertain that there is "discrimination" against both males and females who are physically unattractive only by looking at whether a large number of people deemed unattractive receive rewards commensurate with predicted productivity, though the "unattractive" may not form a conventional social group, a subculture, or a voluntarily created political association.

[9]If, though, the question is whether it is worth investigating whether HIV-positive persons might be subjected to irrational treatment, the answer is plainly that it is. I return to this issue when I discuss in more detail why disability status may matter.

[10]Once more, it would seem that prejudice against those who are HIV-positive is widespread enough, rather than idiosyncratic, that one would think that from this viewpoint, relying on market-based rather than state-based correction for prejudice would be ill advised. Again, we return to this issue.

[11]Thus, for example, a hearing-impaired worker might seek communication devices that permit her to read a supervisor's commands; a blind worker might require a reader or an expensive printer that generated Braille copies of texts that she received.

[12]If the employee can satisfy the decision-maker who is responsible for determining whether she is entitled to prevail in an antidiscrimination suit that she produces as much over the course of her employment as other workers though she works fewer hours, then she is really not asking for an accommodation. Instead, she is claiming that the employer's insistence on "normal" schedules is a form of simple discrimination. (The employer might argue that while she may as an individual produce as much working irregular hours as others produce working more conventionally, permitting atypical schedules imposes costs on others in the firm—either morale costs or administrative costs. If that is the case, then this is an accommodation claim.) Note, more generally, that disability rights advocates quite typically argue, quite persuasively in my view, that the failure to grant accommodations is a form of simple discrimination because the accommodations are not in fact costly, though bigoted or ignorant employers assume that accommodating difference will be. I discuss the demand for accommodation as a separate form of antidiscrimination claim on the supposition that there are situations in which the public accommodations owner or employer is correct that it is more costly to serve some customers or to give them the capital equipment support that permits them to generate the same output their fellow employees do.

[13]There is one serious qualification in this regard, worthy of an entire separate essay. Should an employee who is physically unable to do some particular job without an accommodation, but would be capable of doing a range of other jobs without accommodations, be entitled to one? In formalistic legal terms, the question is whether the plaintiff should be deemed unable to perform a significant life activity when she is able to work if she is unable to perform some subset of activities (e.g. lifting, sitting still as long as one must to perform a particular job) useful for the job the plaintiff most prefers. It strikes me as quite plausible, but by no means obvious, that the accommodation requirement of the ADA was and should be designed to subsidize people who would not otherwise work, not to provide an income-maximizing subsidy. One could argue that the statute was especially directed at overcoming the social isolation and exclusion that accompany joblessness. Moreover, one could argue that an accommodation is unreasonable (even if not especially expensive) insofar as it is far costlier for the particular employer than it would be if the employee chose to work in some other setting. In this sense, we may believe that

a plaintiff who needs accommodation in only a small subset of settings ought to work somewhere where he does not need them. Alternatively, he should pay for them himself if he chooses to receive them though he does not need them in all settings. On the other hand, one can surely hypothesize cases in which a plaintiff would claim that he would be radically underemployed given his skill level, though he could find some work, unless accommodated in his "ideal" setting. The statute was arguably designed to prevent those with strong underlying skills from being unable to exercise them.

[14]Some might claim that they would be distracted; some might claim that they would be exhausted trying to do too many things in a day.

[15]I focus in this essay on the "beneficiary" side. There are substantial questions as well about whether it is appropriate to levy such a regulatory tax on employers or public accommodations owners rather than to spread them more broadly.

[16]*Bragdon* is an especially complex case for reasons I do not have space to detail. HIV-positive persons are victims of both homophobia and conventional phobic prejudice against those with diseases, especially diseases that are poorly understood by significant parts of the population. HIV-positive plaintiffs may both face persistent mistreatment because of aversion to gays and because of aversion to the ill. (Similarly, to anticipate the next argument in the text, they may suffer more from such mistreatment because it demeans them in both group statuses.) While gays and lesbians are clearly subject to all the sorts of harms the antidiscrimination norm is designed to protect against, they are not a congressionally protected class. (Presumably, many legislators believe that persistent mistreatment of them is justified or that stigma is warranted.)

[17]In the hate-speech context, there is widespread agreement that nasty speech is more stigmatizing and damaging when directed at one because of one's group status. It is more controversial whether there is a significant distinction between the stigmatic injury felt by members of historically subordinated groups than dominant groups: Are the stigmatic injuries distinct when African-Americans are called "dumb niggers" rather than when white males are derided as "dumb honkies," assuming both are more stigmatizing than simply being called "dumb"?

[18]I ignore in this piece a host of complex empirical and ethical issues. Would we really know, *ex ante,* the expected effect of spending incremental funds researching a particular disease? If we assume that the research results in a new treatment that alters mortality and morbidity at different ages, do we have any noncontroversial scale to measure the improvements created in terms of improvements in the Quality Adjusted Life Years that people will experience?

[19]There are a number of reasons that one might believe that we should care about the group identity of those to whom we distribute resources (particularly in-kind resources like opportunities). For instance, certain group members may have strongly interdependent welfare functions; the success of some group members may serve to encourage others in the group to higher levels of achievement.

[20]In part, this no doubt reflects the problematic acceptance of the notion that those lacking market skills feel *justifiably* excluded. They lack market productive skills, the most relevant trait that merits higher status in the culture. Thus, even if their exclusion is just as esteem-defeating as the exclusion of group members who require accommodation, the lack of esteem seems irremediable. The view that social groups seeking accommodation deserve esteem equal to that of historically dominant groups is based as well on the supposition that the need for accommodation is caused in significant part by the fact that existing institutions accommodate the dominant. In this view, the expenses of court-ordered accommodation arise simply from the failure to establish work settings favorable to the subordinated group. Thus, flextime schedules are costly when they are atypical; men designed "typical" work-time schedules with their work styles in mind. Persons with physical disabilities cannot use existing capital equipment designed for the able-bodied; the equipment they need is not intrinsically costlier. I am skeptical that this view of the accommodation problem is correct. Whether it is or not fundamentally an empirical issue, though, it is not one that has been subjected to much empirical study.

Biological Normality and the ADA

RON AMUNDSON

DISABILITY, RACE AND REIFICATION

Debates about laws that protect certain groups of people from discrimination cover a wide range of factors. These include the social situation of members of the groups under consideration, the likely consequences of the proposed laws and ethical considerations of rights and justice. One factor that is less frequently acknowledged in legal discussion is the ontological question of the reality (or the kind of reality) of the group itself. What are the differences between members and nonmembers of the group? By this I mean not the practical legal question of how we identify or legally designate group members, but the extralegal question of what constitutes the group and membership in it. What are the relevant facts about the members of the group at issue, and how do they differ from nonmembers?

In many cases these facts are taken to be biological facts or facts of similarly objective scientific status. Even though biological fact cannot entail moral value, debates about the true nature of male-female differences occur at the same time as debates about women's rights, and debates about the true nature of racial differences occur at the same time as civil rights movements for racial groups. Many nineteenth-century advocates of slavery considered Africans and Europeans to be not just separate races, but separate species. This purported fact was relevant to the moral and political issue of slavery. Psychological and biological doctrines about sex differences have been closely associated with differences in legal status between men and women. Modern biological beliefs about racial and sexual differences are as different from those of two hundred years ago as modern civil rights laws are from the racist and sexist institutions of those days.

The Americans with Disabilities Act contains no revolutionary pronouncements about the biological reality of its protected class. But the same is true of laws that protect women and racial minorities. Laws are created against biological background beliefs but need not spell them out. The ADA does reconceptualize disability in comparison to earlier law. Legislation prior to the Rehabilitation Act of 1973 treated the social problem of disability as merely the aggregate of the problematic biomedical conditions of individuals. Disability was to be remedied by treatments applied to each person, and charitable concern for the disadvantage of each individual was an appropriate moral basis for the policy. In contrast, the ADA recognizes that disadvantages involved in disability are created in part by the social and built environment, and the remedies are justified not by charity but by the civil rights claim to equal access to the goods of the society. The change is from an individualistic medical model of disability to what is sometimes called the social model of disability.

This kind of reconceptualization does not necessarily require new discoveries about the biological conditions of individuals. It may simply have come from more careful attention to the social causes of disadvantage. But the new view of disability expressed in the ADA raises a new question. If we assume that social factors are responsible for much of the disadvantage that attaches to disability, we might still wonder about the nature of disability apart from those social factors. After the social causes of disadvantage are accounted for, what is left? Are members of the protected group objectively abnormal and deserving of civil rights protection because of their abnormality? Or is the judgment of abnormality itself merely a part of the social context that creates the disadvantage?

Concepts of race have undergone vast modification since the beginning of the nineteenth century. Early white advocates of protection (if not civil rights) for nonwhite races believed that these races needed protection because of their innate disadvantages of intellect and temperament. Later, coincident with gains in civil rights, nonwhite races were increasingly seen to be equal in endowment and disadvantaged only by social arrangements. Today a more extreme position is held by biologists: human races simply do not exist (Lewontin 1995; Marks 1995; AAPA 1996). This is not to deny the large amount of biological diversity among humans. The fact of diversity does not imply the reality of races. The distribution of variation spreads across humankind and is not partitioned into the neatly packaged "kinds" we call races. The social-scientific study of race is a study not of a biologically natural kind but of the complex social consequences of an outmoded biological doctrine.

Could disability lose its biological underpinnings in the way race has? At first glance, the idea seems absurd. People who cannot see, cannot see, and that is a fact of individual biology. The failure to see is an example of *functional abnormality*. Is it not obvious that blind people are abnormal in biological function?

To the contrary, I will argue that the reality of blindness, paraplegia and other such biological conditions does not entail the biological reality of the categories of normal versus abnormal function. Blindness is real. But the same is true of skin color. Biologists accept the facts of skin color but reject the reality of race. The rejection of race is not a rejection of the diversity of biological traits. It is the rejection of the *kind* "race," a biological category into which human diversity was previously believed to be naturally partitioned. The concept of race served to compartmentalize and thereby to manage human diversity. The category *normal function* is similar. The reality of individual biological traits like blindness and paraplegia does not entail the reality of the contrasting *kinds* normal versus abnormal function, any more than the reality of diversity in skin colors and hair textures entails the reality of the kinds called races.

The belief in the objective biological reality of the categories normal and abnormal function will be termed *functional determinism*. I will argue that functional determinism is false; the categories of normal versus abnormal function are not parts of the biological world. The contrast between normal and abnormal function, like the Caucasian and Negroid races, is based not on biological fact but on social myth.

The rejection of the category of normal function appears to conflict with one common strategy of justifying the ADA and other disability rights laws. The strategy is to drive a wedge between the objective reality of abnormal function and the disadvantages experienced by those who are abnormal. This questions the assumption that disadvantage is a natural consequence of abnormality. The strategy can be seen in the *International Classification of Impairments, Disabilities, and Handicaps* (ICIDH) (World Health Organization 1980). Impairment, disability and handicap are analyzed as three aspects of the social problem of disability. Impairment and disability (which need not be distinguished for present purposes) are conceived to be objective matters of biomedical fact: a person is or is not functionally normal. A handicap, on the other hand, is a disadvantage experienced by a person with a disability *in a given environment.* The handicap is a product of both the disability and the environment; a person with the same disability would not be disadvantaged in a more accessible environment. This analysis is meant to show that the "naturalness" (i.e., the objective status) of the disability does not entail the "naturalness" (i.e., the justice) of the disadvantage. The social system that designed the environment is partly responsible for the disadvantage of the person with the disability.

The inconsistency is only apparent. The ICIDH assumes the naturalness of functional abnormality, but its conclusions do not require it. The analysis shows only that handicaps can be unjust *even if* disabilities are a fact of nature (i.e., that functional normality and abnormality are natural biological kinds). I agree. The ADA should exist even if biological normality is a natural kind. But if normality is *not* a natural kind, our understanding of the basis of the ADA may be different. The Civil Rights Act of 1964 would be important even if races were natural kinds. Nevertheless, our understanding of the law changes when we recognize the conventionality of the concept of race itself. The doctrine of functional determinism is a factor in the oppression of disabled people, just as a belief in the reality of race is a factor in racism.

Diversity of function is just as true of the human race as is diversity of skin color or hair texture. Normality of function is a myth of the same sort as race, a myth involved in the social management of diversity. The next section will sketch some evidence from biological sciences that throws into question the concept of functional normality. Later sections will show how a commitment to the objective reality of functional normality can lead to analyses of the disadvantages of disabled people that are inconsistent with the understanding of disability embodied in the ADA.

FUNCTIONAL DETERMINISM

Christopher Boorse gave the most influential philosophical argument for functional determinism (Boorse 1975, 1997). Boorse's work is important because of its influence on biomedical ethics, as will be discussed in the following section. His main interest is in concepts of disease, but his analysis covers disabilities (blindness, paraplegia, loss of a limb) as well, and these are the traits of interest here. Boorse states that the *normal function* of an individual's body part is a statistically typical contribution of the part to the individual survival and reproduction of members of the individual's species. His account commits him to an empirical claim about the functional uniformity of species members. It is that members of a given species are similar enough that unusual or atypical bodily conformations are few, poor in function and, so, identifiably abnormal. Boorse bases his claim on his reading of the literature of pathology. There is indeed a tendency towards functional determinism in that literature. I believe, however, that it arises from the pragmatics of diagnosis and medical education rather than from a scientific consensus on the reality of normality. Criticisms of functional determinism are not hard to find in other areas of biomedicine.

Boorse's view has been most widely criticized from the standpoint of Darwinian evolutionary biology, which holds that genetic diversity characterizes all natural species (for his response, see Boorse 1997, 33ff). The human species contains a very great deal of genetic diversity. Studies of a group of four hundred functionally diverse but related fish species in Africa have shown that there is less genetic variation between those four hundred species than within the single human species (Stiassny and Meyer 1999). Additional grounds to doubt the uniformity of function within a species comes from developmental biology and embryology. The processes of development are flexible and make allowances for variations during growth. Adults that arise from these processes are not cookie-cutter identical. They function, but they do not function identically. Evolutionary biologist John Maynard Smith describes a well-studied case of a goat born without front legs. The goat learned to walk bipedally and developed musculature and a torso shape that was appropriate to its human-like gait. "The relevance of such developmental flexibility is that a single major change—for example the loss of the fore legs—instead of being a disaster may be compatible with life" (Maynard Smith 1975, 317). It is important to recognize that developmental flexibility is not a special emergency process that only rescues "abnormal" individuals. It functions in the developmental construction of every organism, whether the eventual outcome is typical or atypical of members of its species. To call a typical or average species member "normal" is to assume a blueprint in the developmental process that simply does not exist.

Less dramatic accommodations to developmental contingencies exist in very large numbers. Hundreds of anatomical examples are now available online at the *Illustrated Encyclopedia of Human Anatomic Variation* (Bergman, Afifi and Miyauchi 1999). The authors accept as "normal" any variant possessed by a living (and therefore viable) organism no matter how unusual. (Surprisingly few individuals are entirely anatomically "usual.") They observe: "Man is not machine made but rather more subjectively fashioned with many developmental and environmental factors intervening in the process." Similar points have been made with respect to physiology by pathologist Jiří Vácha (Vácha 1978, 1985). Vácha criticizes the common view that what is frequent is normal and therefore healthy. Extreme values of physiological parameters are associated with disease in many individuals but are compensated for in others. Indeed, the constellation of other parameters in an individual may directly require the extremeness of a particular character for good health. "Immense variability has been found in the manner in which individuals in the population attain health" (Vácha 1985, p. 339).

Taking into account this information from the diverse fields of evolutionary biology, developmental biology, anatomy and physiology, it certainly cannot be said that the science of biology has established the reality of the distinction between normal and abnormal function. (For more detailed discussion of these and other cases, see Amundson, in press.)

NORMALITY ASSUMPTIONS IN HEALTH CARE ETHICS

Boorse's functional determinism is influential in philosophical discussions of health care policy. Norman Daniels argues that the preservation and restoration of normal function is a primary goal of health care, citing Boorse as the authority on the objectivity of normal function: "[T]he kinds of [health care] needs picked out by reference to normal species functioning are objectively important because they meet this high-order interest persons have in maintaining a normal range of opportunities" (Daniels 1987, 301). The goal of normality is seen as especially legitimate, because it is fixed by nature rather than by human convention: "we can take as fixed, primarily by nature, a generally uncontroversial baseline of species-typical [i.e., normal] functioning" (Daniels 1987, 303). Since the normality of function implies the normality of opportunity range, it would appear that the normal opportunity range is just as fixed by nature as is normal function. And so must be the reduced opportunities of abnormals. The unemployment of disabled people appears as a simple fact of nature.

The tight linkage between normality and opportunity reappears in Dan Brock's analysis of the concept of quality of life. "[Q]uality of life must always be measured against normal, primary functional capacities for humans" (Brock 1993, 308). Brock cites Daniels on the observation that the "normal opportunity range" is available to only functionally normal humans. He draws additional conclusions about the quality of life of the abnormals. Just as opportunities are (naturally) lower for abnormals, so must be their quality of life.

One might think that quality of life would be measured by the satisfaction and fulfill-ment actually experienced by the people living those lives. This would allow an empirical test of the hypothesis that quality of life correlates with functional normality. If the linkage were empirically verified, then functionally atypical people would report low qualities of life. But in fact the data do not support this hypothesis. Atypical people typically report a high quality of life. There is a great deal of empirical evidence that people with even serious disabilities report a quality of life averaging only slightly lower than that reported by nondisabled people. Physicians, in particular, estimate the quality of the lives of their dis-abled patients to be much lower than do the patients themselves (Bach and Tilton 1994).

Brock is aware of the mismatch between biological normality and the reported quality of people's lives. But he does not treat it as an empirical test of the identification of normal-ity with quality of life. Rather, Brock concludes that since normality does not correlate with subjectively reported quality of life, subjective reports of happiness do not measure quality of life! In order to protect from refutation the link between normality and quality of life, Brock distinguishes *ad hoc* between the subjective and objective aspects of quality of life (Brock 1993, 306). Subjective aspects are the degree of happiness and satisfaction that a person experiences. Objective aspects include the person's own objective abnormality and the opportunity losses associated with it. Abnormal people who report a high quality of life are simply mistaken about the quality of their own lives. Their quality of life is merely *sub-jectively* high. Objectively, it is low.

How does Brock account for the mismatch between high subjective quality and low normality-defined ("objective") quality? He offers only one explanation. Functionally abnormal people who report a high quality of life have lower expectations than function-ally normal people do. Lowered expectations are more easily satisfied. The easy satisfaction of low expectations yields a high "subjective" quality of life. But this, to Brock, is not *real* quality of life: "To be satisfied or happy with getting much less from life, because one has come to expect much less, is still to get *less* from life or to have a less good life" (Brock 1993, 309). I am greatly discomforted by Brock's confident judgment on this matter. As a happy resident of small-town Hawaii, I am sometimes bewildered that people can find happiness while living in large mainland American cities. But when they tell me that they do, I believe them. I do not assume that their standards must be lower than mine.

The important point here is not Brock's inability to imagine a full but functionally abnormal life. It is the consequences he draws from the doctrine of functional determin-ism. He asserts a linkage from objective normality, through objective opportunity, and on to objective quality of life. The linkage is not treated as a falsifiable hypothesis. In the face of counterexamples (reports of high life-quality submitted by abnormal people), the link-age is defended from refutation by *defining* high quality of life as necessarily involving bio-logical normality. It is not a discovery but a semantic stipulation that only the normals experience high quality of life. Keep in mind that quality-of-life assessments are intended by some to play a role in the allocation of health care. An assessment of quality of life that systematically discriminates against "abnormal" people may have very serious implications for their access to health care.

UNFASHIONABLE FUNCTION

Functional diversity can be conceived in two different ways, which have been called *level* and *mode*. Level is a quantitative aspect of a functional performance outcome, measured by weight lifted, speed traveled or some similar metric. Mode is the manner or fashion in which a particular performance level is achieved. Silvers revealingly points out that the social biases surrounding disability are directed more intensely at functional mode than functional level (Silvers 1998, 101ff). Unusual functional modes are more strongly stigmatized than reduced functional level. Some people who experience progressive impairments, such as the loss of hearing or mobility, refuse to use tools that would make their disability more apparent even though the tools would greatly enhance their level of function. The fact that individuals try to hide their disability has usually been interpreted patronizingly, as evidence of the failure to accept one's own limitations. It should instead be seen as recognition on the part of disabled people of a deep social prejudice against them. Cosmetic normality at the cost of functional performance has been an acknowledged goal of many rehabilitation programs. In the past, many schools for deaf people suppressed the use of sign language in favor of oralism (lipreading and the attempt to produce spoken speech). Oralism is an extremely limited means of communication for most profoundly deaf people. But the poorly functioning oralist mode is cosmetically more normal than sign language (Davis 1995, p. 84 ff.).

Wheelchair use is another example of the stigmatization of an unfashionable performance mode. Many people with mobility impairments are taught not to use wheelchairs if there is any way to avoid it. This is true even if shunning the wheelchair means walking with difficulty, pain and very low efficiency. Depending on the environment and the task at hand, a wheelchair user can function at or above the level of a person with bipedal mobility. The world's record for a marathon race is 45 minutes faster for a wheelchair user than for a runner. Nevertheless "wheelchair-bound" and "confined to a wheelchair" are used as synonyms for paralysis. The irony is that wheelchairs are tools of mobility, not confinement devices. The people who are genuinely confined are paraplegic people who do not *have* a wheelchair or who have one but live in an environment filled with barriers to its use. The stigmatization of wheelchairs shows how a higher level of performance is sacrificed to the cosmetic normality of functional mode. Upright walking is socially approved over wheelchair use no matter how painful and inefficient the walking or how convenient and efficient the wheelchair.

The doctrine of functional determinism can be seen at work in how both philosophers and social scientists discuss the quality of life of people with mobility impairments. Brock discusses approvingly an assessment instrument called the Health Status Index (HSI), which is designed to measure what he describes as "functions of the 'whole person'" (Brock 1993, 28ff). The HSI actually measures something quite different. It has separate scales for "physical activity" and "mobility." Each illustrates the bias towards fashionable normality of mode over level of functional performance. The "physical activity" scale scores 4 points for walking freely, 3 points for walking with limitations (using a cane or crutches) and 2 points for moving independently in a wheelchair. A walking person scores higher in physical activity than a person who uses a wheelchair even if the walker manages only slow and painful steps and the wheelchair user is a marathon racer. Cosmetic normality wins over functional performance.

The "mobility" scale of the HSI awards 5 points for using public transportation alone, 4 points for requiring assistance to use public transportation and 3 points for needing assistance to go outside. Consider how a physically fit paraplegic wheelchair user would score on this assessment. If there were barriers between her living quarters and the street (e.g., stairways without elevators), she would score 3. If there were no such barriers but her city's public transportation was inaccessible to wheelchairs, she would score 4. If her living quarters and her public transportation were both wheelchair-accessible, she would score 5.

Does this scale measure "functions of the whole person"? Obviously not. It measures the barriers that exist in her environment. It then treats *as an attribute of the person* whatever degree of immobility her environment imposes on her.

The HSI gives an operationalization of "mobility," the results of which are attributed to an individual person. People familiar with the ADA will recognize the distortion in this attribution. It is not a property of an individual being measured but the accessibility of her environment. The measurement could have been named "accessibility" and attributed not to her but to her living quarters and city transportation system. Nevertheless, this misconceived "mobility" is exactly what Brock refers to as an "objective" component of quality of life (as opposed to subjective components such as happiness). The objective naturalness of a paraplegic person's inability to leave her apartment was derived from Boorse's functional determinism, via Daniels's identification of opportunity with normality. The paraplegic woman who lives in inaccessible housing and an inaccessible city is said to be disadvantaged by her own abnormality, not the designed inaccessibility of her environment. If the ADA does nothing else, it forces us to recognize that a fallacy has been committed here.

INTERPRETING THE ADA

In the account I have just given, the doctrine of functional determinism is the foundation on which an anti-ADA interpretation is made of the causes of disadvantage associated with disability. Boorse asserts the objective reality of functional normality, Daniels infers from that to the objective reality of normal opportunity (and the naturalness of lower opportunity for abnormals), and Brock infers the "objectively" low quality of life of abnormals from their naturally low opportunity range. It seems that the social causes of disadvantage, such as inaccessible environments, are unnoticed because of the sheen of objectivity that attends functional determinism.

Even though the ADA allows us to see that a fallacy has been committed, it does not tell us where to locate the fallacy. I have located it in functional determinism itself. But it might be argued that the fallacy lies not in functional determinism but in the uses to which it was put. Perhaps Boorse was correct about the reality of abnormality, and the fallacy was only the inference from abnormality of function to the naturalness of reduced opportunity. Here are a few considerations that count towards my view.

First, as was argued above, biology and biomedicine do not give the kind of support that has been claimed for the reality of normality. Second, the social stigmas and biases that explain mistaken anti-ADA assumptions such as "normal opportunity range" seem no different from those that support "normal walking abilities." The preference for the usual modes of function can be seen in functional determinism itself, and not just in the social inferences about normal opportunities. A preference for fashionably normal functional modes is clearly tied not to goal achievement but to typicality. As the wheelchair discussion showed, the only way objectively to link performance mode with goal achievement is by deciding in advance that one *environment* is more "normal" than another. But it is not the job of biomedical scientists to decide whether stairways or ramps are more "normal" environments. Any scientist who does so commits the very fallacy that we have recognized in the writings of Daniels and Brock.

Third, we must ask ourselves what the use is of functional determinism in the age of the ADA. If it no longer licenses discrimination (as it formerly did), what purpose has it? Antidiscrimination laws do not require the objective inferiority of the protected groups.

Belief in the objective inferiority of women and certain ethnic groups is a part of the history of discrimination. As women and ethnic minorities gained protection, the beliefs in inferiority lost credence. When disadvantages are recognized to be social in origin, theories about inherent inferiority are of questionable social value, at least in the absence of real scientific support of their claims.

If functional determinism is a factual mistake, the ADA can still be seen to protect against discrimination based on functional differences, rather than functional abnormality and categorical inferiority. If the social understanding of the ADA proceeds in a way that parallels other antidiscrimination laws, this is the understanding that will eventually develop. It is not the understanding now current in the legal community. Three Supreme Court decisions in June 1999 imply that the group protected by the ADA is defined by functional inferiority and not by functional difference (Silvers 2000). As with many popular but outmoded notions about the reality of race, the assumptions behind this ruling deserve critical examination.

ACKNOWLEDGMENTS

Portions of this work are reprinted from Ron Amundson: "Against Normal Function," *Studies in History and Philosophy of Biology and Biomedical Sciences,* v. 31C, March 2000, with permissions from Elsevier Science.

REFERENCES

American Association of Physical Anthropologists. "Statement on Biological Aspects of Race." *American Journal of Physical Anthropology* 101 (1996) 569–570.

Amundson, Ron. "Against Normal Function." *Studies in the History and Philosophy of Biological and Biomedical Sciences,* v. 31C, March 2000.

Bach, John R., and Margaret C. Tilton. "Life Satisfaction and Well-Being Measures in Ventilator Assisted Individuals with Traumatic Tetraplegia." *Archives of Physical Medicine and Rehabilitation* 75 (1994): 626–634.

Bergman, Ronald A., Adel K. Afifi and Ryosuke Miyauchi. *Illustrated Encyclopedia of Human Anatomic Variation.* Iowa City: University of Iowa, 1999. http://www.vh.org/Providers/Textbooks/AnatomicVariants/AnatomyHP.html

Boorse, Christopher. "On the Distinction Between Disease and Illness." *Philosophy & Public Affairs* 5 (1975): 49–68.

Boorse, Christopher. "A rebuttal on health," in *What Is Disease,* eds. James M. Humber and Robert F. Almeder. Totowa, NJ: Humana Press, 1997, 3–134.

Brock, Dan W. *Life and Death.* Cambridge, UK: Cambridge University Press, 1993.

Daniels, Norman. "Justice and Health Care," in *Health Care Ethics,* eds. Donald VanDeVeer and Tom Regan. Philadelphia: Temple University Press, 1987.

Davis, Lennard J. *Enforcing Normality: Disability, Deafness, and the Body.* London: Verso, 1995.

Lewontin, Richard C. *Human Diversity.* New York: W.H. Freeman, 1995.

Marks, Jonathan B. *Human Biodiversity: Genes, Race, and History.* New York: Aldine de Gruyter, 1995.

Maynard Smith, John. *The Theory of Evolution.* 3rd ed. Cambridge, UK: Cambridge University Press, 1975.

Silvers, Anita. "A Fatal Attraction to Normalizing," in *Enhancing Human Traits: Ethical and Social Implications,* ed. Erik Parens. Washington DC: Georgetown University Press, 1998.

Silvers, Anita. "The Unprotected: Constructing Disability in the Context of Antidiscrimination Law," this volume, 2000.

Stiassny, Melanie L. J., and Axel Meyer. "Cichlids of the Rift Lakes." *Scientific American* 280, no. 2, (1999): 64–69.

Vácha, Jiří. "Biology and the Problem of Normality." *Scientia* 113 (1978): 823–846.

Vácha, Jiří. "German Constitutional Doctrine in the 1920s and 1930s and Pitfalls of the Contemporary Conception of Normality in Biology and Medicine." *Journal of Medicine and Philosophy* 10 (1985): 339–367.

World Health Organization. *International Classification of Impairments, Disabilities, and Handicaps.* Geneva: World Health Organization, 1980.

Impairment and Embodiment

MARY CROSSLEY

When Congress enacted the Americans with Disabilities Act in 1990, disability rights advocates acclaimed it as the "second generation" of legislation protecting the rights of persons with disabilities.[1] In contrast to its forebear, the federal Rehabilitation Act of 1973, the ADA significantly expanded the types of actors subject to the federal nondiscrimination mandate and made explicit that a failure to provide reasonable accommodations to persons with disabilities was one of numerous forms of prohibited discrimination. When it came to defining who were the individuals with disabilities protected from discrimination under the ADA, however, Congress by and large cloned the definition already existing in the Rehabilitation Act. As under the Rehabilitation Act's definition, an individual with a disability protected by the ADA is a person (a) who has a physical or mental impairment that substantially limits one or more of the person's major life activities, (b) who is regarded as having such an impairment, or (c) who has a record of having such an impairment.[2]

Because Congress simply imported an existing statutory definition of disability into the ADA, and because that definition had previously engendered little controversy over who fell within the definition, the phenomenal growth in litigation in the second half of the 1990s over which individuals can claim the ADA's protections has come as something of a surprise. But there it is: more than half of the ADA cases litigated in the mid- to late 1990s have involved the question of whether the plaintiff legally had a disability, and the question has occupied the Supreme Court in both of its past two terms. Commentators, including authors in this volume, have offered various explanations for the increasing attention paid to the question of who is an individual with a disability. Whatever the precise reasons, however, I believe this surfeit of litigation reflects a profound societal uncertainty regarding just which members of our society should be able to lay claim to the protections of disability discrimination law.

This essay focuses on impairment as one aspect of defining disability. Under the ADA, the existence of an impairment is a threshold question in the determination of disability. It is only when an actual, perceived or past impairment substantially limits a major life activity that disability will be found. But what types of bodily characteristics qualify as impairments? What is it about a person's body that lays the foundation for a finding of disability? Better understanding the concept of impairment will not end our inquiry as to the meaning of disability (at least as that term is defined in the ADA), but it would provide a worthy beginning.

Once we begin looking at the body of an individual seeking to invoke the ADA, though, deciding whether that individual has an impairment (which may or may not substantially limit a major life activity—a separate question) is often less straightforward than one might anticipate, for several reasons. First, the definition of impairment provided by the regulatory agencies charged with enforcing the ADA offers more breadth than precision and differs in its sense from the dictionary definition for the term. The Equal Employment Opportunity Commission's (EEOC) regulations define physical impairment as: "any physiological disorder, or condition, cosmetic disfigurement, or anatomical loss affecting one or more" of an extensive list of body systems.[3] This definition, on its face, is extremely broad: it appears that "any condition . . . affecting" one of the listed body systems qualifies as an impairment. Is the muscle soreness I experience after working out for the first time in months a condition affecting my musculoskeletal system and thus an impairment? One might so conclude. But if so, under such a literal reading, could not the strength I develop after working out regularly also qualify as a condition affecting my musculoskeletal system?

By contrast, the common usage of the term "impairment" and the dictionary definition of the word and its verb form "to impair" reflect a different understanding of the term. These nonlegal definitions associate impairment with a deterioration in strength or value—some kind of injurious lessening—rather than simply an effect on a body system. Some courts, faced with deciding whether a plaintiff has an impairment, have been unable to distance themselves from what they have understood as the term's plain or common meaning and have rejected the idea—at least implicitly suggested by the regulatory definition—that the effect of a condition or disorder on the bodily system need not necessarily be negative.[4]

Second, beyond the potential for divergence of the legal definition of impairment from the common understanding of that term, the immense variety found in human bodies makes it quite difficult to draw a bright line between those bodily characteristics that are considered impairments and those that are not. Human bodies come in a boundless diversity of shapes and sizes, and human beings display a broad spectrum of levels of functioning and degrees of good and ill health. Given the seemingly limitless gradations of health and disease, function and dysfunction, how are we to establish boundaries that demarcate those who are in the "individual with an impairment" group from those who are not?

Third, the attempt to identify physical impairment is an exercise in attaching a legally significant label to bodily characteristics, and this exercise's focus on the body should accordingly recognize the subjective experience of embodiment and the cultural embeddedness of the body. The nature of an individual's body and its parts cannot simply be objectively described and assessed by another, for it is the individual's very body that situates the person in relation to the material world and that mediates the individual's experience of reality.[5] In other words, a characteristic that medical science objectively describes as uniform—for example, loss of a limb—may be subjectively experienced quite differently by individuals living in different economic, social and familial contexts. Similarly, the social meaning attached to physical characteristics in different cultures affects our understanding of which bodily traits are impairments and which are "normal." Cultural practices and expectations certainly play a role in whether and how an impairment impacts an individual's ability to perform her or his major life activities, but culture can also mediate the prior concept of impairment.

In light of these factors, the difficulty that the courts have experienced in assessing even the threshold question of whether an ADA plaintiff has an impairment becomes somewhat more understandable. The remainder of this essay probes the complexity of the impairment inquiry by focusing on how the courts and agencies interpreting the ADA have struggled to divine the term's meaning as applied to two groups of plaintiffs: pregnant women and obese persons.

PREGNANCY

When a pregnant (or formerly pregnant) woman files suit alleging discrimination under the ADA, the court must decide whether the plaintiff is (or was) an individual with a disability. The first step of that analysis is to decide whether the woman's pregnancy qualifies as an impairment. At first blush, a straightforward reading of the regulatory definition of impairment would appear to include pregnancy as a "condition . . . affecting . . . [the] reproductive [system]." Nonetheless, in interpretive guidelines explaining its regulations, the EEOC—apparently ignoring the disjunctive between "disorder" and "condition"—has concluded that pregnancy is not an impairment because it is "not the result [of a physiological disorder."[6] In an attempt to clarify the question further, the EEOC has explained that, while pregnancy plain and simple is not an impairment, complications resulting from pregnancy *are* impairments, presumably because they do reflect some physiological disorder.[7]

By and large, courts presented with plaintiffs claiming pregnancy discrimination have followed the EEOC's rejection of pregnancy, in and of itself, as an impairment. Moreover, a number of courts have lumped "pregnancy and related medical conditions" together, finding that all such bodily changes aggregated do not constitute an impairment, at least in the absence of "unusual circumstances."[8] For example, one court found that a plaintiff, who during her pregnancy complained of morning sickness, stress, nausea, back pain, swelling and headaches, did not have an impairment because her pregnancy was not unusual or abnormal. This court relied on the EEOC's interpretive guidelines regarding pregnancy, and reasoned: "Pregnancy is a physiological condition, but it is not a disorder. Being the natural consequence of a properly functioning reproductive system, pregnancy cannot be called an impairment. . . . All of the physiological conditions and changes related to a pregnancy also are not impairments unless they exceed normal ranges or are attributable to some disorder."[9] Courts adopting this approach to exclude pregnant women from the ADA's coverage have often reassured the plaintiff by reminding her that the Pregnancy Discrimination Act (PDA) and Title VII prohibit adverse employment actions based on pregnancy, by treating pregnancy discrimination as a form of sex discrimination rather than disability discrimination.[10]

But does this line of reasoning mean that pregnant women have no prospect of claiming the ADA's protection when they are discriminated against? Not necessarily. A few women experiencing pregnancy-related conditions have managed to circumvent this line of cases by characterizing their disability not as their pregnancy, or even as pregnancy plus its manifestations, but instead as a separate condition which just happened to accompany their pregnancy. For example, one woman alleged that severe back pain—which she suffered as a result of her pregnancy and the aggravation of a prior back injury—was her impairment and that it substantially limited her ability to sit at work for extended periods of time. While noting the line of case law holding that the ADA does not recognize pregnancy as a disability, the court found that the woman could proceed under the ADA because she alleged her disability to be severe back pain.[11] Thus, by cleaving the disabling result of a pregnancy from the pregnancy itself, this woman was able to convince the court that her case really was not about pregnancy.

Somewhat more recently, several courts have built on this willingness to focus the impairment inquiry away from the simple state of pregnancy and onto its side effects, but have done so by distinguishing between "normal, uncomplicated pregnanc[ies]" and the complications that can arise out of a pregnancy. In one such case, a woman alleged that her experience of spotting, leaking, cramping, dizziness and nausea during pregnancy qualified as disabilities. In allowing the woman's ADA claim to proceed, the court embraced the distinction between an uncomplicated pregnancy and pregnancy complications as supported by medical science—specifically, a statement by the American Medical Association that most women with uncomplicated pregnancies could work until labor commenced, but that certain "substantial complications" might disable the pregnant woman from further work. The court emphasized that the case did not involve "an entirely normal, healthy pregnancy," and concluded that the woman had indeed alleged a disabling impairment.[12]

So under this approach, a pregnant woman might be able to lay claim to the ADA's protections if she can convince the court that her pregnancy-related complication(s) can be seen as a disorder or as abnormal (so that it might be deemed an impairment), notwithstanding that the complication is inextricably part of her experience of pregnancy (which is deemed not an impairment). In assessing one woman's argument that her premature labor was a disabling impairment, the court explained its reasoning:

> Pregnancy is not considered a physiological disorder under [the EEOC regulations]. . . . However, the regulation does not explicitly exclude pregnancy-related impairments, provided they are the result of a physiological disorder. "Physiologic" is defined as "characteristic of or conforming to the normal functioning or state of the body or a tissue or organ." . . . Thus, a physiological disorder is an abnormal functioning of the body or a tissue or organ. Clearly, plaintiff's condition was not a function of a normal pregnancy. It was a physiological disorder.[13]

Thus, these recent cases endeavor to draw the line between "impairment" and "not impairment" by distinguishing between pregnancies that are normal and those marred by abnormal complications.

If we take a step back from the cases and regulations regarding a pregnant woman's ability to claim the ADA's protection, though, how does the law look? It looks as if the EEOC and the courts are attempting to draw lines between the majority of pregnant women, who cannot complain under the ADA if they are discriminated against based on the bodily and emotional changes that accompany pregnancy, and those few women who experience conditions that deviate so far from what is considered normal for a pregnancy that the women are found to have an impairment under the ADA. This effort at line-drawing is seen throughout the case law, whether it takes the form of an "unusual circumstances" or "abnormal complications" standard; the courts essentially demand a finding that something is wrong with or abnormal about a pregnant woman's body before they will acknowledge an impairment. This reluctance to find impairment is premised on the understanding that a pregnancy itself represents the proper functioning of a healthy reproductive system; it also probably rests on a common perception that pregnant women are not typically viewed as having a disability.

Disability theorists, however, have argued that disability is constructed not simply by barriers in the physical environment but also by social expectations of what a body should be able to do[14] and cultural ideals of what a body should look like.[15] If that is the case, deciding whether pregnancy discrimination should be treated as a form of disability discrimination requires a more careful focus on why pregnant women experience discrimination. When an employer (or other actor covered by the ADA) discriminates against a woman based on her pregnancy and related conditions, it may be likely that the discrimination is consciously or unconsciously prompted, at least in part, by the deviation of the pregnant woman's body from cultural ideals of what the body should look like and how it should perform. And if that is the case, discrimination based on pregnancy seems quite similar to discrimination based on disability.

As noted above, a number of courts have found that pregnancy discrimination is discrimination based on gender, not disability, and it should be treated accordingly. But can these two possible bases for adverse treatment really be so easily untangled? Does the employer who terminates a woman "based on her pregnancy" really do so primarily because she is female (after all, only females become pregnant)? Perhaps, for it certainly rings true that discrimination based on pregnancy, like the public regulation of pregnancy, is prone to reflect social attitudes regarding sexuality and motherhood as aspects of femaleness.[16] On the other hand, though, might the employer's termination of the woman be primarily motivated by the facts that she's been late to work (because of morning sickness), missed several days (when she experienced spotting and her doctor put her on bed rest) and is often eating at her desk (in order to keep up her blood sugar and prevent nausea)? Or might all these elements come into play in a single decision?

While the out-of-hand conclusion that pregnancy discrimination is remediable only under a sex discrimination analysis fails to attend to possible similarities between pregnancy discrimination and disability discrimination, the steps that a number of courts have taken to allow some pregnant women to claim protection under the ADA clearly reflect a medicalized view of disability. These rulings have depended either on isolating an impairment such as back pain or morning sickness from its cause, or on viewing the complications of pregnancy as impairments. Such an approach effectively demands the artificial cleavage of an impairing condition from its source (the woman's pregnancy) and considers the condition in isolation from the bundle of other physical changes experienced by a pregnant woman. In so doing, this approach reflects a medicalized understanding of human experience as something best described in terms of symptoms and disorder in discrete bodily systems or organs, rather than as a complexly integrated experience of the whole body in context. This medicalization of pregnancy in the search for impairment is even more explicit in the recent cases that have relied on the "current state of medical knowledge" to draw a line between pregnancies that are normal and those that are not because of complications.[17] This approach appoints the medical profession as the arbiters responsible for drawing lines between normal and abnormal (or "complicated") pregnancies.

Such granting of authority to the medical profession and the medicalization of personal experience, however, have been rejected by disability theorists as ignoring the true social and cultural roots of disability. Under this view, disability should be understood not simply as a problem located in a person's body (i.e., the "medical model" of disability), but as the constellation of social, economic and political disadvantages experienced by persons whose bodies deviate from social and cultural norms (i.e., the "social model" of disability). If we so understand disability, then the quest to identify impairment in a pregnant woman's body by isolating abnormal (or "complicated") pregnancies is wrongheaded. Instead, in assessing when pregnancy should be considered a disability, the proper questions would be how women subjectively experience their pregnancies and all the accompanying changes— without attaching labels like "complicated" or "abnormal" or "unusual"—and how those changes affect women's lives and ability to participate fully in the workplace and society. This approach would validate the significance of embodiment and accord with the efforts of the women's health movement over the past several decades to demedicalize pregnancy and childbirth and wrest control of those experiences from the predominantly male medical profession.[18] It would be a sad irony, however, if the struggle to have pregnancy and childbirth understood as normal, healthy experiences rather than as medical problems were to contribute indirectly to leaving remediless those pregnant women who are discriminated against because of their physical condition.

Similarly, the courts' desire to compartmentalize cases in which pregnant women complain of discrimination into instances of sex but not disability discrimination seems to reflect an inability or unwillingness of the courts to recognize the frequency of dual discrimination encountered by women with disabilities. It is not always a satisfactory answer to say, as the courts often have, that pregnancy discrimination is indeed prohibited, but under the Pregnancy Discrimination Act rather than the ADA. Granted, the PDA prohibits differential treatment based on pregnancy, but, unlike the ADA, it does not impose any obligation to provide accommodations for an employee whose pregnancy-related conditions affect her ability to perform her job in the manner required by her employer.[19] Given this difference, the question bears addressing: If one of the ADA's purposes is to enable persons whose bodily differences result in functional limitations to obtain and retain employment by requiring employers to accommodate those limitations, does not the reasonable accommodations requirement make equal sense as applied to pregnant women? It is also worth noting that the PDA provides an alternative avenue of protection only in the employment context; it does not protect pregnant women discriminated against by public accommodations or public entities. Thus a greater judicial willingness to find that pregnancy and its accompanying physical and mental changes qualify as impairments (and thus possibly disabilities) under the ADA would not simply duplicate protection already existing for pregnant women.

These criticisms of how the EEOC and the courts have employed the concept of impairment in addressing the claims of disability discrimination brought by pregnant women, however, do not necessarily settle the question of whether some pregnant women *should* be viewed as having a disability and thus be entitled to the ADA's protections. To better answer that ultimate question, however, itself requires a different set of preliminary questions. Perhaps we should be asking not whether a woman's pregnancy is characterized by some physiological dysfunctioning or abnormality, but instead whether pregnant women, like people with disabilities, have been subjected to social oppression primarily because of their bodies' deviations from cultural norms.[20] Or we might ask whether pregnancy significantly affects a woman's daily life and whether pregnant women present themselves to the world as disabled people.[21] Ultimately, the questions become how much alike and how different from disabled people—in terms of the nature and origin of disadvantages experienced—are women whose pregnancies prompt discrimination, and whether the gender-based norms associated with pregnancy provide the overriding basis for the discrimination. This approach to the question does not avoid the need to draw lines between those persons who are deemed disabled for purposes of the ADA and those who are not; it simply demands that the lines be drawn based on a close examination of the social reality that people subjectively experience, and not simply on objective medical classifications.

OBESITY AND OVERWEIGHT

Cases in which plaintiffs assert violations of disability discrimination laws by alleging discrimination based on their weight provide another example of how the medical model of disability influences legal application of the ADA's definition of disability. Plaintiffs have sought to characterize weight discrimination as disability discrimination in two types of cases. In the first, a morbidly obese individual (medically defined as someone weighing 100 percent or more over her ideal body weight) alleges that discrimination occurred and either that her obesity was an actual disability or that her employer (or other actor covered by the ADA) perceived her obesity to be a disability. In the second type of case, the complaining individual is not morbidly obese and may not even be obese (defined as 20 percent or more over ideal body weight); nonetheless, the plaintiff has suffered some adverse outcome as a result of a failure to meet weight guidelines or standards adopted by an ADA-covered entity. These individuals say they are the victims of discrimination based on a perception that their failure to meet the standards makes them disabled.

These weight cases pose even more starkly than the cases involving pregnancy the difficulty of drawing lines on any kind of principled basis. We have all heard that "there's no such thing as a little bit pregnant"; by contrast, we all know from experience that while variations in weight among a group of people may be large, the increments by which variation occurs are small. Thus these cases present directly to the agencies and courts the question of how to establish and maintain boundaries between "impairment" and "not impairment" when it comes to weight.

The EEOC's interpretive guidelines take the position that the term "impairment" does not include "physical characteristics such as eye color, hair color, left-handedness, or height, weight or muscle tone that are within 'normal' range and are not the result of a physiological disorder."[22] In its Compliance Manual, the commission goes on to explain that "[b]eing overweight, in and of itself, generally is not an impairment. . . . On the other hand, severe obesity . . . is clearly an impairment. . . . In addition, a person with obesity may have an underlying or resultant physiological disorder, such as hypertension or a thyroid disorder. A physiological disorder is an impairment."[23] Thus the EEOC asserts that while a person's weight generally will not be deemed an impairment, it may be in two circumstances: (1) when the weight is attributable to or results in some physiological disorder, or (2) when the weight falls outside the "normal" range, as in cases of morbid obesity.

Courts interpreting the ADA's definition of disability in the context of weight-discrimination claims have generally followed the EEOC's approach to assessing when weight can be an impairment. *Cook v. Department of Mental Health, Retardation, and Hospitals*[24] provides an example of a morbidly obese plaintiff challenging an adverse employment action. Bonnie Cook was denied a job working as an attendant at an institution for persons with mental retardation. At the time she applied for the job, Cook weighed over 320 pounds and stood five foot two inches tall, which classified her as morbidly obese. In turning down her application, the institution asserted that Cook's weight could affect her ability to evacuate residents in the event of an emergency and that her weight also created risks for her own health, which might lead to repeated absences and worker's compensation claims. Cook sued, claiming that her rejection violated disability discrimination law and arguing that although she was capable of doing the job in question, the defendant perceived her as having a disability. The jury found for Cook and awarded her $100,000 in damages.

On appeal, the court affirmed, finding that the evidence supported the jury's verdict. In the course of assessing the evidence, the court concluded that the jury could reasonably have found that Cook had a physical impairment: "[A]fter all, she admittedly suffered from morbid obesity, and she presented expert testimony that morbid obesity is a physiological disorder involving a dysfunction of both the metabolic system and the neurological appetite-suppressing signal system, capable of causing adverse effects within the musculoskeletal, respiratory, and cardiovascular systems."[25] So because she met the medical definition of morbid obesity and produced expert medical testimony that her obesity was a physiological disorder, Bonnie Cook was able to recover for weight-based discrimination as a form of disability discrimination.

By contrast, in a case decided just a few months before *Cook*, a morbidly obese woman lost on her claim of disability discrimination when the California Supreme Court more narrowly circumscribed when obesity could be deemed an impairment.[26] After a health food store declined to offer Toni Linda Cassista a job, several employees expressed concern to her about whether her weight would affect her ability to do the job. So Cassista sued, claiming that she had been denied employment because the store *perceived* her to be disabled because of her morbid obesity.

The court, however, rejected the proposition that simply showing that the store failed to hire Cassista because of a belief that her weight disqualified her was enough to show perceived disability. Instead, the court reasoned, because the "regarded as" prong of the disability definition refers back to the type of impairment that can give rise to a finding of actual disability, only a condition qualifying as an actual impairment can support a perceived disability claim. Moreover, the court interpreted regulations and case law under the ADA and Rehabilitation Act as standing for the proposition that weight unrelated to a "physiological, systemic disorder" cannot be a disability. As a result, the court concluded that in order to succeed on a perceived-disability claim based on weight, a plaintiff has to show that the defendant perceived her weight to be in the nature of a physiological disorder.[27] Because Cassista had not presented evidence that her obesity was the result of a physiological condition or disorder affecting a body system, she could not succeed in her claim. Thus, under this approach, even morbid obesity—a condition that falls outside the range of "normal" weights—cannot be an impairment unless it results from some physiological disorder.

The requirement of evidence of some sort of physiological disorder as a prerequisite to making a showing of an impairment also shows up in the handful of cases in which persons who are not morbidly obese challenge weight standards used by employers. In these cases, the plaintiffs have claimed that they were fully able to perform their desired jobs, but that their employers' use of weight tables or weight guidelines as a basis for disciplining them showed that the employers perceived the plaintiffs to be disabled by their excess weight. In each of these cases the plaintiffs have failed, with each court following a basic line of reasoning.

For example, in one case a firefighter was suspended for repeatedly failing to keep his weight under a maximum acceptable weight established by a height and weight chart. The court acknowledged that to succeed on a perceived-disability claim, the plaintiff did not have to show that he had an actual disability. The court went on, though, to say that the plaintiff could succeed on a perceived disability claim only if he could show that the employer believed (albeit erroneously) that he suffered from a condition that, if it in fact existed, would qualify as an impairment under the actual-disability prong. An individual cannot proceed based on the employer's simple belief that a physical characteristic such as weight makes the plaintiff unable to do the job. And finally, this court concluded, because the plaintiff's weight was not an impairment unless it related to a physiological disorder, no claim lay against the city that took disciplinary action because the firefighter failed to meet weight guidelines.[28]

Courts following this line of reasoning justify dismissing the overweight plaintiff's claim not only in terms of adherence to the EEOC's interpretation of the ADA, but also in terms of furthering that statute's broad purposes. The courts seem to fear that permitting suits that allege discrimination based on simple (albeit socially undesirable) characteristics such as excess weight will fling wide open the floodgates of specious ADA claims. Interpreting the ADA to cover such claims, as one court opined: "would make the central purpose of the statute[ ], to protect the disabled, incidental to the operation of the 'regarded as' prong, which would become a catch-all cause of action for discrimination based on appearance, size, and any number of other things far removed from the reasons the statute [was] passed."[29]

In sum, reading together the cases challenging employer-imposed weight limits with those alleging discrimination based on actual or perceived morbid obesity, the courts have generally agreed with the EEOC that a person's weight will be considered an impairment only if it reaches the level of morbid obesity (or is otherwise outside the normal range) or is related to a physiological disorder of some sort.[30] Does this choice of boundary markers stand up to critical scrutiny? On closer examination, it appears that two bases on which the EEOC and the courts have chosen to segregate those people who can claim weight as an impairment are, respectively, arbitrary and medicalized.

First, a person may successfully assert weight as an impairment if that person is morbidly obese or her weight is otherwise beyond the "normal" range. But this boundary raises questions of its own. Disability theorists have asserted that the very idea of normalcy is itself socially constructed and therefore socially and culturally relative. Rather than being easily divisible into two distinct categories of "normal" and "abnormal" (or "nonnormal," "deviant" or whatever term is used), the range of human physical and mental traits and functioning lies spread across a wide spectrum. That being so, any demarcation of what is "normal" from what is not requires a shared understanding of where lines are appropriately drawn, an understanding that may be rearranged over time and among different cultures.[31] How, then, is "normal" weight to be determined? Should it be defined as less than a specified deviation from the ideal weights established by a particular height and weight chart? But it becomes difficult to argue that assessments of normalcy should be based on ideal benchmarks when about 25 to 30 percent of Americans weigh 20 percent or more over their ideal weights.[32]

Even if lawmakers were to decree that only weight rising to the level of morbid obesity deviates from the normal range enough to be deemed an impairment, a logical problem remains: Why should someone whose weight is 100 percent more than her ideal weight be found to have an impairment when someone whose weight is a mere 99 percent over her ideal weight does not have an impairment?[33] Under this approach, we cannot escape the fact that morbid obesity (an impairment) is distinguished from lesser levels of obesity (not impairments) simply by additional weight. What logic justifies attaching legal relevance to the surpassing of an arbitrary threshold such as the criterion for morbid obesity?

The second basis for drawing lines around weight-based impairments that the EEOC and the courts have used is more logical, but shows how firmly entrenched those lawmakers are in a medicalized understanding of disability. Here, the EEOC asserts that "physical characteristics such as . . . weight . . . that . . . are not the result of a physiological disorder" do not fall within the definition of impairment, implicitly suggesting that weight that *is* the result of a physiological disorder is an impairment.[34] As in the earlier discussion of pregnancy and related conditions, recognition of impairment here depends on finding something medically and diagnosably wrong with the obese individual's body. Only if the fat[35] person submits herself to medical care and produces expert testimony regarding the cause of her obesity can she claim protection against weight-based discrimination.

From the perspective of disability studies, this basis for line-drawing, too, is arbitrary and likely to produce unfair results. If disability is properly understood as a social rather than medical phenomenon, then why should Bonnie Cook (who produced a diagnosis of what causes her morbid obesity) receive protection from employment discrimination when Toni Linda Cassista (who produced no evidence of a diagnosis) does not? Regardless of what caused these women's morbid obesity, the social effects that they experienced were nearly identical: they were denied employment opportunities because employers believed that a fat applicant could not do the job.

Moreover, simply delegating to medical professionals the responsibility for determining who has obesity attributable to a physiological disorder and thus has an impairment and may (if the impairment substantially limits a major life activity) be qualified for ADA protection is particularly problematic given the high level of medical uncertainty regarding the causes of obesity. Medical science still knows little about the etiology of obesity[36] and thus is often incapable of stating with certainty whether a particular person's obesity is or is not the result of some physiological disorder. In addition, the courts' insistence on identifying an underlying physiological disorder may reflect a societal desire to avoid according legal protections to persons whose obesity can be attributed to their own sloth, gluttony or lack of self-discipline rather than any "medical" cause. Thus we see not only social and cultural but also moral understandings playing a role in constructing which physical characteristics *in which people* will be deemed an impairment.

So we come back to our original question: Does the law's insistence on a finding of either physiological disorder or "abnormal" weight as a basis for finding impairment make good sense in light of an understanding of disability as a socially rooted phenomenon? More bluntly, why should the phrases "physiological disorder" or "morbid obesity" matter? Both social science research and everyday experience demonstrate that fat people are commonly stigmatized and discriminated against based on their weight.[37] Some portion of this discrimination likely flows from myths and stereotypes about how obesity affects a person's physical capabilities. Some of the discrimination, however, is undoubtedly based on what Harlan Hahn calls "aesthetic anxiety"—the anxiety and discomfort provoked by the presence of a person who deviates from cultural norms of physical attractiveness.[38]

The contrasting experience of persons, particularly women, with extremely low weight bears out the observation. While extremely fat women are often dismissed or ridiculed in our society, extremely thin women may be held up in popular media as ideals of female beauty. The lack of lawsuits claiming discrimination based on thinness is not surprising in light of the idealization of thinness. Yet the reason that thin women are praised rather than disparaged is not necessarily because their bodies are less deviant or less disordered than the bodies of fat women; indeed, many extremely thin women may suffer from anorexia nervosa—a psychiatric disorder that would seemingly clearly qualify as an impairment—or some other eating disorder. Instead, very thin people do not face the social and economic disadvantages of very fat people because the former's bodies conform to our culture's ideals of physical attractiveness.

Each of the reasons for weight-based discrimination noted above is closely akin to the reasons that disability theorists identify as explaining why disability discrimination occurs. So we could conclude that the disadvantages experienced by fat persons are indeed quite similar to those experienced by persons with disabilities, and on that basis argue that fat people should have access to the same legal protections. This conclusion, however, begs a question of its own: *How fat* must a person be before her weight will be considered an impairment and thus potentially a disability? And how can a line be drawn in a fashion any less arbitrary than the lines drawn by the courts and the EEOC? Ultimately, we must concede that all line-drawing ventures separating persons into categories based on physical characteristics or functioning are inevitably arbitrary to some degree. This is true whether we are talking about degrees of fatness, or weakness, or visual or hearing impairment. Nonetheless, an attempt to draw lines based on how greatly persons have experienced social exclusion and disadvantage as a result of physical characteristics may be a preferable basis for creating categories—however arbitrary their boundaries might be—than is the medicalized approach currently employed.

REFLECTIONS

Examining the legal treatment of pregnant women and fat people who have sought to invoke the ADA's protections prompts several observations regarding the courts' interpretation of "impairment." First, it is apparent from the foregoing discussion that defining impairment, like defining the larger concept of disability for which impairment is a building block, unavoidably presents questions about where lines should be drawn. At what point and on what basis should a physical characteristic be considered an impairment? The legal assessments of impairment discussed above suggest two possible responses. A certain level of deviance from normal bodily characteristics is one possible basis for drawing lines, one that the EEOC employs in determining when a simple physical characteristic such as height or weight can be an impairment. As discussed above, however, trying to draw a dividing line between normal and deviant anywhere along the spectrum of bodily characteristics is artificial and ultimately arbitrary.

Another possible basis for drawing lines between characteristics that are impairments and those that are not is to draw the lines based on medical diagnoses of disorder and dysfunction. An examination of the regulatory definition of impairment suggests, at first blush, that determining the existence of impairment simply involves an objective assessment of the physical body, which then produces a clear cut response. Indeed, this is part of the appeal of a medicalized approach to impairment: simply let the doctor take a look at the plaintiff and perform objective tests, and the doctor can validate the existence or confirm the nonexistence of impairment. Thus, under an approach to impairment consistent with the medical model, the line-drawing dilemma is obscured, for the sheen of straightforward objectivity attaches to medical decisions.

But a medicalized approach to determining impairment has its own problems. Medical judgments are often far less precise, less certain and more influenced by the physician's subjective biases than is popularly appreciated. While physicians are undoubtedly able to make definite diagnoses in some cases, medical "science" is often quite tentative in its assessments.

Thus neither a deviance approach nor a medicalized approach to identifying impairment is problem-free. In addition, a characteristic that the two approaches share is that they each address the question of impairment purely from an external viewpoint and ignore the particular or subjective experience of the individual whose bodily characteristic is alleged to give rise to a disability. Admittedly, once an impairment is found and the inquiry shifts to whether it substantially limits a major life activity, the inquiry is individualized to ask whether a major life activity of the particular plaintiff is limited. And although it is not typical in employment cases, in some instances courts have even taken into account the plaintiff's own subjective experience of limitation in the assessment of impacts on major life activities. For example, in *Bragdon v. Abbott,* when the Supreme Court considered whether Sidney Abbot's HIV infection substantially limited her major life activity of reproduction, it took into account her subjective decision to forgo childbearing in light of the risk of transmitting HIV infection to her child.[39]

But because an impairment must be found before the impact on major life activities is even assessed, using a medicalized, objective approach to identifying impairment may exclude from the ADA's protections those individuals whose experience of a bodily characteristic is atypical. The difference in experience could be the result either of an individual's subjective response to the bodily characteristic or of the reaction found in the individual's particular social, economic or cultural surroundings. In either event, an individual experiencing significant disadvantage flowing from a trait that is deemed not to be an impairment is left without recourse.

This outcome—that an individual who is subjected to discrimination based on a physical characteristic finds no protection under the ADA—results from an understanding that people with disabilities must have bodies either that are notably different from "normal" people's or that have something wrong with them. That is what the impairment requirement has come to mean. And perhaps that is what Congress had in mind when, in the legislative findings included in the ADA, it described people with disabilities as a "discrete and insular minority."[40] We can certainly imagine a disability-law regime in which only individuals who fit into set, externally defined categories receive protection against discrimination.

But the cases in which the impairment requirement has functioned to deny protection to individuals who claim to have been discriminated against because of a physical characteristic present us with a question: Is that the kind of disability-law regime we want? Do we find the action of an employer who terminates a fat person because of her weight any less objectionable because the weight does not rise to the level of morbid obesity and has not been shown to be the result of a "physiological disorder"? If not, perhaps that is a sign that a broader understanding of disability is in order—an understanding that includes persons who suffer significant social and economic disadvantage because of bodily characteristics without requiring those characteristics to be classified as deviant or diagnosable. It might even suggest an understanding that recognizes the role that embodiment—the subjective and particular experience of living in a body—plays with respect to disadvantage. Ultimately, the cases denying pregnant women and fat people protection under the ADA for lack of impairment may serve to cause us to question the appropriateness and utility of continuing to use the concept of impairment, as currently understood, in determining the existence of disability.

ACKNOWLEDGMENTS

Many of the points in this essay were first made in "The Disability Kaleidoscope," 74 *Notre Dame L. Rev.* 621 (1999), copyright Notre Dame Law Review.

NOTES

[1] Robert L. Burgdorf, Jr., "The Americans with Disabilities Act: Analysis and Implications of a Second-Generation Civil Rights Statute," *Harv. C. R.-C. L. L. Rev.* 26 (1991): 413–522.

[2] 42 U.S.C. § 12102(2).

[3] 29 C.F.R. § 1630.2(h)(1).

[4] For example, *Runnebaum v. Nationsbank of Maryland,* 123 F.3d 156 (4th Cir. 1997) (en banc).

[5] Peter Halewood, "White Men Can't Jump: Critical Epistemologies, Embodiment, and the Praxis of Legal Scholarship," *Yale J. L. & Feminism* 7 (1995): 1–36.

[6] 29 C.F.R. App. § 1630.2(h).

[7] Equal Employment Compliance Manual (CBC) 2 (1995) § 902.2(c)(3).

[8] For example, *Villareal v. J.E. Merit Constructors,* 895 F. Supp. 149, 154 (S.D. Tex. 1995).

[9] *Gudenkauf v. Stauffer Communications, Inc.,* 922 F. Supp. 465, 473–74 (D. Kan. 1996).

[10] For example, *Johnson v. A.P. Products, Ltd.,* 934 F. Supp. 625, 627 (S.D.N.Y. 1996).

[11] *Patterson v. Xerox Corp.,* 901 F. Supp. 274, 278 (N.D. Ill. 1995).

[12] *Cerrato v. Durham,* 941 F. Supp. 388, 393 (S.D.N.Y. 1996) (citing "Council on Scientific Affairs, Effects of Pregnancy on Work Performance," 251 *JAMA* 1995 (1984)).

[13] *Hernandez v. City of Hartford,* 959 F. Supp. 125, 130 (D. Conn. 1997).

[14]Susan Wendell, *The Rejected Body: Feminist Philosophical Reflections on Disability.* New York: Rout-ledge, 1996.

[15]Harlan Hahn, "Antidiscrimination Laws and Social Research on Disability: The Minority Group Perspective," 14 *Behavioral Sciences & the Law* 41 (1996).

[16]Reva Siegal, "Reasoning from the Body: A Historical Perspective on Abortion Regulation and Questions of Equal Protection," 22 *Stanford L. Rev.* 261 (1992).

[17]*Cerrato,* 941 F. Supp. 388, 393.

[18]Barbara Katz Rothman, *In Labor: Women and Power in the Birthplace.* New York: W.W. Norton, 1991; Julia Epstein, "The Pregnant Imagination, Fetal Rights, and Women's Bodies: A Historical Inquiry," 7 *Yale J. L. & Human.* 139 (1995).

[19]Pamela S. Karlan & George Rutherglen, "Disabilities, Discrimination, and Reasonable Accommo-dation," 46 *Duke L. J.* 1(1996).

[20]Harlan Hahn, "Feminist Perspectives, Disability, Sexuality and Law: New Issues and Agendas," 4 *S. Cal. Rev. L. & Women's Stud.* 97 (1994).

[21]Carol J. Gill, "Questioning Continuum," in *The Ragged Edge: The Disability Experience from the Pages of the First Fifteen Years of "The Disability Rag."* Louisville, KY: Avocado Press, 1994.

[22]29 C.F.R. App § 1630.2(h).

[23]Compliance Manual, 902.2(c)(5)(ii).

[24]10 F.3d 17 (1st Cir. 1993).

[25]10 F.3d at 23.

[26]The California court was actually interpreting the term "physical disability" found in California's Fair Employment and Housing Act. That term's statutory definition tracks the EEOC's regulatory defi-nition of "impairment."

[27]*Cassista v. Community Foods, Inc.,* 5 Cal. 4th 1050, 1065–66 (1993).

[28]*Francis v. City of Meriden,* 129 F.3d 281 (2d Cir. 1997).

[29]*Francis v. City of Meriden,* 129 F.3d at 287.

[30]E.g., *Fredregill v. Nationwide Agribusiness Insurance Co.,* 992 F. Supp. 1082 (S.D. Iowa 1997).

[31]Lennard J. Davis, *Enforcing Normalcy: Disability, Deafness, and the Body.* London: Verso, 1995; Gina Maranto, "On the Fringes of the Bell Curve, the Evolving Quest for Normality," *New York Times,* May 26, 1998, at F7.

[32]Jane Byeff Korn, "Fat," 77 *B.U. L. Rev.* 25 (1997).

[33]Korn, at 42.

[34]29 C.F.R. App. § 1630.2(h).

[35]Many individuals favor the use of the word "fat" over "obese," which has medical connotations, or "overweight," which imposes societal notions of weight norms. Christian Crandall, "Prejudice against Fat People: Ideology & Self-Interest," 66 *Journal of Personality and Psychology* 882 (1994).

[36]Korn, at 45.

[37]Karen M. Kramer & Arlene B. Mayerson, "Obesity Discrimination in the Workplace: Protection Through a Disability Claim under the Rehabilitation Act and the Americans with Disabilities Act," 31 *Cal. W. L. Rev.* 41 (1994).

[38]Hahn, *Behavioral Sciences* at 54.

[39]*Bragdon v. Abbott,* 118 S. Ct. 2196 (1998).

[40]42 U.S.C. § 12101(a)(7).

The Supreme Court's Nearsighted View of the ADA

ARLENE MAYERSON AND MATTHEW DILLER

When the Americans with Disabilities Act was signed into law, President Bush declared that "every man, woman and child with a disability can pass through once-closed doors into a bright new era of equality, independence and freedom." For many people with disabilities, recent rulings of the Supreme Court slam the door that Congress and President Bush opened.

The 1999 Supreme Court decisions on the definition of disability under the ADA put up new barriers to individuals whose disabilities are mitigated or controlled by technological aids or medical treatment. Unfortunately, a critical legal issue was decided based on facts that could obscure the gravity of the impact of the decision. Two women with poor vision that was fully corrected by eyeglasses were turned down by United Airlines as pilots because they did not meet United's vision standards unless they wore glasses.[1]

Although it may seem a simple and unsurprising result that people with myopia are not entitled to claim "disability," the Court's reasoning has profound implications for many people who face persistent discrimination and whom Congress meant to protect. The ruling that the term "disability" in the ADA is determined by examining the individual claiming discrimination in their "corrected" state, even if the employer's reason for not hiring or firing was the underlying uncorrected condition, leads to the perverse result that a person with a disability who avails him- or herself of the benefits of technological and medical advances thereby risks losing protection from job discrimination.

For example, if an individual with epilepsy or diabetes manages through medication and discipline to control the effects of the condition, he or she may have a hard time bringing an ADA case even if he or she was fired from the job simply because of the condition and even if the condition has no impact on job performance. In other words, the employer is free to act on every bigoted and irrational impulse that it may have toward a particular disability. Make no mistake about it, this danger is not imagined—many employers respond to conditions such as epilepsy and diabetes in precisely this way. A person with controlled epilepsy is five times as likely to be unemployed as his or her nonimpaired counterpart.

The Americans with Disabilities Act, of course, was intended to put an end to this kind of discrimination. It was drafted as a civil rights statute, a break from the "hopeless, helpless, protect and pity" model of disability. The ADA is a celebration of the "new" disabled man or woman—independent, free, loud and proud. The recognition that people with disabilities can excel in all kinds of functions and roles is at the heart of the statute.

The crabbed interpretation delivered by the Supreme Court puts a rejected applicant with a disability in the untenable position of emphasizing all the things he or she cannot do in order to claim ADA protection, and then, once through the courthouse door, downplaying limitations in order to prove he or she is qualified for the job. It is important to realize that establishing that you are disabled under the ADA does not get you the job. It just means that you get your day in court to challenge an adverse employment decision that was based on your physical or mental impairment. By attempting to limit the ADA to the "truly disabled," the Supreme Court continues to look at disability as a matter for pity rather than equality. In essence, the Supreme Court condones exactly the behavior Congress sought to eradicate. When it comes to the ADA, the Court just does not "get it."

In order to make the breadth of the statute clear, the Congress included in the definition of disabled an individual who is "regarded" as disabled but has no actual incapacity at all. The Court's decisions could allow an employer to argue that it did not regard an individual to be "disabled" because (take a deep breath) he or she can work elsewhere. The fact that other employers have not adopted the same exclusionary policy based on medical conditions can actually serve as a defense, because if someone will hire you, you are not "disabled" enough to claim nondiscrimination protections. Thus the more irrational the discrimination, the more unassailable it is.

Imagine this logic in any other area of civil rights and it does not pass even the laugh test. "No we don't hire women, Jews (fill in the blank) but you can get a job somewhere else, so what's the beef?" The ADA is about equality of opportunity, which means a fair opportunity to perform all jobs for which an individual is qualified.

These absurd results are not required by the statute. Congress made clear that it intended the ADA as a broad and comprehensive protection against the irrational exclusion of people with disabilities from jobs and public programs. The Court ignored both the clear legislative history on this point as well as the view of the federal agency charged with interpreting the statute. As the eloquent dissent by Justices Stevens and Breyer explains, the majority's "miserly" interpretation is a disservice to the law.

Despite the ruling, ligation will continue on the issues left open by the Court. Ironically, in its attempt to curb litigation, the Court spawned a whole new generation of litigation on the question of who does or does not fit within the definition of "disability." People with disabilities will continue to work to redeem the promise of the ADA. They and their allies have fought too long and hard to let this law go undefended.

NOTE

[1] *Sutton v. United Airlines, Inc.,* 1999 U.S. LEXIS 4371 (1999).

The Unprotected
Constructing Disability in the
Context of Antidiscrimination Law

ANITA SILVERS

INTRODUCTION: THE RATIONALE FOR PROTECTION

How broadly and thoroughly should citizens be protected against discriminatory practices? U.S. policy in the second half of the twentieth century made the widening of such protection the preeminent strategy for advancing social justice. Repeatedly during this period, legislation has been crafted to protect groups of people whose distinctive characteristics have been stigmatized and who for that reason have been condemned to social disadvantage. Fueled by the faith that individuals' competence and courage must be enabled to surmount whatever disadvantage inferior social status inflicts, legislative and judicial action has aimed to identify and reform practice which is so biased as to derail the achievement members of socially stigmatized groups otherwise would enjoy.

Thus, during the last fifty years, justice for individuals with dark skins and female sexual characteristics has been pursued through programs to eliminate social impediments that bias has imposed on the realization of their talents. Bias against such people usually issues from falsely equating the group's distinctive characteristics with weakness and limitation. To illustrate, such erroneous correlations seem to have been a crucial factor in the suppression of the talents of women. Women's physical differences were imagined to be a "disability that demands rest and withdrawal from ordinary activities."[1] What ensued is a history in which "woman's imputed physical and mental frailty became the grounds for refusing her any civil or legal rights."[2] This is clearly a history of how false beliefs about the limitations of females' courage and competence not only disadvantaged individual women but deprived society as a whole of the benefit of their contributions. To counter this history, feminists initially insisted on portraying women as able to demonstrate the same character and competence as men, if given the opportunity to do so. Subsequently, they argued that women's distinctive virtues and capabilities are different from men's but are equally deserving of recognition and respect. Similar strategies—first the promotion of integration, and subsequently the politics of difference, or "identity politics"—were devised by advocates of racial and ethnic minorities.

Prompted by such strategic responses to history, the construction of protected classes during the first forty years of the civil rights era aimed to elevate groups whose achievements and contributions had been artificially depressed by a history of unequal treatment impelled by false beliefs about the limitations of the groups' members. The 1990 Americans with Disabilities Act pressed this program further. The ADA advanced the proposition that individuals whose achievement not only is artificially attenuated by hostile social arrangements, but is naturally constricted by their biology as well, are also owed effectively equitable opportunity to achieve success. On this reading of how justice should promote the realization of talent, the mere fact that someone's physical prowess or cognitive proficiency is less versatile or replete—and consequently is narrower or more limited—than is commonplace neither diminishes the duty to afford meaningful opportunity to the person nor reduces the value of doing so.

In the "Findings" that preface the ADA, Congress affirmed that: "unfair and unnecessary discrimination and prejudice denies people with disabilities the opportunity to compete on an equal basis and to pursue those opportunities for which our free society is justifiably famous, and costs the United States billions of dollars in unnecessary expenses resulting from dependency and nonproductivity."[3] To preserve continuity with earlier discrimination law, which understands the protected classes' prior lack of achievement to be the product of social oppression, Congress emphasized in the "Findings" that: "society has tended to isolate and segregate individuals with disabilities, and . . . such forms of discrimination . . . continue to be a serious and pervasive social problem."[4] From a perspective on limitations that is consistent with the analysis presented in the "Findings," being unable to execute fully some important physical or mental activity does not obviate the importance of opportunity nor render it futile. Despite this truth, the "Findings" declare, social practice has evolved so as to bar people whose physical or mental activity is more limited than is usual from much of the range of opportunity that is pursued through equitable social participation.

Its emphasis on the competence of people with disabilities to participate in society and be productive notwithstanding, the ADA appeals to a notion of limitation to elucidate "disability." An individual is disabled if he or she has "a physical or mental impairment that substantially limits one or more of the major life activities of such individual" (or has a history of or is regarded as having such an impairment).[5] Notice, however, that the way the ADA limns disability does not specify whether the dysfunction occasioned by impairment is biological or social. So what this rendering of "disability" for the purposes of civil rights law leaves unclear is whether the natural biological limitations of people with disabilities or, instead, the artificial and arbitrary restrictions imposed by social arrangements disadvantageous to them constitute the primary reason their talents have been unrealized and therefore the primary basis on which they are owed protection.

How we respond to this question about the ground for extending civil rights protection to the disabled affects whether the foundational premise of earlier discrimination law is preserved in the shield we erect against disability discrimination. For traditional antidiscrimination law presumes that once freed of socially imposed impediments, protected class members are competent to turn opportunity to good account. But it is hard to see how this presumption can be extended to the class of people with disabilities if class members are defined as quintessentially malfunctional individuals rather than as individuals who have been erroneously imagined to be so.

By equivocating instead of coming to grips with the implication of identifying disability with inescapable biological dysfunction, we invite construals of the group to be protected by the ADA that are retrogressive in relation to the accomplishment of the civil rights project of the past half-century. By doing so, we abandon the central strategy of the civil rights movement, namely, the delineation of protected classes as those whose members have been subjected to socially embedded fabrications of their incompetence and thereby made extraordinarily vulnerable to having their talent disregarded or suppressed. Moreover, by doing so, we fail to protect people who are presently not dysfunctional but whose impairments threaten to be the occasion of dysfunction unless they are protected from disability discrimination. In failing these people, I argue, we safeguard no one—

neither the incontrovertibly nor the contestably disabled—from disability discrimination. Consequently, I propose, the ADA can accomplish the purpose traditionally assigned to civil rights legislation only if its functional definition of disability gives primacy to the social over the biological dimensions of functioning.

SETBACK FOR PROTECTION, ONSET OF CONFUSION

The values expressed in the language of the "Findings" make it seem as if the ADA was meant to sweep away social practice that arbitrarily relegates people to inferior treatment or outcomes based on their being physically or mentally impaired, just as earlier civil rights legislation aimed at sweeping transformations of practices that fostered race-based or sex-based disadvantage. The prevalence of this impression among people with physical or cognitive impairments accounts for the feeling of disorientation that pervades their complaints about the Supreme Court's June 1999 decision to restrict the ADA's protection against disability discrimination. A press release from the National Council on Disability, a federal agency, exemplifies the dismay the decision provoked: "the U.S. Supreme Court totally missed the mark last week in three cases construing the definition of 'disability' in the Americans with Disabilities Act (ADA). The Supreme Court has left . . . millions of . . . Americans with significant mental or physical impairments unprotected against egregious discrimination."[6]

In the three cases in which this diminution of protection was iterated—*Kirkingburg, Murphy* and *Sutton,*[7] applicants whose work record inarguably demonstrated their ability to perform the essential tasks of the relevant position were denied employment because, according to the employers' standards, they were physically inadequate for the positions. Broadly, in these cases individuals with not-uncommon impairments (amblyopia resulting in monocular vision, high blood pressure, and severe myopia, respectively) were denied employment because of standards that explicitly made these impairments disqualifying. The plaintiffs argued that their demonstrated ability to deliver the products or outcomes of the job with as much success and safety as unimpaired individuals showed that the employers' standards violated the ADA Title I prohibition against "utilizing standards, criteria, or methods of administration that have the effect of discrimination on the basis of disability."[8]

However, the Court ruled that, although the plaintiffs' impairments eventuated in curtailment of their opportunity to fill the positions in question, no discrimination had occurred because the plaintiffs were not sufficiently disabled to invoke the protection of the law. If individuals' impairments are or are regarded as mitigated or surmounted, the majority of justices reasoned, they are not disabilities. The bewildering prospect is that to pursue mitigating or compensating for or surmounting one's impairment is to risk being propelled into the ranks of the unprotected. In other words, being competent despite being impaired threatens an impaired individual with loss of legal protection against biased attributions of incompetence.

But the Court's approach to understanding disability appears insensitive to the relevant contexts. A common idea, to which the Court clings, is that disability is fixed to defective biological states, and that overcoming such defects disposes of disability. Yet, as we shall see, the dimension and degree of an impairment's interference with an individual's life activity, as well as the line of substantial diminishment of significant performance, are relativized to social arrangements rather than fixed to biological states. Therefore, whether an individual's impairment crosses the threshold of substantial diminishment of significant performance cannot be determined solely or even primarily by reference to either unmitigated or surmounted biological fault. To nevertheless insist on doing so vitiates protection against disability discrimination not only for people whose limitations may seem to some to be insufficiently severe to deserve special safeguards but also for people whom nobody contests are disabled. Carefully untangling these ideas about how biological deficits and social limitations curtail the opportunities of people with disabilities thus is critical to the project of extending civil rights protection to this group of people.

Constructing a Protected Class

One challenge to fixing on who deserves protection from disability discrimination is that, unlike classes of people sorted according to sex or race, the population of the class constructed of individuals substantially limited by physical or mental impairments shifts, because whether each individual is a member is a transient fact. While some, but relatively few, of its members are born into the class of the disabled, illness or accident can precipitate membership at other points in persons' lives. Attempting to interpret the statute in a way that recognizes the permeability of the class but fixes the qualifications for membership in it, the Court specified that only currently functionally limited individuals, not potentially or hypothetically limited ones, are protected.[9] But because acquiring as well as relinquishing membership in this narrower group—currently dysfunctional people—is relativized to both social and personal factors, construing eligibility for protection this way is likely to generate at least as many borderline cases as central ones. And as we also shall see, this theory about class membership promotes controversial and unworkable conclusions about who shall be protected.

In this regard, Lambda AIDS Project Director Catherine Hanssens observed: "The Court rulings endorse a Catch-22 for many people with disabilities. The Court suggests that the ADA's safeguards against workplace discrimination vanish when people with disabilities find ways to overcome their limitations and make themselves more employable. These rulings strike at the very core of important civil rights protections for people with disabilities."[10]

In a *Boston Globe* column entitled "The Court's Nearsightedness," Ellen Goodman wrote: "But let us remember that the law against gender discrimination also protects men. And the law against racial discrimination is also used by whites. . . . Civil rights are supposed to be universal. The ADA was written for all of us. In the workplace, it said that we're supposed to be judged on just one ability—the ability to do the 'job.'"[11] For the analysis that follows, I will assume that the justice of Goodman's thesis—namely, that assessments of prospective employees should be commensurate with their qualifications and demonstrated competence—is evident and compelling.[12] Further, it seems inequitable and paternalistic to protect people with substantial limitations from the imposition of unfairly arbitrary physical criteria but condone holding less limited people to such an unfair standard. The majority opinion states that: "an employer's physical criteria are permissible as long as they do not cause the employer to make an employment decision based on an impairment, real or imagined, that it regards as substantially limiting a major life activity."[13] This reading of the law suggests that for an individual to have legal protection against disability discrimination, the individual must be regarded by whoever perpetrates allegedly discriminatory action as having reached the threshold of being substantially limited. Shortly after the Court's decision was announced, the journalist John Hockenberry wryly remarked:

The Court said that if a disability can be corrected or mitigated, employers can conclude that an impairment does not amount to a "substantial limitation." This is something of a revelation. I have a job. I have a family. I travel all over the world. By this definition the fact that I use a wheelchair to mitigate my paraplegia suggests I am not disabled. Someone should tell the doctors working on a cure for spinal cord injury they are wasting their time. The Supreme Court just beat them to it.[14]

Growing Confusion While Trying to Cure It

It might be thought, of course, that the line between the significant impairment marked by Hockenberry's need to use a wheelchair to mobilize, and the unremarkable impairment marked by the *Sutton* plaintiffs' need to use corrective lenses to see, is precisely where the Court's clarification lies. Whereas lenses restored the myopic Suttons to 20/20 vision, the wheelchair compensates for, but cannot correct, Hockenberry's impairment. Separated from the wheelchair, he cannot mobilize, a limitation he would not have if his injured spinal cord could be repaired or its operation reproduced by an implanted mechanical device. Perhaps the line the Court drew is meant to differentiate integral repair of a limiting physical condition from partial peripheral prosthetic intervention.

To see whether the distinction does this work, we should look at how it is explained in the majority's opinion. According to the Court, diabetes exemplifies an impairment that should not usually be deemed a disability because usually it is biochemically mitigated by administering medication, while impairments requiring the use of medical equipment such as wheelchairs are paradigmatic of disability for the Court. Although "if [diabetics] failed to monitor their blood sugar levels and administer insulin, they would almost certainly be substantially limited in one or more major life activities," the majority opines, "a person whose physical or mental impairment is corrected by medication . . . does not have an impairment that presently 'substantially limits' a major life activity. To be sure, a person whose physical or mental impairment is corrected by mitigating measures still has an impairment, but if the impairment is corrected it does not 'substantially limi[t]' a major life activity."[15]

On the other hand, in the language of the Court, "the use of a corrective device does not, by itself, relieve one's disability."[16] People who use adaptive equipment to function do not cease to be disabled on this view, for "individuals who use prosthetic limbs or wheelchairs may be mobile and capable of functioning in society but still be disabled because of a substantial limitation on their ability to walk or run. The same may be true of individuals who take medicine to lessen the symptoms of an impairment so that they can function but nevertheless remain substantially limited."[17]

However, closer examination of these examples suggests they have the effect of blurring precisely the line they are supposed to bring into focus. What the Court is obviously reaching for is a functional definition of disability.[18] In estimating the size of the class Congress meant to protect, the Court declares that the number of Americans with disabilities specified in the "Findings" prefacing the law is derived from a functional definition of disability rather than by compiling the numbers of people with conditions that compromise normal health.[19] This conclusion is taken to mean that the disabled to whom the ADA refers must be individuals who are not functional. But the simple, unqualified equation of disability with currently manifested dysfunction will not accomplish the requisite conceptual work.

Dysfunction Is Relative to the Height of Expectation. This unqualified identification of disability with significant dysfunction is unworkable because a variety of contextual factors can disconnect being so impaired as to be substantially limited in performing an activity from being dysfunctional in respect to the purposes that make the activity significant. That is because what scope and degree of physical or mental impairment are experienced as substantially (as opposed to moderately or minimally) limiting an activity depend on what outcomes the activity is usually expected to attain, and these change as the prevalent social, political and economic arrangements and objectives and cultural values, alter. So an impairment may be experienced as negligible in a context in which the activities it precludes are unimportant, but as substantially limiting in a context in which those same activities are crucial to flourishing. For example, it is well known that mild mental retardation is negligibly limiting to women in low-technology societies in which a woman's role is to clean, cook and bear children but substantially limiting in high-technology societies in which women also need literacy and computational skills. That is because the activities that are significant for women in low technology environments do not demand high levels of cognitive performance, while those significant for women in advanced technology environments do so.[20]

It is, further, not always, or even often, clear whether devices that correct impairment thereby eliminate dysfunction. Corrective devices are quite commonly effective in some circumstances but less so in others. For example, a prosthesis might "relieve" an amputee's inability to run for short distances but be ineffective (because of the injurious way running with the prosthesis impacts the stump) for long distances. Whether or not the prosthesis fully corrects the individual's physical impairment or leaves him or her substantially limited in respect to the major life activity of running thus turns on whether his or her activities include sprinting or, instead, running marathons. Broadly, whether he or she is considered to function in a normal rather than a limited way will depend on whether he or she finds him- or herself in a context in which distance running is a normal expectation. So in a sedentary society an individual with a prosthetic lower limb who is not substantially limited in walking or running is easily conceivable.

This brings us to a related reason why a functional definition of disability does not sustain a clear line between correctable and irreparable impairments. The statute itself does not define what counts as a major life activity. It is evident that how important anyone considers an activity to be results from a confluence of social ideals with personal life plans. For example, not everyone in every society views the ability to dress oneself as vital. In societies arranged to indulge the rich and highly ranked, these kinds of persons are freed by the labor of others from having to do so. In such a society, dressing oneself would be a peripheral activity reserved for unimportant people, much as the activity of killing one's food is not given a thought by most people in our society. It is unlikely, in such a society, that being unable to dress oneself would be viewed as limiting important activity. And if neither anomalously limited individuals nor those who engage with them experience the limitations as defects or losses, it is hard to understand why they should be designated "disabilities." This example indicates how contextualized to both personal and interpersonal purposes and practices the attribution of disability is.

Learning is an important activity for youngsters, but is it always a major life activity? Limitations on how much and what we can learn commonly appear as we age, although they do not always do so. Nor is this considered abnormal, for in our culture (unlike some others), elderly people are seldom called on for demonstrations of erudition or wisdom. From a social point of view, then, whether learning is a major life activity is relative to age, but that relativity is itself relative to culture.

Of course, some people do savor lifelong learning, and for these individuals learning is constantly a central element of their life plans. Any such person will count herself to be substantially limited in respect to a crucial life activity if impaired memory or intellect abridges her capability to learn. But many others, perhaps the majority of our citizens, find no need for learning once youth is past, nor any joy in doing so. They prefer to rely only on previously acquired knowledge and skills. For such citizens, becoming unable to learn is a negligible difficulty. Learning is by no means a major life activity for them, nor do increasing limitations on executing it disrupt their life plans. Consequently, even substantial limitations on their learning are not disabilities.

Yet it seems peculiar to think of some elderly people who have become unable to learn as disabled while others, equally limited in respect to learning, are not disabled, and to allow that this kind of difference between then depends upon how consistently learning has been central to their life plans. Yet not to do so appears to mean that depending on the centrality of learning in their prior lives, some elders with substantial reductions in learning ability would be protected against disability discrimination in virtue of their impairment while others with the same impairment would not be. Implications like this argue against thinking that, for the purposes of disability discrimination law, we can simply observe whether an individual is dysfunctional and thereby easily clarify whether the person is disabled.

Dysfunction Is Relative to the Price of Opportunity. So far we have seen that whether an individual with a physical or mental impairment is to be counted as being substantially dysfunctional is contingent on both personal and social expectations. Judgments of functionality thereby are relativized to the kind and level of activity required for common social practices, to the individual's own life plan, and to such variables as the individual's age and station in life. Yet another consideration likewise contextualizes how significantly physical or mental impairments limits activity and achievement. Agreement about this matter is hard to achieve wherever there are differences about what scope of opportunity is desirable or indispensable for flourishing.

Whether an individual overcomes impediment to execute fully an activity hampered by her impairment often depends on what the cost, to the individual or to society, of doing so happens to be. On the Court's criterion that direness of impairment is to be assessed in respect to an individual's present rather than potential conduct, is such an individual—who can run to save her life, but reasonably does not do so absent life-threatening circumstance because it is so painful or difficult—substantially limited in performing a major life activity? The Court's view in its first ADA case, *Bragdon v. Abbott,*[21] suggests that she may be if her hesitation to overcome the limitation is reasonable. The Court found the plaintiff to be disabled because her HIV infection substantially limited her in respect to the major life activity of reproduction. While the infection had not impaired her reproductive organs and she was physically able to conceive, the circumstances it created—increased risk of infecting a partner, of transmitting illness to the child, and of inflicting the costs of partner's and child's medical treatment on the state—seemed to the Court to be sufficient to deter a responsible individual from motherhood and thereby to preclude her from engaging in a major life activity. For an HIV-infected individual to engage in reproductive activity seemed to the Court to be "dangerous to the public health" and potentially costly to the public coffer as well.

Thus other-regarding reasons influence whether an impairment remains substantially limiting even if it can be mitigated. An individual who can mitigate an impairment and thereby function still is limited, and consequently disabled, if it is in the public interest for her not to function. To grasp the complexity of deciding this issue, think about whether individuals with lower-limb prostheses are too limited to participate in competitive sports like track. Although at one time lower-leg amputees were deemed noncompetitive because their prostheses made them run too slowly, now they are deemed noncompetitive because their prostheses make them run too fast.[22] New materials and designs have created specially springy sports prostheses that permit their wearers to run faster than can be done with fleshly feet, so using these corrective devices is banned in competitive running to prevent unfairly disadvantaging nondisabled runners in the competition.

There is a further contextualizing condition which also truncates opportunity on the basis of disability but not on the basis of dysfunction. One can be substantially limited, based on being physically or mentally impaired, but at the same time be fully functional physically and mentally. The mere presence of a physical or mental anomaly can shrivel the person's opportunity to engage in those practices that make the activity significant for people's lives. To illustrate, a person with controlled epilepsy is five times as likely to be unemployed as her nonimpaired counterpart.[23] Nor is it unusual, to take another example, for persons who have suffered severely disfiguring facial injuries or burns to be ignored and made to feel unwelcome. As Sander Gilman observes, deformation of the face "[is] the worst thing: [the] discomfort is of the observer not the patient."[24] Suppose such a disfigured individual applies for a position which she is well qualified to fill, but is denied the job because other workers feel discomfort in her presence. Our hypothetical employer thereby echoes the values expressed by the Supreme Court of Wisconsin when it excluded a boy with cerebral palsy from school because he "produces a depressing and nauseating effect on the teachers and school children."[25] Could the rejected applicant in this case qualify for protection under the ADA? She is not unable to execute fully the usual repertoire of human actions, nor is she regarded by the employer as unable to do so. From the view on which individuals are members of the class protected against disability discrimination only in virtue of their being substantially dysfunctional, she is not disabled and therefore not protected. Yet it is hard to see why she is less deserving of protection from disability discrimination than persons whose movement or cognition is substantially limited.

Historically, aversion to physical and corporeal anomalies has been a cause both of judging people to be disabled and of isolating and segregating them in virtue of their disabilities.[26] Undoubtedly, individuals whose impairments discomfort, alarm or sadden others have been prominent among those who meet a standard Justice Ginsburg applied in *Sutton* to determine whether people who exhibit a particular kind of difference deserve heightened protection against discrimination, namely, the standard that they "coalesce as historical victims of discrimination."[27] Moreover, because others find their anomalies alarming, such individuals are especially vulnerable to the isolation and segregation which Congress, in its ADA "Findings," declares must be remedied.

To engage with people who have extraordinary corporeal or cognitive anomalies confronts us with the facticity of being disturbingly different, a threatening dimension of life. Historically, this challenge was deflected by banning such individuals from facilities and programs which would have placed them in the presence of ordinary people. The rationale for doing so was couched in language remarkably similar to that used during the same period to promote the separation of women from professional and commercial endeavors and the segregation of people of color in the use of public facilities. For all three groups— women, people of color and people with disabilities—prohibitions against the presence of their members in various social domains were absolved by appealing to the dispossessed's presumed frailties of corpus, cognition and character, and to the consequent burdens and dangers their presence in public posed both for them and for the common good.

Misreadings of their biological anomalies created a context so hostile to their personal traits as to render them socially dysfunctional. Although their impairments were mitigated, compensated for, or benign, people with extraordinary corporeal or cognitive conditions were (and continue to be) isolated, ostracized, impoverished, institutionalized and denied access to ordinary opportunity, and thereby were substantially limited by society in executing major life activities out of fear of their purported special needs and the imagined burden imposed on the public by their company.

RETROSPECTIVE AND PROSPECTIVE PROTECTION

Having observed that function and dysfunction are complexly contextualized—to personal and social expectations and to the price of pursuing opportunity under conditions of benign or hostile practices, arrangements and environments—we might imagine that the solution to the conceptual quandaries we have observed so far is to understand that judgments about protected class membership must be individualized. Justice O'Connor points out that the statutory definition of "disability" is said to be "with respect to an individual," and takes this phrase to mean that "whether a person has a disability under the ADA is an individualized inquiry."[28] But an individualized inquiry as to whether a person meets a standard cannot escape measuring the person under scrutiny against some prototype. Some procedure of generalized reference to the distinguishing features of disability therefore seems unavoidable.

Citing the Court's earlier discussion of this matter in *Bragdon v. Abbott,* Justice O'Connor in *Sutton* quotes: "The determination of whether an individual has a disability is not necessarily based on the name or diagnosis of the impairment the person has, but rather on the effect of that impairment on the life of the individual."[29] The problem with categorizing according to diagnosis, she believes, is that it "would create a system in which persons often must be treated as members of a group of people with similar impairments, rather than as individuals."[30] Because Justice O'Connor insists that no diagnosis is definitive of disability, she would presumably extend her principle so as to agree that no one is disabled simply because he has an injury such as a severed spinal cord or an impairment such as blindness. To decide whether a physical or mental condition is disabling, we must investigate whether it has a substantially negative effect on how that individual leads his life.

As we have seen, however, making this determination is not simple. Nor can it be as easily restricted to evidence about the present moment as the majority's language suggests.[31] That is because whether medication or corrective devices are effective in repairing or compensating for an impairment often depends on the prevailing environment. Individuals with diabetes that is completely controlled by medication very often require that accommodating working conditions be maintained: a work schedule and work site that permits frequent testing of blood sugar level and the administration of effective medication, permission to keep certain food products at the workplace, the opportunity to comply with a rigid schedule for meals, and so on. As long as the employer permits these arrangements, the employee's condition is fully remediated and the individual is, on the Court's criterion, not legally protected against disability discrimination.

But suppose a new manager disturbs the arrangement. On the Court's analysis, the individual whose diabetes is mitigated by medication is not protected and so has no legal recourse against changes in the work environment that vitiate the effectiveness of her medication. On this interpretation, the ADA cannot help her to deflect or dodge environmental transformations that threaten to send her diabetes out of control. Once that happens, of course, her current state of health will be one limited by serious illness, at which point, after the fact of the onset of dysfunction, presumably the act's protection will embrace her.[32]

What needs to be recognized, of course, is that individuals whose impairments are controlled, corrected or compensated for in a favorable environment nevertheless are extremely inelastic in respect to maintaining function when the arrangements on which they rely are altered. In such circumstances, the environment transforms from benign to hostile. This is true not only of individuals whose impairments can be mitigated, but also of those whose impairments are unalleviated but do not presently interfere with their execution of activities of major importance to them.

Protecting Those Vulnerable to Dysfunction

Noticing that the ADA explicitly directs that barriers created by past practice be removed, it is reasonable to ask whether protection against the unnecessary imposition of dysfunction on the basis of impairment should not be prospective as well as retrospective. If barriers that presently occasion dysfunction are vehicles of disability discrimination, it is hard to see how initiating new barriers could escape being equally discriminatory. It thus is reasonable to expect that protection against disability discrimination should extend beyond (the effects of) practices that now make people with impairments substantially more dysfunctional than they need be to (the effects of) practices that threaten to do so in future.

It follows from this prospective aspect of antidiscrimination protection that people who have not yet suffered from discrimination but who are especially vulnerable to it reasonably expect to be included in the protected class. People whose impairments make them extraordinarily vulnerable to being made dysfunctional by seemingly innocuous alternations in their environments are substantially limited simply in virtue of their hypervulnerability. This point drives to the conclusion that individuals who are currently functioning because their biological deficits have been mitigated or surmounted but whose corporeal or cognitive impairments leave them unusually vulnerable to socially induced dysfunction are something more than hypothetically disabled.

The same conclusion is reached by analogy. People of color and women are protected against race and sex discrimination even if they have not (yet) personally been denied opportunity on the basis of their race or sex. Nor are they properly described as being merely hypothetically or potentially diminished by racial or sexist discrimination or as hypothetical or potential members of the classes protected against it.

Vulnerability to Dysfunction

Why would antidiscrimination law distinguish invidiously between persons who are extraordinary vulnerable to being made dysfunctional by biased practice, and persons who are already dysfunctional, at least in part because of biased practice? One explanation is that the courts tend to implement prohibitions against discrimination so as to favor paradigmatic members of the protected class. But should individuals who do not presently suffer from disability discrimination be bereft of protection against it because they insufficiently approximate both the paradigm of being functional and the paradigm of being dysfunctional? As Kimberle Crenshaw has perspicaciously argued, protecting people against oppression should not be limited by "the extent that their experiences are recognizably similar to those whose experiences tend to be reflected in antidiscrimination doctrine."[33] The ADA's emphasis on individualized inquiry cited by Justice O'Connor draws on an understanding about the impact of discrimination that has long existed in civil rights law. For instance, in 1978, in determining that it is discriminatory to make pension benefits more costly for individuals who happen to be women than for individuals who happen to be men, the Supreme Court explained: "The [Civil Rights Act] statute's focus on the individual is unambiguous. It precludes treatment of individuals as simply components of a class. . . . Even a true generalization about the class is an insufficient reason for disqualifying an individual to whom the generalization does not apply. It is equally true . . . that all individuals in the respective class do not share the characteristic that differentiates average class representatives."[34]

Antidiscrimination protection surely should not be limited just to people whose experience reiterates that which initially or centrally prompted the protective policy. Contemporary young women need to be as thoroughly safeguarded by the law against sexist practices as their grandmothers are, although their suffering is quite different and their opportunities much less drastically curtailed by bias against women than their grandmothers' losses and constricted options. And immigrants from Africa and tenth-generation African-Americans have similar needs to be secured against racism, although members of these two groups do not equally suffer the residual effects of the American practice of slavery.

Individuals have standing in a class protected against racial or sexual discrimination in virtue of their extraordinary vulnerability to that kind of discrimination. By having such standing, they can seek redress for harms visited upon them by specific racist or sexist acts. By analogy, then, we would expect individuals who are especially susceptible to the constrictions disability discrimination imposes on confidence and ambition not to be excluded from the class that has standing to seek redress—that is, not to be unprotected against disability discrimination.

We have seen so far that whether or not individuals are disabled by their impairments—in the sense of being made dysfunctional and unable to engage successfully in the activities requisite to their being productive and fulfilled—is importantly contingent upon their being positioned in an environment that supports mitigating or surmounting the impairment. People who can be confident of maintaining such an environment are less likely to be debilitated by awareness of their vulnerability to disability discrimination than people whose assurance of stability and security is negligible. Consequently, they will be less susceptible to stifling of the ambition that is needed to energize activity pursuant to achieving major life goals.

Protecting Those Vulnerable to Disability Discrimination

Who are these people, the ones who, though impaired, can rely on enjoying an environment that supports their performance, however dependent on corrective or compensatory measures their functioning may be? Answering this question is crucial to determining how to delineate the class of individuals extraordinarily vulnerable to and therefore deserving of protection against disability discrimination. We begin to answer by considering whether the impact impairments have on the execution of life activities fluctuates in concert with random alterations in the social environment, or whether there is a pattern to how changes in social arrangements aggravate any deleterious impact of physical and mental impairments. Is there a basis for predicting that people with certain kinds of impairments will only rarely be made dysfunctional by how the socially manipulated environment is arranged, while people with other kinds of impairments have a heightened susceptibility to dysfunction occasioned by disadvantageous social practices and policies? If such correlations can be discerned, protection can be better directed toward people whose impairments make them likely victims of disability discrimination.

It is useful to notice in regard to this point that in *Sutton* the Court supposed population statistics to be of relevance in determining the scope of the disability class, despite the fact that these data do not differentiate between corrected and unmitigated impairments. The Court notes that a hundred million Americans (more than one third of the population) have visual impairments, fifty million suffer from hypertension, and 28 million are hearing-impaired. Justice Ginsburg cites Congress's intent "to restrict the ADA's coverage to a confined, and historically disadvantaged, class." She continues: "And persons whose uncorrected eyesight is poor, or who rely on daily medication for their well-being, can be found in every social and economic class; they do not cluster among the politically powerless, nor do they coalesce as historical victims of discrimination."[35]

One premise of this remark clearly is correct. Generally, we do not think of every physical and mental limit as an impairment. For example, although running a mile in under four minutes is within human capacity, people who cannot do so are not considered to be impaired. That is because most people cannot do so. Further, not only do we eschew establishing practices that require us to be four-minute-mile runners in order to be functional, but we have also developed prostheses—commonly known as cars—to facilitate traveling a mile in less than four minutes without having to run.

The lesson here seems to be that the environment we fashion for ourselves facilitates common modes of performance, especially if these advance the ambitions of the majority who can execute them, even at the price of disregarding or disadvantaging minorities. To illustrate, the sighted majority's mild preference for pictures over text overshadows the blind minority's urgent need for text rather than pictures, with the result that the supplanting of computer program menus by graphical interfaces shrank employment for blind people even in a worker-hungry job market in which employment for other historically out-of-work groups shot upward.[36]

Jim Cox, product planner for the Encarta line of reference titles at Microsoft, exemplifies how the majority population's tastes trump considerations of inclusiveness and productivity for the entire population in the development of technology. Asked why the Encarta line still does not include the accessibility for visually impaired users that Microsoft incorporated in the Windows 98 operating system with the "active accessibility" feature, he replied:

> The . . . Encarta product line has been a tremendous success in part because it creates an environment that is inviting, comfortable, intuitive, and beautiful for our sighted users. In a very short time, it became clear that a significant part of Encarta's success has been due to the fact that the custom interface gives us a unique identity. Over the past few years, we have struggled with accessibility issues. We feel that we cannot simply scrap our custom look and feel and adopt a standard Windows user interface. To do so would take away a large amount of reason that sighted users like our product and prefer it over our competition.[37]

What these observations suggest is that another of Justice Ginsburg's premises is faulty. We cannot presume that the current collective socioeconomic success of persons who are physically or mentally impaired in a specific way demonstrates a reasonably strong probability of their continued thriving.

Some commentators explain the special vulnerability to exclusion imparted by impairments as being the natural consequence of being biologically flawed. For instance, Norman Daniels and his followers believe that: "we can take as fixed, primarily by nature, a generally uncontroversial baseline of species-typical functioning."[38] The thought here is that the way the species typically functions constitutes a natural and therefore a neutral standard to which the public can assent. Were this the case, we would seem to have biological authorization to adopt whatever practices enhance the modes of functioning that typify our species, even if these exacerbate the disadvantage of individuals who fall below the natural human standard. For example, because we naturally communicate by speaking to each other, the dominance of the practice of telephoning might be thought to reflect no social choice but simply our instinctive preference for amplifying the oral performance that is natural to our species.

If there are natural modes and levels of human performance that characterize our species, then the functioning of individuals whose corporeal or cognitive impairments preclude their engaging in the relevant kinds and degrees of activity will be less than normal. On this account, the biological limitations of those who are impaired make it naturally difficult for them to flourish. It is this unfortunate circumstance that renders them especially susceptible to exclusion, for social practice evolves to facilitate using the full range of species-typical proficiencies. Individuals whose performances fail to achieve normal levels or to be executed in normal modes thus need protection from the consequences of their personal lack of competence.

But there are problems with this account. For it seems odd to think that some technological practices are natural to us, while others are not. Telephoning, which disadvantages deaf people, is no more natural an activity than teletyping, even though we learn to talk before we learn to type. Telephoning now is being superseded by e-mailed typed text. To take another example, we naturally pump our legs when we walk. But it would be ludicrous to insist that bicycling gives us a more natural technology for mobilizing than donkey-riding or auto-driving do.

Further, Daniels to the contrary, the influence of social context defies determining what level of performance is natural to the species. Among human males, strong competitors are supposed to reproduce more abundantly than weak ones, so their inheritable traits should become typical of the species. As we have seen, however, the kind of performance crucial to being a strong competitor is relative to the demands levied and compensations made available in the artifactual environment. As an environment becomes physically forgiving (for example, requires less physical prowess and endurance to thrive), the typical levels of performances involving strength and stamina are reduced; the reverse is true if an environment turns unforgiving and harsh.

This last discussion shapes a response to our initial question about the rationale for extending the protection of the law to safeguard people against disability discrimination. Corporeal and cognitive impairments dispose individuals to dysfunction, which, in turn, occasions susceptibility to disability discrimination and the accompanying unfair deprivation of opportunity. But it is equally important to recognize that impairment is neither identical to nor entails dysfunction. To specify a biological standard below which dysfunction occurs and above which it is absent seems to be unworkable because the difference between being disposed to dysfunction and actually being dysfunctional often turns on the hostility or benignity of the socially organized environment. Consequently, there is no degree of biological limitation that serves as the fixed line between being extraordinarily vulnerable to disability discrimination and being normally safe from it. Because we cannot even say, apart from considerations of social context, whether corporeal and cognitive deficiencies will narrow opportunity, their natural biological limitations do not appear to be why people need nor why they deserve protection against disability discrimination.

PROTECTING THE DISABLED MINORITY

If no modes and levels of performance are authorized by nature as preeminent, why are some of them—such as keen hearing, 20/20 vision, energetic walking and running—so influential in shaping our practices along lines that disadvantage individuals whose biological limitations detract from these common proficiencies? Here the global adoption of graphical interfaces—operated using a computer mouse—suggests an explanation. Clicking on icons is no more effective a method of entering computer commands than typing in texts. But clicking on icons requires less effort—in learning and in executing—than typing texts. Although most people can do either, their predilection for effortless exercise propels the weight of their numbers behind the seemingly easier activity. And the prospect that altering a practice to please the majority would relegate a minority of people—those with certain impairments—to the margins of opportunity is hardly ever cause for hesitation in the marketplace.

Were a majority rather than a minority of users mobility- and hearing-impaired, the initial designs of public transportation and communication systems would have accommodated them, making unnecessary the remodeling expenditures needed to include them later on. To project how living with a particular impairment would be different had history been otherwise and different social practices or arrangements had obtained is an exercise of the imagination I have elsewhere called "historical counterfactualizing."[39] This exercise permits us to assess whether an exclusionary practice is the arbitrary instrument of majority power. Such historical counterfactualizing facilitates our identifying what features of our artifactual environment persist because of the pervasive belief that people with physical, sensory or cognitive impairments, being a minority, have no claim on social participation. It helps us see what components of practice exist because people with certain physical and mental conditions have traditionally been, as described in the section of Congress's "Findings" to which Justice Ginsburg refers, in "a position of political powerlessness in our society, . . . resulting from stereotypic assumptions not truly indicative of the individual ability of such individuals."[40]

Not all outcomes of historical counterfactualizing lead to this result. Consider the following application. Although responsive to the historical exclusion that makes employment available to a smaller percentage of individuals with disabilities than of any other U.S. minority, the ADA does not mandate the provision of compensatory income for people with disabilities. Is this equitable to a group that historically has been penalized in the workplace? Here counterfactualizing reveals nothing arbitrary nor inequitable if society supplies no such compensation. For there is no reason to think that, were the disabled the majority instead of the minority, they could command compensatory income. Were most people disabled, it would surely be very difficult for the able-bodied minority to care for and sustain so many people with disabilities. Were the nondisabled in the minority, it is less rather than more likely that they could guarantee to provide subsistence for the disabled. Thus testing hypotheses by counterfactualizing helps us distinguish between what is denied people with disabilities because they perform differently from the majority of the population, and what is denied because of their biological conditions.

Counterfactualizing also helps us to apply the Ginsburg test by distinguishing between impairments correlated with powerlessness, and impairments that are not. Although we have examined some of the difficulties with the Court's reasons (in *Sutton*) for denying that corrected myopia is not a disability, we still may have an hunch that impairments amenable to correction with common types of lenses (spectacles or contact lenses) are not disabilities *per se*. When we counterfactualize, we understand better why they are not.

Which of our practices would be different if the majority of people used glasses or contact lenses? Nothing substantial would be different. So many people now correct their vision with lenses that enormous support for doing so is diffused through our culture. For instance, to keep spectacles intact, a convention warns us against hitting guys with glasses. Our shops are replete with the paraphernalia of lenswear: cases for spectacles and contacts, cleaning cloths and cleaning chemicals, and a variety of implements to facilitate wearing them. All this is to say that corrective lens wearers form a formidable market force. So it seems unlikely that myopics are much disregarded in commercial and civic organizations.

Compare the situation for people with diabetes. If most of us had diabetes, many things would be different. Most processed foods would be made without sugar. Work sites would offer privacy for employees to engage in necessary medical procedures, and work schedules would allow for a systematic approach to meals. Individuals would be facilitated in sitting rather than standing for their work, so they would not exacerbate the neuropathies or ulcers that often accompany diabetes.[41] Notice that because these reforms are compatible with productivity, social reorganization to create an environment more supportive of the pursuit of opportunity for people with diabetes does not curtail opportunity for other people. Here counterfactualizing indicates the heightened susceptibility of people with diabetes to disability discrimination, shown by the pervasive disadvantages our predominant social arrangements now impose on them, whereas no similar indications of majority-imposed disadvantage appeared when we counterfactualized by hypothesizing that people who correct their vision with lenses (contacts or spectacles) were in the majority.

But disadvantage is not tantamount to discrimination. To be so, the identified disadvantage must unfairly reduce opportunity below the level most people expect and enjoy, as occurs when inflexible workplace regulations prevent individuals, on the basis of their having diabetes, from participating in employment and contributing to society. By historical counterfactualizing, we can discover which people have the kinds of impairments that make them especially vulnerable to unfairly reduced opportunity and therefore to disability discrimination.

People with disabilities deserve protection not because they suffer from unfortunate biological limitations that make them unequal, but rather because they suffer from artificial and arbitrary social arrangements that treat them as unequal.[42] Historical counterfactualizing helps reveal not only those practices that are oppressive, but also the groups of people most vulnerable to them. Of course, it is unlikely that any court would be fully satisfied by such a purely conceptual inquiry as historical counterfactualizing. Consequently, historical counterfactualizing needs to be supplemented by empirical investigation of the historical development of practices and institutions that impose exclusion based on disability.

As Mary Crossley points out: "Courts will still have to draw lines if asked to apply a standard like 'physical characteristic associated with social, cultural, or economic disadvantage.' They will still have to answer questions such as: How serious must the disadvantage be?"[43] However, this question is simply a more generalized and theorized version of the inquiry that, according to Crossley, "echo[es] the questions that courts are struggling with today regarding, for example, how limited a person's employment options must be in order to be substantially limited."[44] No doubt, pursuing this inquiry demands we pay thorough and thoughtful attention to our understanding of both the mandates and the limits of achieving equality in civic and commercial life.

For instance, while democratic morality frowns on practice that has a disparately negative impact on minorities, little agreement exists as to the degree to which a group may be disadvantaged before special statutory protection for it is required. Should a practice's mild benefits for the majority weigh sufficiently to justify dismissing the profound difficulties it poses for the minority? Adding closed captioning to television does not compromise and sometimes enhances the majority's experience of the programs. As the cost of doing so is not great, relative to the full costs of production and transmission, it seems unfair not to modify practice so as to add text to talk on television to prevent the minority of deaf people from being excluded.

In contrast, requiring everyone to be bilingual by knowing both a spoken language and sign language appears to some to carry a great cost for the non-Signing group, although it is worthwhile noting that an analogous transformation was executed in the reestablishment of French as the official language of Quebec. In respect to this last example, Charles Taylor argues that justice requires cultivating openness to a fusion of horizons that has the power to take us beyond "our own limited part in the whole human story."[45] (Parenthetically, it is not the ADA that first prompted concern about the social costs extracted by having to learn, transform and compromise in order to accommodate the variations in performance modes of different kinds of people. Many of us are old enough to recall the obfuscatory fuss directed at the imagined costs of equalizing employment opportunities for women. Objections ranged from the expense of providing uniforms and equipment in women's sizes, to the liability of their being in stressful and strenuous positions when their hormones reputedly rage uncontrolled, to the disruptions of commercial practice resulting from the inability to conduct crucial business in the men's room. These memories should warn us against rushing to assess the price of social change as exorbitant absent a plausible scheme for computing the expense of accepting and engaging with difference.)

CONCLUSION: PROTECTING NO ONE

Establishing who is disabled is a threshold decision only. This verdict merely permits an individual to seek a further verdict, namely, a determination as to whether disability discrimination has actually occurred. Does pursuing an approach focused on the plaintiff's potential for being arbitrarily excluded to a substantial degree from civic and commercial activity promise greater clarity than the alternative focus on the current magnitude of the plaintiff's deficiencies? Even if each approach generates its share of borderline cases and controversial decisions, we should notice that there is an element of the latter that commentators on the *Sutton* decision who take a disability perspective view with special alarm.

Speaking for the National Council on Disability, Andrew Imparato warns: "Under the decisions last week, people bringing ADA claims will need to emphasize the negative about their impairment and how it affects them, as if they were applying for disability retirement benefits. The evidence they submit to demonstrate their disability can and will be used against them when they seek to demonstrate their qualifications for the position they are seeking." As Arlene Mayerson and Matthew Diller point out: "The crabbed interpretation delivered by the Supreme Court puts a rejected applicant with a disability in the untenable position of emphasizing all the things he or she cannot do in order to claim ADA protection, and then once through the courthouse door, to downplay limitations in order to prove he or she is qualified for the job. . . . By attempting to limit the ADA to the 'truly disabled,' the Supreme Court continues to look at disability as a matter for pity rather than equality."[46]

This gets to the argument for the preferability of constructing the class the ADA protects in terms of vulnerability to arbitrary social exclusion based on corporeal or cognitive impairment, rather than constructing it in terms of personal deficiency. Unlike earlier policies protecting people against other kinds of discrimination, enforcement of and litigation conducted under the ADA has focused not on competence but on dysfunction. But as the federal report that established the need for new civil rights legislation to protect people with disabilities pointed out: "For persons who have spent many years of their lives stressing their abilities rather than their limitations . . . the need to prove that one is a 'handicapped individual' can be very undesirable."[47]

Traditional civil rights laws do not make people claiming the right to equal opportunity meet the threshold requirement of establishing membership in a protected class.[48] By safeguarding from disability discrimination only those seen as deficient and as requiring protection because they are pitiable, rather than covering all those whose competence is compromised by the deficiencies of social practice biased against individuals with impairments, the courts threaten to make enfeeblement the price of protection under the ADA. That is, they require individuals damaged by a stereotype to accede to that stereotype in order to be protected against it. In effect, they deny the intelligibility of extending the tradition of equal protection for minorities against arbitrary practice based on stereotyping to the ADA's definitive protected class. In doing so, they leave even individuals incontestably included in the ADA's protected class unprotected.

NOTES

[1]Susan Sherwin. *No Longer Patient.* Philadelphia: Temple University Press, 1992, 182.
[2]Rosalind Miles. *A Women's History of the World.* London: Michael Joseph, 1988, 187.
[3]42 U.S.C. § 12101(a)(9).
[4]42 U.S.C. § 12101(a)(2).
[5]42 U.S.C. § 12102(2).
[6]The National Council on Disability (NCOD) is an independent federal agency with a board appointed by the President of the United States and confirmed by the U.S. Senate. Its purpose is to promote policies, programs, practices and procedures that guarantee equal opportunity for all people with disabilities and to empower people with disabilities to achieve economic self-sufficiency, independent living, and inclusion and integration into all aspects of society. The quotation is from an NCOD press release dated June 28, 1999.
[7]*Albertsons, Inc. v. Kirkingburg,* 1999 U.S. LEXIS 4369 (1999); *Murphy v. United Parcel Service, Inc.,* 1999 U.S. LEXIS 4379 (1999); *Sutton v. United Airlines, Inc.,* 1999 U.S. LEXIS 4371 (1999).
[8]42 U.S.C. § 12111(b)(3).
[9]1999 U.S. LEXIS 4371, at *22.
[10]Press Release from Lambda Legal Defense and Education Fund, "Disappointing ADA Rulings Threaten Protections for Workers with Disabilities: 'Catch-22' Created for People Who Are Able to Overcome Their Impairments," New York, June 23, 1999
[11]Ellen Goodman, "The Court's Nearsightedness," *Boston Globe* Sunday, June 27, 1999. F7.
[12]See Iris Young's "Disability and the Definition of Work," this volume, for a discussion of the impact of violating this thesis.
[13]1999 U.S. LEXIS *35–36.
[14]John Hockenberry, "Disability Games," *New York Times,* June 29, 1999. A19.
[15]1999 U.S. LEXIS *22.
[16]1999 U.S. LEXIS *31.
[17]1999 U.S. LEXIS *32.

[18]Legislative history shows that in debating the language to be adopted in the ADA, Congress rejected defining disability by reference to a list of characteristics or diagnoses. This approach was eschewed largely to avoid an underinclusive protected class, for some conditions—especially those not yet diagnosed—would be absent. A secondary consideration is the desirability of avoiding hypermedicalized litigation focusing on conflicting assessments of the plaintiff's medical condition. See Mary Crossley, "The Disability Kaleidoscope," *Notre Dame L. Rev.* 74 (1999): 621–716.

[19]1999 U.S. LEXIS *29.

[20]Christopher Murray and Allan Lopez, eds. *The Global Burden of Disease.* Cambridge, MA: Harvard School of Health, 1996, 33.

[21]524 U.S. 624 (1998).

[22]For discussions of similar cases, in which accommodating a mobility-impaired golfer with golf cart transport and accommodating a manually impaired bowler with a bowling ball ramp were claimed to privilege the disabled sports participant unfairly, see Anita Silvers and David Wasserman, "Convention and Competence: Disability Rights in Sports and Education," Report from the Institute for Philosophy and Public Policy, vol. 18. no. 4 (Fall 1998): 1–7, 5.

[23]Arlene Mayerson and Matthew Diller, "The Supreme Court's Near-Sighted View of the ADA," this volume.

[24]Quoted by Jonathan Cole, "Stealing Beauty," *Times Literary Supplement,* no. 5023, July 9, 1999, 8–9, 9, in a review of Sander Gilman's *Making the Body Beautiful: A Cultural History of Aesthetic Surgery,* Princeton: Princeton University Press, 1999.

[25]Cited in Record of Senate Hearings, testimony supporting the passage of the ADA was filled with narratives about how disabled citizens were expelled from auctions (because they were "disgusting to look at"), from theaters ("I don't want her in here"), from zoos (because they "upset the chimpanzees"), and a bank (because the customer "did not fit the image the bank wished to project"), and from other commercial, educational and recreational sites to which the rest of the public was welcomed. Americans with Disabilities Act: Record of Senate Hearings, May/June 1989. See also 117 Cong. Rec. 45,974 (1971) (remarks of Rep. Vanek).

[26]Trent. *Inventing the Feeble Mind.* Berkeley: University of California Press, 1994, chaps. 1–4, pp. 230, 253, 298. Also see "Mpho ya Modimo—A Gift From God: Perspectives on 'Attitudes' Toward Disabled Persons," where Benedicte Ingstad describes how institutionalization in Africa similarly debilitated the productivity of a cognitively disabled individual. In the case she reports, the individual was institutionalized at age eight at the behest of rehabilitation professionals. After repeated requests while he grew to adulthood, the family was able to bring him home, but only on condition that he be locked up. He was unable to communicate and was often violent. However, over the years they were unable to maintain his incarceration. As he was less and less restrained, he acquired communication skills, began to perform work around the house—sweeping and chopping and, eventually, took up life as a goatherd. This was the kind of work people with cognitive impairments often performed in the U.S. prior to the institutionalization movement. In *Disability and Culture,* eds. Benedicte Ingstadt and Susan Reynolds White. Berkeley: University of California Press, 1995, 246–266.

[27]1999 U.S. LEXIS 4371, at *42 (Ginsburg, J., concurring).

[28]1999 U.S. LEXIS 4371, at *22.

[29]1999 U.S. LEXIS 4371, at *23.

[30]1999 U.S. LEXIS 4371, at *23–24.

[31]Notice that Justice Ginsburg's concurring reference to the historical association between kinds of impairments and the social disadvantage and political powerlessness associated with the impairment lies very uneasily alongside the majority's emphasis on determining the present degree of correction of any impairment.

[32]Further consideration of this example reveals the precipitateness of the downward slope on which the Court's approach has set protection of workers with disabilities. Even after the illness of the employee in this example becomes uncontrolled, the employer could maintain she is not disabled because she is not precluded from the class of job she heretofore has executed. She is, in fact, precluded only from working for employers who arbitrarily prohibit her maintaining the necessary medication schedule. Because there are hypothetical reasonable employers for whom she could work if they exist, she is not substantially limited in a major life activity and therefore is not disabled according to the Court's interpretation. Thus, the employer could argue, there is no requirement to accommodate her by

modifying workplace rules to permit her to monitor her condition and administer the corrective medication. Notice that this line of argument unfairly places several burdens on employees with disabilities. To obtain accommodations necessary to the continued correction of their disabling condition, they must prove that other employers do not make accommodations so there is no other place they can work. This means that the success of workers in gaining accommodation at a few places of employment defeats broader access to employment in the class of jobs and segregates workers with the impairment to just a few worksites. Such an outcome surely is antithetical to the intent of Congress to end the segregation of people with disabilities. Further, to suggest that employers can defend against having to accommodate an otherwise qualified worker by hypothesizing that someone else might do it defeats Congress's clear intention to assign responsibility for the social inclusion of individuals with disabilities to those who most directly interact with them. A system in which such responsibility is passed to a third party quickly devolves into one that identifies specialists in dealing with the disabled and special places where such dealings may occur—that is, into precisely the kind of institutional isolation and segregation Congress intended the ADA to vanquish.

[33]Kimberle Crenshaw. "Demarginalizing the Intersection of Race and Sex: A Black Feminist Critique of Antidiscrimination Doctrine, Feminist Theory, and Antiracist Politics," in Jaggar, Alison, ed. *Living with Contradictions: Controversies in Feminist Social Ethics.* Boulder, CO: Westview Press, 1994, 39–52, 45.

[34]*Los Angeles Department of Water and Power v. Manhart,* 1978.

[35]1999 U.S. LEXIS 4371, at *42 (Ginsburg, J., concurring).

[36]Anita Silvers, David Wasserman, and Mary Mahowald. *Disability, Difference, Discrimination: Perspectives on Justice in Bioethics and Public Policy.* Lanham, MD: Rowman & Littlefield, 1998, 107–110, for an account of how public action can intervene beneficially in such market-driven processes.

[37]E-mail to Kelly Ford on file with the author. Parenthetically, when the majority population's interests are served, Microsoft does acknowledge the presence of people with impairments in the group of users. "When new techology is first introduced, it is often pretty cumbersome," says Greg Lowney, director of the Accessibility and Disabilities Group at Microsoft: "Mainstream audiences aren't willing to try it and quickly give up in frustration because the inconvenience outweighs the benefit it provides them. Microsoft relies on early adopters—such as . . . people with disabilities—to teach us how to make our products usable." Lowney listed voice recognition, artificial speech, ergonomic keyboards and portable devices as having been invented to serve as adaptive technology and as now being developed by Microsoft for the general market. "Technology Pioneered by and for People with Disabilities Benefits Everyone," Press Release from Microsoft, Redmond, Washington, July 26, 1999. On file with the author.

[38]Norman Daniels. "Justice and Health Care," in Donald Van DeVeer and Tom Regan, eds., *Health Care Ethics: An Introduction.* Philadelphia: Temple University Press, 1987, 290–325, 303.

[39]I introduced the technique of historical counterfactualizing in "Reconciling Equality to Difference: Caring (f)or Justice for People with Disabilities," *Hypatia: A Journal of Feminist Philosophy* 10 (Special Issue on Feminist Ethics and Social Policy), ed. Patrice DiQuinzo and Iris Marion Young, no. 1 (Winter 1995): 30–55. The usefulness of this way of testing whether the specifics of a practice are nothing more than responses to the preferences of the most populous or dominant group is explored further in *Disability, Difference, Discrimination,* 129–131. Historical counterfactualizing is an instrument for heightening the scrutiny of practices disadvantageous to minorities who have not enjoyed equality of protection. Its purpose is to free our imaginations from the constricting routine of institutionalized behaviors so that we are not misled into assuming that the familiarity of a practice signals its biological or economic necessity. Historical counterfactualizing is sometimes misread as being a technique for positive policy guidance, or a recipe for fair distribution of resources, or a method of articulating a political ideal. Historical counterfactualizing is only a test for discerning the effects of political exclusion or oppression. But justice does not equate to the absence of political exclusion or oppression, so historical counterfactualizing does not offer a recipe for justice, nor is it any more appropriate than other instruments of heightened scrutiny for resolving conflicts of distributive interest.

[40]42 U.S.C. § 12101(7).

[41]It is not uncommon for employers to require individuals in certain kinds of jobs, such as retail sales, to remain on their feet when not waiting on customers, even if they have diabetes, a condition in which nonhealing ulcers result from pressure on the feet.

[42]In *City of Cleburne v. Cleburne Living Center, Inc.*, 473 U.S. 432 (1985), the Supreme Court declined to acknowledge that the mentally retarded are a "quasi-suspect" class. One reason given is that "if the large and amorphous class of the mentally retarded were deemed quasi-suspect, . . . it would be difficult to find a principled way to distinguish a variety of other groups who have perhaps immutable difficulties setting them off from others . . . and who can claim some degree of prejudice from at least part of the public at large. One need mention in this respect only the aging, the disabled, the mentally ill, and the infirm. We are reluctant to set out on that course, and we decline to do so." Two comments are useful here. First, in *Cleburne* the Court went on to state that the mentally retarded are not without protection because legislation cannot pick them out for invidious treatment unless the legislation furthers a legitimate government purpose. Yet in *Sutton* the Court permits employers to treat individuals with certain impairments invidiously regardless of whether the unequal treatment serves a legitimate employment purpose. Second, the *Cleburne* Court also argued that the mentally retarded are not politically powerless, and thus do not display a traditional characteristic of classes whose protection requires heightened scrutiny. To address this view of the matter, Congress included the following language in its findings: "individuals with disabilities are a discrete and insular minority who have been . . . subjected to a history of purposeful unequal treatment, and relegated to a position of political powerlessness." Robert Burgdorf, "The Americans with Disabilities Act: Analysis and Implications of a Second-Generation Civil Rights Statute," *Harv. C. R.-C. L. L. R.,* 26; 2 (1991): 413–522, 436.

[43]Mary Crossley, "The Disability Kaleidoscope," *Notre Dame L. R.* 74 (1999): 621–716, 713–714.

[44]Ibid., 714.

[45]Charles Taylor, Amy Gutmann, Stephen Rockefeller, Michael Walzer and Susan Wolf, *Multiculturalism and "The Politics of Recognition."* Princeton: Princeton University Press, 1992. See also Andy Lamey, "Francophonia Forever: The Contradiction in Charles Taylor's 'politics of recognition'." *Times Literary Supplement,* 5025 (July 23, 1999): 12–15, 13.

[46]"The Supreme Court's Near-Sighted View of the ADA," this volume, pp. 124–125.

[47]National Council on the Handicapped, *Toward Independence.* Washington, D.C.: Author, 1986, A22, 23.

[48]Robert Burgdorf, "Second-Generation Civil Rights Statute," 413–522, 442. See also National Council of the Handicapped, *Toward Independence,* 1986, "Proof of class membership is not required under other types of nondiscrimination laws, and statutes guaranteeing equal opportunity for persons with disabilities need not have such a requirement either. Such laws should focus upon the demonstration of discrimination 'on the basis of handicap' rather than requiring proof of membership in a protected class." A25.

Stigma without Impairment
Demedicalizing Disability Discrimination

DAVID WASSERMAN

INTRODUCTION

During oral argument in *Murphy v. U.P.S.* (1999), a case in which the Supreme Court was asked to decide whether the ADA covered individuals whose impairments are largely mitigated by assistive devices or medication, Justice Scalia removed his glasses and waved them in the air (Greenhouse 1999). He was making the point that if mitigation were ignored, he, along with millions of other Americans, would be swept into the category of "disabled," swelling its ranks far beyond the 43 million recognized by Congress when it adopted the statute a decade ago.

Justice Scalia's gesture nicely evokes a broader dispute about the scope of the ADA: between those who see it as limited to the relatively small proportion of the population marked by their functional limitations, material privation and social exclusion, and those who see the statute as applying to a broad and loosely bounded range of people stigmatized by physical and mental differences. The former believe that a narrow definition of disability is critical for preserving the moral urgency and popular support of the ADA; the latter fear that restricting the ADA to severe disability excludes many who are also subject to invidious discrimination.

The ADA appears to embody both these conflicting tendencies. It is prefaced by congressional findings that emphasize the exclusion and poverty of people with disabilities (Section 2(a)(6)) *and* their large and growing numbers (Section 2(a)(1)). It designates people with disabilities as "a discrete and insular minority" (Section 2(a)(7))—a legal status conferred on social groups that have faced pervasive oppression and exclusion—yet it offers a definition of disability that leaves its boundaries vague and elastic. On the one hand, it defines a disability as a "physical or mental impairment that substantially limits one or more of the [individual's] major life activities" (Section 3(2)(A)), suggesting that the protected class is confined to those with significant functional limitations. On the other hand, its definition of disability includes "being regarded as having such an impairment" and "having a record of such impairment" (Section 3(2)(C), (B)), thereby encompassing impairments that are falsely perceived as substantially limiting and, arguably, conditions falsely perceived as impairments (so long as they are also perceived to be substantially limiting).[1] The ADA thus recognizes social perception as well as functional limitation as a source of disability.

The narrower view of the ADA prevailed in the recent Supreme Court decisions in *Murphy* and *Sutton v. United Airlines* (1999), which held that "disability" does not include impairments that are substantially limiting only in the absence of corrective devices or medication. For a majority of the Court, people who can achieve normal functioning simply by putting on glasses or taking a pill do not belong to the highly vulnerable and disadvantaged group the ADA was intended to protect. As Justice Ginsburg observed in her concurrence:

> [P]ersons whose uncorrected eyesight is poor, or who rely on daily medication for their well-being, can be found in every social and economic class; they do not cluster among the politically powerless, nor do they coalesce as historical victims of discrimination. (1999, 2152)

Justice Stevens, in dissent, did not deny Justice Ginsburg's claim that people with correctable impairments are generally less vulnerable and disadvantaged than people with severe disabilities. Nonetheless, he argued that this difference provides no reason to deny them protection from discrimination:

> When faced with classes of individuals or types of discrimination that fall outside the core prohibitions of antidiscrimination statutes, we have consistently construed those statutes to include comparable evils beyond Congress' immediate concern in passing the legislation. Congress, for instance, focused almost entirely on the problem of discrimination against African-Americans when it enacted Title VII of the Civil Rights Act of 1964. . . . But that narrow focus could not possibly justify a construction of the statute that excluded Hispanic-Americans or Asian Americans from its protections—or as we later decided . . . Caucasians. (1999, 2157)

It may, however, be more difficult in the case of disability than race to decide what classes of individuals face evils comparable to those addressed by the statute's "core prohibitions." Construing the 1964 Civil Rights Act to include Hispanic-Americans, Asian-Americans, or Caucasians appears (at least in retrospect) straightforward, because it is clear that people of any racial, ethnic, or national-origin group can be treated as moral inferiors by virtue of their membership in that group. In contrast, the justices in *Sutton* disagreed about whether discrimination against individuals with minor and correctable impairments was an evil comparable to discrimination against individuals with more severe, less tractable impairments. For the majority it was not, because the former, unlike the latter, are not a discrete and insular minority, left poor and powerless by a long history of exclusion and neglect. Because of this difference, the majority held an employer was "free to decide that physical characteristics or medical conditions that do not rise to the level of an impairment—such as one's height, build, or singing voice—are preferable to others, just as it is free to decide that some limiting, but not substantially limiting, impairments make individuals less than ideally suited for a job" (1999, 2150). The dissent, however, saw in such preferences just the kind of "stereotypic assumptions" about competence that confront people with more severe impairments, assumptions that the ADA was intended to overcome (1999, 2159).

Before *Sutton* and *Murphy,* several commentators had argued that the ADA should cover a variety of conditions less limiting than paradigm cases of disability (e.g., Burgdorf 1997; Mayerson 1997). Not only should correctable impairments be included, but also impairments that are substantially limiting only in a narrow range of activity, such as a specialized kind of work, or that are substantially limiting only by virtue of the discriminatory response they elicit, such as the denial of a job or service. And at least one commentator took the argument a step further, proposing the outright elimination of the "substantial limitation" requirement (Eichhorn 1999). If, as Justice Stevens argued in his *Sutton* dissent, "the purpose of the ADA is to dismantle . . . barriers based on society's accumulated myths and fears" (1999, 2159), it should protect all people with impairments, since those myths and fears are not confined to impairments that are, or are perceived to be, substantially limiting.

After *Sutton* and *Murphy*, these arguments for enlarging the scope of the ADA can no longer be made within the confines of the existing statute. Whether or not they were correct as statutory interpretation, I believe they are correct in articulating what the central purpose of the ADA *should* be: to challenge discrimination based on physical or mental difference, not to protect a vulnerable class of people bearing the most salient or substantial differences.

By the same token, however, I believe that these arguments require a more radical revision of the ADA than their proponents acknowledge. The reasons for extending the protection of the ADA to persons whose impairments are not substantially limiting also justify extending these protections to persons with atypical physical or mental conditions that are not (and are not regarded as) impairments at all. A revised statute, I shall argue, should protect anyone with a disfavored physical or mental variation: it should apply to those who are overweight but not morbidly obese, short but not achondroplastic, unattractive but not disfigured, and "dull-witted" but not mentally retarded.

The expansion of the ADA to include all disfavored physical and mental variations would treat people with substantially limiting impairments not as a discrete and insular minority, but as some of the most salient and aggrieved victims of prejudice and stereotyping that adversely affect most Americans at some point in their lives. Perhaps the class protected by this extended statute should not be referred to as "Americans with disabilities," reserving the term "disability" for those who have, or are regarded as having, functionally significant impairments. Then again, retaining the name would be a useful reminder that people with "normal" structural and functional imperfections can be disabled by aversion, contempt and stereotyping. I am less concerned about the statute's name than with its scope.

This further extension of the ADA would doubtless be opposed by many who favor the liberal interpretation or outright elimination of the substantial-limitation requirement. Justice Stevens himself, in arguing for the inclusion of mitigated impairments, made it clear that he did not "mean to suggest, of course, that the ADA should be read to prohibit discrimination on the basis of, say, blue eyes, deformed fingernails, or heights of less than six feet. Those conditions, to the extent that they are even 'impairments,' do not substantially limit individuals . . . and thus are different in kind from the [substantial but mitigated] impairment in the case before us" (1999, 2158). My first task, then, is to show that a variety of normal imperfections, from short stature to excess weight, are not "different in kind" from many substantially limiting impairments, and that the discrimination faced by people with these conditions is sufficiently similar to that faced by people with major impairments and substantial limitations to be covered by the same statute.

THE EXPERIENCE OF STIGMA

Clearly, some common imperfections elicit hostility and contempt as intense as that elicited by many substantially limiting impairments. Consider the case of Deborah Birdwell, as described by Ruth Colker, an opponent of narrow eligibility requirements in antidiscrimination law:

> Birdwell is obese and had wanted to see a movie with her niece. Knowing that she could not fit into a movie theater seat, she called ahead to ask if she could bring her

own chair and use it in the wheelchair section. She was told that she could. But when she went to the theater with her chair, she was rudely informed that she would not be able to use it. Birdwell sued under the public accommodations section of the ADA and the case was settled. (Colker 1996, 176)

There is little doubt that Birdwell was discriminated against on the basis of a disfavored physical difference;[2] it is unlikely that someone who needed extra space because he was seven feet tall would have met with such a rude response. Fat people, unlike tall people (at least tall men), are stigmatized; they are widely regarded as self-indulgent, undisciplined and indolent. The myths and stereotypes they face are arguably no less invidious than those facing people in wheelchairs. The question for disability discrimination law is how far beyond the impairment category such stigmatization extends.

Defenders of the impairment requirement in the ADA might contend that cases like Birdwell's seem appropriate for a disability discrimination statute just because conditions like obesity are on the cusp of impairment; indeed, Birdwell might well be classified as impaired by a health professional. They would argue that the biomedical classification of impairment and the social creation of stigma are parallel processes. Both impose a sharp dichotomy on a continuum of functioning: health professionals attach the label "impaired" to functioning below a given threshold, typically two standard deviations from the mean on a normal distribution, while society draws similar, if less consistent lines. As the U.S. Civil Rights Commission observed in its influential report on *Accommodating the Spectrum of Individual Abilities*, "instead of perceiving the range of individual abilities, society categorizes people either as blind or sighted, either epileptic or not epileptic, either handicapped or normal" (1983, 89). Even if they diverge in specific cases, as they may in Birdwell's, biomedical and social classifications correspond closely enough to make it appropriate to limit disability discrimination to people with, or regarded as having, physical or mental impairments.

But this argument rests on a misconception of both the biomedical classification of impairment and the social creation of stigma. First, it involves a mistaken or incomplete view of biomedical classification. Although some impairments are defined statistically, in terms of standard deviations from a mean, many, if not most, are defined by the presence of an underlying pathology (see Wachbroit 1998). To take a familiar example from the bioethics literature, a very short child deficient in human growth hormone will be classified as impaired, while an equally short child without any hormonal deficiency will not be.[3]

More important for our purposes, the argument rests on a mistaken or oversimplified view of the social perception of, and response to, physical and mental differences. The Civil Rights Commission is surely right that in categorizing people as "handicapped," "disabled," or "impaired," society imposes a rigid dichotomy on a spectrum of functioning.[4] But one does not need to be classified as impaired to be stigmatized on the basis of a physical or mental difference. It is doubtful that Birdwell was seen as handicapped, disabled, or impaired; indeed, the theater's rude response appears to reflect an implicit contrast between her condition and a "true handicap." Yet her condition was similar to a perceived handicap in evoking an array of adverse behavioral generalizations and stereotypes, and in dominating her interaction with strangers.

This suggests the more expansive view of stigma taken by Erving Goffman (1963), who introduced the notion to modern social science. For Goffman, a person is stigmatized by "his possessing an attribute that makes him different from others . . . and of a less desirable kind." This attribute can be a physical deformity, a character flaw, or membership in a particular racial, ethnic, national, or religious group (3–4). Although he recognized the pervasive effects of stigma on routine social interaction, Goffman declined to restrict the notion to "those who possess a flaw that uneases almost all their social situations." Rather, he regarded stigmatization as a threat to almost all people some of the time: "The most fortunate of normals is likely to have his half-hidden failing, and for every hidden failing there is a social occasion for which it will loom large. . . . Therefore, the occasionally precarious and constantly precarious form a single continuum" (127). For Goffman, this continuity reflects the nature of the prevailing norms:

> [W]hile some of these norms, such as sightedness and literacy, may be commonly sustained with complete adequacy by most persons in the society, there are other norms, such as those associated with physical comeliness, which take the form of ideals and constitute standards against which almost everyone falls short at some stage in his life. And even where widely attained norms are involved, their multiplicity has the effect of disqualifying many persons. For example, in an important sense there is only one completely unblushing male in America: a young, married, white, urban, northern, heterosexual Protestant father of college education, fully employed, of good complexion, weight, and height, and a recent record in sports. . . . Any male who fails to qualify in any of these ways is likely to view himself—during moments at least—as unworthy, incomplete, and inferior. . . . The issue becomes not whether a person has experience with a stigma of his own, because he has, but rather how many varieties he has had within his own experience. (128–131)

A stigma, then, is not the marker of a discrete and insular minority, but a universal human condition.

Now, it may be that in emphasizing the "precariousness" of the normal, Goffman understated the disparity in social attitudes toward the normal deviant and the significantly impaired. There may well be differences, in kind as well as degree, in attitudes towards different kinds of deviance—differences which, for some purposes, eclipse the underlying commonalities that Goffman found. Those deviating from an ideal "which almost everyone falls short of at some stage in his life" may be stigmatized far less severely or pervasively than those displaying a rare and conspicuous physical or mental abnormality. The "myths, fears and stereotypes" (ADA Interpretive Guidance, 1630.2(1), 1995) associated with impairments in general, or with certain kinds of impairments, may be more invidious, and more recalcitrant, than those associated with mediocrity and garden-variety deficiency. However unworthy, incomplete, or inferior a male may judge himself, or be judged by others, if he falls below the norm of WASP excellence Goffman sketches, his stigmatization may be qualitatively different from that experienced by someone who deviates from less ideal, more categorical norms, such as those involving human morphology. Goffman begins *Stigma* (1963, n.p.) with a letter to Miss Lonelyheart from "Desperate," a 16-year-old girl with a "nice shape" and "pretty clothes" but no nose, whose ostracism from her peer group has driven her to thoughts of suicide. The failed WASP can take comfort in, and expect commiseration from, friends and neighbors with kindred imperfections; the girl without a nose will evoke a kind of visceral aversion the failed WASP never experiences, and will find commiseration as rare as dates.

One might argue, then, that the stigma associated with striking cosmetic anomalies, serious limb deformities and neuromuscular disorders, profound retardation, and the impairment of multiple senses is distinct from, and worse than, any stigma associated with physical and mental variations not regarded as impairments. But this is hardly true of all substantially limiting impairments. It would be difficult, for example, to claim that the exaggerated solicitude displayed toward people with serious cardiovascular or lower-back impairments is more invidious than the revulsion and contempt displayed towards Deborah Birdwell.

The substantially limiting impairments covered by the ADA elicit a broad range of social responses and are subject to a wide variety of myths, fears and stereotypes, from the intense aversion and anxiety provoked by leprosy, epilepsy, AIDS and schizophrenia to the constricting solicitude and overprotectiveness triggered by cardiovascular and lower-back problems.[5] The ADA recognizes that even more "benign" responses to impairment, involving the exaggeration of frailty and dysfunction, contribute to the exclusion and devaluation of the people who have those impairments. But many physical and mental differences not classified as impairments elicit equally contemptuous, dismissive, patronizing and oversolicitous responses, that can be equally handicapping. People with normal imperfections are often relegated to inferior roles and places, if not excluded outright, by the false assumption that their conditions limit their suitability for various tasks or activities. Short, fat and unattractive people are widely assumed to be less intelligent, competent and reliable. A large body of research, for example, finds that people regarded as unattractive are also regarded as less competent and intelligent (see, e.g., Jackson et al. 1995).

One might nevertheless argue that conditions classified or perceived as impairments are stigmatized in a distinct manner, warranting special legal protection.[6] The symbolic significance of impairment status is suggested by the slightly hysterical reaction to the revised body-mass guidelines, which reclassified many overweight people as clinically obese. It is difficult to see what besides the threatened stigma would account for the fierce resistance to this reclassification, based on accumulated evidence of medical risk. But the fact that there is a further stigma in being classified as obese, rather than merely overweight, does not mean that the stigma of being overweight is significantly less damaging. Public attitudes toward the impairment classification are ambivalent, and there are advantages as well as disadvantages to having one's differences so designated: an increase in perceived deviation may be offset, at least in the eyes of the designee, by a decrease in perceived responsibility.

Moreover, the example of weight classification highlights the arbitrariness of basing discrimination protection on medical classification. There were presumably good (if debatable) medical reasons for shifting the boundaries of the "obese" and "severely obese." Those reasons concerned the risk of death and disease that people face at various weights, not their vulnerability to discrimination. A medical sociologist might conclude in retrospect that the reclassification revealed, and in some small way contributed to, changing sensibilities about weight and body size. But it would display considerable skepticism about the objectivity of medical judgments in this area to treat them primarily as indicators of shifting public attitudes. And although people may be unhappy to see themselves reclassified as impaired, that reclassification is unlikely to affect the way they are perceived and treated by other people—except, perhaps, their doctor.

While a scheme for classifying the bodily, personal and social consequences or correlates of health conditions, such as the International Classification of Impairment, Disease, and Handicap (ICIDH and ICIDH2), may be properly anchored in a medical taxonomy, the biological status of stigmatized differences should be of less concern in a statute designed to reform social attitudes and practices. Homosexual orientation hardly ceased to be a stigmatized difference when it was "declassified" as a psychiatric impairment, even if a general decline in stigmatization contributed to its declassification.[7]

There may, however, be a more general reservation about eliminating the impairment requirement in disability discrimination law. Although that requirement may exclude some highly stigmatized people and conditions, it lays down a reasonably clear boundary for the protected class. If we cannot restrict the protected class in that way, how can we restrict it at all? How do we decide whether a person falls sufficiently below a standard "against which almost everyone falls short" to be "truly stigmatized"? How unattractive must he be to be stigmatized as ugly, how overweight to be stigmatized as fat, how uncoordinated or ill-proportioned to be stigmatized as ungainly? It would be difficult to draw, let alone justify, any line on the continuum from the occasionally to the constantly precarious. But without such a line, we are left with a statute that protects us all from unwarranted and exaggerated responses to our minor imperfections. The defender of an impairment requirement would argue that such a statute would trivialize disability discrimination, because discrimination on the basis of minor imperfections is far more benign than discrimination on the basis of impairments—it is simply not a comparable evil.

I think this concern has some moral force, but much less than may initially appear. First, the harm or wrong of trivializing disability discrimination—of "debasing the high purpose of the statute" (*Forrisi v. Bowen,* 1986, 934) must be weighed against the harm or wrong of denying legal protection to people profoundly stigmatized by physical or mental conditions that are not classified or regarded as impairments. Second, I believe that discrimination against minor and widespread imperfections is not a trivial offense. The concern about trivialization derives spurious force, I suspect, from two false assumptions about the moral character of discrimination against a large majority of the population— that such discrimination is more benign in its consequences, because it involves merely the failure to confer a discretionary advantage on the majority enjoyed by the minority, and that such discrimination is less invidious, because we cannot sustain aversion and contempt toward a large majority of the population, particularly when that large majority may include us.

The first assumption surfaces in a recent review article on the association between attractiveness and presumed competence. The authors assert that this association "is cause for concern insofar as it results in liabilities for the less attractive," but conclude that "existing research . . . does not permit us to answer definitively whether attractiveness is an asset or . . . unattractiveness is a liability" (Jackson et al. 1995, 118). This, however, is a distinction without a moral difference in any setting where attractiveness is not an appropriate criterion for allocating scarce resources. To the extent that the comparatively less attractive, however large a proportion of the population, are disadvantaged by irrelevant criteria, they have grounds for complaint.

The second assumption is that the prevailing attitudes toward a relatively disfavored majority will necessarily be more benign than those toward a relatively disfavored minority. It might be supposed that, with the exception of a few practiced misanthropes, people cannot sustain the kind of aversion and contempt for a large majority that they often display for a small minority; that the larger the share of the population devalued, the less devalued it is. This strikes me as extremely naive. We are familiar with a multitude of caste and apartheid systems that consign a majority of a society, or of humanity, to a subhuman status. And while our own society has strong democratic and egalitarian sentiments, our attitudes toward older people—consistently found to be among the most stigmatized groups (e.g., Tringo 1970)—should suggest that we are quite capable of despising what we are, or are likely to become. Leslie Fiedler (1996) argues that the "cults of slimness and eternal youth" are profoundly demeaning and oppressive to the vast majority of Americans who embrace them. It may be not only conceptually possible, but fairly common, for most people in a democratic society to regard themselves as unworthy or morally inferior.

Even if we are not quite as suffused with self-loathing as Fiedler imagines, a preference for the young and beautiful can be unfair and cruel, denying older and less attractive people meaningful work and rewarding social experience. Moreover, a preference for the young and beautiful may reinforce, or evolve into, an aversion to the old and ugly. For these reasons, the law would not trivialize its condemnation of discrimination against the constantly precarious by banning discrimination against the occasionally precarious as well.

DISTRIBUTIVE IMPLICATIONS

There is, however, another basis for objecting to the extension of the ADA to people with minor impairments and normal imperfections, arising from the distributive implications of that extension. Even if the ADA does not have a distributive purpose—an issue still subject to debate—extending its coverage might well have perverse distributive effects, reducing the resources available to those who most need the statute's protection.

It is clear that Congress regarded the deprivation and disadvantage of people with disabilities as giving moral urgency to the antidiscrimination mandate of the ADA. The statute is prefaced by the finding that people with disabilities are, as a group, among the least advantaged members of society (Section 2(a)(6)).

It is, however, a familiar and perhaps unavoidable feature of modern civil rights law that its primary beneficiaries are often among the more advantaged, and sometimes among the less oppressed, members of the protected groups. As several commentators have observed, the primary beneficiaries of the ADA are the "disability elite"—those individuals with disabilities who possess indisputable competence, which they are prevented from displaying by structural or attitudinal barriers (Burkhauser 1992; Mudrick 1997). This, however, is the "trickle-down" pattern we have come to expect from the enforcement of laws against race and gender discrimination; it does not offer the same reproach to a statute designed to eliminate discrimination as it would to a statute designed to improve the material condition of the worst-off or least advantaged.

At the same time, there would be strong reason to reject the extension of the ADA if it significantly exacerbated this disparity in impact—if it resulted in even less being done to increase the social participation of the most impaired or stigmatized individuals. This concern arises most concretely with respect to the ADA's provision for reasonable accommodation (ADA I Section 101(9)). Whether or not reasonable accommodation has a distributive purpose,[8] it has distributive effects, which are relevant to the proposed expansion of the class of people entitled to demand it. As a quadriplegic man wrote to the *New York Times* (Sorani 1999) concerning *Sutton*: "the effect of diluting the definition of disability by including nearly half of the population would ultimately have hurt those who need accommodation the most." In particular, the statutory exception holding that accommodation need not be provided if it imposes "undue hardship" (ADA I Section 101(10)) may be more frequently available the larger the class of people who can claim accommodation. It would certainly seem unjust if an employer were not required to accommodate a severely impaired employee because she had already accommodated a slightly impaired one.[9]

While that perverse result could be avoided by permitting the claims of the severely impaired to trump those of the slightly impaired, such a priority scheme would hardly be better, forcing employees and prospective employees to compete for accommodation on the strength of their varying impairments. Alternatively, such competition could be mitigated, if not avoided, by public funding of employee-specific accommodations, as Sue Krenek (1994) proposes.[10] But public funding might not be politically possible, and even if it were, it would surely blunt the perception of the ADA as an antidiscrimination statute and reinforce the already strong tendency to perceive reasonable accommodation as a special benefit.

The problem of perverse distributive effects, however, will arise under any statute that, like the present ADA, covers individuals who vary widely in the severity of their impairments and the magnitude of their disadvantage. It is unlikely that the proposed expansion of the ADA would make the problem much worse, since it should not give rise to many additional claims for costly accommodation. The barriers faced by people with many normal imperfections, such as homeliness and short stature, will be predominantly attitudinal rather than structural. People with slightly deviant shapes and sizes do face some structural inconveniences, for instance, in reaching switches and ordering clothes, but the more substantial barriers they face arise without structural mediation, from the attitudes and assumptions of other people. While attitudinal barriers can sometimes be lowered by structural modifications, such as the restructuring of a job to reduce public contact, such modifications would often be seen as accommodating the very prejudices the ADA was intended to eliminate. Further, most of the site improvements that people with normal imperfections may require, such as lower electrical switches, will already have been mandated for people with substantially limiting impairments. Finally, any individual accommodations that might be required, such as an adjustable chair or a more flexible work schedule, would probably be less expensive on average than the individual accommodations required for people with impairments.

Still, the cost of accommodating an individual will not always be proportionate to the magnitude of his physical or mental differences, and the accommodation of people with normal imperfections or minor impairments may sometimes limit the resources that are available for accommodating people with more severe impairments. It would be naive to expect that the extension of the ADA would have no adverse effects on some of those who now enjoy its protection.

A legal ban on discrimination against all disfavored or stigmatized physical and mental differences may also impose less tangible costs. These range from the administrative burdens faced by a judicial system required to field a vast array of new complaints arising from a broad and vaguely formulated proscription, to the erosion of public support that may result from extending protection against disability discrimination far beyond the "truly handicapped." Critics who regard the United States as litigation-crazed and rights-obsessed will raise the specter of short, fat and homely people clogging the courts with petty complaints that reveal nothing more than the increasing incidence of the "disability" of thin skin. More ominously, they will see an oblique assault on the very idea of merit; on practices and institutions that celebrate beauty, strength and intelligence.[11] I shall address these concerns in turn, arguing that they are greatly exaggerated but not entirely baseless. The ultimate question is whether the risk of additional expense, litigation and public hostility is justified by the moral and practical value of extending the statute's protections.

IMPACT ON LITIGATION

However credible the threat of exploding litigation may be in general—and many leading scholars of contemporary litigation doubt that there has been more than a modest increase in any area except intra-business lawsuits—that specter seems particularly remote here. As

Justice Stevens remarked in his *Sutton* dissent: "it is hard to believe that providing individuals with one more antidiscrimination protection will make any more of them file baseless or vexatious lawsuits" (1999, 2160). The very awkwardness of raising claims of discrimination on the basis of excessive weight, short stature, or physical unattractiveness would serve as a powerful deterrent to anyone lacking a strong grievance. Moreover, the elimination of the substantial-limitation requirement would eliminate one of the most litigated issues under the present ADA.

Research on ADA claims suggests that much current litigation is attributable to disputes about whether an impairment is substantially limiting (e.g., McNeil 1993). Those disputes would arise less frequently under the revised statute, which would focus not on the severity of the condition but on the social response to it, for example, did the reassignment of a worker with a lower-back or heart problem reflect myths and fears about her frailty or weakness, or a prudent avoidance of risk? Of course, issues about the severity of such conditions would continue to arise in considering such issues as the reasonableness of a proposed accommodation or the existence of a safety threat. But it would no longer be necessary to establish the severity of the condition as a prerequisite for accommodation. If employers and service providers were less confident about their ability to sustain a threshold challenge to eligibility, they might be more willing to make accommodations without judicial intervention.

The revision of the statute would also reduce the incentive for the kind of fraud that has preoccupied disability policy-makers (Bickenbach 1994). The pressure to obtain false medical evidence arises from the need to establish impairment and substantial limitation, a need that the proposed revision largely eliminates. The corrupting pressure to "diagnose disability down" would be relieved by a statute that demanded no medical evidence of impairment or substantial limitation. It is possible, of course, to imagine litigants fattening up to claim weight discrimination, or putting on unflattering makeup and clothes to claim unattractiveness discrimination, but such stratagems would hardly be more deceptive than much routine trial preparation. And they would be of no avail in satisfying the most difficult element of proof for all such claims: not that of establishing a disfavored difference, but of establishing that discrimination occurred on the basis of that difference.

Admittedly, litigation would arise over the scope of the expanded statute, about whether a particular type of physical or mental difference is actually subject to social prejudice or stigma, and about whether it should be covered by the statute if it is not. For example, while left-handed people may once have been subject to a variety of myths, fears and stereotypes, they do not appear to face them in turn-of-millennium America. It is doubtful that any current or residual stereotyping or animus explains the absence of left-handed mail-sorting devices or "crossover" training complained of by Daniel de la Torres, a discharged mail sorter whose claim of disability discrimination was dismissed for want of an impairment (610 F.Supp. 593). The court may have reached the right result in that case, not because left-handedness is not an impairment, but because it is not stigmatized. Then again, the lack of accommodation for left-handed people might well create a risk of stigmatization, by making them appear incompetent as they struggle in a world of right-handed equipment.[12]

The one question that might seem to demand case-by-case resolution concerns how much of a disfavored difference an individual must have to be eligible for statutory protection. While there is no doubt that widespread prejudice exists against physically unattractive people, there may be considerable doubt that an individual is unattractive enough to face such prejudice. The removal of the apparently objective threshold imposed by the requirement of a physical or mental impairment might seem to compel the courts to make awkward threshold judgments about physical appearance.

As I argued earlier, however, an antidiscrimination statute should not limit itself to differences that fall below some vaguely defined social benchmark for an "acceptable" appearance or physique. To be discriminated against on the basis of physical appearance, a person need not be unattractive, just insufficiently attractive to satisfy the job-irrelevant preferences of an employer. If an employee of average appearance could actually show that he was denied a promotion because he did not meet his employer's high aesthetic standards, he would have a valid claim of discrimination under the revised statute. The claim that "I would have been promoted if I were better-looking" would state a cause of action, because an employer who places an unwarranted premium on beauty devalues the plain-looking as well as the homely.

Although this expansive view would, in theory, open the courthouse door to virtually anyone with an adverse employment outcome and a physical or mental imperfection, I do not think a flood of "baseless and vexatious lawsuits" would result. It would not only be very unpleasant to claim discrimination on the basis of such an imperfection; it would be extremely difficult to prove such a claim. A plaintiff would be likely to prevail only against an employer who was remarkably indiscreet or emphatic about his illicit preferences. The great majority of counterfactuals of the sort "I would have been hired if I were better-looking" will be unprovable even if true, and the obvious difficulty of proving them should keep the floodgates closed against all but the most serious grievances.[13]

It may seem a dubious recommendation for the proposed extension of the ADA that it would be virtually unusable by those it was intended to protect. But this overlooks the fact that a few cases can have a major impact on social practice. A judicial decision that Deborah Birdwell had a right to reasonable accommodation would have both symbolic and practical value, condemning the indignities visited on people with ordinary physical differences (as well as making life easier for overweight moviegoers). A single administrative ruling that a law or advertising firm could not defer to its clients' preferences for good looks in hiring its professional staff would increase employment opportunities for homely and plain-looking professionals, although it would hardly eliminate the advantages of physical attractiveness. As many commentators have noted, the law casts a broad shadow, and the benefits to people with ordinary imperfections would be more likely to arise from preemptive measures than from specific judicial or administrative orders.

A QUIXOTIC STATUTE?

Nevertheless, the very difficulty of proving specific instances of a kind of discrimination we believe to be ubiquitous may suggest that there is something quixotic about the revised statute. Precisely because physical appearance has such a pervasive impact on social judgment, and because norms of beauty are so deeply enmeshed in social practice, it might be argued that a law against discrimination on the basis of physical appearance would be either wildly impractical or unreasonably demanding. We are willing to accept the sometimes awkward formalities imposed on job searches by affirmative action guidelines as an acceptable price to pay for purging the great evils of race and sex discrimination. Similarly, we may accept the relentless institutional self-scrutiny and small monetary expense involved in making jobs and activities more broadly accessible, to end the wholesale exclusion and isolation of people who are blind, deaf, or paraplegic. But the effort to purge ourselves of "lookism" may seem to require greater sacrifice and contortion for a less urgent objective.

Thus, Robert Post argues that a proposed Santa Cruz ordinance that bans discrimination on the basis of "physical appearance" would require an almost inconceivable abstraction and impersonality in routine interactions:

> The Santa Cruz ordinance demands that employers interact with their employees in ways that are blind to almost everything that is normally salient in everyday social life. It is not clear, however, what such blindness actually entails. We can conceive what it would mean to treat someone in a way that renders their race irrelevant, we think we know (though I have my doubts) what it would mean to treat someone in a way that renders their sex irrelevant, but I suspect that we have almost no idea what it would mean physically to encounter a person and nevertheless treat him in a way that renders irrelevant his face, voice, body, and gestures. In what sense does a person without an appearance remain a person? (2000, 12)

Of course, we *can* conceive, particularly since the advent of electronic communication, extended and, in some respects, intimate interaction with a person in which her appearance (and ours) has only marginal relevance. Post is well aware of such possibilities, but he appears to view them as temporary, artificial, and somewhat desperate expedients. Thus, speaking of blind auditions as a means of limiting appearance discrimination in hiring, Post declares:

> [T]he audition screen itself is an essentially artificial device, serviceable only in discrete, bounded, and exceptional circumstances. It cannot be generalized. Once hired, a musician must step from beneath the screen, disclose her body and gender, and live her professional life in the full glare of social visibility. (2000, 16)

This almost sounds as if the musician were auditioning for a topless bar, not a symphony orchestra. It is not necessary to ignore the pervasive effects of gender and sexual attraction on face-to-face interaction to believe that those effects can be limited or contained in the workplace by such simple measures as chaste clothing and norms of conversational privacy, and that their sway can be significantly reduced by more intrusive means at such "critical stages" as hiring and promotion decisions.

Post is not necessarily denying this; he appears to be responding to what he takes to be the law's ambition to eliminate rather than control the effects of gender, sexual attraction and appearance. But disability discrimination law has always had more modest ambitions. As many commentators have noted (e.g., Karlen and Rutherglen 1996), it does not demand "blindness" about physical and mental impairments; not only does it recognize that those impairments may in some circumstances be relevant to qualification, it also requires a reasonable effort to accommodate those impairments. The spirit of disability discrimination law has always been more pragmatic than the "dominant conception" of discrimination law described by Post.

This pragmatism can be preserved in the extension of disability law to normal imperfections. For example, the law (or its accompanying regulations) might require that face-to-face interviews be deferred until the final stage of the hiring process (Note 1987). At the same time, it might decline to bar face-to-face interviews altogether, recognizing that it would be unduly burdensome to forgo the information such interviews could yield. In this pragmatic spirit, the law would seek to limit the sway of powerful aesthetic preferences, but not aspire to eliminate them entirely.

There is reason to hope that we can reform social practices to reduce the importance of physical and mental differences, as we have reduced the importance of race and gender. Over the past three decades, we have learned that much of what we value in our public as well as private lives, such as humor and spontaneity, can flourish within the strictures of antidiscrimination law. I believe that, with experience and good will, we can endow the now alien, and alienating, procedures for limiting the sway of aesthetic preferences with a patina of familiarity and grace. But I realize that others may not share my optimism, and I want to conclude with what I think is the most compelling reason for extending the ADA to all disfavored physical and mental differences: that it is better than the alternatives.

Proponents of a broader interpretation of the present ADA have argued persuasively that the necessity of proving substantial limitation frustrates the enforcement of the statute and demeans those seeking its protection (Burgdorf 1997; Mayerson 1997). Even worse, defining the protected class in terms of the limitations of its members reinforces the false impression that the ADA is an "entitlement" statute bestowing special benefits on people with disabilities by virtue of their incapacity.

Eliminating the substantial-limitation requirement, however, leaves the question of whom the statute protects. Some commentators argue that there is no need to define "disability" or "people with disabilities"; they suggest that the ADA should simply ban discrimination "on the basis of disability" and leave it at that, just as older civil rights statutes ban discrimination "on the basis of" race or gender, without defining race or gender (e.g., Burgdorf 1997). But how can we decide if a person is discriminated against "on the basis of" a disability? It would no longer be necessary that the person be regarded as substantially limited by an impairment. Would she have to be regarded as "disabled" in some less stringent, more conventional sense? We appear to have a commonsense understanding of what it is to be "disabled." But protecting only those people regarded as disabled in this sense would narrow the scope of the ADA far more than the most conservative readings of the current statute. It would likely exclude many serious, substantially limiting, medical conditions that are now covered (because they are commonly seen as illnesses rather than disabilities), as well as many stigmatized conditions that are not. To treat someone with aversion, contempt or condescension as the result of a physical or mental difference, it is hardly necessary to regard that difference as a disability.

This leaves the proposal to limit the ADA to those with impairments or perceived impairments, whether or not these impairments are substantially limiting. While this has the advantage of extending legal protection against discrimination to many people who are now unprotected, it shares many of the problems that its proponents find in the substantial-limitation requirement. It preserves a dichotomy between protected and unprotected individuals based on the biomedical classification of their physical and mental differences, or on mistaken beliefs about that classification. It thereby reinforces the false impression of the ADA as an entitlement statute for the medically impaired and appears to locate the source of disability exclusively in the individual rather than in social attitudes. And it creates a distorting pressure to medicalize various ordinary imperfections and limitations in order to qualify for statutory protection.

In contrast, a broadly inclusive statute, focused on stigma rather than impairment, would not rely on medical classification to determine who should be protected against discrimination. It would challenge, rather than reinforce, the sharp dichotomy between the disabled and able-bodied that the U.S. Civil Rights Act Commission (1983, 161) saw as the core of disability discrimination. If we are all susceptible to impairment and limitation, as proponents of a universal model of disability have long maintained, we are all vulnerable to stigmatization. The Americans with Disabilities Act should be for "us," not for "them." It should command broad popular support not only because it seeks to protect some of the least advantaged and most stigmatized members of society—its capacity to do so will not, I have argued, be significantly diminished by its extension—but because it seeks to protect all of us from our disabling habits of thought and social practices.

NOTES

[1] The tension between these approaches surfaces not only in the debate about mitigating and assistive devices, but in another issue now under judicial review: whether a person impaired but only perceived as substantially limited is entitled to reasonable accommodation by the person who so perceives him (e.g., Dudley 1999; Moberley 1998). The conservative approach limits reasonable accommodation to individuals with "actual" disabilities, who require environmental modifications to function effectively; the liberal approach sees reasonable accommodation as, in part, a corrective for the "myths, fears and stereotypes" (ADA Interpretive Guidance, 1630.2(l), 29 C. F. R. pt. 1630 (1995)) that make impairments seem more limiting than they actually are, and favors modifications that permit the impaired individual to dispel those myths, fears and stereotypes by more fully displaying her proficiency.

[2] It is possible, of course, that the theater was merely displaying timidity or scruple about the scope of reasonable accommodation, based on the belief that Birdwell, however inconvenienced by her weight, is not "truly handicapped," and so is not entitled to reasonable accommodation.

[3] Some philosophers of science would argue that the underlying pathology must also be understood in statistical terms, but others would deny this (Boorse 1977; Wachbroit 1998).

[4] Gliedman and Roth offer a striking illustration in the contrasting responses to a person with a limp, depending on whether he turns out to be wearing a cast or a metal brace: the former is immediately seen as normal but temporarily injured; the latter as handicapped (1980, 20).

[5] The range of impairments, and the differences in their stigmatization, are suggested by a study of impairments and social distance conducted by Gary Albrecht and his colleagues (1982). Their factor analysis of the perceived social distance of corporate managers from individuals with 27 stigmatized conditions yielded four groups: severe, visible, physically disabling conditions such as paraplegia, amputation and Parkinson's disease; "social disabilities" such as prior imprisonment, mental illness, drug addiction and juvenile delinquency; visible conditions not typically degenerative or functionally incapacitating, such as scars, acne, stuttering and obesity; and less visible but serious medical conditions, such as cancer and asthma. Albrecht's study suggests that the degree of stigmatization (to the extent it can be captured by, or measured as, "social distance") a person is likely to experience is only loosely correlated with the functional magnitude of his impairment.

[6] It may well be that Albrecht's subjects would have perceived less social distance from people with normal imperfections, just because of the familiarity and "stability" of their conditions.

[7] This suggests that homosexual orientation (but not conduct) would be protected under a revised ADA as a stigmatized mental difference. While this might be objectionable to those who regard homosexuality as a legitimate choice rather than a non-voluntary physical or mental variation, their objections would reflect the larger debate about the character of sexual orientation or preference. Arguably, non-white race and female gender could be treated as stigmatized physical differences. While it would certainly be awkward to place race or gender under the rubric of disability, it would have the desirable effect of imposing a requirement of reasonable accommodation. Indeed, Karlen and Rutherglen (1996) propose to treat race and gender discrimination as disability discrimination for just that reason.

[8] The requirement of reasonable accommodation is seen by some commentators as insinuating a mandate for distributive justice into an antidiscrimination statute (e.g., Karlen and Rutherglen 1996; Van de Walle 1998). 1 think, however, that it is better seen as a heuristic for approximating the arrangements that would prevail in a society no more egalitarian than our own, but in which people with disabilities were not stigmatized; as a corrective for the effects of stigmatization on the physical and social organization of our present society.

Reasonable accommodation is simply not up to the task of achieving distributive justice among people with and without disabilities. The ADA mandates far less structural modification than most accounts of distributive justice, sketchy as they are, would require, while allocating the cost of accommodation in a manner that would seem arbitrary from the standpoint of distributive justice. Reasonable accommodation does require some redistribution, but it does so to eliminate discrimination.

The ADA is informed, not by the assumption that people with disabilities need special compensation, but by the conviction that discrimination against them is typically expressed in the neglect of their needs and interests in designing physical structures and social practices—in the fact that "public and private environments, customs, and institutional structures are all designed for people with normally functioning bodies and minds" (Kavka 1992, 271). The core evil the ADA addresses is not the hardship caused by this neglect, but the aversion and contempt that underlie it. "[R]easonable accommodation is not a special service for individuals with disabilities. It is a method for eliminating discrimination that inheres in the planning and organization of societal opportunities based on expectations of certain mental and physical characteristics" (Burgdorf 1997, 553).

⁹The impact of additional claimants will not be as great if the accommodations requested are permanent site improvements rather than employee-specific modifications, a distinction made by Sue Krenek (1994). (Karlen and Rutherglen [1996] make a similar distinction, between "wholesale" and "retail" improvements.) While an expansion in the number of people entitled to request ramps or wider doorways would increase the odds that the employer would have to install them, those improvements could serve an indefinite number of employees. In contrast, customized equipment, readers, or interpreters might have to be obtained for each employee requesting them, and a more flexible work schedule for one employee might mean more rigid or inconvenient schedules for others.

¹⁰More comprehensive public funding is proposed by Moss and Malin (1998).

¹¹A distinct concern has been raised about the burden on a person seeking redress because of a disfavored but medically unrecognized difference such as homeliness or short stature. Kavka (1992, 282) suggests that having to establish that one is ugly or dull-witted would be profoundly demeaning. But this is not equally a problem for all normal imperfections—it is easy and relatively painless to establish short stature; easy, if not painless, to establish mild obesity. And it is not a problem limited to people with normal imperfections; it is a familiar and unavoidable dilemma for many of those seeking to correct or modify the social response to deviance. What Kavka describes is one horn of the "dilemma of difference" that also confronts many people with substantially limiting impairments: in order to obtain appropriate treatment, they must establish their impairments and emphasize their debilitating aspects. Kavka, however, appears to deny that the marginal burden is as great for people with substantially limiting impairments as for people with normal imperfections—he claims that most disabilities are "readily discernible." But many disabilities are hidden, and many that are manifest have limiting effects that are not obvious to the observer. While medical evidence or certification of many impairments is readily available, its display in a public forum may be quite painful for the impaired individual, and the practical burden of proof will vary considerably, as it would for normal imperfections. It would, of course, rarely be a pleasant experience to raise a claim that one was discriminated against on the basis of being short, fat, or ugly. But the availability of a legal remedy might provide some comfort, and even some leverage, to those understandably reluctant to pursue it.

¹²The case for coverage is even weaker with respect to "favored" variations in some physical variables such as height and body composition. While men who are seven feet tall, for example, do not face aversion or adverse stereotyping on the basis of height, they do suffer countless inconveniences because of the poor fit between their height and standard design. If we are troubled that a man five feet tall can demand accommodation in the placement of shelves or switches, but a man seven feet tall cannot demand accommodation in the placement of ceilings, it may be because we persist in thinking of reasonable accommodation as a measure to achieve distributive justice, not to reduce discrimination.

It might also seem odd if a five-foot (or five-foot-two) woman could not demand the same accommodation as a man of the same height, since her difference was not stigmatized. The way to avoid this anomaly would be to extend reasonable accommodation to gender discrimination, as Karlen and Rutherglen (1996) propose. The placement of various instruments at heights inconvenient or inaccessible for many women is due in part to the fact that in the design of standard workplace features, women were not regarded as among the people whose varying dimensions needed to be accommodated; and to the fact that such placement tends to reinforce the stereotype of women as clumsy or inefficient workers.

An issue might also arise about physical variations that appear to be under the control of the individual, such as hair length. While long-haired males have been subject to widespread animus and adverse stereotypes for several generations, this is a social prejudice that can be avoided by a trip to the barber. I think, however, that it would be unwise to make an exception for voluntary differences, because of the difficulty of assessing voluntariness in light of the myriad social pressures and psychological constraints that individuals face and the difficulty of drawing appropriate lines.

[13]This is not to deny that some issues under the revised statute would be frequently litigated. There might, for example, be disputes about the admissibility of evidence on the average height, weight, or other easily-measured attribute of the workforce, offered to support or rebut a claim of discrimination. But there is precedent for resolving issues such as these in the case law on gender and race discrimination.

REFERENCES

Albrecht, G. L., Walker, V. G., & Levy, J. A. "Social Distance from the Stigmatized: A Test of Two Theories." *Soc. Sci. Med.* 16 (1982): 1319–1327.

Bickenbach, J. E. "Voluntary Disabilities and Everyday Illnesses," in *Disability Is Not Measles: New Research Paradigms in Disability,* eds. Marcia Rouix and Michael Bach, Toronto: Roehrer Institute, 1994.

Boorse, C. "Health as a Theoretical Concept." *Philosophy of Science* 44 (1977): 542–573.

Burgdorf, R. "'Substantially Limited' Protection." *Villanova Law Review* 42 (1997): 481–585.

Burkhauser, R. V. "Beyond Stereotypes: Public Policy and the Doubly Disabled." *American Enterprise* 3(5) (1992): 60–69.

Colker, R. *Hybrid: Bisexuals, Multiracials, and Other Misfits under American Law.* New York: New York University Press, 1996.

Dudley, A. "Right to Reasonable Accommodation under the Americans with Disabilities Act for 'Regarded As' Disabled Individuals." *George Mason University Law Review* 7 (1999): 389–416.

Eichhorn, L. "Major Litigation Activities Regarding Major Life Activities: The Failure of the 'Disability' Definition in the Americans with Disabilities Act of 1990." *North Carolina Law Review* 77 (1999): 1469–1477.

Fiedler, L. *Tyranny of the Normal: Essays on Bioethics, Theology & Myth.* Boston: Godine, 1996.

Forrisi v. Bowen, 794 F.2d 931, 1986.

Gliedman, J., & Roth, W. *The Unexpected Minority: Handicapped Children in America.* New York: Harcourt Brace Jovanovich, 1980.

Goffman, E. *Stigma: Notes on the Management of Spoiled Identity.* Englewood Cliffs, NJ: Prentice-Hall, 1963.

Greenhouse, L. "Justices Wrestle with the Definition of Disability: Is It Glasses? False Teeth?" *The New York Times on the Web,* April 28, 1999.

Jackson, L. A., Hunter, J. E., & Hodge, C. N. "Physical Attractiveness and Intellectual Competence: A Meta-Analytic Review." *Social Psychology Quarterly,* 58, no. 2 (1995): 108–122.

Karlan, P. S., & Rutherglen, G. "Disabilities, Discrimination, and Reasonable Accommodation." *Duke Law Journal* 46 (1996): 1–40.

Kavka, G. S. "Disability and the Right to Work." *Social Philosophy & Policy* 9, no. 1 (1992): 262–290.

Krenek, S. A. "Beyond Reasonable Accommodation." *Texas Law Review* 72 (1994): 1968–2014.

Mayerson, A. B. "Defining the Parameters of Coverage under the Americans With Disabilities Act: Who Is 'An Individual with A Disability'?" *Villanova Law Review* 42 (1997): 587–612.

McNeil, J. M. "Americans with Disabilities: 1991–1992." *Current Population Reports* (1993): 70–33.

Moberly, M. D. "Letting Katz Out of the Bag: The Employer's Duty to Accommodate Perceived Disabilities." *Arizona State Law Journal* 30 (1998): 603–638.

Moss, S. A., & Malin, D. A. "Public Funding for Disability Accommodations: A Rational Solution to Rational Discrimination and the Disabilities of the ADA." *Harvard Civil Rights–Civil Liberties Law Review* 33 (1998): 197–236.

Mudrick, N. R. "Employment Discrimination Laws for Disability: Utilization and Outcome." ANNALS, AAPSS, 549 (1997): 53–70.

Murphy v. United Parcel Service, 119 S. Ct. 2133 (1999).

Note, "Facial Discrimination: Extending Handicap Law to Employment Discrimination on the Basis of Physical Appearance." *Harvard Law Review* 100 (1987): 2035–2045.

Post, R. "Prejudicial Appearances: The Logic of American Antidiscrimination Law." *Calif. L. Rev.* 88 (2000): 1–40.

Sorani, M. "Are the Rights of the Disabled in Jeopardy?" *The New York Times,* June 23, 1999, Section A, Page 16.

Sutton v. United Airlines, Inc., 199 S. Ct. 2133 (1999).

Torres v. Bolger, 610 F. Supp. 593 (1985).

Tringo, J. L. "The Hierarchy of Preference toward Disability Groups." *Journal of Special Education* 4 (1970): 300.

U.S. Commission on Civil Rights. *Accommodating the Spectrum of Individual Abilities,* Clearinghouse Publication 81. Washington, DC: U.S. Government Printing Office, 1983.

Van de Walle, J. M. "In the Eye of the Beholder: Issues of Distributive and Corrective Justice in the ADA's Employment Protection for Persons Regarded as Disabled." *Chicago-Kent Law Review* 73 (1998): 897ff.

Wachbroit, R. "Health and Disease, Concepts of." *Encyclopedia of Applied Ethics* 2 (1998): 533–538.

Practical Applications
Work, Health, Congress and the Courts

Part C of this volume takes up three of the most important practical applications of the ADA: employment, health care and the relative roles of Congress and the courts. Employment and health care are two central components of the well-being of individuals, disabled or not: employment for its role in individuals' being self-sufficient, contributing members of the community, and health care for its role in maintaining physical and mental well-being. The activities and relative powers of Congress and the courts are central both to how the ADA is interpreted and to what possibilities for reform of the statute might exist.

Employment, the subject matter of Title I of the ADA, has occasioned the greater part of ADA litigation. The 1999 decisions of the United States Supreme Court significantly limited the range of plaintiffs who can claim ADA protection to those who experience substantial limits on major life activities when their conditions are assessed in their corrected states. These same decisions also signaled deference to employer discretion in such areas as setting and assessing job qualifications.

The papers in **Section 1 of Part C** represent a range of positions about employment discrimination and the ADA. Iris Marion Young argues that interpretations narrowing the ADA represent a failure to challenge the power of employers to determine the conditions of work. Gregory S. Kavka defends the right of people with disabilities to work as being central to the primary good of self-respect. Michael Ashley Stein argues that the difficulties in achieving increased levels of employment for people with disabilities can be explained as a function of market failure and not by the supposed inefficiency of ADA requirements.

In exploring what she views as the recent perverse narrowing of the scope of the ADA as it applies to employment, Iris Marion Young begins with the dilemma of difference identified by Martha Minow. Equality appears to require setting difference aside, but to be neutral with respect to a difference such as disability ignores ways in which differences are relevant. The ADA, in Young's view, has encountered this dilemma head-on, for it both requires equal treatment and recognizes that in some circumstances equal treatment may demand reasonable accommodations. The solution, Young argues, is to recognize that the judgment that an accommodation is "special" takes place against the background of the existing structure of the workplace. If employers were not simply assumed to have the power to set that structure, but instead the background assumption were a humane workplace environment for all, accommodations would not be erroneously perceived as special.

In a now classic paper, reprinted here, Gregory S. Kavka argues that people with disabilities in advanced modern societies have a strong *prima facie* moral right to work. The justification for the right to work is contractarian, Kavka maintains. He explores Rawlsian contractarianism, on which social institutions should work to the advantage of the disabled

163

because they are among the worst-off in society (see Pogge's essay in Part A for another discussion of Rawlsian theory). Hobbesian contractors differ from Rawlsian contractors because they are positioned to take their own life circumstances into effect when making choices about social arrangements. They, too, would select practices that work to the advantage of the disabled, both because they would want to protect themselves against the eventuality of becoming disabled and because they would want to protect their loved ones against the possibility. In addition, Kavka argues, a sufficient number of contractors would opt for the right to work to guarantee its incorporation in the legal system. Anticipating the objection that people should insure themselves against the effects of disability if such insurance is sufficiently important to them, Kavka replies that this option is insufficiently protective because many people are disabled before they have a reasonable opportunity to acquire insurance. To the objection that his contentions apply equally to those who are disabled and those who suffer other forms of bad luck, his answer is that people with disabilities are generally more systematically worse-off and that, in any case, society both has and should move towards distributive justice for other forms of disadvantage as well.

Two criticisms of Title I of the ADA are its alleged inefficiency from the point of view of the employer, and its purported ineffectiveness, at least up to this point, in improving employment statistics for people with disabilities. Michael Ashley Stein attributes these phenomena to market failure. The ADA is not inefficient; the problem is that employers misjudge and overestimate the expenses of hiring workers with disabilities. Because they assume the "medical" model of disability, employers tend to attribute costs to workers themselves rather than to the structure of the work environment.

Peter Blanck, a leading scholar of the employment picture for people with disabilities, presents recent data that complement Stein's claims about market failure. Blanck paints a picture of enhanced participation in the workforce by people with disabilities. One very encouraging development is the success of Manpower, Inc., a company that provides temporary staffing services, in training and providing transition opportunities for people with disabilities to move into the permanent workforce. Another study, this one of Sears, Roebuck, demonstrates that most reasonable accommodations are very low-cost (on average, $30), and that the indirect benefits such as worker retention are quite high. Blanck concludes that there is no evidence that the ADA has been counterproductive or has promoted the employment of the undeserving.

Protection from discrimination in health care occurs in all three titles of the ADA. Title I prohibits employers from discrimination on grounds of disability in conditions of employment, an important example of which is health benefits. Nonetheless, employers are permitted to charge a premium for health insurance which is actuarially fair, an allowance likely to have significant disparate impact on people with disabilities who have expensive health care needs. Title II prohibits discrimination in the provision of public services, an important aspect of which is publicly provided health care services. And Title III's prohibition of discrimination in public accommodations encompasses health care facilities, including physicians' offices. The writers in **Section 2 of Part C** take different positions on what counts as discrimination in health care for people with disabilities. Dan Brock defends limited forms of rationing that apply to people with disabilities with expensive health care needs. David Orentlicher differs, arguing that the ADA requirement of reasonable accommodations prohibits most such rationing of health care and that utilitarian criteria are inequitable to persons with disabilities. Joel Feinberg's careful analysis of the concepts of illness and disease provides guidance for deciding what is health care, an inquiry of particular relevance in the area of mental health. The final selection in Section 2, a classic piece by Norman Daniels reprinted here, discusses the justification for treating mental and physical disabilities with parity under the ADA.

Finally, Congress and the courts will play major roles in the ultimate impact of the ADA on American life. Some writers in **Section 3 of Part C** criticize courts for a lack of activism in the protection of disability rights—an approach ironically characterized as "benign neglect." Some also fault Congress for not framing the ADA to parallel other civil rights statutes. Nevertheless, they unite in the recognition that the ADA has brought important gains for people with disabilities. Harlan Hahn, opening the section, challenges the courts' not-so-benign neglect of the analogy between people with disabilities and other minorities who have suffered from discrimination. According to Hahn, courts have tolerated far more compromise in the recognition of rights for people with disabilities than in the recognition of rights for other minorities. Like Hahn critical of the medical model of disability, Richard Scotch views the ADA both as a traditional civil rights statute and as transformative social policy. Measured against these goals, the ADA has been a modest success. Supporters of further gains for people with disabilities, Scotch contends, must look beyond the law to education and political mobilization.

It was predictable, Andrew Batavia explains, that the ADA would not prove a panacea for people with disabilities, nor was it designed to be one. Batavia's concern is that other federal disability policies are at odds with the ADA, and the tensions among them retard progress for people with disabilities. Income maintenance programs linked to eligibility for health insurance, for example, discourage people with disabilities from entering the workforce. Training and education programs, on the other hand, are more closely aligned with the ADA.

Title III of the ADA, the public accommodation title, provides the most direct protection for the right of people with disabilities to be in the world. Yet, Ruth Colker argues, it embodies a deeply troubling compromise. In exchange for broad coverage, Congress limited the remedies available under Title III. The result is a cycle of diminished incentives to litigate violations of Title III. Lori Andrews and Michelle Hibbert take up a specific example of how other legal doctrines may conflict with the goals of the ADA. Lawsuits that are based on the assumption that someone was wronged by the birth of a person with disabilities arguably undermine respect for people with disabilities. Wrongful-birth lawsuits, recognized in a number of jurisdictions, contend that the parents were harmed by a failure of diagnosis or counseling, because with desired information they would have avoided the birth of a disabled child. Wrongful-life lawsuits, infrequently recognized, claim that the child was harmed by being born with a disorder, in contrast to not having been born at all. Even when courts reject such claims, opinions are replete with descriptions of the difficulty and undesirability, rather than the possibilities and promise, of lives of people with disabilities.

In the final piece in this section, Lennard Davis compares the relative invisibility of hate crimes against people with disabilities to the greater visibility of hate crimes based on race. Critical legal theorists would describe this eclipse of disability by race as the problem of "intersectionality." Davis concludes with a call for education about hate crimes against people with disabilities that parallels our growing knowledge about hate crimes based on race. The goal of this volume is to contribute to such education as well as to the ongoing inspection of these and many other policies that affect the lives of people with disabilities.

Work

Disability and the Definition of Work

IRIS MARION YOUNG

The Americans with Disabilities Act is the most important legislation ever passed in the United States recognizing the legitimate expectations of people with disabilities to be included equally in the economic, political and social life of this society. Ten years later, however, many people express disappointment that the law has not had more effect in transforming the status of people with disabilities. Recent Supreme Court decisions seem to indicate, moreover, that the act may be having a perverse effect of narrowing the definition of who may legally count as a person with a disability. In these brief remarks I propose that one explanation for both these outcomes is a failure of both the act and its implementation to challenge the right of employers to define the content, qualifications and performance criteria of work.

DILEMMAS OF DIFFERENCE

Historically, people with disabilities have suffered exclusion from benefits or opportunities because people with power to allocate those benefits or opportunities have judged the people with disabilities as incompetent or despicable. People with disabilities were physically segregated in special services and residences, and socially stigmatized as different and inferior. Social movements have demanded equal respect and dignity for all people with disabilities and their inclusion in all the benefits and opportunities of economic, political and social life.

More than a decade ago, Martha Minow showed that remedies to prejudice and discrimination against marginalized groups typically run into the "dilemma of difference." The stigma of difference may be created both by trying to ignore the facts about persons that contribute to discrimination and by paying attention to them. On the one hand, institutions may adopt a stance of blind neutrality, saying that from now on everyone will be treated the same way without regard for sex, race or ability. Such an "equal treatment" approach risks reinscribing difference, however, because the rules and practices of those institutions were designed with the features of only some people in mind. Recognizing that a stance of neutrality perpetuates historic exclusion and disadvantage, institutions can instead pay specific attention to the attributes and needs of the formerly excluded and accommodate to them. Such a "special treatment" approach also risks reinscribing difference, however, because the people who deserve the special accommodation must be singled out according to criteria distinct from those used to assign benefits and opportunities to others.[1]

Ten years after its passage, it appears that efforts to apply and enforce the Americans with Disabilities Act run squarely into this dilemma of difference. The act legalizes equal rights for people with disabilities. Employers, landlords, governments and other bodies cannot bar access to facilities, positions or activities solely because a person has or is perceived to have a disability trait: moves in a wheelchair, is hearing-impaired, shows symptoms of

Parkinson's disease, and so on. When apartment houses, workstations and information distribution systems have been designed with nondisabled people in mind, however, formally equal treatment of all citizens or applicants perpetuates the exclusion of many people with disabilities. The ADA recognizes this, and thus mandates that employers and public facilities should alter their structures to enable people with disabilities to function in them.

As several of the essays in this book suggest, however, this legal requirement of accommodation has in some cases created a new stigma for people with disabilities. In the perceptions of some prospective employers or landlords, accommodating people with disabilities creates financial or other burdens, and on this account some people probably suffer a more hidden form of discrimination. The law seems to have the effect of reinscribing difference as deviance, moreover, and of freezing the category of disability, because litigants battle over whether a given person is in fact different enough to qualify for the special rights the law calls for. While the provisions of the ADA apply to several types of situations in which people with disabilities may find themselves excluded, I will focus the rest of these remarks on paid employment situations, because these appear to be the most contentious and have generated the most court dispute.

THE POLITICS OF RESENTMENT

It seems that some of the consequences of debate and litigation prompted by the ADA today also fuel what William Connolly and Wendy Brown theorize as a politics of resentment.[2] Groups come together who claim to have been excluded and marginalized, and claim rights to redress their injuries. To make such claims and benefit from redress, these legal rights and remedies require that people position themselves as victims and others as responsible for their harms. Like the dilemma of difference, these legal remedies reinscribe members of the group as deviant and evoke debate about who does and does not fit the status of deserving redress. Members of the group themselves, that is, find that they must speak in the public arena in the voice of resentment and blame.

Especially when redress takes the form of litigation, the logic of such legal remedies fuels resentment from many others. Through its laws the state holds some agents particularly responsible for ensuring the inclusion of the formerly marginalized, and regulates their activities. The laws also encourage complaints and suits against parties whom victims claim have not met their responsibilities. Those parties blamed and held responsible tend to be resentful both of further regulation and the threat of litigation.

Insofar as such legal structures rest on designating injured classes, finally, those not found to be in those classes can develop resentment about what they perceive as special benefits for those in the classes. In response, others may look for their own injuries to formulate as public claims against others. Thus evolves a spiraling "me-too-ism," as more groups claim redress for a victim status. An alternative response of employers and third parties may be to deny that many who claim to belong to a group legally recognized with certain special rights do in fact qualify as members of the group or that their condition qualifies as the harm recognized by law. Resentment fuels attempts to narrow the class of victims.

I think that this sort of analysis goes too far if it intends to imply that individuals and groups should not make claims that they suffer injustice or that other people and institutions should not be held responsible for redress and change. The analysis is nevertheless useful as a reminder that contemporary politics is sometimes unproductively negative and recriminatory, and it can help us understand the backlash and conflict that many political and legal claims produce. Something like the politics of resentment may explain why, so quickly after passage of the ADA, efforts to narrow the definition of who counts as "really" disabled have had some success. It is in the interest of employers to circumvent requirements that they accommodate workers with disabilities by claiming that the limitations these workers evince are not really disabilities of the sort that the law recognizes. Instead, they have individual traits that make them not appropriate for the jobs they want to do.

Potential resentment of other workers may also contribute to the impulse to narrow the category of people with disabilities. Most workers feel put-upon and frustrated by their working conditions and the demands of their employers on their time and energy. They have to stand up all day, or have few bathroom breaks, or work overtime or at night, and their employer refuses to accommodate to their aching backs, their family pressures, their sleeplessness or difficulty in concentrating. Many workers, that is, find the demands placed on them next to overwhelming at times, and they feel barely able to cope. Rarely do they get a sympathetic ear to voice their frustrations, however, and the only agents they are allowed to blame for their difficulties are themselves. It is little wonder that they might resent people that the law requires employers to accommodate in order to enable them better to fit the work situation. I do not mean to suggest that there are not important differences between the situation of those whom the ADA is intended to cover and just plain harried workers. As I will make more thematic shortly, the point is that in either case the employer has the right to specify nearly everything about the terms and conditions of work.

THE UNSTATED ASSUMPTION: EMPLOYERS DEFINE WORK

Disability is a more contestable category than the other categories American law has recognized as naming protected classes—race, sex and, to some degree, age. All are contestable, of course. The variability of condition of people with disabilities is huge, however, and many of those brought together under this label have nothing at all in common in the way of experience, culture or identity. More than the other categories, moreover, disability is a matter of degree, and it is arbitrary where the line is drawn between not disabled enough to warrant accommodation, and disabled enough. A politics of resentment motivates some people to draw that line as far down the extreme end of the continuum as possible so that almost everyone will be legally expected to conform to the *normal* workplace demands.

Under the law, employers have extensive prerogatives in the definition of these "normal" workplace requirements. In this simple fact lies, I believe, the main source of the relative inefficacy of the ADA in bringing people with disabilities into paid employment, the disputes about the extent and meaning of the ADA's mandate, and potential resentments surrounding its application. In the United States, as in most other places, employers have the right to define job tasks and the qualification for being judged able to perform those tasks. Employers define the meaning and measures of productivity and where an individual must fall on these measures to be judged as performing well. Antidiscrimination law, now covering people with disabilities, forbids defining any of these worker attributes in ways that require or rule out suspect categories of people; and it is up to individual claimants to prove that particular qualifications or measures have discriminatory intent or disparate impact on a group.

While unions can negotiate in grey border areas about the definition of jobs or qualifications, and some occasionally do, most labor negotiations concentrate on pay, benefits, hours and working conditions, not on the work process itself. The latter remains the legal prerogative of employers. Labor regulations also concentrate on these factors. For all intents and purposes, employers can hire people to perform any tasks they deem necessary, require whatever qualifications they wish for these tasks, and evaluate their performance according to whatever criteria they choose, so long as these do not explicitly single out protected classes of people for differential treatment. The norms of work are whatever employers define them as, and for many workers in diverse occupations, these are oppressive norms that they have difficulty fitting.

Far from challenging this employer right to define work, case law emerging from the Americans with Disabilities Act seems to be upholding that right. In *Sutton v. United Airlines,* for example, the Supreme Court denied the claim of petitioners that a United Airlines' requirement that persons have uncorrected vision of 20/100 to qualify as pilots for them was impermissible under the ADA. The Court affirmed the right of an employer to specify physical criteria for a job; presumably the decision implies that employers also have a right to specify mental criteria or other qualifications as the employer chooses. If employers have the primary right to define qualifications and performance in these ways, then it is extremely difficult for people with disabilities to prove that they are qualified to do certain jobs if the employer makes reasonable accommodation for their disability. Since employers have the right to determine qualifications in a way specific to their own job context, a person's general training or previous employment will not necessarily be sufficient to demonstrate that she or he is qualified for this job if only reasonable accommodation is made for a disability. In practice, people with disabilities are most likely to be able to demonstrate that they are qualified for a particular job if they have performed that job already, say, before they became disabled.

Martha Minow argues that the source of dilemmas of difference lies in a set of unstated assumptions that lie as background to the judgment and evaluation of people. One is that what makes people different are some attributes intrinsic to their being rather than a comparison between them and others. Other assumptions involve the perspective from which these judgments are made. When people judge some people as different or deviant, they do so from the perspective of a particular, usually unstated reference point or set of norms that are erroneously taken to be neutral, universal or natural. These reference points for what is normal or natural derive from existing social and economic arrangements.

Among such unstated norms of work that have an impact on people with disabilities is the norm of the "hale and hearty" worker. The "normal" worker is supposed to be energetic, have high concentration abilities, be alert to adapt to changing conditions, and be able to withstand physical, mental or interactive stress in good humor. Workers who fail to measure up to one or more of these standards are "normally" considered lazy, slackers, uncooperative or otherwise inadequate. All workers must worry about *failing* in the eyes of their employers, and enough people do fail to keep such worries alive. Part of the necessary discipline of the workplace, from the point of view of most employers, is keeping such fear of failing to "measure up" before the workers. Permanent or temporary inability to conform to the standards and work processes defined by employers for their own purposes is widespread among workers. Just this fact might motivate a narrow definition of legal disability, because recognizing the particular needs and capacities of individuals would entail challenging these unstated norms.

The politics of resentment I discussed above derives at least in part from this context of normalization. Those with power to set standards and establish norms resent infringement on this power, since the structures of the society act as though it is an acceptable and natural power. Those who must measure up to the standards are placed in a competition in which most are destined to lose. Challenging the right of employers to define the content, qualifications and performance criteria of work seems to me the next step toward equal opportunity for people with disabilities. As long as the rules of social institutions and interpretations of disability law assume that employers have the sole or primary right to define work, many people with disabilities will continue to be excluded from workplace opportunities even though litigation cannot prove they suffer illegal discrimination. If the society expects every adult to contribute productively to the society to the best of their abilities, and if engaging in such productive work is a major source of both the esteem of others and self-esteem, then general public discussion and decision should have more influence over what tasks and projects count as work, how those activities ought to be organized, what the qualifications are to perform them competently, and how to evaluate performance.

How might these assumptions be challenged? The language of the Americans with Disabilities Act is broad enough to permit such a challenge, if litigants are willing to mount it. Laws and litigation can only go so far, however. As I have tried to show, all workers have an interest in challenging this employer prerogative, and many workers who do not identify themselves as disabled would likely benefit if they allied with people with disabilities to call for generally more humane and individualized workplace accommodation. Unions, professional associations and other employee organizations have an important role to play in such a campaign. They can foster discussion of these problems among their members and develop strategies for educating and agitating among their employers about the injustice done to workers by normalizing definitions of task performance and evaluation. Unfortunately, however, labor law in the United States gives to employee bargaining agents only limited right directly to negotiate the content of work and its performance evaluation. Thus legal reforms additional to the ADA may be needed to expand workplace opportunities for people with disabilities as well as others.

NOTES

[1]Martha Minow. *Making All the Difference: Inclusion, Exclusion and American Law.* Ithaca: Cornell University Press, 1990, Part I. Minow first articulated the notion of dilemmas of difference in "Learning to Live with the Dilemma of Difference: Bilingual and Special Education." *Law and Contemporary Problems* 48 (Spring 1985): 157–211.

[2]William Connolly. *Identity/Difference: Democratic Negotiations of Political Paradox.* Ithaca: Cornell University Press, 1991; Wendy Brown. *States of Injury.* Princeton: Princeton University Press, 1994. The analysis that follows in this paper is inspired by the ideas of Connolly and Brown, but I am not summarizing and applying their exact formulations.

Disability and the Right to Work

GREGORY S. KAVKA

Philosophers have generally paid little attention to the rights of the handicapped (other than the right to be allowed to die),[1] except occasionally when those rights either support or pose problems for general theoretical claims which these philosophers wish to advance.[2] I hope in this essay partly to remedy this record of neglect by providing persuasive arguments in support of disabled people's possession in advanced modern societies of a key economic right—the right to work. Since certain portions of the Americans with Disabilities Act of 1990 pertain to this right, this essay may be viewed as providing a moral foundation for aspects of this legislation.

DEFINING THE PROBLEM

Do disabled people in advanced modern societies (such as those of North America, Western Europe and the Pacific Rim) have a right to work? Before we can begin to answer this question, we must be clearer about what it means. And this requires some preliminary comments on each of the question's key constituent terms. Of these, the notion of a disability (or handicap) is easiest to deal with, for we may adopt the broad definition contained in the Americans with Disabilities Act, which says a disability is a physical or mental impairment that: "substantially limits one or more of the major life activities of an individual."[3]

Characterizing the right to work, as I intend it, is a complex matter. For present purposes, we may think of rights, in general, as potential claims by (or on behalf of) someone to some thing (an object or a liberty to act) against someone else. These rights are moral or legal, and *prima facie* or absolute, according to whether the underlying rules, principles and standards which ground and justify the potential claims in question are themselves moral or legal, *prima facie* or absolute. (A *prima facie* right is overridable by competing considerations, while an absolute right is not. Among the rights thought to be absolute by some are the right not to be tortured and the right not to be punished for a crime one did not commit.)

The right of handicapped people to work that I argue for is a moral right; it will be justified by appeals to moral considerations. However, since important moral rights concerning economic matters should be protected by and embodied in the law, my arguments will aim at showing that disabled people should be accorded a legal right to work. Disabled people's right to work is *prima facie*, not absolute: it can in principle be overridden by competing rights or other considerations (such as economic feasibility). But it is, I will contend, a *strong prima facie* right: the moral arguments in its favor are substantial enough that it would take competing moral considerations of considerable weight to override it. In particular, I will argue that a small gain in social utility or economic efficiency is not enough to override this right.

Editors' note: this is an abridged version of a previously published work, reprinted with permission from Gregory S. Kavka, "Disability and the Right to Work," *Social Philosophy and Policy* 9: 262–290 (1992).

If the disabled have a moral right to work, against whom is it a right? That is, who bears the moral obligation to offer them jobs or help them obtain employment? The most general answer is society as a whole. But the way this right must be vindicated in practice means that specific obligations generated by the right may fall especially upon governments, particular government officials and certain private employers.

Why this is so becomes clear when we address the critical question of just what handicapped people's right to work is a right to. The "right to work," as I use the term, is the right to participate as an active member in the productive processes of one's society, insofar as such participation is reasonably feasible. A number of aspects of this characterization require comment.

Most importantly, the right to work is a right to *employment;* it is a right to *earn* income, not simply a right to receive a certain income stream or the resources necessary to attain a certain level of welfare.[4] I believe that it is relatively uncontroversial that disabled people in wealthy modern societies have a right to the economic resources (for example, income) necessary for them to have a reasonable chance of achieving a basic minimum level of welfare.[5] This welfare right of the disabled may be derived from a variety of philosophical theories: Rawls's maximin theory of justice, with the disabled treated as the least-advantaged group in society; utilitarianism, under the assumption that a dollar spent on disabled people below the welfare floor tends to raise their utility more than a dollar spent on other members of society; welfare-state theories that ascribe a right to a basic minimum to all citizens; egalitarian theories; and various theories that assert the priority of meeting needs in distributing (or redistributing) the economic output of society.[6]

My "right to work" thesis makes the more controversial claim that disabled people in advanced societies have a right not only to receive a basic income, but to earn incomes at— or above—the basic maintenance level. I will argue for employment as a right, not a duty. I avoid the vexed question of whether disabled people should be forced to work for their basic support income if they do not want to do so. I focus on whether those disabled persons who want to work should be afforded special sorts of opportunities to do so.

What specific sorts of treatment or "special opportunities" are entailed by handicapped people's right to work? First, a right of nondiscrimination in employment and promotion—that people not be denied jobs on the basis of disabilities that are not relevant to their capacities to carry out the tasks associated with those jobs. Second, a right to compensatory training and education, funded by society, that will allow disabled people the opportunity to overcome their handicaps and make themselves qualified for desirable employment. Third, a right to reasonable investments by society and employers to make jobs accessible to otherwise qualified people with disabilities. Fourth, and most controversially, a right to minimal (or tiebreaking) "affirmative action" or "preferential treatment": being admitted, hired or promoted when in competition with other equally qualified candidates. Spelled out in this way, the right of handicapped persons to work is seen to be, in its various elements, a right against society, government and private employers.

In arguing for the disableds' right to work, in this sense, I limit my discussion in two ways to take account of problems of feasibility. I consider only the case of advanced modern societies; for in other societies, the economic resources needed to vindicate this right to any substantial degree are either not present or are very likely to be needed for even more urgent social tasks. And I acknowledge that employment of many people with severe handicaps may not be "reasonably feasible"—that is, it may be impossible or excessively costly.[7] But I will contend that applying a strict economic cost-benefit standard of hiring and training feasibility may be unfair to the disabled.

A final clarification is in order. Why describe the employment of the disabled as a "right" rather than simply a morally significant social goal? I regard the rights terminology as apt here to signal that providing employment opportunities for the disabled is a social goal with the following special features: (1) there are strong moral arguments (offered below) favoring it, hence it should be accorded relatively high priority among social goals; (2) it grounds claims by particular individuals against other individuals and groups; (3) the satisfaction of those claims is urgent and important for the claimants; and (4) the general satisfaction of those claims is quite feasible.

The first and fourth features explain why I limit the disableds' right to work to advantaged societies. In other societies, too many other important social goals might have to be sacrificed to vindicate such "rights." Similar reasoning underlies my reluctance to ascribe a right to work to *everyone* in advanced societies. A job for everyone who wants one is certainly a worthy social goal, but it may not be feasible without excessive sacrifices in economic efficiency. In addition, because the able-bodied unemployed are generally better situated to pursue satisfactions in other realms of life—and achieve self-respect thereby—than are unemployed handicapped people, condition 3 (concerning the urgency for individual claimants) is more clearly satisfied as regards the right to work of the disabled. I conclude, then, that providing employment opportunities for the disabled in advantaged societies is a social goal possessing special features that justify describing it as a "right" while at the same time withholding application of that term to such other worthy goals as employment for everyone in advantaged societies and employment for the disabled in other societies.

EFFICIENCY, JUSTICE AND THE RIGHT TO WORK

In presenting my arguments for a right to work of the disabled, it will be useful to have a foil. For this purpose, I choose a blunt form of objection to that right, derived from the notion that the economic rights of the disabled are strictly limited by considerations of economic efficiency that imply the desirability of a free market in labor in which employers are entitled to hire whomever they regard as best qualified for the jobs they offer.[8] The objection runs as follows: "Society's obligations to the disabled extend no further than the previously assumed obligation to provide a basic welfare minimum. Because of their special medical and equipment needs, this may require a larger cash stipend to most disabled people than would be necessary to support able-bodied persons at the same basic welfare level. But society has a right to provide the necessary economic resources to the disabled in whatever way it deems to be most efficient. Perhaps for some classes of disabled persons, training and continued employment will allow them to achieve (or exceed) the basic welfare minimum at less net cost to society as a whole than if receiving a public stipend. And perhaps private employers can profitably employ disabled workers by exploiting public sympathy for them and successfully charging higher prices for products they have produced. But if society (and private employers) find it cheaper just to pension off the handicapped, because it would cost more to provide handicapped people with special training and equipment and to determine which handicapped people may be profitably employed, this is their prerogative. Disabled people therefore have no more right to work than anyone else does. If they can compete successfully for jobs, if private employers or government agencies want to hire them for specific jobs because of their qualifications, they will be hired. If not, they have a right to support payments, but no right to employment." For ease of reference, I will henceforth refer to the viewpoint expressed in this objection as the Crude Economic Efficiency Position, or CREEP.

What is wrong with CREEP? At least three things that I can think of: it employs an inappropriate notion of efficiency, it fails to attach sufficient importance to self-respect and the means to self-respect, and it ignores key issues involving distributive justice. I now proceed to develop these points into an argument for the right to work of the handicapped, as characterized earlier.

Social Efficiency

CREEP says that the disabled have no right to work and that society should see to their employment only to the extent that society (or individual employers) regard this as economically cost-effective. Though this line of argument seems to be based on a morally respectable utilitarian appeal to social efficiency, this is not really the case. First, CREEP is ambiguous between appealing to efficiency for society as a whole (including the handicapped) and appealing to efficiency for those who are offering aid to the handicapped (employers, the government and taxpayers). The latter position is not a genuinely utilitarian one at all, and is supportable only if one believes that because the disabled are generally in a dependent role in these transactions, their interests are not to be counted (or counted equally) in determining which policies are most socially efficient overall. Second, the notion of "society" deciding the most efficient policies in these areas is ambiguous in a similar way: if efficiency decisions are left entirely to the discretion of particular employers, government bureaucrats and managers, rather than being circumscribed politically, then the disabled (who currently occupy very few of these influential positions) will be effectively prevented from having their interests adequately represented where the relevant decisions are made. Third, by focusing on a narrow economic notion of efficiency rather than a broader utilitarian notion, CREEP ignores the importance of key noneconomic values, such as self-respect, which may justify ascribing to disabled persons a right to work as well as a right to a basic welfare level.

But suppose we interpret CREEP in the most generous way possible, as implicitly relying on a genuinely utilitarian argument that encompasses nonmonetary aspects of utility and gives equal weight to the utilities of the handicapped. Do we not now have a sound argument against a right of employment for the disabled? For instead of ascribing such rights, should we not train and employ the disabled only to the point of social efficiency, where further employment and training for handicapped people who want work would cost more in these genuinely utilitarian terms than disability pensions?

The answer to this last question, even in purely utilitarian terms, is not an unequivocal "yes," for two reasons. First, there is a good indirect utilitarian argument that the disabled have a right to work. If we allow individual employers and educators to apply efficiency criteria, their lack of information about the disabled, their unwillingness to take risks under conditions of uncertainty, and their own discomfort at being around disabled people will probably lead to significant undertraining and underemployment of the disabled overall,[9] even relative to their actual (less than average) productive capacities. Put more bluntly, as long as there is lingering prejudice against the disabled, we cannot rely on free labor markets alone to provide appropriate employment opportunities for the handicapped.

Strong believers in free markets might reply that if employers generally underestimate the productive capacities of disabled persons, there will be room in a free-market system for clever entrepreneurs to move in and make large profits by hiring the handicapped. Thus there will be a long-run equilibrating tendency for disabled workers to be employed and paid commensurate with their actual productive capacities. In the real world of high information costs, grave uncertainties, risk aversion and irrational investors, however, few of us are willing to rely on these theoretically effective mechanisms as sufficient practical safeguards against the unfair treatment of members of generally disadvantaged groups. Furthermore, the basic welfare minimum for the disabled, which we have assumed is morally required in advanced modern societies, could undermine the equilibrium mechanism in the "clever entrepreneurs" argument by weakening the incentives for the disabled to work for low wages.[10] Hence, even a pure utilitarian analysis properly carried out may favor some system of employment rights for the disabled, rather than a system of decentralized hiring decisions governed by utilitarian criteria on a case-by-case basis.

Second, there may be certain desires or "utilities" associated with not hiring the handicapped that it would be inappropriate to count, or count equally, in determining disabled people's work rights, even from a utilitarian standpoint. The presence of a handicapped employee may make customers or other employees of a firm uncomfortable and unhappy. But, as in the case of racial prejudice, we do not normally consider these good reasons not to hire the disfavored but otherwise qualified person.

Indeed, we may be inclined to think that we ought not to count these offensive preferences *at all* in our utilitarian calculus, just as some utilitarians have suggested that malevolent or sadistic pleasures should not count.[11] There are several possible rationales for this. Perhaps we feel (as does utilitarian Richard Brandt) that these preferences would not survive cool, informed reflection on their own origins and the real nature of the preferred states of affairs.[12] Perhaps we believe (as does nonutilitarian John Rawls) that desires incompatible with certain basic moral constraints simply do not deserve to be satisfied, at least from a social viewpoint.[13]

Distributive Justice and Self-Respect

Arguments purely in terms of economic efficiency or social utility, such as CREEP, do not directly address questions of distribution. Once we turn to matters of distributive justice, the moral case for the disabled having a right to work is substantially strengthened. The basic reason for this is that the handicapped are typically, in virtue of their condition, among the most disadvantaged members of advanced modern societies with respect to well-being and opportunities for well-being. By definition, a disability is a substantial impairment of a major life activity such as seeing, hearing, walking or talking. Two features of such impairments make them especially devastating to the welfare and life prospects of those who have them: their permanence and their pervasiveness.

People are often disabled temporarily by disease or injury. But sick or injured people are not treated or regarded as a separate class of persons by society, and their work problems are dealt with by policies designed for "normal" workers—for example, sick leaves and short-term disability insurance. When people speak of the disabled or handicapped, however, they normally have in mind those who are in such a condition *permanently* (or at least for a period of years). It is the economic rights of such people—that is, those suffering long-term disablement—that is the subject of my discussion.

Significant permanent handicaps are usually pervasive, in the sense that their effects are not confined to a single sphere of the affected person's life but tend to have damaging, limiting or stigmatizing effects on all major spheres—family, personal, social and recreational life, as well as economic and professional life.[14] In pointing out the pervasiveness of the difficulties disabled persons face, I do not mean to suggest that the individuals in question are powerless to overcome or ameliorate these difficulties. But doing so generally involves an expenditure of resources of one sort or another—money, time, effort, psychological determination, incurring of obligations to other people and so on. And there is little reason to suppose that most disabled persons have an excess of these resources to expend. The result is that most permanently disabled persons suffer significant disadvantages in all major spheres of life and are correspondingly among the least advantaged members of modern advanced societies. And since some of the extra resources that handicapped people must expend to cope with their difficulties (for example, time and effort) are not readily compensable in kind, there is an added necessity for providing offsetting economic compensation—support payments, job training and employment opportunities.

Special social provision for the welfare of the disabled thus follows from practically any account of social justice—Rawlsian, egalitarian, need-centered, or whatever—that pays attention to how social welfare or resources are distributed and correspondingly prescribes improving the lot of society's least advantaged members. But how does a right to work rather than a right to disability pensions follow from such distributive considerations?

The key mediating concept here is self-respect. Suppose that we agree with Rawls that self-respect is a vital primary good, something of great importance that any rational person is presumed to want.[15] Now, given actual human psychology, self-respect is—to a considerable degree—dependent upon other people's affirmation of one's own worth. And in modern advanced societies, employment, earnings and professional success are, for better or worse, positively correlated with social assessments of an individual's value. Further, beyond the reactions of other people, work and career identifications form significant parts of some people's conceptions of themselves and their own worth; hence these identifications may contribute directly to the creation and sustenance of self-respect, and their absence will frequently have the opposite effect.

To be sure, "economic" criteria are not the only standards of value used by oneself or others to assess one's worthiness. But because of the *pervasiveness* of disability, as noted above, satisfaction of standards of value in other important spheres of life are also usually negatively affected by handicaps. Thus the handicapped are on average likely to be less convenient social companions, more limited in their sports and recreational activities, less able to fulfill nurturing and helping roles within the family, and so on. Thus, nonworkplace bases of self-respect will also be harder for the disabled to fulfill, making it even more important that the workplace bases of self-respect be made available to them. (In addition, employment may foster success—and self-respect based on success—in the other spheres of life, as when one's social life is better because of friends one has made at work.)[16]

In the end, then, the concept of self-respect plays a dual role in my refutation of CREEP. First, it serves as an example of an important aspect of utility that is overlooked in the narrow economic interpretations of CREEP. Once this narrowness is avoided and the "indirect" utilitarian advantages of a social policy of training and employing the disabled are noted, it is evident that there are substantial utilitarian reasons in support of the disabled having a right to work. Second, the handicapped are disadvantaged in obtaining the bases of self-respect, a critically important good. And because of the way the psychology of self-respect interacts with the work ethic present in modern advanced societies, this disadvantage *cannot be rectified by transfer payments,* but (sometimes) can be rectified by training and employment opportunities. Hence considerations of distributive justice, which prescribe easing the plight of society's less fortunate members, provide further support for ascribing to disabled people a right to work.

At a slightly more abstract level, my response to CREEP may be concisely summarized as containing three elements. The distributive-justice element says that we should aim not only at efficient social states but at those in which the plight of the least advantaged—such as the permanently disabled—is ameliorated. The market-failure element says that a key contributor to personal utility for the disabled, self-respect, cannot be efficiently provided by the free market (even if the disabled receive monetary subsidies) because, like love, self-respect cannot be purchased with money.

The informed-preferences element says the justifiability of providing the disabled with opportunities for self-respect through a right of employment need not presuppose an actual present preference of the disabled for more jobs rather than more cash. Many of the disabled may presently undervalue self-respect because, in their current downtrodden circumstances, they place too little value on their own importance and their own attitudes toward themselves and their lives. Suppose it is reasonable to believe that if given sufficient employment opportunities, the permanently disabled would come to value their self-respect more. Once they had jobs and greater self-respect, they would be happy that they had them instead of higher welfare payments. If this is so, the market-failure and distributive-justice elements of my argument support a right to work for the disabled based on the hypothetical *informed* priorities of the disabled.

HYPOTHETICAL CONTRACTS AND INSURANCE SCHEMES

The arguments offered in the last section for the disabled in advanced modern societies having a right to work constitute a mixed bag. But there is a natural way of incorporating them into a unified theoretical perspective. The fundamental idea to be exploited is the contractarian one that certain moral and political rights can be justified by observing that rational people would, under appropriate conditions, agree to have these rights recognized and enforced in a society in which they expected to live. This idea can serve as a useful heuristic in attempting to determine the overall moral status of a right to work for the disabled. In particular, thinking about what practices concerning the disabled we would agree to live under, in the absence of certain information that would inappropriately bias our choices, provides a useful perspective from which we can hope to assess accurately the comparative weight of the various competing considerations mentioned in the last section—economic efficiency, distributive justice, insurance against some of the worst consequences of disability maintenance of self-respect and so on.

There is, of course, considerable disagreement as to whether and why the fundamental contractarian idea—justification by hypothetical rational agreement—is sound. But for present purposes I will ignore these disputes and focus on showing how a right to work of the handicapped might be justified from a contractarian perspective. Actually, I will consider two distinct but related contractarian approaches to the matter. One, which I call "Rawlsian," is included because of its prominence and wide acceptance in the literature, as well as its intellectual attractions. The other approach I call "Hobbesian" because, while it is not Hobbes's own view in every particular, it is based on—and inspired by—his political philosophy.[17]

The two approaches, Rawlsian and Hobbesian, share a number of common features. They both imagine hypothetical rational contractors agreeing on final binding rules to govern the society in which they expect to live out their lives together. They both impose information constraints that deprive the parties of specific information about their own standing in society and their social roles. At the same time, both approaches assume that the parties possess relevant general information—for example, that their society is an advanced modern one that values productivity, that handicapped people suffer disadvantages in various spheres of life, and that self-respect is partly a function of other people's perceptions of one's worth. And both contend that when making a final one-time choice, under uncertainty, of social rules that will substantially affect one's life prospects, it is ratio-nal to choose conservatively in the sense of not sacrificing prospects of acceptable out-comes in risky pursuit of greater gains.

Three differences between Rawlsian and Hobbesian contractarianism are relevant to our discussion. First, the Rawlsian account imposes a stronger information constraint and supposes that the parties lack knowledge of their own personal as well as social characteris-tics. As regards the problem at hand, Rawlsian contractors do not know whether they themselves have been or ever will be disabled, while Hobbesian contractors will know whether they have been disabled up to the point in their lives (presumably some stage of rational adulthood) at which the negotiations take place.

Second, the Rawlsian account regards the parties as purely self-interested, while the Hobbesian account holds that the parties are predominantly egoistic but may have consid-erable concern for the well-being of particular others and significant concern for the well-being of others in general.[18] Third, the Hobbesian account calls for nearly unanimous agreement on the terms of the society-governing contract, while the Rawlsian approach calls for unanimous agreement. Looked at broadly, the difference between the two approaches is this: the severe information constraint of the Rawlsian approach is intended to guarantee the impersonality or impartiality of the resultant rules and to provide a plausible device by which unanimous agreement might be reached among self-interested parties; the Hobbes-ian approach conserves the contractarian insight that social rules are the result of a bargain among differently situated individuals.[19] But it is then forced—due to its thinner veil of ignorance—to "relax" the unanimity and self-interest assumptions to make it plausible that any agreement would be reached.

The Rawlsian hypothetical agreement argument for the right to work of the disabled is rather straightforward. Behind the thick veil of ignorance, the individual parties do not know whether and when they will be disabled. But they have the general information that a high percentage of people suffer permanent disability at some time before death, and that a quite significant percentage do so during (or prior to) their normal working years.[20] They also know that theirs is an advanced modern society which can afford to provide welfare and work rights to the disabled without reducing others in society below a decent eco-nomic minimum. They are further aware of the pervasive disadvantages of handicaps and the relations between self-respect and employment in modern societies which were noted in the previous section. Facing a once-and-for-all choice under uncertainty, a conservative Rawlsian individual will not gamble on the hope of not being disabled during (or prior to) her working years, but will sacrifice some potential wealth by agreeing to having society accord the disabled a right to work of the sort described in my first section. She thus insures herself against the worst outcome of being a disabled person who wants (and may be capable of) gainful employment but is cut off from this avenue (as well as others) of retaining self-respect and participating in the public life of society.[21] In a nutshell, once we note that the permanently disabled may be viewed from a certain perspective as the most disadvantaged major group in society and observe the relationship between work and the key Rawlsian value of self-respect in modem productive societies, a right to work for the disabled follows rather directly from Rawlsian "maximin" reasoning.

The Hobbesian contractarian argument for the right to work of the handicapped is essentially the same as the Rawlsian one—with one complicating wrinkle. The majority of the contractors now know that, so far, they have not been disabled. Why, then, would they agree to a social insurance scheme which they will have to pay for, and which they have less chance of benefiting from than do their disabled counterparts?

Many would so agree, as in the Rawlsian account, to insure against worst outcomes in the case of their own future disablement. Since the Hobbesian account allows substantial altruism toward some others (for example, family members), other parties would sign on to insure against the future disablement of their loved ones and descendants. And as Hobbesian contractarianism allows that some may have significant general benevolence, some parties may agree to the right to work because of sympathy for the disabled, whomever they turn out to be. Others, probably the majority, would agree from some combination of these motives. There might be a small minority of non–risk-averse, non-sympathetic holdouts who would not agree, but Hobbesian contractarianism does not require unanimous agreement.

Both versions of the contractarian argument treat the right to work as a form of insurance against some of the avoidable bad consequences of becoming disabled. But looking at the right this way suggests a significant objection to its justification via the contractarian notion of hypothetical consent. Why, the objection goes, should we accord the disabled a right to work, thus treating them in accordance with some purely hypothetical insurance scheme, when we could treat them in accordance with the actual insurance arrangements they have (or have not) freely made in the real world? In particular, if most people have not chosen to insure themselves against certain of the worst consequences of possible disability (for example, unemployment), why should we force the lucky winners of this gamble to ameliorate the plight of the unfortunate losers?

A full answer to this objection would require a fundamental defense of hypothetical agreement (contractarian) accounts of rights and obligations against actual agreement (libertarian) accounts. I will not attempt such a defense here. But I will make three observations that, in my view, vindicate the application of the hypothetical agreement account to this particular substantive issue. First, many handicapped people are disabled at birth or as children, or before they have a reasonable chance to accumulate sufficient resources to insure themselves against the worst consequences of disability. Second, actual private insurance markets offer only money in the event of disablement, not employment opportunities that may be a necessary means for the sustenance of self-respect among many of the disabled.[22] Third, disability is a condition, like old age, that is not pleasant to think about. Hence people have a natural psychological tendency to avoid thinking about it, to imagine it cannot happen to them and so on. This may not entirely prevent people from insuring themselves against future catastrophes: people do, after all, prefer jobs with good medical insurance, unemployment benefits and pension systems. But it produces a *tendency* toward irrational underinvestment in insurance schemes (for example, pension plans, disability insurance) that would ameliorate these undesirable conditions when they occur.

In sum, the case for *designing policies* in accordance with the dictates of hypothetical *rational* agreement is particularly strong as regards handicapped people's right to work, for market imperfections and systematic irrationalities limit people's opportunities and capacities prudently to protect their long-term interests with respect to potential disabilities.

LUCK AND RESPONSIBILITY

Why should disabilities be treated differently from other disadvantages which render it more difficult for individuals to achieve a given level of well-being? Why should those with handicaps be given special rights and resources by society that are not given to people who suffer other significant forms of bad luck—lack of natural endowments, a poor early environment, possession of wants that are expensive to satisfy, unpredictable changes in consumer demand that render one's investments worthless, and so on?

Some of these questions have recently been discussed in an interesting article by Richard Arneson.[23] Arneson's position is that, in principle, handicaps should not be treated differently from other forms of bad luck that cause people to need extra social resources to attain a given level of welfare. For Arneson, the category or cause of need is basically irrelevant. What does matter is whether (or to what extent) the individual in question is responsible for possession of the special need. If he is—if he voluntarily (or negligently or recklessly) acquired it or risked acquiring it—then society is not obligated to devote extra resources to satisfying his special need. But if his acquisition (and retention) of the need was (and is) beyond his control, society has reason to provide the extra resources he requires to reach an appropriate overall welfare level, regardless of the nature of the need.[24]

Expensive Tastes

Arneson focuses much of his attention on the case of "expensive tastes," such as the sophisticate's taste for fine wines. These expensive tastes are preferences for commodities or experiences that can be satisfied only by relatively large expenditures of resources. Arneson recognizes that treating the handicapped person's special needs on a par with the preferences of the expensive wine enthusiast is counterintuitive. But he contends this is due to two factors: (1) we assume (normally correctly) that the wine enthusiast's expensive preferences are (or were) more under his control than the disabled person's disabilities; and (2) we are aware of much more severe practical difficulties in society accurately determining people's preferences than their disabilities (including the incentives people would have to exaggerate their expensive preferences in hopes of receiving larger subsidies). Thus Arneson poses the rhetorical question: "If we put aside practical difficulties about information gathering and measurement of hypothetical rational preferences, what further good reasons could there be for treating involuntary expensive preferences due to handicaps differently than involuntary expensive preferences due to tastes?"[25]

There are good answers to Arneson's question. First, putting aside measurement difficulties in the way Arneson does distorts the issue. For expensive preferences are not simply less reliably measurable than disabilities: their nonsatisfaction normally has a drastically less severe impact on people's overall welfare than do disabilities. Hence, in the absence of reliable measurability, there is an extremely powerful presumption in favor of treating the amelioration of handicaps as more socially urgent than the satisfaction of expensive preferences for good wine or ocean views.[26]

Second, the formation of expensive preferences can be influenced by persons other than the individual in question—in particular, by the individual's parents. Social subsidies for satisfaction of expensive tastes thus provide an extra incentive (or reduce the disincentive) for parents to inculcate such tastes in their children.[27] This observation holds even though the two sorts of disadvantages in question—handicaps and expensive tastes—are equally beyond the control of the individual in question. The point is that being beyond the control of the individual and being beyond *anyone's* control are different, and the difference matters a great deal in the present context. If society were to treat involuntary expensive tastes on a par with involuntary handicaps, this would encourage parents to inculcate expensive tastes in their children, thus lowering overall social welfare. It would unfairly require some of its members to subsidize the aspirations of others who want their children to live their expensive conception of the good life. This and its differing impacts on overall welfare and the aforementioned "practical" difficulties of accurately measuring preferences constitute fully adequate reasons for society to treat handicaps and expensive tastes very differently and to assign special economic rights to possessors of the former but not the latter.

Other Forms of Bad Luck

What about other forms of bad luck besides expensive tastes? Are there good reasons for compensating the permanently disabled by affording them certain legally protected economic rights without doing the same for victims of other kinds of bad luck? I believe that there is a variety of such reasons; different ones apply depending upon what other form of bad luck we are comparing to handicaps. Among these reasons are (1) the *pervasiveness* of disability (noted in my second section) in typically disadvantaging its victims in all major spheres of life; (2) the counterproductive stigmatization of not-yet-stigmatized victims of bad luck as being "defective" and in need of social support; (3) the greater practical difficulties in identifying the victims of other forms of bad luck; and (4) the practical impossibility or social undesirability of *rectifying* the effects of other sorts of bad luck by ascribing rights parallel to the economic rights that I advocate for the disabled.

Let us briefly illustrate how these differences operate to justify treating handicaps differently from four other important types of bad luck, as regards the ascription of rights like the right to work. Consider first ordinary bad luck in free economic markets: an entrepreneur sinks capital into an enterprise that unpredictably fails, or a worker invests time, money and effort to develop a skill that (again unpredictably) turns out to be no longer needed.[28] Here, the main reason for lesser compensation is that both parties' losses, while not a result of any fault on their part, were "voluntary" in an important sense. The entrepreneur and the worker either knew or should have known that their investments were risky ones and that unpredictable losses might occur. Further, their bearing (most of) their losses is the necessary price of luckier investors making gains from their investments, and the prospect of such gains is necessary in principle for the free market to operate as an effective mechanism of economic growth and productivity. It is worth noting, however, that despite the voluntary risk-assumption inherent in one's investments in financial or human capital, modern free-market societies do ascribe some economic rights to losing investors (in the form of bankruptcy laws, unemployment insurance, retraining programs and other provisions of the welfare state) to protect them from some of the worst consequences of bad luck (and folly). Given the pervasiveness of the effects of permanent handicaps and their generally nonvoluntary nature, it is not unreasonable to afford their victims even more extensive economic rights.

A second kind of bad luck is one whose negative effects are arguably nearly as pervasive as the effects of permanent disabilities: a poor early environment, which for a variety of psychological and cultural reasons apparently disadvantages individuals in their later functioning in the economic, social and familial spheres. As in the case of handicaps, advanced modern societies do have a variety of special programs designed in part to ameliorate the plight of victims of poor early environments. As programs to help those from disadvantaged backgrounds contain provisions essentially like those embodied in the disabled's right to work (for example, training programs and nondiscrimination and affirmative-action laws), there is no substantial ground for the complaint that those with handicaps are arbitrarily treated better than those suffering from this other "life-pervading" form of bad luck.

A third form of bad luck—physical unattractiveness—is worth discussing because it is generally (and properly) not regarded as a grounds of social compensation.[29] Why not?

First, it is relatively unpervasive; it mainly affects (by limiting) an individual's range of options regarding marital and sexual partners, though it can have wider effects on social life. Second, it is thought to be under an individual's control to some significant degree—dressing right and taking care of one's body can, within limits, increase one's degree of attractiveness. Third, the social and psychological costs of identifying—and stigmatizing—some individuals as so unattractive as to need compensation from society would very likely outweigh any benefits gained by these individuals, such as having an extra stipend to spend on dates, clothing or health spas. Fourth, and finally, the remedies for this disadvantage that are analogous to the right to work—for example, nondiscrimination in choice of marital partners—would be unworkable, silly and self-defeating, given the vital necessity of free choice in the spheres of personal, family and sexual life.[30]

The last sort of bad luck to be considered is lack of intelligence or mental capacity[31] A severe deficiency in this regard—mental retardation—is itself classified as a disability, but what of less extreme disadvantages in this realm? Arguably, they are pervasive, reducing one's capacity to cope with the problems of—and hence enjoy and succeed in—family, social and recreational life as well as economic endeavors. So why not compensate for these disadvantages as we compensate for handicaps?

Clearly, stigmatization is one problem: being publicly declared of lesser mental competence would probably do people greater harm than any good they might receive from a compensatory stipend. (Disabilities, by contrast, are usually readily discernible, hence the disabled generally pay stigmatization costs whether or not they are publicly identified as such.) Also, the appropriate remedies here are unclear. Should we have more education for the less mentally able, to help them function better? Should we substantially relax hiring and promotion by qualifications? Should we compensate lesser intelligence with cash payments? None of these options seems at all attractive.

Responsibility for One's Own Handicaps

Arneson's proposal that social compensation for bad luck be tied to lack of voluntariness rather than type of bad luck has another implication bearing on disabilities. His discussion raises the issue of whether an individual's rights are forfeited if she was (partly) responsible for the accident or illness leading to her own disablement. Arneson's voluntariness test suggests that if someone becomes disabled through her own recklessness, negligence or voluntary risk-assumption, then society's obligation to offer special help to that person is correspondingly cancelled (or weakened). Thus he writes: "distributive justice does not recommend any intervention by society to correct inequalities that arise through the voluntary choice or fault of those that end up with less."[32]

To deal with this matter thoroughly would involve delving into fundamental questions about the nature and limits of society's obligations to its individual members and the relevant trade-offs between respecting individual autonomy and promoting individual welfare. Needless to say, I am not prepared for any such undertaking here. But I will offer two observations that count against society treating an individual's "contributory negligence" as grounds for withholding aid needed to alleviate the bad effects of that individual's subsequent permanent disablement.

The first observation relates to the practical difficulties (and distastefulness) of society officially determining which handicapped persons are at fault for their own condition. Institutionalizing this process would doubtless result in the usual bureaucratic inefficiencies, errors and rigidities and would create the unseemly spectacle of professionals—acting on behalf of society as a whole—adding to the woes of handicapped people (and their families) by trying to have them thrown back on their own resources to save the average taxpayer a few dollars.[33]

My second observation concerns equity. Temporary injuries, illnesses, serious loss of property due to natural disasters, unemployment, unwanted pregnancies and drug dependencies are only some of the many serious misfortunes that modern advanced societies invest resources in ameliorating. If "contributory negligence" is to be treated as a ground for denying the permanently handicapped their rights to aid, then fairness requires the same treatment of victims of these other conditions. Until we are ready to deny low-interest government loans to burned-out residents in high-fire-danger areas, to leave careless motorcycle riders lying in the street with untreated broken limbs, and to withhold cancer treatments and heart surgery at government-subsidized hospitals from heavy smokers, fairness prohibits penalizing those permanently handicapped people who are partly responsible for their conditions.

AFFIRMATIVE ACTION

A meaningful right to work for the disabled must entail an obligation not to discriminate against handicapped people (that is, not to count their handicaps against them except when those handicaps render them less able to perform the job in question). But should such a right also include an affirmative-action requirement giving disabled persons some form of preference over others in hiring, promotion and admissions decisions? In this section, I address this difficult question obliquely by considering which of the main arguments for and against affirmative action in the case of women and minorities also apply to the disabled.

There are, as I see it, three major groups of arguments in favor of affirmative action programs in general. First, there are forward-looking utilitarian arguments, emphasizing various good effects of bringing more representatives of the disadvantaged group in question into responsible positions in society. Second, there are error-correction arguments. Third, there are various forms of arguments for compensatory justice, saying that members of disadvantaged groups should be given hiring preference to compensate for past hiring discrimination against them or members of their group or other disadvantages they suffered at the hands of society.

Do these arguments for affirmative action apply as well to the disabled as they do to women and minorities? For the most part, it seems, they do. Consider, first, forward-looking utilitarian considerations. Successful handicapped persons can serve as role models for the many people who are disabled as well as for others who face serious obstacles of other sorts in life. Nor is there any reason to think they would bring a less distinct perspective to their jobs or be less inclined to help others in their situation than are women and minorities.

Application of the error-correction argument is less clear in the case of the disabled. Potential employers are perhaps even more likely to underestimate the relevant abilities of the disabled than to underestimate the abilities of women and minorities, simply because the issue of "potential special problems" is raised by the mere existence of their handicaps. On the other hand, some of the main obstacles that permanently disabled people faced in the past in obtaining their current skills and qualifications—namely, their disabilities—will remain with them through their period of employment and will continue to constitute barriers to peak performance. Further, some of the disabled obtained their main qualifications prior to the onset of their disability; hence their possession of them is no special sign of merit or determination. Different aspects of the error-correction argument, therefore, point in different directions on the question of whether this argument is stronger as regards the handicapped or minorities and women.

When it comes to compensation for past disadvantages suffered by the very individuals to be helped by affirmative-action programs, the handicapped are more deserving in some respects than women or racial minorities and less deserving in others. They are more deserving in the United States, at least, because they have not previously had legal protection against discrimination. This means that the current generation of handicapped people who might be advantaged by affirmative-action programs contains many individuals who may have suffered unfair but legal discrimination. The disabled may also be viewed as more deserving of compensation because of the pervasiveness of their disadvantages, as noted earlier.

The disabled may be less deserving of affirmative action, on the other hand, because their disadvantages are less purely the result of society's misconduct and more the result of simple bad luck. And despite earlier legal protection from discrimination, women and minorities have continued to face discrimination in practice that may equal what the disabled have faced. The force of this last consideration, in particular, depends upon complex empirical matters that I am in no position to sort out.

Turning to arguments against affirmative action, there are four main lines of argument to consider. First, any departures from a pure merit system of hiring will harm economic efficiency. Second, affirmative-action programs tend to help the most advantaged members of disadvantaged groups—for example, the middle-class minority student who is well-educated enough to compete for law school admission. Third, such programs are counterproductive for the very disadvantaged groups they are designed to help, since they undermine confidence and stigmatize even the successful members of those groups as having needed preference to succeed. Fourth, and most important, such programs are unfair to more qualified candidates from groups not singled out for preference, since they are denied positions they would have otherwise obtained.

Do these same objections to affirmative action apply in the case of the disabled as well as women and minorities?[34] The first clearly does, for I have interpreted the disableds' right to work as requiring efforts to employ them beyond the point of maximum economic efficiency. Nonetheless, the aggregate economic costs of the sort of affirmative action for the disabled which I espouse are kept within reasonable limits by three factors. The pool of work-age disabled people who want to work and are able to do so at all is likely to be relatively small (compared to the pool of employable women and minorities). And, as noted in the next section, I limit my advocacy to "tiebreaking" affirmative action for the disabled, which further restricts the effects of the policy. Finally, the argument for the right to work defended here advocates sacrificing some economic efficiency to provide job opportunities to the disabled, but it does not require sacrifices without limits.

The second objection, about *which* individuals in the disadvantaged group would benefit, seems less serious in the case of the disabled. For while it is likely to be the less disabled who would benefit most from preferential hiring, there need be no worry that these people have not been disadvantaged at all, as there might conceivably be in the case of middle-class minorities or women.

Objection three—about the counterproductive psychological and social effects on the members of the disadvantaged group of the affirmative-action policy—appears to apply equally to the disabled and other disadvantaged groups. But it is an especially worrisome objection in the context of my argument, which defends opportunities for employment primarily as means for the disabled to achieve self-respect. Can self-respect be enhanced by receiving a job through government subsidies or affirmative-action programs rather than open competition? Can self-respect be retained in a social environment in which others believe you were hired for reasons other than your qualifications? Can income received for work that is profit-making only with government subsidies be said to be "earned" in a sense that will promote the sense of self-worth of the worker? If the answer to these questions is an unequivocal "no," then the right to work advocated in this paper would be essentially pointless.

I believe, however, that there are good reasons for answering these questions, as they apply to complex modern societies such as ours, in the affirmative. The first point to notice is that the relevant comparison in many cases will be between a member of a disadvantaged group having an "affirmative-action" job rather than no job at all, or a good "affirmative-action" job rather than a worse job. While the former alternative may do less to promote self-respect than a good job otherwise obtained, it may do more to promote self-respect and respect from others than being unemployed or employed in a poor job. This is especially so if unemployment or menial employment—together with membership in a disadvantaged group—is regarded by society as characterizing "low-worth" individuals.

Further, in a world of incomplete information and moral complexity, people judge their own and others' vocational worth by more than the criteria on the basis of which one was hired. Actual performance on the job is probably the most important measure of all, and hiring under affirmative-action programs will give many members of disadvantaged groups opportunities to prove themselves at work that they would not otherwise have had. If, as the error-correction argument suggests, such people will—on average—perform better than their hirers initially expect, they will be able to earn the respect of themselves and others by their performance.

The final objection to affirmative action, which is based on unfairness to the losing but better-qualified candidates, clearly applies to affirmative-action programs for the disabled as well as for other groups. For if you are unemployed or underemployed, it will hardly matter to your well-being whether the job opportunity you lost was to a disabled person or a member of a racial minority group. Further, the observations in my second section about the significance of employment as a support of self-respect in advanced modern societies underscore the force of this objection to affirmative action.

This does not affect our main conclusion, however. For if we review the various lines of argument for and against affirmative action, it turns out that for each line of argument discussed, preferential hiring for the disabled fares *as well or better,* on balance, as preferential hiring for women and minorities. Thus if the latter programs are justified, the former surely are.

THEORY AND PRACTICE

In this concluding section, I briefly spell out some practical conclusions that may be drawn from my arguments, and their limits. As I see it, three basic principles are supported by my analysis. First, as argued in my second section, the disabled have, in virtue of their special disadvantages, a claim on extra resources from society beyond the point of economic cost-efficiency on grounds of both utility and justice. Methodologically, this means that economic cost-benefit analysis should not be regarded as the sole governing criterion of social policy with respect to the handicapped. Second, because of the special connection between employment and self-respect in modern productive societies spelled out in my second section, the disabled have a special claim on employment opportunities, not simply on welfare payments. Third, and finally, because of the contractarian nature of the justification of economic rights for the disabled, which views those rights as part of an insurance scheme that rational agents in an appropriate "original position" would adopt (see my third section), the *cost* of special aid to the disabled should be spread as widely as possible throughout society, That is, as far as possible, the special expenses of aiding and employing the handicapped should not fall in large lumps on the handicapped themselves, their families or particular employers, but should be evened out among all of the members of society.

Various practical implications seem to flow from these three principles and the arguments that support them. Along with nondiscrimination laws, the right of the disabled to work implies tax-supported subsidies for educating and training (or retraining) the disabled as well as subsidies to those who hire the handicapped (or to disabled workers themselves) to cover the expenses involved in modifying workplaces and equipment to make them accessible to and usable by those with disabilities. The idea of the widest possible cost-sharing is the rationale for such subsidies, and the same principle may justify placing stricter requirements on large than on small businesses.[35] If the costs of subsidies are spread widely, few of the nonhandicapped should suffer excessively.

Affirmative action for the disabled is more problematic, partly because it is less feasible to spread the costs of such programs widely and evenly among the nonhandicapped. Yet the comparisons of the previous section suggest that affirmative action for the disabled is no more problematic than affirmative action for minorities and women. In my view, that means there is considerable justification for it in some form.

The drawbacks are economic costs, potential negative effects on the reputations of highly qualified disabled workers and the problem of unfairness to possibly better-qualified candidates who lose out in competition for jobs. This last problem is especially serious from the point of view of the present analysis because of the connections between employment and self-respect (which also apply to nondisabled persons), as well as the lack of wide distribution of the costs involved (which fall mainly on the particular unsuccessful competitors). Perhaps any unfairness suffered by a nonhandicapped person under such programs is a lesser harm or injustice than leaving a more disadvantaged and somewhat less qualified disabled person without a job. But the uncertainties here are great enough that I am inclined to endorse only a weak form of preferential hiring for the disabled: preferring an equally qualified handicapped candidate to a nonhandicapped one. This proposal also has the advantages of lowering the economic costs of affirmative action for the disabled and posing less of a threat to the reputations of highly qualified handicapped workers.

The key practical question that my arguments do not and cannot answer concerns *how much* of a sacrifice of general efficiency society is required to make to aid and employ the handicapped.[36] Some sacrifice is appropriate here, but there are obviously limits to what is reasonable. At a minimum, we want to disallow aid to the disabled that is *collectively counterproductive* for them, in the sense of interfering so much with economic growth and productivity that they suffer more in the long run.[37] And sacrifices well short of this limit may already constitute an unreasonable burden on the rest of society.

The notion of a hypothetical rational agreement may be of some (limited) heuristic use in dealing with this problem. The amount of sacrifice in overall efficiency we should make to help the disabled is the amount it is rational to choose in an original choice position. It seems rational to sacrifice some social efficiency to provide for the possible core interests of those loved ones (including yourself) who might become disabled, and so we could expect general agreement on welfare and work rights for the disabled.

But are there grounds for expecting a rational consensus on the precise rate of trade-off between efficiency and protection of the handicapped? I doubt it. Careful reflection under the appropriate restrictions might well narrow the range of differences, but I see no unique account of rational choice under such conditions that could be expected to yield general consensus on the appropriate trade-off between these values. So perhaps the best contractarianism can do as regards this matter is to (1) specify and justify the economic rights of the disabled in fairly general terms (as I have done); (2) characterize fair political procedures and institutions; and (3) leave it to those procedures and institutions to work out the precise contours of the rights of the disabled.

ACKNOWLEDGMENTS

I am grateful to Eric Cave, Tyler Cowen, Ellen Frankel Paul, the members of the Moral and Political Philosophy Society of Orange County (MAPPS) and others for helpful comments on earlier versions of this essay.

NOTES

[1] In a recent article, Susan Wendell writes: "I decided to delve into what I assumed would be a substantial philosophical literature in medical ethics on the nature and experience of disability. I consulted The Philosopher's Index, looking under 'Disability,' 'Handicap,' 'Illness,' and 'Disease.' This was a depressing experience. At least 90% of philosophical articles on these topics are concerned with two questions: Under what conditions is it morally permissible/right to kill/let die a disabled person and how potentially disabled does a fetus have to be before it is permissible/right to prevent its being born?" "Toward a Feminist Theory of Disability," *Hypatia* 4; 4; 2 (Summer 1989): 104.

[2] See, for example, my own *Hobbesian Moral and Political Theory*. Princeton: Princeton University Press, 1986, 215–216, 242.

[3] Steven A. Holmes, "House Approves Bill Establishing Broad Rights for Disabled People," *New York Times,* May 23, 1990, A10.

[4] The employment need not be with a profit-making firm. Paid work in governmental, nonprofit or charitable organizations could serve the purpose. Even unpaid employment might vindicate a disabled person's right to work if (1) the job is seen by the person and others as tied to the person's skills and abilities, and thus can play a role in promoting self-respect (see the second section of this essay); and (2) the person has adequate financial resources from other sources (for example, from family or government programs).

[5] I say "relatively" uncontroversial because certain hard-line libertarian views might imply otherwise. The position expressed in Robert Nozick. *Anarchy, State, and Utopia.* New York: Basic Books, 1974, which never mentions the disabled, seems to fall in this category.

[6] See, for example, John Rawls. *A Theory of Justice.* Cambridge: Harvard University Press, 1971; Robert Goodin. *Reasons for Welfare.* Princeton: Princeton University Press, 1988; and David Braybrooke. *Meeting Needs.* Princeton: Princeton University Press, 1987.

[7] For examples, see S. J. D. Green. "Competitive Equality of Opportunity; A Defense," *Ethics* 100; 1 (October 1989): 24.

[8] Robert Goodin, "Stabilizing Expectations," *Ethics* 100; 3 (April 1990): 532–553, offers a different sort of argument against income maintenance for the long-term disabled, which might be applied also to the right to work. He writes: "Those who have been permanently incapacitated would be living a lie to persist with their same plans, just as before. . . . Whatever value we see in people's framing plans and projects for themselves is conditional upon their being realistic plans and projects, appropriate to the person's circumstances" (548–549). This argument overlooks the fact that what plans are "realistic" or "appropriate" in a disabled person's circumstances depends partly upon the level and types of social resources (for example, income, training, job opportunities) available to that person. Hence it simply begs the normative question at issue to deny resources to the disabled on the grounds that it is unrealis-

tic for them to expect to achieve the goals those resources would help them achieve. A similar point is made in John E. Roemer, "Egalitarianism, Responsibility, and Information," *Economics and Philosophy* 3; 2 (October 1987): 242–243.

[9]Wendell, "Feminist Theory of Disability," 113–115, discusses why the presence of the disabled makes people uncomfortable.

[10]Because employers cannot count on hiring disabled workers at pay much below the level of their guaranteed stipends, the possibility of large entrepreneurial profits may be greatly diminished.

[11]See, e.g., G. E. Moore. *Prinicipia Ethica.* London: Cambridge University Press, 1962, 209–210.

[12] Richard Brandt. *A Theory of the Good and the Right.* Oxford: Clarendon Press, 1979.

[13]Rawls, *Theory of Justice,* 130–132.

[14]Wendell, "Feminist Theory of Disability," characterizes and discusses this stigmatization of the disabled as a form of oppression.

[15]Rawls, *Theory of Justice,* 440–446.

[16]One might wonder whether the self-respect argument for a right to work applies less strongly to disabled women, since social respect for women has traditionally been less tied to their activities in the world of paid employment. But given the increasingly active role of women in the workforces of modern advanced societies and the difficulties that disabilities pose for women fulfilling other roles (for example, caretaker within the family), this argument seems to apply to disabled women with virtually equal force.

[17]Kavka, *Hobbesian Theory.* On the relationship between Rawlsian and Hobbesian contractarianism, see especially chap. 5.

[18]On predominant egoism, see ibid., 64–80. In chaps. 2 through 4 of that work, I argue that it is unclear whether Hobbes himself was commited to pure egoism, but that the weaker and more plausible doctrine of predominant egoism suffices to ground his famous argument against anarchy.

[19]See David Gauthier. "The Social Contract: Individual Decision or Collective Bargain," in C. A. Hooker, J. J. Leach and E. F. McClennen, eds., *Foundations and Applications of Decision Theory.* Dordrecht: Reidel, 1978, vol. 2, 47–67, and Jean Hampton, "Contracts and Choices: Does Rawls Have a Social Contract Theory?" *Journal of Philosophy* 77; 6 (June 1980): 315–338.

[20]In 1988, 8.6 percent, of the U.S. population aged 16–64 years (and 22.3 percent, of the population aged 55–64) was "work disabled," according to the Bureau of the Census. See their *Statistical Abstract of the United States: 1989.* Washington: U.S. Government Printing Office, 1989, 109th ed., table no. 592.

[21]There are even worse outcomes—for example, being disabled so badly that one is incapable of any meaningful participation in society, regardless of the social resources devoted to one's rehabilitation. But there is little society can do to ameliorate these outcomes, other than to provide for welfare needs.

[22]Would social respect go along with the government-subsidized, affirmative-action jobs for the handicapped advocated in this paper? This important question is taken up in the section below on affirmative action.

[23]Richard E. Arneson. "Liberalism, Distributive Subjectivism, and Equal Opportunity for Welfare," *Philosophy and Public Affairs* 19; 2 (Spring 1990): 158–194. [Ed. note: see also a more recent version of Arneson's position in Part A of this volume.]

[24]Ibid., 185–194. A similar view is put forward in G. A. Cohen, "On the Currency of Egalitarian Justice," *Ethics* 99; 4 (July 1989): 906–944. Both Arneson and Cohen approach the issue from an explicitly egalitarian perspective.

[25]Arneson, "Liberalism, Subjectivism, and Equal Opportunity," 190.

[26]See ibid., 188, where Arneson discusses other aspects of measurability but unaccountably ignores this one.

[27]Thus, Arneson (ibid., 194) is wrong that "the only possible justification for discriminating in the treatment of physical handicaps and other expensive preferences is a perfectionist knowledge of human good." One justification derives from an awareness that other people believe that they have such perfectionist knowledge, and act on these beliefs in raising their children.

[28]Arneson discusses a version of the laborer example. See ibid., 189–190.

[29]For a brief but highly charged discussion of this issue, see Antony Flew. *The Politics of Procrustes.* Buffalo: Prometheus Books, 1981, 101–102.

[30]One of the characteristic features of libertarianism is that it extends this line of argument to cover economic as well as personal life.

[31]I use the term "intelligence" to refer in general to complex mental capacity without assuming that mental capacity is a unitary (rather than multidimensional) competence, or that standard intelligence (IQ) tests are a good measure of it. For some problems concerning IQ testing, see N. J. Block and Gerald Dworkin, "IQ: Heritability and Inequality, Part 1," *Philosophy and Public Affairs* 3; 4 (Summer 1974): 331–409.

[32]Arneson, "Liberalism, Subjectivism, and Equal Opportunity," 176.

[33]Currently, in civil law suits private attorneys will sometimes try to establish that particular handicapped people are responsible for their own handicaps, in order to reduce or eliminate the liability of their own clients. But at least in doing so they are not acting as representatives of society as a whole.

[34]I remain noncommittal on how strong some of these objections are; my primary concern is with their comparative force in the case of the handicapped.

[35]The Americans with Disabilities Act does exempt small businesses from certain requirements. See Holmes, "House Approves Bill," A10.

[36]In addition to this macroallocation issue, there are also microallocation issues about how resources designated for aiding the disabled are to be used and distributed among people with different types and degrees of disability.

[37]See Rawls's discussion of his analogous "difference principle" (*Theory of Justice*, 75–83).

Market Failure and ADA Title I

MICHAEL ASHLEY STEIN

RATIONAL MARKET DECISIONS AND UNEMPLOYED WORKERS WITH DISABILITIES

Legal theorists with faith in the principles of the neoclassical economic model of the labor market assert that antidiscrimination statutes are inefficient and unnecessary. A statute or regulation that preempts an employer's considered personal choice and directs that some other applicant be hired or promoted is characterized as introducing inefficacy into the employment equation. Their core belief in market rationality also leads these commentators to deny that state regulation of hiring decisions can be a corrective policy. Instead, legislative intercession is seen as a needlessly distributive method of addressing imbalances that is inferior both to allowing labor market dynamics to restore a nondiscriminatory balance as well as to nonregulative incentives such as job programs or cost-spreading through the tax system.[1]

As applied by law and economics commentators, the comprehensive normative goal of the neoclassical economic model is to achieve legal regimes whose efficiency mirrors those attained in an ideal market of perfectly competitive equilibrium. Under this scheme, the term "efficient" (or "Pareto-efficient") refers to the most optimal outcome or one having the greatest utility. It is in large part differences about how to determine what solutions are efficient that separate the various approaches within law and economics. Thus the discipline encompasses several distinct strands of thought, including welfare economics,[2] Kaldor-Hicks economics,[3] wealth-maximizing law and economics,[4] feminist law and economics,[5] behavioral law and economics,[6] expressive law and economics,[7] and what may be loosely termed "progressive" law and economics.[8] How each branch confronts a given inquiry will depend upon the relevance and weight that it places on particular preferences as criteria. Thus Richard Posner's study of gender implications in the workplace[9] was considered deficient by Gillian Hadfield for not adequately inquiring into the impact regulations on sexuality have on women's role determinations.[10]

With this interpretation of factors that affect efficiency in mind, I now turn to the question of how well Title I of the ADA conforms to the neoclassical economic paradigm. The assumption that informs Title I, as well as other prohibitions against discrimination in employment, is that imposing these regulations will equalize employment opportunities for their targeted groups. But empirical studies of post-ADA employment effects foreground a phenomenon that is puzzling. Although analyses suggest that employing workers with disabilities can be cost-effective,[11] and despite a burgeoning economy in which the unemployment rate for most categories of workers has plummeted, unemployment of working-age individuals with disabilities appears not to have similarly diminished.[12] From the point of view defined by scholars applying the neoclassical labor market paradigm to Title I, the clearest explanation of this phenomenon would seem to be that the studies reporting the cost-effectiveness of employing the disabled are incorrect or at least overstated.

An earlier version of this essay appeared in the *Berkeley Journal of Employment and Labor Law*.

Following from this explication is the conclusion that selecting workers with disabilities over nondisabled workers is an inefficient practice.

In what follows, I examine and assess the arguments made by proponents of the view that the inefficiency of employing workers with disabilities is a deterrent to their inclusion in the labor market. If these arguments are sound, then rational market forces appear to be inexorably at work to attenuate the strategy embodied by Title I of the ADA. To the contrary, however, I will identify a market failure that prevents certain employers from reaching rational labor market decisions by creating a "taste for discrimination"[13] in which the costs of including people with disabilities in a workforce are perceived as being greater than they really are. Further, I will propose an improved manner for assessing the efficiency of employing workers with disabilities and consider what this method implies regarding the rationality of Title I's strategy. Finally, I will show that the failure of the existing neoclassical economic model, as well as the Title I critiques that rely on it, is attributable at least in part to that model's having societal misconceptions about people with disabilities built into its assumptions. That is, far from being neutral or objective, these critiques sanction and perpetuate the very irrational biases the ADA was designed to correct.

ASSESSING THE NEOCLASSICAL ECONOMIC MODEL

The neoclassical economic model of the labor market begins from the premise that markets for goods and services operate rationally. As part of this postulate, it is assumed that markets set their own prices, free bargaining is the norm, and knowledge is completely and symmetrically disseminated, resulting in correct end values for commodities. Under this theory, market forces discipline employers and their self-destructive tastes against particular groups by driving them from the market. This economic Darwinism occurs because employers' discriminatory practices of declining to hire particular types of employees despite their greater utility adds to business costs and thus diminishes their profit margins. Exercising distaste also raises the net-product margin of nondiscriminatory competitors who engage same-group employees at reduced wage levels.

Resting on this foundation, the neoclassical economic paradigm posits that in the context of a rational labor market, employers hire workers with the greatest net productivity. This utility is calculated by subtracting total labor cost from total production benefit. Since workers with disabilities require costly inputs in the form of accommodations, an employer, if sufficiently unconstrained so that she can act of her own rational preference, would logically choose nondisabled employees.

The most thorough criticism of Title I to be expressed though a law-and-economics perspective was published by Richard Epstein after passage of the ADA but prior to promulgation of its regulations.[14] Although therefore somewhat precipitate, because successive literature closely follows Epstein's position in applying the neoclassical economic labor market model, elucidating his arguments will yield an understanding of how those who make similar assumptions of principle assess Title I. For facility of reference, these views (with his courteous permission) will be attributed directly to Epstein.[15] At the same time, however, my criticisms of Epstein are relevant to other law-and-economics practitioners to the extent that they adopt normative assumptions common to the neoclassical economic model, for example, the belief in a rational marketplace.[16]

Epstein advances three main reasons for believing that the potential benefits associated with reasonable accommodations are inherently less than the costs they engender. First, it is in the nature of disability that those individuals are less productive than their able-bodied counterparts. Second, providing accommodation—that is, giving a disabled worker something her able-bodied peers do not receive as a means of ameliorating her impairments—must be costly. Third, the employment of workers with disabilities extracts yet a further cost when coworkers and customers respond with "awkward" and "unpleasant" feelings, which as "preferences should not be blithely condemned as irrational."[17]

When employers are forced to hire disabled employees against their own considered judgments, these employers are made to internalize costs that they would not have otherwise borne. Consequently, according to Epstein, Title I accommodations are inherently inefficient because they reduce the utility the employer is able to achieve. Title I's requirements are also unfair because they compel private employers to bear the costs of an inefficient social policy. Epstein therefore concludes that the current exclusion of people with disabilities from the employment sphere is the result of rational decision-making, not of prejudice (or of statistical discrimination).[18]

According to Epstein, a better solution toward achieving the same end of altering historical imbalances in the labor market would be abrogating the ADA so as to allow the market to function normally. In this circumstance, employees with disabilities could underbid the true value of their services or decline health insurance coverage as a way of offsetting their accommodation costs. If necessary, the state could create incentives for accommodating disabled workers by spreading those costs through the tax structure or by directly issuing vouchers to employers. Finally, Epstein maintains that specific industries and plant locations could be chosen as "centers" of accommodation. By concentrating workers with disabilities at such sites, there is increased likelihood that physical plant or equipment accommodations will see repeated usage. This last option, "far from being seen as handicap ghettoization, will be regarded as a sensible effort to economize on public funds."[19]

Four principal theoretical flaws undermine Epstein's application of neoclassical economic principles to Title I. First, and in turn undermining each of the subsequent three postulates, is unconditional acceptance of the neoclassical economic labor market model. This paradigm, far from being neutral, adopts and perpetuates many of the same irrational biases the ADA was designed to correct. Second, it is assumed that to employ an individual with a disability requires providing significant accommodations. This conjecture is maintained even though many accommodations involve only minimal or no cost, and some occasion positive benefits. Third, the appraisal presumes that policy-makers ought to factor in the costs of provoking negative feelings even when these are engendered by biased tastes. That is, no consideration is introduced to distinguish costs occasioned by behavior influenced by insupportable or mistaken beliefs from the costs of justified or sustainable ones. Fourth, the analysis is incomplete because it considers only internalized costs associated with workplace accommodations. By so doing, Epstein ignores both concomitant internalized and external benefits.

The neoclassical economic model posits that employers acting rationally will hire and maintain workers with the greatest net product, while those who act irrationally will be disciplined by market forces and driven from competition. This premise, which is taken as a standard economic assumption by many law-and-economics practitioners, has questionable factual and normative elements as applied to the reality of disabled workers' experiences in the labor market. In explaining this assertion, the scholarship of Cass Sunstein[20] and John Donohue[21] is instructive.

A primary objection to applying the neoclassical labor market model to disabled workers is factual. To begin with, the standard neoclassical economic model is premised on complete and symmetrical distribution of information to all actors within a given market. Yet not all markets function equally in this respect. Accordingly, although the neoclassical economic account of disseminating information might be true of financial markets, whose extensive "reporting" requirements are rigorously enforced by the Securities and Exchange Commission (SEC), no parallel structure exists in the labor market. Similarly, the liquidable nature of financial market commodities does not extend to the market for employment services, where the value of individual workers is difficult to disaggregate.

Next, contrary to the neoclassical labor market account, empirical studies conducted both before and after passage of the ADA clearly demonstrate the persistence of employment discrimination as an obstacle to labor-market opportunities for workers with disabilities.[22] In analyzing the effects of employer practices, these studies, which assume information asymmetry in the labor market, glean the effects of nonstatistical (or economically rational) behavior from that caused by prejudice. In other words, they separate the consequences of decisions arising from the use of indicators that substitute reliable generalizations about group characteristics from those that either wrongly assume or overestimate the existence of those characteristics. In the case of workers with disabilities, indicators that are meant to signal appraisals of productivity and accommodation cost are swayed in their estimates by existing misconceptions about disabled workers that substitute for less easily obtainable accurate information. Additionally, even if economically rational indicators were substituted for biased ones, a market failure would continue because employers' discriminatory behavior would be rewarded as efficient (and conversely, a system requiring economically empowered employers rather than economically disempowered employees to bear cost differentials incurred by disregarding rational economic discrimination may arguably be more efficient from a social welfare standpoint). Thus the baseline assumption that employers act in a rational manner while seeking to maximize their own profits appears empirically invalid.

Moreover, the neoclassical economic model asserts that once discriminatory practices are observed, market forces discipline employers who exercise distaste by reducing their profit margins while also increasing that of their nondiscriminatory competitors. As with the first premise, this theorem has not been empirically demonstrated. Indeed, logical application of the neoclassical economic paradigm would assert that prior to 1964, when federal antidiscrimination laws injected inefficiency into the dynamics governing private employment relationships, discriminatory firms were either penalized or driven from competition. I am unaware of any empirical evidence that supports this position. To the contrary, United States markets have historically evidenced various forms of discrimination. Consequently, belief in the self-corrective force of competitive market pressures in the labor field is unproven.

Another objection to utilizing neoclassical economic principles to examine the dynamics of disabled workers' participation in the labor market is normative, for accepting this paradigm would not discipline irrational behavior and restore the employment market to a nondiscriminatory equilibrium. Instead, reliance on competitive pressure as advocated in neoclassical economic analyses would perpetuate market failure by reinforcing the stereotypes Title I was meant to counteract. This is because the neoclassical economic paradigm uses as its baseline a status quo designed by an empowered majority that has already absorbed existing prejudices and made them endogenous to future decision making. Hence any analysis that assumes market neutrality has reflexively erected obstacles to antidiscrimination principles that are entrenched in the same stereotypes those civil rights statues seek to alter. Whether embracing these stereotypes is an unconscious,[23] semiconscious,[24] conscious[25] or cognitively biased[26] decision remains hotly debated, as does the issue of whether preferences are fixed[27] or malleable.[28] For now, however, it is sufficient to say that accepting the neoclassical economic model's view that existing prejudicial preferences built into the marketplace are neutral will only serve to continue those stereotypes.

Within the context of Epstein's Title I analysis, propagation of disability-related biases would result from his recommendation that deference be paid to the distastes of both third parties and employers, even under a regime in which the ADA was itself abrogated.

In the case of third-party distaste, whether arising from coworkers or customers, market pressure would foster discrimination instead of eliminating it. This is because the inclusion of third party distaste into the equation of efficiency will necessarily cause employers to factor into their decisions the very prejudices that Title I endeavors to avoid. Furthermore, it would be unusual, from a methodological standpoint, to defer to preferences of nonmarket third-party actors.

As for employers, Epstein's claim that workers with disabilities could either underbid the value of their services or forego health insurance benefits as a way of capturing accommodation costs would, if heeded, also perpetuate market failure. Working for lower remuneration or benefits might indeed be an inducement for nondiscriminatory employers to engage workers with disabilities; however, it would also reinforce the devaluation of those individuals begot by unfounded stereotypes, and so continue market failure. Acceding to employers' distastes by bribing them through reduced compensation also reduces whatever social good and external benefits can arise from equal pay and occupational dignity. In addition, because the prospects of recovering the costs of education and training are influenced by prevailing market conditions, utility will be lost as the result of reduced willingness among the disabled to invest in their own human capital. Finally, the loss of health care coverage is considered a major disincentive for disabled workers to leave public assistance programs and enter the workplace.[29] This is true to the extent that Congress recently voted to extend the length of time preceding the cutoff of these benefits following gainful employment.[30] Thus having workers with disabilities bargain away insurance coverage as a means of increasing labor market participation would only further sustain an existing market failure.

The second systemic flaw in Epstein's account is the tripartite assumption that because disabled employees are by their natures less productive than nondisabled counterparts, they require accommodations, and that these accommodations are inherently costly.

Empirical studies have not established the prevalence of the need for accommodation among disabled workers across the labor market. It is reasonable to assume that some percentage of employees with disabilities will require accommodations. The size of this group will depend upon the individual circumstances of present or prospective employees, on the degree to which an employer's work site and processes already are accessible, as well as on how the term "disabled" is conceived or measured.[31] There is, however, no reason to suspect that every employee with a disability requires an accommodation, as counterexamples to any such broad generalization are abundant.

Moreover, although this is an area in need of greater and more representative study, available empirical data suggest that accommodating workers with disabilities engenders either minimal or no cost. For example, a study examining five hundred accommodations made by Sears, Roebuck & Co. over the twenty-year period from 1978 to 1997 found that nearly all of the accommodations were made at minimal cost.[32] Results of the Sears study are corroborated by those of the Job Accommodation Network, which reported the typical cost of accommodation as $200,[33] and by other appraisals showing similarly moderate costs.[34] Another analysis concluded that the cost of accommodating disabled workers was equal to that of acclimating nondisabled workers.[35] Nevertheless, the fact that these studies report the activities of only a minority of corporations, when similar practices would compel more widely spread efficient corporate planning, evidences a market failure.

Lastly, it is not accurate to assume that disabled workers are by nature less productive than their counterparts free of disabilities, although this may be true for some individuals with disabilities, just as some nondisabled workers are less productive than the majority of disabled ones. In terms of statutory protection, a disabled worker is not considered "qualified" under Title I unless she can perform the essential job functions of her chosen occupation, either with or without accommodation. A disabled employee who satisfies the requirements of her position without accommodation is clearly equally productive to her nondisabled peers. When accommodations are needed to accomplish integral activities, the question and degree of relatively lower net productivity is affected by the ability of that disabled worker to accomplish nonessential job functions and by the value of those supplementary services to her employer. It bears noting, however, that forty years of pre-ADA empirical studies indicate comparable overall productivity levels among disabled and nondisabled workers.[36] For example, statistics from the U.S. Office of Vocational Rehabilitation indicate that 91 percent of disabled workers were rated either "average" or "better than average," the same rating given to nondisabled workers.[37] This information seems not to be readily known by human resource managers, judging from the shortage of disability awareness[38] and management programs[39] instituted by corporations as part of their business practices. This scarcity further denotes a market failure. For under a neoclassical economic model, companies with access to this information would act on these favorable economic incentives and promote greater employment among the disabled.

A third systemic flaw of the Epstein view is to take coworker and client distaste into account when calculating the costs of employing people with disabilities. This is because, although law-and-economics assessments are expected to take into account all possible costs and benefits when assessing efficiency, it is atypical when calculating social good to find them giving weight to preferences arising from socially undesirable criteria (for example illegal tastes). Consequently, deferring to prejudicial irrationalities about disabled workers is a controversial method of applying conventional law-and-economics criteria. Such inclusion would also result, as was shown above, in continuation of the same biases that Title I was meant to counteract. At the very least, justification is required for this unusual accession to irrational preferences. Furthermore, focusing on disability as being the exclusive cause of distaste felt by one worker for another posits a depth of ignorance about human reactions, as well as an information void, that Epstein claims does not exist in a rational workplace.

Additionally, an information asymmetry exists as to the distastes of employers and third parties towards workers with disabilities. While empirical surveys of Fortune 500 executives,[40] senior executives[41] and coworkers[42] uniformly report favorable attitudes to employing disabled individuals, available data fail to evidence significant increases in the relative employment rate among disabled individuals. Two conclusions can be drawn from this apparent paradox: either cognitive dissonance causes the individuals surveyed to believe they favor disabled employment when in reality they do not, or those interviewed truly do espouse prodisabled sentiments, but because of an information asymmetry this preference does not manifest itself when these individuals act aggregately as corporations.

Fourth, in assessing the efficiency of Title I accommodations, Epstein focuses exclusively on costs affecting individual employers but does not take into account benefits that impact positively the statute's efficiency.[43] The main costs that Epstein associates with Title I are the three set forth above: that (1) disabled employees are naturally less productive than their able-bodied counterparts; (2) workers with disabilities therefore require accommodations; and (3) providing accommodations engenders great expenses, including negative externalities. However, a balanced and complete analysis of Title I should also take into account positive benefits, both directly internalized and arising through externalities, that impact upon disabled employment. The fact that economic analyses have not yet realized the existence of counterweighing factors, which are set forth in the next section, further illustrates the existence of an informational market failure.

BENEFITS FROM EMPLOYING PERSONS WITH DISABILITIES

Positive benefits exist that can be considered when assessing the economic effect a worker with a disability can have upon a given firm. These externalities range from the readily quantifiable to those less easy to measure. Considering the impact of these benefits will not result in all accommodations being seen as economically efficient, but should render a more balanced calculus.

The most immediately quantifiable benefits are those internalized by employers due to savings in recruitment, training and replacement expenses.[44] One federally funded agency found that for every dollar spent on accommodation, on average companies saved some $50 in net benefits.[45] Another survey reported that 60 percent of disabled workers remained with their job placement as opposed to only 40 percent of able-bodied ones, and that the average cost of each job turnover was $2,800.[46] Moreover, empirical evidence corroborates that workers with disabilities have absenteeism rates equal to or lower than their nondisabled peers.[47] The rational economics of hiring workers with disabilities is also validated by anecdotal accounts.[48]

In addition, emanating from accommodations are what Peter Blanck has described as "ripple effects."[49] Among such desirable consequences are higher productivity,[50] greater dedication,[51] better identification of qualified candidates for promotion,[52] fewer insurance claims, reduced postinjury rehabilitation costs,[53] improved corporate culture[54] and more widespread use of available technologies.[55]

External benefits to employers whose direct impacts are less immediately quantifiable are public cost savings, including reduction of disability-related public assistance obligations, which are estimated at $120 billion annually.[56] Hiring people with disabilities has also been shown as beneficial to taxpayers' burdens[57] and the national economy.[58] These economic benefits, which were clearly a congressional concern when passing the ADA,[59] are recognized by a minority of companies.[60]

Finally, intangible benefits also flow from the extension of civil rights protection to disabled individuals. Although their effects upon individual employers are more difficult to quantify, these advantages may nonetheless maximize the collective good. These benefits include placing people with disabilities in a position to exercise all the responsibilities of citizenship,[61] acknowledging that capable individuals have a "right" to work,[62] permitting the disabled to achieve dignity through labor and productivity,[63] and realizing the values of a diverse society.[64] The value of these gains, as well as what any of them is worth to individual employers, is not necessarily negligible even if it is unclear. The expenses extracted for achieving these benefits must therefore be closely evaluated when determining whether to place such costs upon employers rather than spread them through taxes or other state-governed devices. Nevertheless, employers arguably benefit individually from a collective climate in which citizens value the identities they achieve from being productive more than they do the relief of being excused from being productive.

How and when to allocate the costs of maintaining a culture of productivity raises a host of issues, including criticisms of those law-and-economics studies utilizing wealth as a value,[65] the continuing commodification debate,[66] questions about the perspective of policy-makers[67] and differences of opinion on the advantages of investing in human capital.[68] Regardless of their resolution, an account that educates both employers and economists about some of the difficult-to-quantify benefits listed above is far more adequate to our traditional thinking about the personal and social value of productivity than a narrow construal of social motivation on which it is assumed, counterfactually, that the statute "would not be necessary if these [accommodations] were beneficial to employers, as they automatically act in ways that promote their self interests."[69]

MARKET FAILURE AND PEOPLE WITH DISABILITIES

In this section, I show why disability can evoke irrational market behavior with respect to employment. The assertion of market failure within the employment relationship is not unique. Claims that imperfect information undermines the rationality of hiring decisions have arisen from econometric,[70] economic[71] and civil rights[72] sources. Additionally, the issue of whether and when to characterize decisions made in the context of imperfect information based on "indicators" believed to evaluate future performance as statistical (and discriminatory)[73] or rational (and predictive)[74] is at the heart of an ongoing debate.[75] Examples also exist of employers failing to capitalize on other economically beneficial actions[76] which application of the neoclassic economic labor market model would suggest as a matter of course.

The theoretical errors in the neoclassical economic model that informs Epstein's analysis incorporate market failure by reproducing two societal informational flaws about people with disabilities. First, there is the focus on disability as causing reactions that may be ecumenically human. Second, there is an imposition of a medical rather than a social account of disability. Acceptance of these paired misapprehensions is occasioned by a pervasive lack of accurate knowledge about people with disabilities and further exacerbated by the distinctive chronicle of their civil rights empowerment. That these fallacies continue to exist, even to the extent that they are diffused through scholarly discourse, underscores the need for raising social consciousness about Americans with disabilities. Disseminating this information is vital if market failure is to be corrected.

Epstein's view on Title I incorporates society's perception that disability is central to determinations which can also be universally human. One example is the positing of awkward feelings which, it is imagined, will be engendered in nondisabled individuals by having to interact in a work situation with a disabled worker. These feelings could arise when either customers or coworkers have not yet been enculturated to disability. Nevertheless, the way in which a worker approaches her job—her personality and demeanor—are factors irrespective of disability that ultimately determine the comfort of interaction. To illustrate, an able-bodied sadist would function poorly in a customer relations department and associate poorly with peers due to his conduct, not because of physical differences. Similarly, we may expect that the rational responses of others will, ultimately, be influenced by whether individuals with disabilities conduct themselves in the ways that disagreeable people without disabilities do, or whether they behave agreeably. Additionally, reacting negatively to the difference of disability does not appear to be inherently different from parallel historic (now antiquated) responses by the dominant majority to the exclusion of other groups—for instance, the discovery that not all doctors are male and that one is about to be examined by a woman urologist, or that for the first time in your life the professor who will determine your course grade and perhaps your future career is a person of color. As for distaste, one of the (now discarded) arguments for failing to offer women equitable career opportunities in police positions was the distaste expressed by officers' wives at the thought of their husbands spending long hours in a patrol car in the company of another woman. This is another example of how an antidiscrimination measure would have been undermined by the same prejudices it sought to remedy if third-party distaste influenced assessments of that statute's efficacy.

It is also inaccurate to suppose that, in compelling accommodations, the ADA differs wholly from other civil rights statutes and is thus uniquely more expensive. Requiring changes of practice or environment in order to function optimally, even when not economically efficient, is not unique to the disabled, and parallel habituations are made to members of other covered groups. Famously, the inclusion of women in most parts of the military workforce required expenditures to increase inventoried uniforms and equipment. Members of both genders under the Family Medical Leave Act[77] and, under certain religious circumstances, the Civil Rights Act of 1964 (Title VII),[78] are legally entitled to various types of accommodations.[79] To varying degrees, all civil rights integration involves expenditures—for example, the parallel costs incurred by a desegregated all-white firm losing clients and members, a formerly all-male corporation having to build womens' restroom facilities, or a uniformly (acknowledged) heterosexual company extending benefits to same-sex partners. Moreover, because of standard business practice dynamics, workers regularly receive various kinds of accommodations that are unrelated to any recognized civil right—for instance, allowing a parent to attend his daughter's soccer match.

Epstein's analysis also mirrors a perspectival flaw of mainstream society by implicitly adopting a "medical model" of disability.[80] On a medicalized account of disability, people with disabilities are cast in two alternative yet dichotomous roles: the pitiable poster child and the inspirational "supercrip."[81] The pitiable poster child is an image created to inspire the exercise of charity by instilling potential donors with pity for unfortunate children. Because of its emotional appeal, the cute and courageous poster child who smiles through his or her "tragic" fate is the most beloved American symbol of disability. The flip side of the pitiable poster child is the supercrip. If science, supported by telethon money, could not cure the scourge of disability, then society demands the disabled to cure themselves through hard work, determination and pluck. The medical model heavily influenced legislation passed in the earlier part of the century, especially those statutes stressing vocational rehabilitation as a means of "overcoming" disability through productive employment. One notable example is the post–World War I Smith-Sears Act, intended as an ameliorative to disabling war injuries.[82]

The social model, also sometimes called the civil rights or minority model, tracks the empowerment movements of the 1950s and 1960s that sought to eradicate discrimination posited on the biological differences of blacks and women. According to this account, inequalities foisted upon the disabled because of their exclusion from social interaction (including work) have been the result of socially constructed practices rather than the outgrowth of natural phenomena. For example, architectural constructions that exclude a portion of the population—as in rest rooms that are not accessible to wheelchair users—may be viewed as a "natural" condition by the majority nondisabled class. Yet, because there is no absolute reason why a "universal design" which can give access to a rest room for all users should not equally be the norm, the social model perceives the distinction as artificial and the result of an unjust social arrangement.[83]

The ADA's provisions (as well as other legislation affecting people with disabilities), were promulgated in large measure to level a playing field that historically had discriminated against people with disabilities by imposing medicalized stereotypes.[84] In assessing Title I, Epstein asserts that social policy affecting people with disabilities should be driven by philanthropic benevolence. As stated by Epstein, "[h]aving a disability is the source of an enormous level of personal loss" leading to "sympathies" that "tug knowingly at the heartstrings" and inspire "charitable giving and charitable services."[85] It is because people with disabilities are worthy of sympathy that subsidizing their inferior work productivity is considered altruistic. Thus those following Epstein's perspective adopt the medical model's assumption that disability entails dependence rather than the social model's rights-based presupposition that disability does not defeat individuals' entitlement to self-determination. By adopting the medical model into the calculus of what is rational, Epstein and neoclassical economists continue the methods and mythologies that the ADA was intended to cure.

CIVIL RIGHTS CHRONOLOGY OF AMERICANS WITH DISABILITIES

Unlike other marginalized minority groups, disabled Americans were empowered by civil rights legislation prior to there being a general elevation of social consciousness about their circumstances and capabilities.[86] In sum,[87] efforts to achieve the ADA's passage helped transform parallel but uncoordinated efforts of disability-specific advocacy groups and individuals into a unified disability rights movement.[88] Formerly, groups representing many different disabilities promoted their own issues and concerns. For instance, the massive and unyielding protest by students for appointment of a deaf president at Gallaudet University, a higher-learning institution for the hearing-impaired,[89] was unconnected to the advocacy of the developmentally disabled constituency of People First, which sought both integration into mainstream society and greater control for its members over the structure of their own lives. In addition, disability rights groups often clashed with one another. The curb cuts fought for by wheelchair users were opposed by some visually impaired people whose method of distinguishing between sidewalk and roadway was to locate the curb tactilely.

The campaign for the ADA's passage brought these fragmented organizations together.[90] However, because the history of disability rights advocacy is largely one of uncoordinated activity among disparate specifically concerned groups, people with disabilities have not acknowledged a single nationally recognized leadership figure (such as the Reverend Jesse Jackson), nor established a central political congress (like the NAACP) through which to voice their concerns and desires. Consequently, people with disabilities were empowered with civil rights absent the political tools and organization for inducing a general elevation of social consciousness. Thus it is not entirely surprising that popular opinions about people with disabilities do not yet conform to the spirit of the legislative findings of the statute nor the letter of assertions made by disability rights advocates.

Compounding these difficulties is the lamentable reality that insufficient knowledge about the ADA has been disseminated either to the general public or to people with disabilities. Most members of the public assume that an ADA-covered person has a condition that limits her mobility or senses. Nevertheless, the average Title I claimant is a middle-aged woman with a musculoskeletal injury, most frequently her back.[91] Whether this should be the typical Title I plaintiff is a valid question but secondary to the observation that lack of knowledge about the nature of ADA claimants results in resistance to their claims in both academia[92] and the popular media.[93] Finally, it is worth noting that four years after the ADA's passage, one survey revealed that only 40 percent of the disabled people interviewed had either read or heard about the ADA (and, by implication, Title I).[94] This problem is particularly acute among minorities with disabilities, wherein a knowledge gap corresponds to employment differentials within the disabled community.[95] This market failure to disseminate information among those affected by the ADA speaks volumes to the issue of information asymmetry.

CONCLUSION

In this essay I investigated the claim made by some proponents of law-and-economics analysis that it is virtually an oxymoron for an employer to express a rational preference for a worker with a disability over an equally qualified or even a slightly less-qualified worker without a disability. We saw that far from its being irrational for employers to suppress biases against hiring individuals who are disabled, errors that inflate the cost of doing so constitute a market failure that deters employers from reaching and executing rational decisions. It is this irrational failure of the market rather than the imposition of irrational regulation that appears to have undercut the efficacy of Title I of the ADA. The conjectural deficiencies of the market model that imply otherwise reflect a more generalized failure, namely a societywide absence of accurate information about the circumstances and capabilities of people with disabilities. The dearth of facts to inform the private determinations that fall under and thereby are regulated by public nondiscrimination disability policy is due in part to a chronology unique to the disabled. The civil rights empowerment of individuals with disabilities preceded their collective political invigoration and consequently occurred prior to educating the public about the realities, both historical and contemporary, of why protection from discrimination is needed.

NOTES

[1]Excellent exegeses are offered by Stewart J. Schwab, *The Law and Economics Approach to Workplace Regulation in Government Regulation of the Employment Relationship,* Bruce E. Kaufman, ed., Madison, WI: Industrial Relations Research Association, 1997, and by Richard A. Posner, *Economic Analysis of Law,* 5th ed., New York: Aspen Law & Business, 1997, 349–376.

[2]See Allan M. Feldman, "Welfare Economics," in John Eatwell, Murray Milgate and Peter Newman, eds., *The New Palgrave: The World of Economics,* New York: Norton, 1998, 713.

[3]See Allan M. Feldman, "Kaldor-Hicks Compensation" in Peter Newman, ed., *The New Palgrave Dictionary of Economics and the Law,* vol. 2, New York: Stockton Press, 1998, 417.

[4]This strand is primarily identified with academicians from the University of Chicago Law School.

[5]Notably the work of Gillian K. Hadfield, as well as those works featured in the publication *Feminist Economics.*

[6]A comprehensive overview is set forth in a 1998 symposium published by the *Vanderbilt L. Rev.*

[7]See Robert Cooter, "Expressive Law and Economics," 27 *J. Legal Stud.* 585 (1998).

[8]See Susan Rose-Ackerman, "Progressive Law and Economics and the New Administrative Law," 98 *Yale L. J.* 341 (1988).

[9]Richard A. Posner, *Sex and Reason,* Cambridge, MA: Harvard University Press, 1992.

[10]Gillian K. Hadfield, "Flirting with Science: Richard Posner on the Bioeconomics of Sexual Man," 106 *Harv. L. Rev.* 479 (1992).

[11]These studies are discussed below in the third section.

[12]Two recent studies report that the post-ADA employment rate of workers with disabilities has moderately declined relative to that of workers without disabilities. See Daron Acemoglu and Joshua Angrist, "Consequences of Employment Protection? The Case of the Americans with Disabilities Act." National Bureau of Economic Research Working Paper No. 6670, 1998; Thomas DeLeire, "The Wage and Employment Effects of the Americans with Disabilities Act." University of Chicago unpublished mimeograph, 1997.

[13]The seminal writing on "distaste" is Gary S. Becker, *The Economics of Discrimination,* 2d ed., Chicago: University of Chicago Press, 1971, 39–45.

[14]See Richard A. Epstein, *Forbidden Grounds: The Case Against Employment Discrimination Laws,* Cambridge, MA: Harvard University Press, 1992, 480–494.

[15]Unless indicated, as in the case of quotation, what follows is generally derived from pages 480–494 of *Forbidden Grounds.*

[16]I want to stress that I am not imputing Epstein's vision of antidiscrimination laws to all other variations within the discipline of law-and-economics, and especially so the inclusion of distaste. The only implication which should be drawn is that publications which have so far arisen from the field adopt, in large measure, Epstein's position.

[17]Epstein, *Forbidden Grounds,* 486–487.

[18]"In light of the business realities of the situation, the popular treatment of the disabled cannot simply be dismissed as prejudice or bigotry." Id., 487.

[19]Id., 494.

[20]See Cass R. Sunstein, "Why Markets Don't Stop Discrimination," in *Reassessing Civil Rights,* Ellen Frankel Paul, ed., Bowling Green, OH: Bowling Green State University, 1991, 21.

[21]The reasoning, present in several articles, is especially pertinent in John J. Donohue III, "Prohibiting Sex Discrimination in the Workplace: An Economic Perspective," 56 *U. Chi. L. Rev.* 1337 (1989), and in John J. Donohue III, "Is Title VII Efficient?" 134 *U. Pa. L. Rev.* 1411 (1986).

[22]See Marjorie L. Baldwin and William G. Johnson, "Labor Market Discrimination Against Men with Disabilities," 29 *J. Human Resources* 1 (1994); Marjorie L. Baldwin, Lester A. Zeager and Paul R. Flacco, "Gender Differences in Wage Losses from Impairments: Estimates from the Survey of Income and Program Participation," 29 *J. Human Resources* 865 (1994); William G. Johnson and James Lambrinos, "Wage Discrimination Against Handicapped Men and Women," 20 *J. Human Resources* 264 (1985).

[23]See Charles R. Lawrence III, "The Id, the Ego, and Equal Protection: Reckoning with Unconscious Racism," 39 *Stan. L. Rev.* 317 (1987).

[24]See Kimberle Williams Crenshaw, "Race, Reform, and Retrenchment: Transformation and Legitimation in Antidiscrimination Law," 101 *Harv. L. Rev.* 1331 (1988).

[25]See Alan David Freemen, "Legitimizing Racial Discrimination through Antidiscrimination Law: A Critical Review of Supreme Court Doctrine," 62 *Minn. L. Rev.* 1049 (1978).

[26]An especially perceptive approach is Linda Hamilton Krieger, "The Content of Our Categories: A Cognitive Bias Approach to Discrimination and Equal Employment Opportunity," 47 *Stan. L. Rev.* 1161 (1986).

[27]For example, George J. Stigler and Gary S. Becker, "De Gustibus Non Est Disputandum," 67 *Am. Econ. Rev.* 76 (1977).

[28]See Amitai Etzioni, *The Moral Dimension: Towards A New Economics,* New York: Free Press, 1988.

[29]See Marjorie L. Baldwin, "Can the ADA Achieve its Employment Goals?" 549 *Annals AAPSS* 37 (1997); Richard V. Burkhauser, "Post-ADA: Are People with Disabilities Expected to Work?" id., 71.

[30]See Robert Pear, "Senate Approves Health Care for Disabled," *New York Times* June 17, 1999, A28; Testimony Before the Subcommittee on Social Security, Committee on Ways and Means, House of Representatives (Statement of Cynthia M. Fagnoni), Washington, DC: GAO Publication No. GAO/T-HEHS-99-82, March 1999.

[31]A recent and pertinent example is the limitation upon the use of mitigating factors in determining disability expressed by the Supreme Court in its recent troika of decisions. See *Sutton v. United Airlines,* 119 S. Ct 2139 (1999); *Murphy v. United Parcel Service, Inc.,* 119 S. Ct 2133 (1999); *Albertsons, Inc. v. Kirkingburg,* 119 S.Ct. 2162 (1999). Particularly illuminating is Justice O'Connor's numerical discussion in *Sutton.*

³²Specifically, from 1978 to 1992, the average out-of-pocket expense for an accommodation was $121; from 1993 to 1996, that average dropped to $45. Overall, 72 percent of accommodations required no cost, 17 percent carried an expenditure of less than $100, 10 percent cost less than $500, and 1 percent required outputs of between $500 and $1,000. See Peter David Blanck, "Communicating the Americans with Disabilities Act, Transcending Compliance: 1996 Follow-Up Report on Sears, Roebuck and Co.," in *Annenberg Washington Program Reports,* 1996, 42–43.

³³See President's Committee on the Employment of People with Disabilities, Report to Congress on the Job Accommodation Network, July 26, 1995.

³⁴For example, Laura Koss-Feder, "Spurred by the Americans with Disabilities Act, More Firms take on Those Ready, Willing and Able to Work," *Time Magazine* January 25, 1999 (citing James Geletka, Executive Director of the Rehabilitation Engineering and Assistive Technology Society of America for the proposition that most workplace accommodations cost less than $200); Peter David Blanck, "The Emerging Role of the Staffing Industry in the Employment of Persons with Disabilities: A Case Report on Manpower Inc." 1998 (reporting that accommodation costs were "minimal") (see the essay by Blanck, pp. 209–220 in this volume); Rita Thomas Noel, "Employing the Disabled: A How and Why Approach," 44 *Training and Development J.* 26 (1990) (70 to 80 percent of accommodations cost less than $500).

³⁵See Louis Harris & Associates, "The ICD Survey II: Employing Disabled Americans," 1987.

³⁶The literature is reviewed in Reed Greenwood and Virginia Anne Johnson, "Employer Perspectives on Workers with Disabilities," 53 *J. Rehabilitation* 37 (1987).

³⁷See Rick A. Lester and Donald W. Caudill, "The Handicapped Worker: Seven Myths," 41 *Training and Development J.* 50–51 (1987); George E. Stevens, "Exploding the Myths about Hiring the Handicapped," 63 *Personnel* 57–60 (1986).

³⁸See John G. Veres III and Ronald R. Sims, *Human Resource Management and the ADA,* Westport, CT: Quorum Books, 1995; Sheila H. Akabas, Lauren B. Gates and Donald E. Galvin, *Disability Management,* New York: American Management Association, 1992; Frank Bowe and Jay Rochlin, *The Business-Rehabilitation Partnership: An Arkansas Rehabilitation and Research Training Center Project,* Fayetteville: Arkansas Rehabilitation Research and Training Center, University of Arkansas, 1983; Jack R. Ellner & Henry E. Bender, *Hiring the Handicapped: An AMACOM Research Study,* New York: AMACOM, 1980.

³⁹See *The ADA at Work: Implementation of the Employment Provisions of the Americans with Disabilities Act: A Study by Society for Human Resource Management,* 1999.

⁴⁰See Joel M. Levy, Dorothy Jones Jessop, Arie Rimmerman and Phillip H. Levy, "Attitudes of Executives in Fortune 500 Corporations towards the Employability of Persons with Severe Disabilities: Industrial and Service Corporations," 24(2) *J. Applied Rehabilitation Counseling* 19–31 (1994).

⁴¹A 1995 survey of senior corporate executives found that 89 percent supported plans to increase the number of workers with disabilities their companies employed. See the National Organization for the Disabled/Harris survey "Employment of People with Disabilities" 1995.

⁴²In a 1991 survey, 68 percent polled said they would support policies that increase number of disabled workers, 65 percent responded that they would not have any problems with disabled coworkers, and 77 percent said they would not be concerned if their boss was a seriously disabled person. See Louis Harris & Associates, "Public Attitudes towards People with Disabilities," 1991, 13.

⁴³For individuals aged 16 to 64, the Census reported that the overall employment rate of people with disabilities improved 0.3 percent during the period 1991 to 1994, rising from 52.0 percent in 1991 to 52.3 percent in 1994. See Michael Ashley Stein, "Employing People with Disabilities: Some Cautionary Thoughts for a Second Generation Civil Rights Statute," in Peter David Blanck, ed., *Employment, Disability, and the Americans with Disabilities Act: Issues in Law and Public Policy,* Chicago: Northwestern University Press, 2000.

⁴⁴See Peter David Blanck and Mollie Weighner Marti, "Attitude, Behavior and the Employment Provisions of the Americans with Disabilities Act," 42 *Vill. L. Rev.* 345 (1997); Peter David Blanck, "The Economics of the Employment Provisions of the Americans with Disabilities Act: Part I—Workplace Accommodations," 46 *DePaul L. Rev.* 887 (1997).

⁴⁵See President's Committee on Employment of People with Disabilities, *Job Accommodation Network Reports* 1994, 10.

[46]See Blanck, "Emerging Role," 29; Akabas, Gates and Galvin, *Disability Management,* 261.

[47]See Gretchen Adams-Shollenberger and Thomas E. Mitchell, "A Comparison of Janitorial Workers with Mental Retardation and Their Non-Disabled Peers on Retention and Absenteeism," 62 *J. Rehabilitation* 56 (1996); Dolores Ondusko, "Comparison of Employees with Disabilities and Able-Bodied Workers in Janitorial Maintenance," 22 *J. of Applied Rehabilitation Counseling* 19–24 (1991); Rick A. Lester and Donald W. Caudill, "The Handicapped Worker: Seven Myths," 41 *Training and Development J.* 50–51 (1987); J. E. Martin, F. R. Rusch, J. J. Tines, A. R. Brulle and D. M. White, "Work Attendance in Competitive Employment: Comparison between Employees Who Are Non-Handicapped and Those Who Are Mentally Retarded," 23(3) *Mental Retardation* 142–147 (1985).

[48]For example, Shelley Donald Coolidge, "Fewer with Disabilities at Work Since Passage of Civil Rights Act," *Christian Science Monitor* March 7, 1995, describes the experience of Carolina Fine Snacks, which provided pork skins to the 1992 GOP convention. Prior to hiring a disabled worker, the company had an 80 percent turnover rate and a 20 percent absenteeism rate. With more than half the company's workers now having a disability, there exists almost no absenteeism, and the turnover rate has been reduced to 5 percent.

[49]See Blanck, "Emerging Role," 29.

[50]"Savvy employers have figured out that a can-do attitude for employees with impairments is good for profits and productivity." Patricia M. Owens, "Employee Disabilities Needn't Impair Profits," *Wall Street Journal* June 7, 1999, A22.

[51]See Stuart Silverstein, "On the Job with more Technology, More Disabled Join the Work Force," *Los Angeles Times* October 25, 1998 (relating EarthLink's President as saying that "What you find are employees who probably are more focused and more dedicated to doing quality work"). See also John King, "Commercial Support services help Special Workers Gain Sense of Dignity, Independence," *San Francisco Chronicle* November 21, 1998, A17; Stacy Lam, "Business Win Awards for Inclusive Hiring," *The Macon Telegraph* October 7, 1998, 6; Kathryn Moss, "Point-Counterpoint: American Disabilities Act Statute Brings Better Lives to Thousands," *Chapel Hill Herald* August 17, 1997, 5.

[52]See Thomas W. Hale, Howard V. Hayghe and John M. McNeil, "Persons with Disabilities: Labor Market Activity 1994," *Monthly Labor Review* September 1998, 3 (relating that the disabled are less likely to work in high-paying positions relative to nondisabled). Cf. David Charny and Mitu Gulati, "Efficiency Wages, Tournaments, and Discrimination: A Theory of Employment Discrimination Law for 'High Level' Jobs," Harvard Law School Discussion Paper No. 182, March 1996 (finding that current antidiscrimination laws are largely ineffective in altering employers' behavior in promotion to "high-level" jobs, thus causing employees subject to discrimination to alter their goals, and resulting in underinvestment in human capital).

[53]See Blanck, "Communicating the Americans," 16–17.

[54]Id.

[55]See Heidi M. Berven and Peter David Blanck, "The Economics of the Americans with Disabilities Act Part II: Patents and Innovations in Assistive Technology," 12 *Notre Dame J. L. Ethics & Pub. Pol.* 9, 85–89 (1998).

[56]See David I. Levine, "Reinventing Disability Policy," Institute of Industrial Relations Working Paper no. 65, 1, June 11, 1997.

[57]See "The JWOD Program: Providing Cost Savings to the Federal Government by Employing People with Disabilities," February 6, 1998 (reporting that the federal government saved $1,963,206 annually by employing 270 people with disabilities); Taxpayer Return Study, California Department of Rehabilitation Mental Health Cooperative Programs, October 1995 (finding that for every disabled person employed, California taxpayers saved an average of $625 per month in costs).

[58]See Thomas N. Chirakos, "Aggregate Economic Losses from Disability in the United States: A Preliminary Assay," 67 *Milbank Quarterly* (Supp. 2, pt. 1) 59 (1989).

[59]"By giving people the opportunity to become self-sufficient we are . . . decreasing the amount of Federal money being spent to support individuals with disabilities and increasing tax revenue." 136 Cong. Rec. S9684,9688 (1990) (Statement of Senator Durenberger). See also S. Rep. No. 101–116 at 16–17 (1990); 136 Cong. Rec. S9684,9688 (1990); S. Rep. No. 116, 101st Cong., 1st Sess. 4 (1989).

[60]See "Implementation of the Employment Provisions of the Americans with Disabilities Act: A Survey of the Washington Business Group on Health," April 1999 (42 percent of companies surveyed).

[61]Eloquently argued by Judith N. Shklar, *American Citizenship: The Quest for Inclusion,* Cambridge, MA: Harvard University Press, 1991, 63–101.

[62]See Gregory S. Kavka, "Disability and the Right to Work," this volume.

[63]See Mark C. Weber, "Beyond the Americans with Disabilities Act: A National Employment Policy for People with Disabilities," 46 *Buff. L. Rev.* 123 (1998).

[64]Elizabeth Clark Morin, "Americans with Disabilities Act of 1990: Social Integration Through Employment," 40 *Cath. U. L. Rev.* 189 (1990).

[65]Heralded by Ronald Dworkin, Jules Coleman, and Mark Kelman, and exemplified by Jules L. Coleman, *Markets, Morals and the Law.* 1988; and the essays by Dworkin and Anthony Kronman in the March 1980 volume of *J. Legal Stud.*

[66]See Richard Craswell, "Incommensurability, Welfare Economics, and the Law," 146 *U. Penn. L. Rev.* 1419 (1998).

[67]See Susan Rose-Ackerman, "Law and Economics: Paradigm, Politics, or Philosophy," in *Law and Economics,* Nicholas Mercuro, ed., Boston: Kluwer Academic, 1998, 233; Susan Wendell, *The Rejected Body: Feminist Philosophical Reflections on Disability,* New York: Routledge, 1996, 117.

[68]Compare, for example, Gary S. Becker, "Investment in Human Capital: A Theoretical Analysis," 70 *J. Pol. Ec.* 9 (1962); Becker with Ruth Colker, "Hypercapitalism: Affirmative Protections for People with Disabilities, Illness and Parenting Responsibilities under United States Law," 9 *Yale J. L. & Fem.* 213 (1997). For an international perspective, see Clement Fuest and Bernd Huber, "Why Do Countries Subsidize Investment and Not Employment?" National Bureau of Economic Research Working Paper No. 6685, August 1998; and Ruth Colker, *American Law in the Age of Hypercapitalism,* New York: New York University Press, 1997.

[69]Thomas H. Barnard, "Disabling America: Costing Out the Americans with Disabilities Act," 2 *Cornell J. L. & Pub. Pol'y* 41 (1992).

[70]In particular, the sources cited in note 29.

[71]See David Neumark, "Labor Market Information and Wage Differentials by Race and Sex," National Bureau of Economic Research Working Paper No. 6573, May 1998; Sunstein, "Why Markets Don't Stop."

[72]See Richard Delgado, "Rodrigo's Roadmap: Is the Marketplace Theory for Eradicating Discrimination A Blind Alley?" 93 *N. W. U. L. Rev.* 215 (1998).

[73]See Dennis J. Aigner and Glen G. Cain, "Statistical Theories of Discrimination in Labor Markets," 30 *Ind. & Lab. Rel. Rev.* 175 (1977).

[74]See Richard A. Posner, "The Efficiency and the Efficacy of Title VII," 136 *U. Pa. L. Rev.* 513 (1987).

[75]See Stewart J. Schwab, "Is Statistical Discrimination Efficient?" 76 *Am. Econ. Rev.* 228 (1986).

[76]For instance, high-efficiency electrical equipment available through negawatt acquisition programs described by Bernard S. Black and Richard J. Pierce, Jr., "The Choice between Markets and Central Planning in Regulating the U.S. Electricity Industry," 93 *Columbia L. Rev.* 1339 (1993).

[77]29 U.S.C. § 2601 et seq.

[78]Pub. L. No. 88–352, §§ 701–16, 78 Stat. 241, 253–66 (codified as amended at 42 U.S.C. §§ 2000e to 2000e-17 (1994)).

[79]Some would apply this assertion to women under the Pregnancy Discrimination Act. See generally Peter David Blanck and Corinne R. Butkowski, "Pregnancy-Related Impairments and the Americans with Disabilities Act," 25 *Obstet. Gynecol. Clin. North America* 435 (1998).

[80]See Richard Bryant Treanor, *We Overcame: The Story of Civil Rights for Disabled People,* Falls Church, VA: Regal Direct, 1993; Claire H. Liachowitz, *Disability as a Social Construct: Legislative Roots,* Philadelphia: University of Pennsylvania Press, 1988.

[81]What follows is drawn from Michael Ashley Stein, "From Crippled to Disabled: The Legal Empowerment of Americans With Disabilities," 43 *Emory L. J.* 247, 249–52 (1994), and from Joseph P. Shapiro, *No Pity: People with Disabilities Forging a New Civil Rights Movement,* New York: Times Books, 1993, 12–16.

[82]Vocational Rehabilitation Act, ch. 107, Pub. L. No. 65–178, 40 Stat. 617 (1919).

[83]See Colin Barnes, Geof Mercer and Tom Shakespeare, *Exploring Disability: A Sociological Introduction,* Malden, MA: Polity Press, 1999; Mary Klages, *Woeful Afflictions: Disability and Sentimentality in Victorian America,* Philadelphia: University of Pennsylvania Press, 1999; Herbert C. Covey, *Social Perceptions of People with Disabilities in History,* Springfield, IL: Charles C. Thomas, 1998.

[84]Specifically, Congress enacted the ADA as a remedy to the continuing pattern "of unfair and unnecessary discrimination and prejudice" which denied "people with disabilities the opportunity to compete on an equal basis and to pursue those opportunities for which our free society is justifiably famous." 42 U.S.C. § 12,101 (a)(9).

[85]Epstein, *Forbidden Grounds,* 486.

[86]See Jonathan C. Drimmer, "Cripples, Overcomers, and Civil Rights: Tracing the Evolution of Federal Legislation and Social Policy for People with Disabilities," 40 *UCLA L. Rev.* 1341 (1993); Richard K. Scotch, "Politics and Policy in the History of the Disability Rights Movement," 67 *Milbank Quarterly* (Supp. 2, Pt. 1) 380 (1989); Richard K. Scotch, *From Good Will to Civil Rights: Transforming Federal Disability Policy,* Philadelphia: Temple University Press, 1984, 111–116. An especially good personal treatment is Hugh Gregory Gallagher, *Black Bird Fly Away: Disabled in an Able-Bodied World,* Arlington, VA: Vandamere Press, 1998.

[87]What follows is derived from Shapiro, *No Pity,* 184–210, and from Stein, "From Crippled to Disabled," 59.

[88]There is, however, the notable exception of the 1977 San Francisco sit-in to protest delay in promulgating Section 504's regulations. See Scotch, "Politics and Policy," 111–116.

[89]See generally Jack R. Gannon, *The Week the World Heard Gallaudet,* Washington, DC: Gallaudet University Press, 1989.

[90]As noted at the time by ADA lobbyist Liz Savage, "people with epilepsy now will be advocates for the same piece of legislation as people who are deaf. . . . That has never happened before. And that's really historic." See Shapiro, *No Pity,* 126–127.

[91]See Marjorie L. Baldwin and William G. Johnson, "Dispelling the Myths about Work Disability," in *Approaches to Disability in the Workplace,* Terry Thompson, ed., Madison, WI: Industrial Relations Research Association, 1998.

[92]See Gary S. Becker and Guity Nashat Becker, *The Economics of Life,* New York: McGraw-Hill, 1997, 20–22.

[93]See Walter Olson, "Under the ADA, We May All Be Disabled," *Wall Street Journal* May 17, 1999, A27.

[94]See Louis Harris and Associates/National Organization for the Disabled, "Survey of Americans with Disabilities," 1994, 122.

[95]See William J. Hanna and Elizabeth Rogovsky, "On the Situation of African-American Women with Physical Disabilities," 23 *J. Applied Rehabilitation Counseling* 39–45 (1992) (comparing the situation of the 25 percent of African-American women with disabilities who were fully employed, with that of the 44 percent of white women, 57 percent of African-American men and 77 percent of white men with disabilities).

Studying Disability, Employment Policy and the ADA

PETER DAVID BLANCK

At the tenth anniversary of the Americans with Disabilities Act of 1990[1] (ADA), critical questions remain to be documented about the nature, composition and qualifications of the American workforce of the twenty-first century. These questions include:

- What types of work skills and qualifications will be needed for American employers to remain competitive in the U.S. and abroad?
- Will our increasingly diversified and aging workforce include millions of qualified persons with physical and mental disabilities?
- What will be the characteristics and capabilities of the workforce of persons with disabilities?
- What types of job design, training and workplace accommodations will be available to that workforce?
- How will the dramatic public policy changes that have occurred in the last quarter of the twentieth century in disability law and policy and in educational, welfare and technological reform affect that workforce?

This chapter highlights my and my colleagues' empirical investigations of these and related questions as they affect the emerging workforce of persons with disabilities.[2] The need for a body of research on disability law and policy from varied scientific and social science disciplines is crucial given the revolutionary shift in just the past fifty years from a model of charity and compensation to medical oversight and then to civil rights, culminating in the passage of the ADA.[3]

An overarching theme of the studies highlighted in this chapter is to document the ways in which disability law and policy are enhancing the equal labor-force participation of qualified persons with disabilities and in reducing their dependence on governmental entitlement programs.[4] Despite advances, there is little definitive evidence that disability laws and policies alone have resulted in substantial increases in qualified persons with disabilities participating in the workplace.

SUBSTITUTING DATA FOR MYTHS ABOUT DISABILITY, THE ADA AND WORK

Systematic study of the work lives of persons with disabilities is lacking. The promise of the ADA and related antidiscrimination laws to prevent the exclusion from society of millions of qualified Americans with disabilities makes this lack of information troubling. In assessing our empirical studies, Senator Bob Dole has commented:

> Some people think that evaluating the ADA is irrelevant, given that its purpose is to establish certain rights and protections. But I believe that we have an obligation to

make sure our laws are working. At the very least, we need to know that all people affected by the ADA are aware of their rights and responsibilities and that its remedies are in fact available and effective.[5]

The research studies highlighted in this chapter have three goals:

1. *Dialogue:* to foster a meaningful dialogue about the hiring, equal employment and career development of qualified persons with disabilities;
2. *Awareness:* to raise awareness about persons with disabilities in terms of their work capabilities and qualifications, and value to employers and the American economy; and,
3. *Fairness:* to enhance the effective implementation of the ADA and related antidiscrimination laws by providing information to facilitate employers' understanding of the law and of initiatives in educational, health care and welfare reform.

Over the past ten years, my colleagues and I have attempted to further these goals through our studies of job applicants, workers with disabilities, employers, assistive technology and workplace accommodation strategies. The following sections review several of our studies on ADA implementation in these areas.

Study 1. The Hiring of Persons with Disabilities: The 1998 Manpower Study

In 1998, my colleagues and I released a case study of Manpower Inc., the nation's largest staffing employer.[6] Manpower provides temporary employment opportunities to almost two million people worldwide. Manpower's revenues have nearly doubled since 1991, with sales of $8.9 billion for 1997. The U.S. Bureau of Labor Statistics estimates that between the years 1994 and 2005, temporary employment opportunities will grow by 55 percent.

The Manpower study examines the employment opportunities available to persons with physical and mental disabilities. The study explored the importance of hiring and job training opportunities as strategies that provide a bridge to full-time employment for qualified persons with disabilities. Interviews of Manpower employees with a range of serious impairments, who worked for various employers across the United States, suggest the company's investment in individualized training programs, job skills assessment techniques and career development strategies has been a critical element of its success in hiring and retaining workers with disabilities.

The study identifies aspects of Manpower's corporate culture that foster equal employment opportunities for persons with disabilities, including a belief that (1) there are no unskilled workers; (2) every individual has job skills and aptitudes that can be measured; and (3) every job may be broken down into essential tasks. The study identifies the ways in which the staffing industry supports the employment of workers with disabilities, showing that (1) individualized training and job placement are available; (2) above-minimum wages and health insurance benefits are provided; and (3) there is opportunity for career advancement, self-advancement, self-learning and transition to full-time employment.

The Manpower study highlights one important bridge from unemployment to employment for qualified workers with disabilities. The preliminary findings of the study may be summarized as follows:

1. *Prompt transition from unemployment to employment:* manpower effectively transitions people with disabilities from unemployment to employment. Ninety percent of the individuals studied were at work within ten days of applying to Manpower.

2. *Workplace accommodation costs are minimal:* the direct costs of accommodating workers with disabilities is low. There were minimal direct costs to Manpower or its customer companies in accommodating the workers studied.
3. *Staying at work:* sixty percent of the individuals studied moved from no employment to permanent employment. Annually more than 40 percent of Manpower's entire workforce transitions to permanent work that is the direct result of the temporary job placements.
4. *Safety at work:* for the employees with disabilities studied, there were no incidences of work-site injury and thus no additional costs to the employer due to workplace safety issues.
5. *Choice in work:* ninety percent of the individuals studied were placed in a job or industry in which they expressed an interest, and job placements were consistent with individualized work skills.
6. *Retaining work that pays:* ninety percent of the employees studied remained in the workforce from the time of their first job assignment, earning above the minimum wage, either through a series of temporary job assignments or permanent employment.

The findings suggest ways for policy-makers, employers, health professionals and others to expand equal employment opportunities for individuals with disabilities consistent with the ADA's goals.

Study 2. Labor Market Trends of Persons with Disabilities: 1990–1998 Longitudinal Research

Since 1990, my colleagues and I have been studying the labor market trends of more than five thousand persons with mental retardation and related impairments living in Oklahoma.[7] The investigation focuses on changes in the participants' employment and economic positions as indicators of progress during ADA implementation. Several measures assess employment and economic trends, including personal and educational backgrounds; job capabilities, qualifications and training; involvement in community, citizenship and advocacy activities; and perceptions of ADA effectiveness.

The investigation's core findings may be summarized as follows:

1. *Attaining employment, integration into competitive employment and retention of employment:* from 1990 to 1998, somewhat less than half of the participants (42 percent) remained in the same type of employment; roughly half (47 percent) engaged in more integrated and competitive employment; and somewhat more than one tenth (11 percent) regressed into less-integrated employment settings.
2. *Employment of a new generation of workers with disabilities:* younger relative to older participants and those individuals with better job skills showed substantial gains in employment.
3. *Drop in unemployment levels:* relative unemployment levels for all participants declined by 23 percent, dropping from 37 percent in 1990 to 14 percent in 1998.
4. *Income growth:* from 1990 to 1998, the gross and earned income of participants rose substantially, with younger participants showing substantial increases in income. Better job skills, greater independence in living and more involvement in self-advocacy activities related to higher earned income levels.

5. *Substantial individual growth:* from 1990 to 1998, participants improved substantially in their job capabilities and qualifications, lived in more integrated settings, became more involved in self-advocacy and citizenship activities, and reported enhanced accessibility to society as defined by the ADA.

6. *Black hole effect:* three out of four (75 percent) of those participants not employed or employed in segregated settings in 1990 remained in those settings in 1998.

Though encouraging, these findings suggest that a good deal of work lies ahead to ensure equal employment opportunity for workers with serious mental and physical impairments. The gains in employment, income, individual growth, independent living and ADA awareness, however, reflect "a core, common cause—the drive for independence and integration of people with disabilities."[8]

Study 3. Economics of Accommodating Persons with Disabilities: The 1994 and 1996 Sears Studies

One aspect of the ADA that has received extensive attention involves the law's effect on employers' ability to provide workplace accommodations for qualified job applicants and employees with disabilities.[9] Critics suggest that the ADA's accommodation provision creates for persons with disabilities an employment privilege or subsidy and imposes upon employers an affirmative obligation to retain less economically efficient workers. Others argue the costs of accommodations are high for large employers, who may be held accountable for extensive modifications because of their greater financial resources.[10]

The research to date does not show that the ADA's accommodation provision is a preferential treatment initiative that forces employers to ignore employee qualifications and economic efficiency. Our studies illustrate that companies that are effectively implementing the law demonstrate the ability or "corporate culture" to look beyond minimal legal compliance in ways that enhance their economic bottom lines. The low direct costs of accommodations for employees with disabilities produce substantial economic benefits in terms of increased work productivity, workplace injury prevention, reduced workers' compensation costs and workplace effectiveness and efficiency.

We have conducted a series of studies at Sears, Roebuck and Co., a company with more than 300,000 employees, examining more than six hundred workplace accommodations provided by the company during the years 1978 to 1998.[11] Our findings show that most accommodations sampled required little or no cost—more than 75 percent required no cost; somewhat less than one quarter cost less than $1,000; and less than 2 percent cost more than $1,000. The average direct cost for accommodations was less than $30.

The following implications may be drawn from the Sears studies:

1. *Compliance linked to culture, attitudes and ADA transcendence:* the degree to which Sears and other companies examined comply with the ADA's accommodation provision appears to have more to do with their corporate cultures, managers' attitudes and business strategies than with meeting the law's minimal obligations.

2. *Benefits of workplace accommodations outweigh costs:* the indirect cost of not retaining qualified workers is relatively high, with the average administrative cost at Sears per employee replacement of $1,800 to $2,400—roughly forty times the average of the direct costs of accommodations for qualified workers. Sears also provides accommodations that require minor and cost-free workplace adjustments which are implemented directly by an employee and her supervisor. Sears is realizing positive economic returns on the accommodation investment by enabling qualified workers

with disabilities to return to or stay in the workforce, reducing the risk of workplace injury and lowering worker absenteeism.

3. *Economic benefits to employers, workers without disabilities and workers who may become disabled in the future:* accommodations involving universally designed technology enable employees with and without disabilities to perform jobs productively, cost-effectively and safely (for example, reducing the potential for workplace injury). The costs associated with the technologically based accommodations studied (for example, computer voice synthesizers) enabled qualified employees with disabilities to perform essential job functions. These strategies create a corporate "ripple effect," as applications increase the productivity of employees without disabilities. The direct costs attributed to universally designed accommodations are lower than predicted when their fixed costs are amortized over time.

The findings from the Sears studies suggest that many economic and social benefits and costs associated with the ADA's accommodation provision remain to be discovered and documented. Studies such as the Sears and Manpower ones illustrate that companies expend large sums of money accommodating the needs of workers without disabilities (for example, through flexible scheduling of work hours, child care support and employee assistance programs), and these costs are substantially greater than those associated with accommodations for workers with disabilities. Analysis of these strategies shows that they complement cost-effective accommodation strategies for workers with disabilities.

Study 4. Resolving ADA Disputes: The 1996 Sears Study

Another major critique of the ADA is that it fosters unintended and costly employment litigation. It has been suggested that a large source of indirect costs associated with ADA implementation is related to expenses for administrative, compliance or legal actions.

The Sears study examined both the formal ADA Title I charges filed with the Equal Employment Opportunity Commission (EEOC) against Sears from 1990 to mid-1995 and informal disability-related disputes raised by employees.[12] The findings include the following:

1. *Formal ADA charges:* almost all of the formal charges filed with the EEOC (98 percent) were resolved without resort to extensive trial litigation.
2. *Informal ADA disputes:* more than three quarters (80 percent) of the informal disability-related disputes were resolved through informal dispute processes that enabled qualified employees with disabilities to return to productive work.
3. *Nature of impairment:* almost half (41 percent) of the employees who filed charges with the EEOC evidenced an impairment before their employment at Sears; more than one quarter (29 percent) who filed charges were injured on the job; and 18 percent who filed charges were injured off the job. The findings do not support the view that the charges reflect issues that would otherwise be raised under traditional workers' compensation laws.
4. *Settlement:* of the formal ADA charges studied, the average settlement cost to Sears was $6,193, exclusive of attorneys' fees.

The findings highlight that analysis of the costs and benefits associated with ADA implementation, compliance and related litigation is needed on a national scale. Nevertheless, discussion limited to EEOC charges associated with ADA implementation tends to focus analysis on the failures of the system as opposed to efficient and fair workplace strategies that enhance the equal workforce participation of persons with disabilities.

Study 5. Unintended Economic Consequences of the ADA:
A Case Study of Technological Innovation and Inventive Activity

Independent of the civil rights guaranteed by the law, estimating the costs and benefits of ADA implementation is a complex undertaking.[13] To illustrate the importance of studying the unintended consequences of ADA implementation, we conducted the first study of economic activity in the assistive technology (AT) market, using data derived from the United States Patent and Trademark Office (PTO).[14]

The findings suggest but do not yet prove that ADA implementation is fostering technological innovation and economic activity in the AT consumer market. As the regulatory shifts imposed by the ADA expand the market for goods that improve accessibility to society, inventors, employers and manufacturers are responding to meet the needs of consumers with disabilities.

The core findings include the following:

1. *Economic activity:* assistive technology patent numbers have shown substantial annual increases since 1976.
2. *ADA awareness:* although reference to civil rights legislation is atypical of patent records, from 1990 through mid-1998, the number of patents citing the ADA has increased substantially, totaling 139.
3. *Unintended economic benefits:* inventors who cite the ADA are a geographically diverse group, many unaffiliated with large corporations. From 1990 to mid-1998, patents were granted for a wide range of assistive devices with uses for a wide array of consumers with disabilities.

The findings are consistent with those suggesting that the ADA is affecting the AT consumer market, including persons with and without disabilities, in economically positive ways and is creating profit-making opportunities that were unanticipated when the law was passed.

Study 6. Social Construction of Disability and the ADA:
An Historical Investigation of Conceptions of Disability

In a large-scale historical investigation, we continue to explore the underpinnings of law and policy affecting persons with disabilities, as exemplified today by the ADA. The historical investigation explores the ways in which public acceptance and reaction to the inclusion into society of persons with disabilities in late-nineteenth-century America were, like today, driven at least as much by political, economic, social and attitudinal factors regarding conceptions of disability as they were by law and policy themselves.[15]

We explored the profound aftereffects on American society of the emergence of the large class of disabled Civil War veterans and the ways in which they changed conceptions of disabled persons in American society. Three preliminary hypotheses were tested:

1. The severe criticism in the press directed against disabled veterans in particular, and against the pension system in general, will have *at least as much to do* with party politics of the day as with the workings of the pension system.
2. The perceived legitimacy of and stigma toward veterans' disabilities will have *at least as much to do* with the provision of pensions as with the severity of disabilities.
3. Social characteristics of the veterans, such as occupational status, will have *at least as much to do* with the provision of pensions as with the severity of disabilities.

Examination of these hypotheses supported the view that attitudes about disability, as illustrated in the context of the empirical studies described above, often have less to do with the operation of law and policy than with underlying attitudinal and political views toward disabled persons. These conclusions are based on findings from the first wave of the data collected from U.S. military archives involving approximately 6,600 Union Army veterans from four Northern states—Illinois, New York, Ohio and Pennsylvania.

The preliminary findings refine prior suggestions about the profound influence of political, economic and social forces on the evolution of conceptions of disability. Deep-seated attitudes about disability and nineteenth-century patronage politics contributed to the negative attitudes toward a then-new social category of individuals with disabilities. Targeted criticisms in the press scapegoating disabled veterans as "illegitimate" and "unworthy" occurred despite evidence that the pension system was performing gatekeeping functions. Negative public attitudes occurred at a time when social norms about disability had not developed and advocacy for the disabled was nonexistent or in its infancy.

The investigation confirms the contemporary view that partisan and attitudinal factors unrelated to disability contributed to the legacy disability policy. Professor Harlan Hahn's seminal articulation of the minority group model is instructive in this regard. Hahn suggests that negative social attitudes are the primary source of barriers to equal participation in society confronted by disabled people.[16] Hahn believes that "disability *is defined* by public policy."[17]

The findings also highlight that conceptions of disability held by examining surgeons' applying late-nineteenth-century diagnostic methods may have been a factor in development of the long-lasting "medical model" approach to disability. The dominance of the medical approach to disability was to last well into the next century.

IS THE PAST A PROLOGUE TO THE FUTURE OF PEOPLE WITH DISABILITIES?

One hundred years after the height of the Civil War pension system in 1890, critical reactions to passage of the ADA included widespread allegations that the law is aiding "gold diggers" with illegitimate disabilities and that it is having a chilling effect on the hiring and employment of "truly" disabled persons.[18] Others argue that the costs of ADA workplace accommodations far exceed the benefits, that there are high numbers of frivolous ADA lawsuits brought by "undeserving" plaintiffs, and that, because of all of this, there have been negative economic consequences from the ADA from "fraudulent or overly bureaucratic programs."[19]

Proponents argue that negative trends in the labor-force participation of people with disabilities to date have less to do with ADA implementation than with macroeconomic trends when the law was passed and with structural inefficiencies and disincentives in existing disability and health insurance policies.[20] Critics respond that a decline or lack of growth in labor-force participation by persons with disabilities, combined with an increase in applications for entitlement benefits, suggests that the ADA may not be helping those it was intended to serve.[21]

The themes articulated by critics come down to the view that the ADA is not serving and indeed is hurting the interests of all Americans. A 1999 *San Francisco Chronicle* article concludes that: "history is littered with laws that not only did not work, but did exactly the opposite of what was intended. The Americans with Disabilities Act appears, sadly, to be one."[22] A 1998 *Reader's Digest* article describes the ADA as "A good law gone bad."[23] Professor Andrew Batavia comments that some critics believe that people with disabilities "have done something morally wrong to deserve their predicament and that they should be assisted only through charity."[24]

The debate pits supporters who stress the civil rights guaranteed by its antidiscrimination provisions against critics who cast the law as broad, inefficient and as a preferential treatment initiative.[25] The debate is cast in ideological terms, as liberal efforts to enlist the federal government in the inclusion of the disabled into society versus conservative attempts to allow the power of economic markets to assist disabled persons.[26] The debate inevitably, like that over social welfare programs generally, comes down to a view about the role of the federal government in the lives of disabled citizens.

The program of study highlighted in this chapter illustrates that attitudinal, economic and political forces affected public views about disability law and policy one hundred years ago as they do today. Because study about persons with disabilities is lacking, much of the criticism has focused on whether certain groups of disabled persons are a "deserving" class.[27] News coverage reflects skepticism and cynicism about the definition and "legitimacy" of disabilities claimed and covered by the ADA. Some commentators have interpreted the negative press as an ideological effort to intentionally deflect meaningful discussion of disability law and policy.[28]

Widespread criticism of the ADA illustrates a growing ideology that, knowingly or unknowingly, perpetuates attitudinal barriers and unjustified prejudice toward disabled Americans in employment, education, housing and daily life activities.[29] Evaluation of attitudes about disability and the operation of disability law and policy is needed for several reasons.

First, study of the equal participation in society of persons with disabilities will aid in long-term evaluation of emerging policies in areas of welfare, educational, health care and dispute resolution reform.[30] Second, study is needed of the extent to which the ADA has enabled persons with severe disabilities to enter the mainstream of society, particularly in education and employment.[31] Third, research from a variety of disciplines is needed to inform policy-makers, employers and members of the disability community about the emerging issues related to prejudice and long-term ADA implementation.[32]

In his classic article, "The Right to Live in the World," Professor tenBroek argued that the disabled have a right to live under a national policy of "integrationalism," which is full and equal participation in society.[33] Integrationalism as a national policy may have commenced formally as early as 1920, when Congress adopted the national Vocational Rehabilitation Act.[34] The gradual shift toward integrationalism may be one legacy of the Civil War pension system—from its early beginnings as policy of charity, to compensation, to the medicalization of disability.[35] In 1990, the modern view of disability civil rights was articulated in passage of the ADA. This new paradigm emphasizes an individualized and socially contextual approach to civil rights enforcement.[36]

CONCLUSION: STUDY OF THE ADA AND THE EMERGING WORKFORCE OF PERSONS WITH DISABILITIES

A new generation of empirical evaluation of the legal, policy and economic implications associated with the emerging workforce of persons with disabilities and ADA implementation is needed. As discussed in this chapter, study of the labor-force participation of persons with disabilities will aid in long-term ADA implementation and other policy initiatives.

Study is needed of the extent to which ADA implementation has coincided with larger numbers of persons with severe disabilities entering the labor force. In 1996, the U.S. Census Bureau released data showing that the employment-to-population ratio for persons with severe disabilities increased from roughly 23 percent in 1991 to 26 percent in 1994, reflecting an increase of approximately 800,000 additional people with severe disabilities in the workforce.

This chapter has highlighted that, despite encouraging trends, study is required of the underlying causes of high unemployment levels facing persons with disabilities. A 1998 survey by the National Organization on Disability (NOD) and the Harris Organization found significant participation gaps between people with and without disabilities in employment and other aspects of life.[37] Of the persons with severe disabilities surveyed, more than two thirds (approximately 67 percent) were unemployed and out of the work-force, compared to less than 10 percent of all Americans. Forty percent of the individuals with disabilities surveyed lived below the poverty line, versus 18 percent of all Americans.

To continue to address the issues, meaningful discussion among scholarly disciplines is needed to inform policy-makers, employers, members of the disability community and others about the issues related to ADA implementation in ways that articulate the values and goals of the nation's policies affecting persons with disabilities.

Of course, the conclusions from any single research study, or even from series of studies, are insufficient for drawing sweeping conclusions about persons with disabilities and employment law and policy. Future large-scale research and case studies are required to provide a springboard for discussion about evolving disability law and policy.

In this last regard, my colleagues and I, with support from the National Institute on Disability Research and Rehabilitation (NIDRR), have established a Rehabilitation Research and Training Center on workforce investment, employment policy for persons with disabilities, and ADA implementation.[38] The center's goals include conducting stud-ies on the effects of federal and state policies on the employment of persons with disabili-ties, such as the ADA and the Workforce Investment Act.

One example of a new research project at the center is a study of self-employment and entrepreneurial activities of people with disabilities.[39] Self-employment is examined as a growing option for joining the workforce. The research explores how the Iowa's Entre-preneurs with Disabilities program enables individuals with disabilities to pursue self-employment. The report uses in-depth interviews, observations and archival data sources to examine the entrepreneurs program. The overarching goal of this research is to stimulate discussion of self-employment techniques and policy initiatives that address the unem-ployment problem faced by millions of Americans with disabilities who want to work and who are capable of and interested in self-employment.

The preliminary findings illustrate that self-employment provides an alternative for people with disabilities to move from unemployment or underemployment to productive employment. Self-employment initiatives provide assessment, technical assistance, train-ing and funding for prospective entrepreneurs, allowing them to pursue self-employment. The self-employment programs studied provide entrepreneurs with opportunities to estab-lish businesses, acquire start-up and expansion funding, build credit histories, enhance their self-esteem, become involved in their communities, interact with suppliers and cus-tomers, and earn income. Through empirical and policy analysis of the kind highlighted in this chapter, the center's goal is to expand and improve disability and generic policy to impact positively equal employment opportunities for Americans with disabilities.[40]

At bottom, useful and credible information about the issues that I have highlighted, and many others, must be derived from study of core values related to our sense of indi-vidual worth and identity, self-respect, fairness and economic common sense. The articula-tion of these values by persons with and without disabilities will shape the lives of the next generation of children with disabilities who have experienced integrated education and who will become part of the competitive workforce of the next century.

One hundred years ago, and today, at the tenth anniversary of the ADA, disabled people were and are portrayed as shirkers, malingerers, freeloaders and undeserving. One hundred years ago and today, some claimed and claim that disabled people seeking protection under the law pose a moral challenge to the notions of fairness in American law and policy.[41] Over the course of the twenty-first century, our challenge is to strive toward national policies that promote inclusion into society for all persons, with and without disabilities.

ACKNOWLEDGMENTS

The program of research described herein is supported, in part, by grants from the University of Iowa College of Law Foundation; the National Institute on Disability and Rehabilitation Research, the U.S. Department of Education; The Great Plains Disability Business and Technical Assistance Center; and Iowa Creative Employment Options. This chapter is derived, in part, from Professor Blanck's statements on October 5, 1998, before the U.S. House of Representatives Committee on Education and the Workforce, and on November 12, 1998, before the U.S. Commission on Civil Rights Public Hearings on the Americans with Disabilities Act.

NOTES

[1] 42 U.S.C. §12101 et. seq.

[2] The research sources discussed are drawn, in part, from Peter David Blanck, *The Americans with Disabilities Act and the Emerging Workforce*. Washington, DC: American Association on Mental Retardation, 1998.

[3] See John Parry, "Civil Rights for Persons with Mental and Physical Disabilities," in *ABA Blueprint for Disability Law and Policy*, Washington, DC: American Bar Association Commission on Mental & Physical Disability Law, 1999.

[4] See Dick Thornburgh, "Ensuring Equal Opportunity for Individuals with Disabilities Through the ADA," in *ABA Blueprint for Disability Law and Policy*, Washington, DC: American Bar Association Commission on Mental & Physical Disability Law, 1999.

[5] Bob Dole, "Are We Keeping America's Promises to People with Disabilities?—Commentary on Blanck," 79 *Iowa L. Rev.* 927, 928 (1994).

[6] See Peter David Blanck, *The Emerging Role of the Staffing Industry in the Employment of Persons with Disabilities: a Case Report on Manpower Inc.* Iowa City, IA: University of Iowa Law, Health Policy, and Disability Center, 1998.

[7] For a review, see Peter David Blanck, note 2.

[8] Bob Dole, note 5. See also Tom Harkin, "The Americans with Disabilities Act: Four Years Later—Commentary on Blanck," 79 *Iowa L. Rev.* 936 (1994) (commenting that "Our challenge, as I see it, is to reach the participants in Blanck's 'black hole' and to continue the positive momentum that he charts.").

[9] See Peter David Blanck, "Transcending Title I of the Americans with Disabilities Act: A Case Report on Sears, Roebuck and Co.," 20 *Mental & Physical Disability L. Rep.* 278 (1996).

[10] See Peter David Blanck, "The Economics of the Employment Provisions of the Americans with Disabilities Act: Part I—Workplace Accommodations," 46 *DePaul L. Rev.* 877 (1997).

[11] See Peter David Blanck, "Communicating the Americans with Disabilities Act, Transcending Compliance: A Case Report on Sears, Roebuck & Co.," Annenberg Washington Program Reports. Washington, DC: Annenberg Washington Program in Communications Policy Studies of Northwestern University, 1994; Peter David Blanck, "Communicating the Americans with Disabilities Act, Transcending Compliance: 1996 Follow-Up Report on Sears, Roebuck & Co.," Annenberg Washington

Program Reports. Washington, DC: Annenberg Washington Program in Communications Policy Studies of Northwestern University, 1996.

[12]See Peter David Blanck, note 11, Follow-Up Report on Sears, Roebuck & Co. (studying 141 formal EEOC charges and 20 informal disputes).

[13]Susan Schwochau and Peter David Blanck, "The Economics of the Americans with Disabilities Act—Part 3: Does the ADA Disable the Disabled?," *Berkeley J. Employ. & Lab. L.,* forthcoming.

[14]Assistive technology is any item, piece of equipment, or product system—whether acquired commercially, modified or customized—that is used to increase and improve the functional capabilities of individuals with disabilities. See Heidi M. Berven and Peter David Blanck, "The Economics of the Americans with Disabilities Act, Part II—Patents and Innovations in Assistive Technology," 12 *Notre Dame J. L. Ethics & Pub. Pol'y* 101 (1998); Heidi M. Berven & Peter David Blanck, "Assistive Technology Patenting Trends and the Americans with Disabilities Act," 17 *Behavioral Sciences and the Law* 47–71 (1999).

[15]Peter David Blanck, "Civil War Pensions, Civil Rights, and the ADA," forthcoming.

[16]Harlan Hahn, "The Potential Impact of Disability Studies on Political Science (as Well as Vice-Versa)," *Policy Stud. J.* (Winter 1993), 741. See also Hahn's essay, pp. 269–274 in this volume.

[17]Harlan Hahn, "Disability Policy and the Problem of Discrimination," 28(3) *Amer. Behav. Sci.* 294 (1985) (emphasis added).

[18]See, e.g., Russell Redenbaugh, *Out of Control: Ten Case Studies in Regulatory Abuse,* Arlington, VA: Lexington Institute, 1998 (arguing that the implementation of the ADA has harmed the interests of persons with disabilities and calling the ADA "The Americans with Minor Disabilities Act"); Editorial, "Americans with Minor Disabilities Act," *Washington Times* Feb. 20, 1999, C2 (quoting Redenbaugh's remarks on the ADA). Cf. Albert R. Hunt, "The Disabilities Act is Creating a Better Society," *Wall Street Journal* Mar. 23, 1999, A23 (commenting that ADA "doomsayers were almost totally wrong" and that the ADA "has won widespread acceptance from the public and most businesses, and has significantly elevated the awareness of and respect for millions of Americans with disabilities.").

[19]Cf. Andrew Batavia, "Ideology and Independent Living: Will Conservatism Harm People with Disabilities," 549 *Annals AAPSS* 14–15 (Jan. 1997).

[20]Cf. Michael Ashley Stein, "Questioning the Assumptions Underlying Law & Economics Evaluations of Title I of the Americans with Disabilities Act," *Berkeley J. Employ. & Lab. L,* forthcoming.

[21]See, e.g., Daron Acemoglu and Joshua Angrist, "Consequences of Employment Protection? The Case of the Americans with Disabilities Act," *National Bureau of Economic Research, Inc., Working Paper* July 1998, 6670 (finding that ADA has a negative effect on the employment of the disabled); Thomas DeLeire, "The Wage and Employment Effects of the Americans with Disabilities Act," *University of Chicago Working Paper,* Dec. 1997 (same).

[22]Carolyn Lochhead, "How Law to Help Disabled Now Works Against Them," *San Francisco Chronicle* Jan. 3, 1999, 7; 1999 WL 2677104 (citing data from economic studies of the ADA).

[23]Trevor Armbrister, "A Good Law Gone Bad," *Reader's Digest* (May 1998) 145 (also claiming that a flood of frivolous ADA lawsuits have clogged the courts). As another example, see also Editorial, "Laws Protecting Disabled Too Susceptible to Abuse," *Atlanta Journal and Constitution* Feb. 9, 1999, A10, 1999 WL 3749474 (commenting that "[h]istory may record the Americans with Disabilities Act as one of the most costly and abused pieces of legislation ever brought forth.").

[24]Batavia, "Ideology and Independent Living," 549 *Annals,* note 19, at 17.

[25]See, e.g., Peter David Blanck, "The Economics of the ADA," in Peter David Blanck, ed., *Employment, Disability, and the Americans with Disabilities Act: Issues in Law, Public Policy, and Research,* Evanston, IL: Northwestern University Press, 2000 (discussing the need for interdisciplinary study of the ADA).

[26]See Mark Kelman and Gillian Lester, *Jumping the Queue: An Inquiry into the Legal Treatment of Students with Learning Disabilities* 1997, 203 (discussing this dichotomy).

[27]Cf. David Matza and Henry Miller, "Poverty and Disrepute," in R. Merton and R. Nisbet, eds., *Contemporary Social Problems* 4th ed. 1976, 601 (discussing stigma associated with "undeserving" poor).

[28]Cf. Dole, note 5, 927–928.

[29]See generally Blanck, *Emerging Workforce,* note 2, 3–10 (discussing attitudinal biases and myths toward persons with disabilities); Peter David Blanck, "Civil Rights, Learning Disability, and Academic Standards," 2(1) *J. Gender, Race, & Jus.* 33–58 (1998), 3 (same). See also Douglas Martin, "Disability

Culture: Eager to Bite the Hand that Would Feed Them," *New York Times,* June 1, 1997, sec. 4, 1, 6 (discussing the view that it is offensive to disabled persons to argue that "cure" would integrate them into society).

[30]John Parry, *The ABA's Blueprint for Disability Law and Policy,* American Bar Association, Washington, DC (1999) (reviewing ABA's disability law and policy agenda).

[31]See Peter David Blanck, "Empirical Study of Disability, Employment Policy, and the ADA," 23(2) *Men. & Phys. Dis. L. Rep.* 275–280 (1999) (discussing future research agenda); Peter David Blanck and Patrick L. Steele, *Self-Employment and Entrepreneurial Activity of People with Disabilities: A Case Study of Iowa's Entrepreneur's with Disabilities Program,* Law, Health Policy & Disability Center Reports, 1999.

[32]See, e.g., Simi Linton, *Claiming Disability: Knowledge and Identity,* New York: New York University Press, 1998, 2147 (discussing emerging field of disability studies as "an interdisciplinary field based on sociopolitical analysis of disability and informed both by the knowledge base and methodologies used in traditional liberal arts, and by conceptualizations and approaches developed in areas of the new scholarship").

[33]Jacobus tenBroek, "The Right to Live in the World: The Disabled in the Law of Torts," 54 *Calif. L. Rev.* 841–919, at 843 (1966).

[34]tenBroek, note 33, 843.

[35]See C. Esco Obermann, *A History of Vocational Rehabilitation in America,* Minneapolis: T.S. Denison, 1965 (describing development of rehabilitation system and relation of system to provision of services for veterans, and noting that prior to 1920 "rehabilitation" meant payment of pensions).

[36]Paul Steven Miller, "Disability Civil Rights and a New Paradigm for the Twenty-First Century: The Expansion of Civil Rights Beyond Race, Gender, and Age," 1(2) *U. Pa. J. Lab. & Empl. L.* 511–26, 26 (1998) (discussing traditional and new disability civil rights paradigms).

[37]See the 1998 *National Organization on Disability/Harris Survey of Americans with Disabilities.* (Washington, DC: National Organization on Disability, 1998).

[38]See Michael Morris, Peter David Blanck, Robert Silverstein, Carl Van Horn and Duke Storen, *Project Overview of the Rehabilitation Research and Training Center on Workforce Investment and Employment Policy for Persons with Disabilities,* Community Options Working Papers, Washington, DC (1999).

[39]See Peter David Blanck and Patrick Steele, *Self-Employment and Entrepreneurial Activity of People with Disabilities: A Case Study of Iowa's Entrepreneurs with Disabilities Program,* note 31 (using case studies and empirical analyses to track program's efforts).

[40]See Albert R. Hunt, "The Disabilities Act is Creating a Better Society," *Wall Street Journal* Mar. 23, 1999, A23.

[41]Cf. Ruth Shalit, "Defining Disability Down," *New Republic,* Aug. 25, 1997, 16 (discussing remarks concerning students with disabilities by President of Boston University). Cf. Hunt, "The Disabilities Act is Creating a Better Society," note 40, A23 (commenting that "the most significant contribution of the ADA is that it has clearly changed the perception of the disabled"), with Mona Charen, "Frenetic Guidelines Straight from the EEOC," *Washington Times* July 31, 1997 (commenting that the ADA "has gone far beyond the benevolent intentions of its designers . . . [it] has accomplished nothing less than to undermine our traditional understanding of character, behavior, and personal responsibility").

Health

Health Care Resource Prioritization and Discrimination against Persons with Disabilities

DAN W. BROCK

In 1990 the landmark Americans with Disabilities Act (ADA) became federal law with the express purpose to "establish a clear and comprehensive national mandate for the elimination of discrimination against individuals with disabilities."[1] The act includes separate titles prohibiting discrimination on the basis of disability in employment, public services, transportation and public accommodations. Since it prohibits discrimination on the basis of disability in both public and private services and programs, in health care "it applies to programs provided by the government, benefits provided by employers, and services provided by physicians."[2] Moreover, the ADA defines disability broadly to include "any chronic medical condition, physical or mental, that substantially limits one or more of the major life activities of (an) individual," although the Supreme Court has ruled that to be covered by the ADA, a person's limitation must persist despite use of available corrective measures.[3] Thus typical chronic medical conditions that even with treatment significantly limit function, such as chronic obstructive pulmonary disease (COPD), congestive heart failure, and AIDS, as well as congenital- or injury-caused functional limitations are covered by the ADA.

Shortly before the ADA was passed, another landmark effort in health policy began— the development by the state of Oregon of an explicit process to prioritize and ration health services within its state Medicaid program. Medicaid is the joint federal-state program initially established in 1968 to fund health care services for the poor who otherwise lack and cannot afford health insurance. However, largely as a result of budget pressures created by rapidly rising health care costs during the decades of the 1970s and eighties, most states significantly tightened the eligibility requirements for their Medicaid programs. In particular, income eligibility requirements were either reduced or not adjusted for inflation, so that by the time Oregon began its Medicaid changes, a majority of Americans with incomes below the federal poverty level nevertheless earned too much to qualify for their state Medicaid programs. While the benefits package for persons who qualified for Medicaid remained relatively generous, many in need were not eligible to receive those services; in addition, low reimbursement rates often made it difficult for Medicaid recipients to secure services. In effect, the practice of the states had been to ration people, by limiting eligibility for the Medicaid program, rather than rationing services available to members of the program.

Oregon proposed two major changes in its Medicaid program—to expand income eligibility to 100 percent of the federal poverty level, with further increases in the income limit to follow over time, and to prioritize and limit the health care services available under its Medicaid program.[4] They proposed to ration services rather than people, arguing that with limited resources it was more rational and equitable to provide the most important

223

services to all in need rather than a broader range of services to some, but none to others, in need. This change promised to increase the overall health benefits that the limited pool of resources available for Oregon's Medicaid program would produce and to treat more equitably those Oregon citizens unable to afford health care or insurance by providing the same package of services to all. It was hard to argue that this would not be overall a change for the better for indigent Oregon citizens without access to health care.

A remarkable feature of the Oregon plan was its open and explicit acknowledgment that resources available for health care, like resources available for all other goods and services, were limited and so it was necessary to ration some potentially beneficial health care. One consequence of the traditional practice of pretending health care was an unlimited good was the irrational and inequitable status quo Oregon set out to change—no longer would it be denied that rationing health care already takes place nor that it should take place. But of course this only raised the question of how health care services should be prioritized and rationed—by what procedures and according to what standards.

Broadly, Oregon sought to combine substantial public input with appropriate professional expertise in a process that would be open and accountable. The Oregon Health Services Commission (OHSC) was established to carry out several tasks. It was to hold a series of public meetings to attempt to determine relevant values of Oregon citizens on health care priorities. However, since the principles and values developed in the public meetings were quite general, their impact on the process appears to have been limited. The OHSC was also to develop a prioritized list of the services then provided under the state's Medicaid program. Specifically, it was to establish a prioritized list of treatment/condition pairs, that is types of treatment given to patients with a particular condition. If a particular treatment had substantially different outcomes and benefits when given to patients with different conditions, it could appear more than once on the list; for example, the initial list distinguished neonatal intensive care for infants below 500 grams and for infants between 500 and 2,500 grams birthweight because of the much worse outcomes in the former group, a case to which I shall return below. The initial list of treatment/condition pairs was prioritized by what was essentially a cost-effectiveness standard, reflecting the very common—indeed, to many health policy experts and others self-evident—principle that limited resources for health care should be used to maximize health benefits for the population served.

To measure the health benefits of different treatments the OHSC adapted the Quality of Well Being Scale (QWB) developed by Kaplan and Anderson.[5] Oregon citizens were asked in telephone surveys how much particular kinds of impairment of health-related quality of life—described in terms of "physical or emotional symptoms and of different degrees of impairment in mobility, physical activity, and social activity"—would reduce quality of life, measured on a scale from 0, equivalent to death, to 1, equivalent to full, unimpaired quality of life; thus each level of impaired function was assigned a specific value from 0 to 1. Health professionals were used to match patients with various medical conditions to appropriate levels of function on the QWB scale both before and after treatment, making possible a quantitative measure of the degree of improvement in health-related quality of life typically produced by each treatment/condition pair. By adding the typical duration of the gain in quality of life from treatment, the overall benefits—essentially in terms of Quality Adjusted Life Years (QALYs), a measure that combines the two main types of benefit from health interventions of extending life and improving quality of life—of each treatment/condition pair were calculated. Using state Medicaid data on the costs of different treatments, the cost-effectiveness of each treatment/condition pair was calculated. The list of treatment/condition pairs was then prioritized from those which produced the most to the least benefits for the resources they required.

For reasons that are not central to my purposes in this paper, the initial list was rejected by the OHSC. Taking account of differences in costs of treatments, as any cost-effectiveness analysis (CEA) does, allows a treatment that produces a small benefit but is relatively inexpensive and so can be given to many people to receive a higher priority than a treatment that produces a very large benefit but is much more expensive and so can be provided to only a few patients for the same overall costs; the example that received the most attention was that capping a tooth for exposed pulp was ranked just above an appendectomy for acute appendicitis, a life-threatening condition, because an appendectomy was estimated to be 150 times as expensive as capping a tooth. Some commentators argued that the values of the adapted QWB scale that Oregon employed failed to give sufficient weight to saving life in comparison with improving quality of life,[6] or that it ignored the so-called "rule of rescue," and that a revised scale would better reflect the high relative importance people give to saving life as opposed to improving of quality of life. Others argued that the counterintuitive ranking arose because ordinary people's rankings of the relative importance of different health services is a one-to-one ranking; in the example above, one tooth capping compared with one appendectomy.[7] In any event, Oregon fundamentally revised its methodology from a cost-effectiveness standard to what was essentially a relative-benefit standard, with cost differences employed only as tiebreakers between treatment/condition pairs producing roughly the same benefit, and revised its priority list accordingly.[8] The OHSC also made many "by-hand" adjustments in the ranking to correct what looked to be "mistakes."

Since Medicaid is a joint federal-state program with a variety of federal requirements, Oregon had to apply to the Health Care Financing Administration (HCFA), the federal agency that administers the Medicaid program, for waivers of a number of regulations in order to put its new program into effect. Although a publicly run health plan that would explicitly and openly ration care was obviously ethically and politically controversial, HCFA's initial rejection of Oregon's waiver request surprised most observers who had been following Oregon's effort. Then the Secretary of the U.S. Department of Health and Human Services, Louis Sullivan, denied the waiver request on the grounds that Oregon's proposal would violate the ADA, using language and analysis prepared by the National Legal Center for the Medically Dependent and Disabled.[9] That analysis imagined the following scenario: a person is injured and two alternative treatments are recommended. Both treatments cost the same and are equal in every other respect—except that after Treatment A the person will live, but after Treatment B the patient will not only live but will also regain the use of his legs as a result. The state has enough money to fund only one treatment and it chooses to fund Treatment B because it provides the greatest improvement in the person's function for the same amount of money.[10]

The National Legal Center granted that this would not be discriminatory, but then posed a different scenario:

> Patient A and Patient B are both injured in an accident. Treatment A is recommended for Patient A while Treatment B is recommended for Patient B. However, Treatment A will sustain Patient A's life, but will not restore the abilities A lost after the accident (such as an ability to walk), while Treatment B will sustain B's life and restore his ability to walk. If the basis for funding B but not A is a quality-of-life judgment that being able to walk is of greater benefit than not being able to walk,

for example, then a decision to deny treatment to A would be discrimination based on A's resulting level of disability. In effect, B's life would be considered more valuable than A's life because B will regain an additional function while A would not. Under the second scenario, a distinction between two effective treatments would be based not on treatment effectiveness, because both treatments would sustain life, but on an inappropriate assessment of the underlying quality-of-life each patient will have after treatment. This scenario describes the Oregon plan.[11]

Some considered Secretary Sullivan's rejection of the Oregon plan as inconsistent with the ADA to be a smoke screen to avoid accepting a highly controversial rationing plan soon before the 1992 presidential election, but whatever political motives may have been involved, I believe Sullivan and the National Legal Center did identify a deep conflict between the ADA and any prioritization of health care services based on either their cost-effectiveness or their effectiveness or relative benefit without regard to cost. Yet any prioritization that ignores differences in the benefits produced by different services would appear to be irrational and deeply problematic. This conflict had not been well appreciated before Secretary Sullivan's decision in part because there had been so few public and explicit efforts to prioritize and ration health care before Oregon, and there have been none since in the United States with the systematic character of Oregon's effort.

However, although few today are willing to prioritize and ration services as openly and explicitly as was Oregon, with the dominant force in health policy now to control health care costs, health plans, insurers and providers inevitably must and regularly are making decisions about what care to provide or cover and what to deny. Probably the dominant public concern about the growth of managed care is that it will deny patients needed and beneficial care. And there is no reason to believe that these provision and coverage decisions do not take into account, even if not systematically, the costs and benefits of different services. So while there are no comparable open conflicts like that between the Oregon plan and the ADA today, the issues raised by that conflict have hardly disappeared. It is those issues that I will explore in the rest of this paper. Before doing so, however, I want to note that Oregon revised its prioritization process and list to meet Secretary Sullivan's objections, and the revised plan was subsequently approved. I shall consider those revisions below when I explore alternative strategies for avoiding the conflict between the ADA and rational priority setting.

The National Legal Center's example of discrimination based on disability that was cited by Secretary Sullivan in his initial rejection of Oregon's waiver request was a specific scenario, but I want to generalize the different forms of discrimination against persons with disabilities that either a cost-effectiveness or relative-benefit standard will produce. For convenience in exposition I will use QALYs as the measure of benefit of health interventions, but I believe the same issues arise with other benefit measures; QALYs might be calculated using the QWB, as in Oregon, or any of a number of other health-related quality-of-life measures.[12] In what ways does priority setting conflict with ADA?

First, when health interventions are lifesaving, the QALYs produced will depend on the life expectancies of the patients who receive them. Since many, although of course not all, disabilities such as cystic fibrosis (CF) or AIDS cause patients to have shorter life expectancies, the years of life saved and QALYs produced by lifesaving interventions will be fewer with such disabled patients than with otherwise similar nondisabled patients. Note that this will be true even if the intervention is unrelated to the disability—for example an appendectomy performed on a person with CF or AIDS. Second, since disabilities by definition under the ADA substantially limit one or more major life activities, they will reduce an individual's health-related quality of life. For this reason as well, lifesaving interventions will produce fewer QALYs with a disabled patient, for example with COPD or impaired vision, than with an otherwise similar nondisabled patient, and again, even if the intervention is unrelated to the individual's disability. Third, benefit measures like QALYs will often discriminate against persons with disabilities with health interventions that protect or improve the quality of life. When a preexisting disability in effect acts as a comorbidity, it can make a treatment less effective in improving a patient's health-related quality of life. Patients with COPD or advanced CF, for example, have substantial limitations in mobility and ability to carry out a variety of activities requiring physical exertion; this would reduce the benefit they would otherwise have to carry out physical activities. Fourth, the disability may not be preexisting but the result of treatment being less effective or itself causing a new functional limitation. To take an example mentioned earlier that arose regarding the initial Oregon proposal, neonatal intensive care for extreme-low-birthweight newborns (less than 500 grams) typically leaves them with various substantial disabilities, whereas neonatal intensive care for low-birth-weight newborns (500 to 2,500 grams) is typically associated with much less or no resultant disability; extreme-low-birthweight newborns typically have greater long-term disabilities even with, and in part caused by, treatment.

Therefore the QALYs produced by treating a typical low-birthweight newborn will be substantially greater than those from treating an extreme-low-birthweight newborn. This last example also illustrates a fifth way in which disabled individuals will be discriminated against when the standard for prioritization is cost-effectiveness, not just relative benefit. The presence of a disability or a more severe disability can often make a treatment more complex or extended—and so more expensive—than it would be with no or a less severe disability; for example, the typical costs of neonatal intensive care for extreme-low-birthweight newborns are much greater than for low-birthweight newborns. Since cost-effectiveness prioritizes on the basis of relative cost as well as relative benefit, it will give higher priority to the less expensive treatment.

I have illustrated these different ways in which prioritization of health interventions by their cost-effectiveness or by their relative benefits will discriminate against the disabled in order to make clear that the discrimination will be systematic and far-reaching, not a minor and rare occurrence. However, often, probably usually, health interventions will be equally cost-effective and beneficial for persons with and without disabilities since the interventions will treat other conditions and not be affected by the presence of a disability. In other cases the health care needs of the disabled will receive higher priority when disabled persons' function can be effectively restored or ameliorated either by treatment of their disability or by treatment which reduces their disability in the course of treating a different condition. So it would be a mistake to believe that persons with disabilities will always fare worse in prioritization of health resources, but the ways and frequency with which they will fare worse are extensive. And, importantly, the cause of the disabled faring worse than the nondisabled is not unrelated to their disabilities.

Instead, it is precisely as a result of their disability that cost-effectiveness or relative-benefit standards give treatment of people with disabilities lower priority in each of the five forms of discrimination I have illustrated above—it is the disability itself that reduces the benefit and/or increases the cost of treatment, and so places persons with disabilities lower down on the priority list for treatment. Not every disadvantage, however, is unjust, nor is being placed lower on a priority list always unjust discrimination. Is this disadvantage and lower priority unjust? (I do not address whether it is legally in violation of ADA.)

The answer to this question is controversial. Some commentators have argued that it is not unjust, that this disadvantaging of persons with disabilities is an inevitable and acceptable consequence of a rational priority-setting process. For example, David Hadorn writes: "Banning consideration of quality of life and ability to function is counterproductive; moreover, it is inconsistent with the massive effort to facilitate and fund health outcomes research—the lion's share of which deals with quality of life and ability to function."[13]

However, we are concerned with the use of quality of life and ability to function specifically for the purpose of prioritizing between—or selecting among—different persons or groups in allocating scarce health care resources. Even if we rejected such use there, outcomes research would still be important to determine which among alternative health interventions would most benefit a given patient or group of patients; this would be the first of the two kinds of funding decisions distinguished by the National Legal Center, which they granted would not be discrimination based on disability.

Paul Menzel, too, has defended this use of quality-of-life considerations in priority-setting, despite acknowledging that it can disadvantage the disabled:

> Quality of life considerations as well as likelihood of medical success sometimes do get associated with disabilities (though not only with disabilities). Such considerations must not be seen as biased against persons with disabilities just because they catch disabilities in their net. They ought to be regarded as inconsistent with the ADA only if we would reject them as legitimate considerations at all were they not sometimes to deny care to persons with disabilities. This is a tough distinction for many to accept, for it means that even with the ADA, particular disabled individuals will end up disadvantaged. It is, however, a distinction utterly essential to maintain if we are going to have any significant rationing at all. . . . Rationing that considers quality of life must be allowed to go forward even if at times it happens to disadvantage persons with disabilities. Indeed, it is questionable whether we could ever devise a system of priority setting that was not informed in some measure by assessments of quality of life.[14]

One argument why use of quality-of-life considerations in priority-setting is unjust to the disabled is that it appears to imply that the lives of disabled persons are worth less than the lives of nondisabled persons, thereby violating the equal moral concern and respect that all persons are due. Hadorn and Menzel would apparently deny this claim. The relevant moral standard, they argue, is maximizing health benefits with limited resources, and it is merely a contingent and unintended effect of the use of this rational and acceptable standard that it sometimes results in lower priority to treatment of persons with disabilities. This is no more unjust discrimination against the disabled, they might argue, than giving a scarce intensive care bed to the sickest patient is unjust discrimination against the less sick patient. But the morally problematic implication in the case of disabilities is not difficult to find, and it is clearest in the case of lifesaving treatment. We use QALYs to measure the value of health benefits; because persons with disabilities have a lower quality of life, we produce less valuable benefits in QALYs by saving their lives than by saving the lives of persons without disabilities. It is a less good or valuable outcome if the person with a disability survives than if the person without a disability survives because the person with a disability has a less good—and so, less valuable—life. This seems to imply that the lives of persons with disabilities are worth less or have less value than the lives of persons without disabilities—worth less because of their disabilities—and so to be incompatible with their equal moral worth as persons.

Why else might this disadvantage that persons with disabilities will suffer in prioritizing health care resources by cost-effectiveness or relative-benefit standards be thought unjust? One line of reasoning, setting aside cases where persons are responsible for causing their disabilities, is that having a disability is a morally undeserved disadvantage. It would only compound that undeserved disadvantage to use it as the basis for giving disabled individuals lower priority than otherwise similar nondisabled individuals for health care treatment, especially when the treatment is unrelated to the disability. Frances Kamm expresses this idea as the "non-linkage principle"—"the fact that some undeserved bad thing has happened to you [should] not make it more likely that another bad thing will happen."[15] A different line of reasoning appeals to a moral principle of equality of opportunity. Equality of opportunity has a deep place in American moral and political culture, although its precise meaning and requirements are contested.

In the most well-developed theory of justice in health care, Norman Daniels has argued that the importance of health care for justice is its role in countering the diminishment of opportunity caused by disease and disability.[16] If disabilities are conditions that substantially limit one or more major life activities of persons, as ADA understands them, then disabilities by definition will reduce individuals' opportunity from that which otherwise similar nondisabled persons enjoy, thereby denying them equality of opportunity with nondisabled individuals. Any of these three lines of argument would need much spelling out to establish fully that the disadvantages disabled persons suffer in prioritization of health care resources are indeed *unjust*, but I shall not pursue those details here.

At the core of these moral objections to practices that discriminate against the disabled is using or allowing an undeserved disadvantage—the disability that limits a person's function—as grounds to disadvantage that person further with regard to some other good or benefit. In the case of health care resource prioritization, it is using or allowing people's undeserved disabilities as the ground for denying them care they would otherwise be eligible for or for giving them a lower priority for care than they would otherwise have. But it is important not to assume that every case of discrimination in this sense is necessarily, all things considered, unjust. The ADA requires employers, for example, to make reasonable accommodations to enable persons with disabilities to hold employment positions. But it does not require always ignoring disabilities in distributing scarce goods such as desirable jobs. Airlines are not required to hire people with severely impaired vision as airline pilots. Their disability prevents them from performing this job at an acceptable level, and the good of the safety of others takes precedence over allowing them an equal chance to become pilots. So if ignoring or accommodating a person's disability would require too great a cost in the good we seek to produce in a particular activity—here, transporting people safely—then denying the person with a disability the benefit sought—here, the job of airline pilot—is not, all things considered, unjust. Likewise, if the good of health care, simplistically put, is health, then using disability as a ground for denying persons care, or for giving persons lower priority for care, may not necessarily be, all things considered, unjust if not doing so would produce too great a cost or sacrifice in furthering the goal of health care.

I want now to explore some standards other than cost-effectiveness and relative benefit for health care resource prioritization that might avoid disadvantaging persons with disabilities in unjust ways. How did Oregon revise its ranking standard to avoid the apparent conflict with ADA, and secure waivers from HCFA to implement its new Medicaid plan? In part by combining some treatment/condition pairs that had been held to be discriminatory when distinguished; for example, neonatal intensive care for newborns below 500 grams and between 500 and 2,500 grams were combined into a single treatment/condition pair, thereby avoiding the apparent discrimination against extreme-low-birthweight newborns by grouping them with low-birthweight newborns who have much better treatment outcomes. More generally, they abandoned explicit evaluation of outcomes in terms of length and quality of life and now assessed them by "the probability (percent of the time) that within five years the average person with a particular condition receiving a specified treatment would (1) die, (2) have significant residual effects (symptoms) because of or in spite of treatment or (3) become asymptomatic."[17] This largely avoids the first two forms of discrimination I noted above with life-sustaining treatment by ignoring the expected length of survival beyond five years and by not adjusting those surviving life years for differences in quality of life.

However, the new second and third criteria still would apparently give lower priority to treatments for patients left with residual disabilities than to treatments that leave patients asymptomatic. This still gives weight to differences in outcomes in terms of patient quality of life and so is still open to the charge of discriminating on the basis of residual disability. On the other hand, since the prioritization standard essentially looks to whether or the extent to which a treatment works (as measured by five-year survival and the continued presence or absence of symptoms which the treatment causes or for which it is intended), it does not discriminate based on differences in life expectancy and quality of life caused by a disability that is unrelated to treatment. Oregon's new criteria substantially, but apparently not completely, avoid the forms of discrimination against the disabled that I noted earlier. However, we need the reasons why particular criteria are or are not morally acceptable—a principled account of when and why disadvantaging of the disabled is and is not unjust. We need to look further.

A radical position that would avoid all the forms of discrimination I distinguished above would be to abandon all appeal to assessments of the impact of treatments on quality or length of life (or to differences in their costs) when prioritizing resources for different persons, so as to avoid differences in these impacts that result from or in disabilities in some patients. This would still be compatible with attending to differential impacts of alternative treatments on length and quality of life in selecting treatments for the same patient or group of patients. However, this position would prevent us from taking any account of the differences in benefits between treatments in prioritizing. If the aim of health care is, again simply put, to promote health, then completely to ignore the different impacts on health of different health interventions would be irrational. Even if taking account of the different impacts of different treatments was shown to be always unfair to those who needed the treatments providing lesser benefits, the opportunity costs in lost health benefits from ignoring all differences in benefits would be sufficiently great to override the unfairness at least sometimes. But taking account of differences in benefits has not been shown to be always unfair.

To explore a different response to this problem of discrimination, consider first prioritizing life-sustaining treatments. Suppose two patients, of whom one is blind but who are otherwise similar, each need a lifesaving organ transplant, and there is only one available organ. Should the disability and lower health-related quality of life of the blind patient, which will result in fewer QALYs produced if she receives the transplant, give her lower priority for the transplant? Many would say it should not, and so, presumably, does the ADA. Why? Frances Kamm has argued that from the subjective point of view of each patient, his or her own survival is far more important than another's survival; even if the quality of life of the blind patient is not as good as the nondisabled patient's, her survival would still be more important to her.[18] From this deontological perspective, morality must take some account of the subjective point of view of individual persons, not just how matters look from an impersonal objective point of view. If, from the subjective standpoint of each individual, the benefit of surviving is not substantially different because one is blind, then each should be given an equal, or at least some significant, chance to live, and the difference in their quality of life should be ignored. Each stands to get, as Kamm puts it, "the major part of what both stand to get"—their life.[19]

Moreover, each stands to lose everything—her life—and each equally needs the transplant for life. Since one individual would prefer an outcome where she survives in full health to one where she survives blind, we can grant that in this respect the former is a better outcome. But this difference in outcomes when two different patients each need lifesaving treatment is insufficient to justify the very great difference in how they would be treated—one lives and one dies—if we select the patient who will be returned to full health with treatment.

Each of the ways that I have put above the reason for ignoring this difference in the quality of life of patients when lifesaving is at stake does not imply that all such differences should be ignored, nor that the position is fully subjective in the sense that if each cares more about her own survival than the other's, that is sufficient to require ignoring the difference in outcomes. Kamm calls her position "sobjective" to indicate that it combines the subjective point of view with an objective impersonal point of view which considers degree of benefit without regard to whether one gets it oneself. Each might not get the major part of what each stands to get if the difference in quality of life were very great, and if it were very great it might be sufficient to justify our saving one and letting the other die. A fully subjective view would have unacceptable implications. To take an extreme example, polls of the public have shown that around 10 percent of people would want treatment to sustain their lives even if they were in a persistent vegetative state (PVS), and to some or most of these 10 percent, it could well be more important to them that they survive even if they were to be in PVS than that another survive in full health. A fully subjective view might then imply that if such a person came to be in PVS, he should receive an equal chance for a scarce lifesaving treatment with a person who could be returned to full health. But few would accept this position; this difference in outcomes is sufficiently great to justify letting the PVS patient die and saving the other.

Roughly the same line of argument can be applied to differences in life expectancy between patients needing lifesaving treatment and, in turn, the differences in expected QALYs that treating them would produce. That Patient A would be expected to survive ten years with treatment and Patient B, twenty years is insufficient to justify the very great difference of saving B and letting A die, and we would expect that it would be more important to each from their subjective point of view that he or she survive. On the other hand, if the difference in expected survival was that A would live for two days and B for twenty years, this difference is sufficient to justify how we would treat each if we save B and let A die. In this case, it might not be more important to A that she be saved instead of B, but even if it were, as Kamm argues, this sacrifice of the loss of two days of life is sufficiently small that A should be morally expected to accept it in order for B to gain twenty years of life.[20]

None of the above reasoning is precise about when a difference in outcomes between patients or between types of treatments is sufficiently great that it can be used to decide who lives and who dies in cases of lifesaving. Nor have I argued here whether significant but not sufficiently great differences in outcome should be ignored and patients given equal chances to obtain the treatment they need to survive, or whether some scheme of proportional chances should be used in which the patient who would get the worse outcome would get some but a lesser chance to survive.[21] If in the case of lifesaving treatment, some but not all differences in outcome of quality or length of life should not be used to prioritize patients or treatments, then some but not all disadvantage based on disability in resource prioritization is unjust. I have not distinguished when a preexisting disability results in a difference in outcomes of lifesaving treatments from when the difference is caused by the treatment; some would hold that intuitively, the former are more plausibly cases of unjust discrimination based on disability, but the basis for this view is not clear.

The third and fourth forms of discrimination against the disabled concerned treatment whose purpose is to improve or protect patients' health-related quality of life and which is less effective either because a preexisting disability acts as a co-morbid or complicating factor in treatment or because some nondisabling difference between patients leaves one but not the other with a disability after treatment. Notice that these forms of discrimination cannot be avoided by the proposal some have made to look only at whether treatments are effective, not at any background conditions of disability, since it is precisely a difference in treatment effectiveness that generates these two forms of discrimination. We may be able to use roughly the same strategy here as sketched above regarding lifesaving treatment—with a significant qualification. If we again want to take some account of the subjective point of view of individual patients, for each of whom their getting needed treatment will be most important despite a disability-related difference in treatment effectiveness and benefit, then we cannot simply prioritize by the degree of benefit different patients would receive from treatments.

Small differences in benefits will not be sufficient to justify treating or funding the cost of treating some, but not treating or funding the cost of treating others. The small difference in benefit would, in this context, be what Kamm has called an irrelevant utility or good, though I think characterizing it as an insufficient good or benefit more clearly directs attention at what it is insufficient or irrelevant for, namely justifying treating the patient(s) who would receive the greater benefit.[22] The qualification is that since the difference in outcome between patients treated or not treated in the case of lifesaving treatment is typically much greater—one lives and one dies—than in the case of treatment that protects or improves quality of life—both live, but only one gets an improvement in quality of life from treatment—with quality-of-life treatments, smaller differences in outcomes of treatments can often justify treating the patient who will benefit more. Here again, with quality-of-life treatments, some but not all disadvantaging of persons with disabilities because their disability will result in their benefiting less from treatment will be unjust.

A different way of thinking about the treatment of persons with disabilities in resource prioritization is as one species of the more general problem of what priority the worst-off should receive. Disability discrimination will not fully fit into a priority to the worst-off framework because, as Kamm points out, sometimes having a disability would not make one worse off than another.[23] Kamm's example is the case of two people with a life-threatening illness, one of whom has just become disabled and so would have a worse quality of life in the future if saved; neither has had a worse health-related quality of life until now (Kamm's backward-looking conception of need), and each will die equally soon without treatment (Kamm's forward-looking sense of urgency). Neither is worse-off measured by her sense of either need or urgency, yet it would be wrong not to treat the disabled person because her future quality of life would be lower; that would be an insufficient or irrelevant good.

There is no reason, however, to believe that disability discrimination always raises the same moral concern, and usually our moral concern for the disabled may be for how their disability makes them worse off than others. If disabilities are understood as limitations in one or more major life activities, as stated in the ADA, then their moral significance may be that this disadvantage, other things being equal, makes persons with disabilities worse off than persons without them, and that it is more important morally to help the worst-off. The question raised by persons with disabilities for health care resource prioritization then will be: What priority should be given to the worst-off? This is a large, complex, and unresolved issue that I cannot pursue here, but I can at least distinguish three different components of the broader issue.

The first component—who are the worst-off for purposes of health care resource prioritization—has special importance for how a priority to the worst-off framework applies to resources for the disabled. Two aspects of this component are important here: Should the worst-off be understood as the sickest, or as those with the worst level of overall well-being, of which health is only one component? Should the worst-off be understood as those worst-off at a point in time or over their lifetimes? If the sickest is the proper focus, then to the extent that where one falls on a health-related quality-of-life scale roughly corresponds to how disabled one is, those who are worst-off will roughly correspond to the most disabled. On the other hand, if the concern for the worst-off should be for those whose overall level of well-being is worst, then some with significant disabilities may nevertheless have a higher level of overall well-being than others without any disability and so receive less, not more, priority. Moreover, even if the proper perspective is how sick people are, whether that means now, over their lifetimes, or possibly some combination of both, will often determine which individuals or groups are the worst-off or most disabled.

The second component of the issue of priority to the worst-off is why—for what moral reason—the worst-off should receive some priority in health care resource prioritization. There are several different possible answers: for example, in order to reduce inequality, in order to increase equality of opportunity, because reducing greater deprivation has greater moral importance, because getting treatment will be subjectively most important to the sickest, or because the sickest have the greatest health needs. Some of these reasons would most plausibly apply to those whose overall well-being is worst, others, to the sickest.

The third component of the issue of priority to the worst-off in health care resource prioritization is how much priority they should receive, which will be determined in part by why they should get priority. Even assuming a compelling moral reason for such priority, it would be implausible to give the worst-off absolute priority. Doing so would raise what has been called the "bottomless pit" problem: for persons with very serious disabilities whom we can only make slightly better-off, but at enormous cost in resource use, assigning their needs absolute priority would excessively drain off resources for very little gain that could be used to produce much greater benefits for others less badly off. Here again, priority to the worst-off or disabled must be balanced against other moral considerations, including treatment effectiveness or benefits.

I cannot pursue here any of these three components of the priority to the worst-off issue, but progress on them may be necessary for us to make progress on the issue of what priority the disabled should receive. One reason for thinking the priority to the worst-off may be the right framework for much of our moral concern for persons with disabilities is that it fits well with two natural intuitive ideas that are quite common in thinking about what we owe persons with disabilities generally. In each case, these ideas explicitly involve the rejection of benefit maximization, as embodied in cost-effectiveness or relative-benefit standards, in order to meet specific moral claims of the disabled. First, in the service of equality of opportunity, access to job opportunities and public facilities through special transportation, access ramps and so forth must be provided to persons with disabilities even when those resources could be used elsewhere to provide greater benefits to others who are not disabled. Second, it is very common to think that because disabilities are undeserved disadvantages, compensation is required in order to remove or reduce the disadvantage; moral claims for compensation in general are grounded in desert, not in whether meeting them is the use of resources that will produce the most benefits.

CONCLUSION

It was the confluence of the passage of the Americans with Disabilities Act and the effort by the state of Oregon to prioritize and ration health care in its Medicaid program that focused the problem of discrimination against persons with disabilities in health care resource prioritization. I have sought here to lay out that problem and to explore some, but by no means all, possible standards for prioritization that may avoid unjust discrimination against persons with disabilities. I have only been able to scratch the surface of the issues, in part because the problem of health care resource prioritization for the disabled raises deep, complex and unresolved issues of health care resource prioritization more generally. The issues of health care equity and justice as they affect both the disabled and others have only begun to be seriously explored, and there is much work to be done.

ACKNOWLEDGMENTS

This paper draws in places on and extends the analysis of my "Justice and the ADA: Does Prioritizing and Rationing Health Care Discriminate Against the Disabled?" *Social Theory and Practice* (1995) 159–185.

NOTES

[1] 42 U.S.C. § 12101(b)(1).
[2] David Orentlicher, "Rationing and the Americans with Disabilities Act," *Journal of the American Medical Association* 271 (1994) 308–314.
[3] *Sutton v. United Airlines,* 119 S.Ct. 2139 (1999).
[4] I draw on Michael J. Garland, "Justice, Politics, and Community: Expanding Access and Rationing Health Services in Oregon," *Law, Medicine, and Health Care* 20 (1992) 70.
[5] Robert Kaplan and John Anderson, "A General Health Policy Model; Update and Applications," *Health Services Res.* 23 (1988) 203–235.
[6] David Hadorn, "Setting Health Care Priorities in Oregon: Cost-Effectiveness Meets the Rule of Rescue," *Journal of the American Medical Association* 265 (1991) 2218–2225.
[7] David Eddy, "Oregon's Methods: Did Cost-Effectiveness Analysis Fail?" *Journal of the American Medical Association* 266 (1991) 2135–2141.
[8] Hadorn, op. cit.
[9] Unpublished letter from Secretary of Health and Human Services Louis W. Sullivan to Governor Barbara Roberts of Oregon, August 3, 1992.
[10] Unpublished letter from Thomas I. Marzen and Daniel Avila, National Legal Center for the Medically Dependent and Disabled, Inc., to Representative Christopher H. Smith, U.S. House of Representatives, December 5, 1991.
[11] Ibid.
[12] See Dan W. Brock, "Quality of Life Measures in Health Care and Medical Ethics," in *The Quality of Life,* A. Sen and M. Nussbaum, eds. Oxford: Oxford University Press, 1993.

[13]David Hadorn, "The Problem of Discrimination in Health Care Priority Setting," *Journal of the American Medical Association* 268 (1992) 1454–1459.

[14]Paul T. Menzel, "Oregon's Denial: Disabilities and Quality of Life," *Hastings Center Report* 22 (1992) 21–25.

[15]Frances Kamm, "Deciding Whom to Help, the Principle of Irrelevant Good and Health-Adjusted Life Years," unpublished.

[16]Norman Daniels, *Just Health Care.* Cambridge, UK: Cambridge University Press, 1985.

[17]*New York Times,* March 20, 1993, 8.

[18]Kamm. "Deciding Whom to Help." See also her *Morality/Mortality Volume 1: Death and Who to Save from It.* Oxford: Oxford University Press, 1993.

[19]As Kamm notes, this might be interpreted as "the biggest part quantitatively of what either can get" or "the meaningful minimum that it is crucial that someone have."

[20]Kamm, "Deciding Whom to Help" and *Morality/Mortality.*

[21]Dan W. Brock, "Ethical Issues in Recipient Selection for Organ Transplantation," in *Organ Substitution Technology: Ethical, Legal, and Public Policy Issues,* Debra Mathieu, ed. Boulder, CO: Westview Press, 1988, 94.

[22]Kamm, *Morality/Mortality.*

[23]Ibid.

Utility, Equality and Health Care Needs of Persons with Disabilities

Interpreting the ADA's Requirement of Reasonable Accommodations

DAVID ORENTLICHER

When health care resources are rationed, a common moral concern involves the trade-off between utility and equity. On one hand, we want to use our limited resources wisely and allocate them in a way that yields the greatest overall benefit (with benefit typically measured in terms of lives saved, improvement in quality of life and the number of years for which life is extended or the quality of life improved). On the other hand, we also want to treat everyone fairly and ensure that resources are allocated in a way that avoids unfair discrimination against persons who are disfavored in society. When health care is being rationed, we might worry that less care will be given to the aged, the poor, members of minority groups[1] or persons with disabilities.[2]

When the Americans with Disabilities Act (ADA) was drafted to protect persons with disabilities from unfair discrimination, it clearly reflected the tension between utility and equity. Concerns about equity are most obviously captured in the basic prohibition against discrimination on the basis of disability. Utility comes in with the protection against discrimination being limited to those persons with disabilities who are "qualified individuals" for the job or service at stake. If a disability prevents an individual from being able to perform the duties of a job or to benefit from the provision of a service, the ADA permits the employer or the service provider to discriminate on the basis of the disability. In other words, the idea of a qualified individual takes into account the fact that discrimination because of disability is sometimes acceptable. People's disabilities may in fact be relevant to their eligibility for a job or service. A person who uses a wheelchair is fully qualified to serve as a telephone operator, but would not be able to carry out the responsibilities of many construction jobs. Similarly, when deciding whether to transplant a heart into a patient with heart failure, it should not matter whether the recipient is hearing-impaired or visually limited, but it may well matter if the patient is dying of metastatic lung cancer or is permanently unconscious.

In this chapter, I will discuss the trade-off between the moral values of utility and equity in the context of protecting the disabled from unfair discrimination in the allocation of health care resources. In doing so, I will argue that the ADA's requirement of reasonable accommodations should be used by the courts as an important vehicle for drawing the appropriate balance between utility and equity.

UTILITY VERSUS EQUITY

Generally, when health care resources are being rationed, commentators worry about the potential conflict between achieving the greatest good with our limited health care

236

resources (utility) and showing equal respect for all persons (equity). For example, a utilitarian will ordinarily want to give a heart or liver transplant to the patient who will live for ten years instead of the patient who will live for five years after the transplant. Similarly, a utilitarian will want to give a heart or liver transplant to a patient who will be fully functional instead of a person who will live as long but be confined to a long-term care facility. With both preferences, it is argued, society achieves better outcomes. More years of life or greater improvements in quality of life are achieved.

Yet an egalitarian might respond, this kind of allocative decision-making shows insufficient respect for the patient who will live for five years, the patient who will be confined to a long-term care facility or other patients who derive a smaller amount of benefit from treatment. In particular, utility-based allocation will often disadvantage persons with disabilities. Organ transplants and other life-sustaining treatments will extend life for fewer years and/or at a lower level of functioning for many persons with disabilities.[3] However, in an egalitarian view, all lives have equal worth, and differences in expected benefit are not always a morally valid basis for treating people differently.

While I agree with the egalitarian position that purely utilitarian approaches are problematic, we must refine the analysis further to make the case against assigning priority for treatment to the patients who will gain more benefit from the treatment. As Dan Brock and others have observed, it is not so clear that giving treatment to the person who will benefit the most from treatment is disrespectful of other persons. That is, even on egalitarian terms, we can invoke an argument that would result in preference for the patient who would live longer or who would have a higher level of functioning (i.e., the nondisabled person).

To see how this is so, consider what might be viewed as the most egalitarian method for choosing the recipient of a heart or liver transplant—a random lottery among all in need of the transplant. Everyone with severe heart or liver failure would be eligible for transplantation, and physicians would employ a random process to choose the transplant recipient. The patient who will live the shortest time with a transplant would have the same likelihood of being chosen as the patient who will live the longest with the transplant.[4]

But, Brock writes, if we want to rely on a random lottery, we arguably do so when we employ utilitarian criteria to rank candidates for organ transplants or other medical treatments. For, according to one view, it is essentially a random process that determines which persons happen to become diseased and in need of an organ transplant.[5] It is a matter of chance whether I am someone who craves fresh, wild mushrooms and inadvertently picks and eats a poisonous mushroom that destroys my liver. Similarly, it is fortuitous whether I instead cannot stand either to harvest my own food or to eat mushrooms. Did I receive the genes and environment that encourage mushroom foraging and eating, or did I receive the genes and environment that discourage those activities? It is also an essentially random process that decides the particular characteristics of patients that influence their ability to benefit from a heart or liver transplant. Whether I have a lung disease that makes me a poor surgical candidate or whether I have strong, healthy lungs that make me likely to survive the rigors of organ transplant surgery is also determined by the random operation of the biological and social lottery.[6] I may have been born with good genes or bad genes, to a wealthy family or a poor family, but it was all a matter of good luck or bad luck.

Under this view, it does not matter whether we have a human-designed lottery to determine which person with heart or liver failure receives a transplant or a genetic and environmental lottery to determine which persons will end up with heart or liver failure and be favored by a system that allocates organs according to utilitarian criteria. The only difference is whether the lottery operates before people get sick (i.e., a biological and social lottery) or after they get sick (i.e., a rationing lottery). Either way, a lottery decides who will have priority for organ transplants. Or, to put it another way, whether we choose heart and liver recipients by lottery or according to utilitarian criteria, some patients will receive a needed transplant and other patients will not. As long as we are going to have some winners and some losers, we might as well make sure the winners will live as long as possible with their new organs.[7] In short, the use of utilitarian criteria to identify organ transplant recipients or to make other rationing decisions with health care may be perfectly consistent with egalitarian considerations.

This view in favor of utilitarian criteria arguably fits in well with the principles underlying the ADA. When the ADA prohibits discrimination against persons because of their disabilities only if they are "qualified" individuals, the act recognizes that physicians and hospitals can take into account disabilities to the extent that the disabilities are relevant to the decision at hand. Just as an employer need not hire applicants whose disabilities prevent them from performing the job duties adequately, a physician need not provide a treatment to patients whose disabilities prevent them from appropriately benefiting from the care. For example, in one case, a federal court indicated that, if a patient's HIV disease would turn an elective surgical procedure from safe to unsafe for the patient, a physician could refuse to perform the surgery without thereby being in violation of the ADA.[8]

Accordingly, if we are to reject purely utilitarian criteria for health care rationing under the ADA, we need a further argument to show the inequity to disabled persons of utilitarian criteria. The argument I will make can be summarized as follows: the inequity rests in the fact that we do not have a random biological and social lottery to determine who develops heart or liver failure or other illnesses, nor do we have a random lottery to determine whether one will be a good or bad candidate for medical treatment. Rather, the biological and social lottery is very much skewed in its operation and effects.

THE UNFAIR BIAS IN SOCIETY'S BIOLOGICAL AND SOCIAL LOTTERY

The bias in the biological and social lottery of life that makes utilitarian criteria suspect rests in an important understanding about the nature of disability. As many commentators have observed, the disabling effects of a disability are a function of both the inherent qualities of the disability and the interaction between the disability and the social environment.[9] A person who needs a wheelchair for mobility is much less constrained when buildings have ramps and elevators in addition to stairs to get from one level to another. Moreover, as Congress recognized when it enacted the ADA, society has developed its structures and policies on the basis of the needs of persons without disabilities. For example, people who use canes may have trouble crossing the street because the green light does not last long enough for them to cross; or consider people whose psychiatric problems result in poor compliance with their medical regimen and therefore ostensibly make them poorer candidates for organ transplants and other complex therapies. Psychiatric illness interferes with the person's ability to follow routines and keep to schedules. Consequently, like children, people with psychiatric illness need more external guidance in exercising control over their lives. Very likely, these individuals would have better compliance if they were able to live in a more structured environment.

Although people with psychiatric problems have to rely more on external structure than on internal structure, our society has evolved with a low level of external structure because most people can muster high levels of internal structure.[10] We could have developed a more structured environment, and people needing external structure would be less disabled. In short, much of the disadvantage of a disability is not inherent in the disability but is a result of society's attitudes, policies and institutions being erected around the norm of a person without disabilities.[11] If we had designed our society with the needs of people with disabilities in mind, we would have a society in which disabilities have much less of an impact on a person's ability to function. Accordingly, if we employ utilitarian criteria and thereby allow distinctions when disabilities have a real effect on a person's ability to benefit from an organ transplant or other medical treatment, we do nothing to counteract the fact that our social structures are inherently biased against people with disabilities. Treating people with disabilities equally when they start out with an unfair disadvantage simply perpetuates the original disadvantage.

Still, one might say, whether one is favored or disfavored by the social environment is all a matter of chance. Even if the environment perpetuates or aggravates the effects of a disabling condition, we do not necessarily violate egalitarian principles if it is random whether one is favored or disfavored by the social environment.

The egalitarian concern arises because the social factors that affect disability are not natural or inevitable but are often employed because they serve the interests of some segments of society at the expense of others. How a societal norm develops may depend more on considerations of popularity or political power than on alternative visions of distributive justice that have greater moral weight. Social norms develop not because they are preordained but because they serve the needs of social groups that are dominant either in numbers or in power.

For example, whether someone develops a disabling condition may be a consequence of societal commissions or omissions that are biased in favor of politically influential persons. Social forces cause disability by commission when environmental pollution leads to lung diseases or cancers, when lead-based paint damages the neurologic systems of children and when unchecked violence results in traumatic injury. And it is not at all random who is at higher risk for these kinds of injuries. Landlords in poorer neighborhoods are less likely to remove lead-based paints. Similarly, industrial companies are much more likely to locate toxin-emitting factories in poorer communities.[12]

An important way in which social organization causes disability by omission occurs when priorities are established for medical research. Some illnesses, like heart disease and cancer, are the subject of vast research expenditures; other illnesses receive little attention from federal research funds.[13] As a result, preventive and curative measures are developed unevenly. People with coronary artery disease are saved by surgery from disability, while people with multiple sclerosis cannot be helped very much by medical care. In other words, there may be discrimination not only between people with and without disabilities, but also among people with different kinds of disabilities. In part, disparities across different disabilities may exist because it may be easier to treat disabilities like coronary artery disease than disabilities like multiple sclerosis. Moreover, since more people suffer from coronary artery disease than from multiple sclerosis, it has made sense to devote more resources to research on coronary artery disease. However, how research dollars are allocated turns not only on the responsiveness of the disease to treatment or the number of people affected but also on the political influence of the people with the disease. Research on coronary artery disease has a strong constituency both because it is a major killer and because it is a major killer of successful professionals in their fifties and sixties (i.e., an age by which people have amassed substantial wealth). Similarly, when persons with (or at risk for) HIV disease mobilized and lobbied for greater funding, resources for HIV research and treatment jumped and did so in a way that may not have been justified by the severity of the threat from HIV disease.[14]

Consider another example in which skewed research efforts may have led to better success rates in treating some patients than others. Persons with chronic lung disease (a disabling condition) who also suffer from coronary artery disease (a second disabling condition) do not do as well with bypass surgery for their coronary artery disease as persons with normal lung function and coronary artery disease. Consequently, they are less likely to be viewed as appropriate candidates for bypass surgery. Yet the difference in likelihood of success may reflect not simply the fact that chronic lung disease inevitably complicates treatment of coronary artery disease but also the fact that techniques for bypass surgery were developed around the prototype of a patient with normal lung function.

If treatment for coronary artery disease had been developed on the assumption that patients with the disease also have chronic lung disease, then different surgical techniques or even altogether different treatments would have been developed—techniques or treatments that would be more successful than current treatments for patients with chronic lung disease (although perhaps less effective than current treatments for patients with normal lung function). For example, there might have been a greater emphasis on nonsurgical therapies than on surgical therapies, since persons with chronic lung disease are much better able to tolerate nonsurgical than surgical therapies. Or there might have been quicker development of minimally invasive surgical techniques. Again, this would be problematic in terms of equity if the tendency to design research around the norm of the person without lung disease reflects in part the greater political power of such people. In fact, we might suspect that people with chronic lung disease lack political power either because lung disease is more common in poorer persons or because having chronic lung disease makes one more likely to be poor (e.g., because it is difficult for people to carry on with their employment once they develop lung disease).

THE REQUIREMENT OF REASONABLE ACCOMMODATIONS

Because reliance on utilitarian criteria entails unfair bias against persons with disabilities, it is important that courts interpret the ADA to compensate for the biases. The requirement of reasonable accommodations suggests two ways in which the courts can do so. (According to the ADA's requirement of reasonable accommodations, if a disability compromises a person's ability to qualify for a service, the service provider must make reasonable modifications in its service to accommodate the disabled person, unless the modifications would "fundamentally alter the nature of the services" or impose an "undue burden" on the service provider.[15])

First, courts can interpret the requirement of reasonable accommodations in its traditional way to overcome some of the problems with the use of utilitarian criteria. While the courts have not done much with the requirement in deciding health care cases,[16] courts have developed the requirement of reasonable accommodations in nonmedical contexts.[17] For example, the U.S. Court of Appeals for the Tenth Circuit has held that, within reason, primary public schools must provide special education services and adopt modifications of their educational programs to ensure that children with disabilities receive an education appropriate to their needs.[18]

If the principle of reasonable accommodations were applied to rationing decisions as it has been applied in nonmedical contexts, we could anticipate some obligation for physicians and hospitals to compensate for the effects of disability on the success of medical treatment. For example, consider the fact that poor compliance with therapy can disqualify a patient from eligibility for an organ transplant.[19] Transplant recipients have many responsibilities to carry out to prevent their body from rejecting the transplanted organ,[20] and those responsibilities may not be feasible for a disabled person alone. Disabled persons therefore may find themselves ineligible for an organ transplant. However, compliance for these individuals may be feasible if the transplant program provides support services. Some transplant centers seem to be able to overcome compliance problems by having frequent contacts with their patients.[21] If interpreted as it has been in nonmedical contexts, the principle of reasonable accommodations would likely require the provision of those support services as long as it would not be unduly burdensome for the transplant program to have to provide them.[22] Or if a person has psychiatric problems that can be kept under control with counseling, there would probably be an obligation to include the counseling as part of the treatment program, as long as the expense of the counseling was not unduly burdensome.[23]

Interpreting the requirement of reasonable accommodations for rationing decisions as it has been interpreted for nonmedical decisions will help overcome the biases against persons with disabilities. However, there are limits to the extent to which additional measures can compensate for the unfairly disadvantaging effects of utilitarian criteria. It may be possible to change immediately the way some health care services are delivered so that persons with disabilities gain the same kinds of benefits as persons without disabilities (e.g., by providing psychiatric counseling to organ transplant recipients when necessary). Still, in many situations, medical treatments will provide more benefit to persons without disabilities, or treatments for some disabilities will be more successful than treatments for other disabilities.[24] Primary reliance on measures of outcome such as increases in length of life or improvements in functional capability will disfavor persons with disabilities and those with some disabilities especially. And it will do so unfairly because of the contribution of biases in social structure to the existence of disability and to the responsiveness of disability to treatment.

To compensate for the social biases in the greater effectiveness of treatments for persons without disabilities (or the greater effectiveness of treatments for some disabilities), we would want to say that differences in outcome among different patients are not necessarily a reason for preferring one patient over another—that these differences may have resulted from unfair biases in social structure. If health care is rationed in terms of biased measures, then the rationing simply perpetuates the unfair bias. Accordingly, differences in utilitarian criteria should be discounted. We should not prefer one patient over another just because the first patient will realize more benefit from the care. Rather, we should place greater emphasis on other criteria for allocating care (e.g., whether one patient's need for care is more urgent than another patient's, or whether one patient has been waiting for care longer than another patient).

Not only would such an approach help compensate for society's structural biases against persons with disabilities, it would also create a strong incentive for society to begin the process of creating more equitable social structures. If the public realizes that treatments will be given to people whose disabling illnesses limit their ability to benefit from the treatment, then the public may make greater efforts to eliminate the structural biases against persons with disabling illnesses (e.g, by making greater efforts to understand and treat those illnesses) so that greater benefit will be realized when treatment is given to persons with disabling illnesses. In other words, because people want society to realize the greatest benefit possible from its limited health care resources, they will try to ensure that the recipients of treatment gain as much benefit as possible.

CONCLUSION

The Americans with Disabilities Act can play a critical role in properly balancing concerns about utility and equity when society rations its health care resources. Because of unfair biases in social structure, the application of utilitarian criteria results in inequitable allocations of health care. The criteria themselves are neutral with respect to equity, but they perpetuate preexisting inequities in social structure. The ADA can compensate for these inequities because its requirement of reasonable accommodations was designed to compensate for unfair biases in social structure. To fulfill the promise of the ADA, courts should give appropriate recognition to the requirement of reasonable accommodations when physicians allocate scarce health care resources.

NOTES

[1]Council on Ethical and Judicial Affairs, "Black-White Disparities in Health Care," 263 *JAMA* 2344–2346 (1990).

[2]David Orentlicher, "Destructuring Disability: Rationing of Health Care and Unfair Discrimination Against the Sick," 31 *Harv. C.R.-C.L. L. Rev.* 49 (1996).

[3]Paul Menzel has observed that persons with disabilities may benefit when considerations of utility come into play. Since the disabled individuals start at a lower level of functioning, treatments that work by improving the level of functioning rather than by extending life have more to offer for them than for able-bodied persons. Paul T. Menzel, "Some Ethical Costs of Rationing," 20 *Law, Medicine & Health Care* 57, 61 (1992).

[4]Of course, even the strongest advocate of egalitarianism might object to transplanting a liver into a patient who will die anyway in a few days or weeks. John Cubbon, "The Principle of QALY Maximisation as the Basis for Allocating Health Care Resources," 17 *J. Medical Ethics* 181, 182 (1991). A modified egalitarian position would establish a minimum threshold of benefit from treatment, with a lottery to decide the recipient from those who meet the minimum threshold.

[5]Dan W. Brock, "Ethical Issues in Recipient Selection for Organ Transplantation," in *Organ Substitution Technology: Ethical, Legal, and Public Policy Issues,* Deborah Mathieu, ed., Boulder, CO: Westview Press, 1988, 86, 95. See also Brock's essay in this volume, pp. 223–235.

[6]Even if smoking led to my lung disease, the biological and social lottery can be held responsible to a substantial extent. Did I grow up in a community where cigarette smoking was common, and did I have genes that facilitate addiction to nicotine, or did I have neither influence in my life?

[7]One might analogize to dietary laws in Judaism. The requirements of a kosher diet exclude meat from pigs but permit meat from cows. According to one view, the purpose of distinguishing between kosher and nonkosher animals is to set limits, to remind people that one should not always yield to the desires of the flesh, and also to remind people of the divine role in making food available. With such a purpose, one could just as easily permit the eating of pigs and forbid the eating of cows. However, as long as one is going to draw a distinction, better that the distinction exclude the less healthy meat and permit the more healthy meat. Since people eating pork historically risked trichinosis while people eating beef did not, it made sense to prefer beef over pork rather than pork over beef.

[8]*Glanz v. Vernick,* 756 F. Supp. 632 (D. Mass. 1991). The U.S. Supreme Court has also held that there may be grounds for denying treatment to a patient with HIV disease when the treatment would pose "a direct threat to the health or safety of others." *Bragdon v. Abbott,* 524 U.S. 624 (1998) (citing 42 U.S.C. § 12182(b)(3)).

[9]Jerome Bickenbach, *Physical Disability and Social Policy,* Toronto: University of Toronto Press, 1993, 11; Harlan Hahn, "Antidiscrimination Laws and Social Research on Disability: The Minority Group Perspective," 14 *Behavioral Sciences and the Law* 41, 45 (1996); Anita Silvers, "Disability Rights," in Ruth Chadwick, ed., *Encyclopedia of Applied Ethics,* San Diego: Academic Press, 1998, 781, 785–786.

[10]Low levels of external structure also reflect this society's valuing of individual liberties. Nevertheless, the point stands that the trade-off between the advantages and disadvantages to the individual of a structured environment looks very different from the perspective of the nondisabled person than from that of the person who is disabled with psychiatric illness.

[11]Martha Minow, *Making All the Difference: Inclusion, Exclusion, and American Law*, Ithica, NY: Cornell University Press, 1990, 21; Cass R. Sunstein, "Why Markets Don't Stop Discrimination," in *Reassessing Civil Rights*, Ellen Frankel Paul, Fred D. Miller, Jr. and Jeffrey Paul, eds., Cambridge, MA: Blackwell, 1991, 22, 23 (discussing how "markets incorporate the norms and practices of advantaged groups"); Susan Wendell, *The Rejected Body: Feminist Philosophical Reflections on Disability*, New York: Routledge, 1996, 39.

[12]Poorer communities are not only more likely to become the site for polluting factories, they also become even poorer after the factories are built. Vicki Been, "Locally Undesirable Land Uses in Minority Neighborhoods: Disproportionate Siting or Market Dynamics," 103 *Yale L. J.* 1383 (1994). And whether one is wealthy enough to escape a relatively unsafe community depends not only on whether one was fortunate enough in the biological and social lottery but also on laws and other social rules that politically powerful people enact to preserve their wealth.

[13]In fiscal year 1989, federal spending for research on, education about and prevention of cancer exceeded that for Alzheimer's disease by a factor of ten ($1.45 billion versus $127 million).

[14]For example, by 1990, federal funding for HIV research exceeded the budgets for cancer or heart research even though one tenth as many people died from AIDS as from either heart disease or cancer. Robert M. Wachter, "AIDS, Activism, and the Politics of Health," 326 *New England Journal of Medicine* 128, 129 (1992); Dick Thompson, "The AIDS Political Machine," *Time Magazine*, January 22, 1990, 24.

[15]42 U.S.C. § 12182(b)(2)(A).

[16]The U.S. Supreme Court recently interpreted the requirement of reasonable accommodations in the context of institutional placement for persons with mental disorders. *Olmstead v. L.C.*, 527 U.S. 581 (1999). However, that decision does not offer much support for rejecting a physician's rationing decision. In *Olmstead*, the Court required the states to provide community-based treatment instead of institutional commitment when, among other things, "treatment professionals determine that such placement is appropriate." Id., 2190.

[17]See, e.g., *New Mexico Association for Retarded Citizens v. New Mexico*, 678 F.2d 847 (10th Cir. 1982); *Prewitt v. United States Postal Service*, 662 F.2d 292, 305 (5th Cir. 1981).

[18]See *New Mexico Association for Retarded Citizens*, 678 F.2d at 854–855.

[19]James L. Levenson and Mary Ellen Olbrisch, "Psychosocial Evaluation of Organ Transplant Candidates: A Comparative Survey of Process, Criteria, and Outcomes in Heart, Liver, and Kidney Transplantation," 34 *Psychosomatics* 314 (1993).

[20]For example, transplant recipients must take drugs as long as the organ is functioning to suppress their body's immune response against the organ.

[21]S. Takemoto and P.I. Terasaki, "A Comparison of Kidney Transplant Survival in White and Black Recipients," 21 *Transplantation Proceedings* 3865, 3866 (1989).

[22]See Philip G. Peters, Jr., "Health Care Rationing and Disability Rights," 70 *Indiana L. Rev.* 491, 529 (1995) (arguing that the principle of reasonable accommodations should impose such a requirement). See also Tom L. Beauchamp and James F. Childress, *Principles of Biomedical Ethics*, 3rd ed., New York: Oxford University Press, 1989, 295–296 (making the same argument from principles of justice).

[23]See, e.g., *New Mexico Association for Retarded Citizens*, 678 F.2d at 854–55 (requiring school system to provide additional services for children with disabilities to ensure that they receive a meaningful education as long as the financial burden of the additional services would not be excessive).

[24]I mentioned previously the example of treatment for coronary artery disease being more effective than treatment for multiple sclerosis.

Disability and Illness

JOEL FEINBERG

Her face has turned a bright green, and she has lost all her hair. During the next few weeks doctors in this city find that thirty or forty people have reported the same symptoms, and the pattern of symptoms is absolutely invariant. Fortunately, after ten days or so the symptoms weaken and then suddenly disappear. The principal investigator for the laboratory, a doctor Greene, in the report later published in the *New England Journal of Medicine*, calls the new disease he has discovered, "Greene's disease." The authorities rename it "Greene's syndrome." If Dr. Greene had reported a single symptom only, and a common one at that (such as high temperature), his discovery would not have warranted a name of its own. If, on the other hand, the single symptom were very unusual, like the green complexion, perhaps it could be called "Greene's complexion symptom" or the like. What Greene did describe was a regular pattern of serious, standardly recurring symptoms. The medical term for such a pattern is "syndrome," a group of signs and symptoms that occur together and characterize a particular abnormal condition. Dr. Greene's discovery should be called "Greene's syndrome."

[Editors' note: the definition of illness is important in many decisions that are relevant to the application of the ADA. Consider, for example, Title II of the ADA, which prohibits discrimination in publicly provided services but which does not require accommodations that would fundamentally alter the nature of the services offered. Suppose health care services are defined as services to prevent, treat or ameliorate the symptoms of illness. An understanding of "illness" would then be central to differentiating "health care services" from other kinds of publicly provided services, such as assisted living.

Or consider the definition of "disability" itself in the ADA. "Disability" requires a "physical or mental impairment" that "substantially limits" a major life activity. "Impairment" is not the same concept as "illness"; as many writers in this volume emphasize, "impairment" refers at least in part to bias in the construction of the environment in which the disabled person lives. Nevertheless, an appreciation of the differences between impairment and illness should be informed by a careful analysis of the latter concept. Moreover, the concept of "illness" itself may be evaluative and relative to features of the social or natural environment.

The piece that follows, never before published, presents just such an analysis. It was not written especially for this volume, but it provides important conceptual tools for understanding disability, impairment and illness. These tools are of particular practical importance in the mental health arena, where individuals invoking the protection of the ADA on the basis of a mental impairment are met with the challenge that they suffer only from difference, deviance or unfortunate traits of personality. Feinberg's piece begins with a careful analysis of concepts such as disease, illness, and syndrome. It then delineates the interplay of factual, socially relative and normative judgments in the use of these concepts.

In the final section, Feinberg turns this analysis to categorizations of mental illness found in DSM-IV. He argues that normative judgments figure in some of the categorizations. But judgments that a condition is an illness may be critical to conclusions about whether it is a disability or whether treatment for it is paid for on a health plan. If Feinberg is correct, therefore, these conclusions are themselves normative.]

244

What would have to be added to Greene's syndrome to make it worthy of the more impressive sounding name "Greene's disease"? Well, first of all, a disease is one class of illness, so the first question to ask is: What must be added to a syndrome for it to be an illness? Then we can turn to the distinction between illness and disease. The latter distinction may be the easiest. As a matter of mere custom, the custodians of medical nomenclature have used the words "syndrome" and "disease" in assigning names, particularly proper names, to newly discovered sicknesses. The medical profession simply does not use words like "Parkinson" to go with "illness" or "sickness." If the sickness is to be named after James Parkinson or Lou Gehrig, it will have to be called "Parkinson's disease," or "Lou Gehrig's disease," not "Parkinson's sickness" or "Gehrig's illness." And a good thing this usage is! Without the convention we would never know whether phrases like "Parkinson's illness" referred to the disease Parkinson was the first to describe or to some particular malady that the historical James Parkinson himself suffered from.

In summary, we have the following terms to apply to medical maladies:

1. *Malady:* a conveniently vague generic term covering all the others.
2. *Symptom:* an indication of the presence of a bodily discord. It is sometimes restricted to subjective evidence of the presence of a disorder—a rational ground for suspicion.
3. *Syndrome:* a group of signs and symptoms that occur together and characterize a particular [functional] abnormality.
4. *Sickness or illness:* a disordered, weakened or unsound condition.

That leaves one more concept, "disease," to fit into its proper place. A disease is an illness with a particular known etiology—that is, an understanding of the cause or origin, for example, a certain strain of invading bacteria or specific virus (e.g. HIV), or at a different level, excessive exposure to the sun's rays (skin cancer) or excessively fatty diet (heart disease). By and large this is an accurate account of the medical ways, but it is subject to so many exceptions that it would be absurd to attach any important to it. One clear exception, for example, is Parkinson's disease, which is officially listed as a depletion of the neural transmitter dopamine from unknown causes. Apparently the desire to honor the great Scottish researcher, James Parkinson, outweighed the requirements that a person's name should attach only to those sicknesses that are diseases and that have well understood etiological explanations.

THE SERIOUSNESS OF MENTAL ILLNESS

To many Americans, "mental illness" still has a frivolous sound. It is likely to be associated in many minds with the practical problems of middle-class neurotics who are long on money and short on wisdom. Psychoanalysis provides the practical wisdom and wraps it in the language of medicine. Wise practitioners then borrow the authority of science and much of its vocabulary. This is to use what is called "the medical model," whereas what is needed by neurotic "patients," and in some cases actually provided by gifted psychoanalysts, is more understanding of the sources of their personal problems and thoroughly well-informed advice enabling patients to cope more successfully with their everyday problems. Everyone could use good advice from sagacious counselors, people are likely to think. But we can hardly charge the bill to insurance companies or a National Health Service. We must decide, the argument then concludes, that what is called "mental health" is a kind of overpriced luxury not worth its cost, and that inclusion of psychotherapy among the forms of sickness covered by Medicare would be frivolous.

Almost as many American families have been afflicted with mental illness as with alcoholism or AIDS, and the results are virtually as damaging. Congressional legislators have vulnerable relatives too. The list includes a sister of John F. Kennedy, a niece of Senator Alan Simpson, a brother of Senator Paul Wellstone, and on and on. The "symptoms" in most of these cases include intense and enduring anxiety or depression leading frequently to suicide, or to homicide and then suicide, or a bodily wasting away in the patient, or serious cognitive impairment and disorientation. *Mental illness can be devastating:* that is the first and most important fact about it that a writer should know before dealing with conceptual riddles. Even the U.S. Senate came to grasp this point in its recent debate over Medicare. In May 1996 the United States Senate voted 100 to 0 for a health care reform bill that "would among other things, require insurers to cover mental illness as fully as they cover medical problems like heart attacks and strokes."

Mental illnesses, like their physical counterparts, are a diverse and miscellaneous bunch. Following the leadership of the clinical psychologists, the custodians of psychiatric nomenclature seem to be becoming more cautious, often speaking of "syndromes" instead of "diseases," for example, when there is little agreement over etiology. The various syndromes, however, can be grouped and classified in a more or less systematic way.

The National Institute of Mental Health in 1980 published data on the numbers of victims in each of the six main categories of mental illness. Put in a diagram form, the results were as follows: some of these syndromes are defined in terms of the constituent elements of the sickness, and some in terms of its causes. Another distinction cuts across this one. Some of the constituent elements are predominantly mental states, dispositions or capacities. Similarly, some of the traceable causes are mental, and others, physical. Thus we have four classificatory pigeonholes resulting from overlap of two distinctions.

1. *Mental constituent:* anxiety, depression, failed memory.
2. *Physical constituent:* constant vomiting, sleeplessness, severe involuntary movement disorders.
3. *Mental causes:* resentment or hatred of parent, sibling, or spouse.
4. *Physical cause:* schizophrenia, hormonal imbalances, or any other factor when aggravated by concurrent abuse of alcohol, tranquilizers or other drugs.

Both quantitatively and qualitatively, the figures released by the directors of the National Institute of Mental Health in 1980 disclose problems of enormous seriousness. More than 20 percent of Americans suffered from mental illness. The study claims that 23 million suffered from disorders in the anxiety-related category. This is not a reference to the simple and unavoidable "stress" from which we all suffer when in challenging situations. If that were all that is meant in the chart by anxiety, 100 percent of us would be sick in this way. Twenty three million is bad enough! And qualitatively the study is even more alarming. Some years ago, a pioneer mental health researcher, Karen Horney, wrote that "anxiety can be so intense, even when unsupported by reason, that it rivals even intense pain in the suffering it can bring . . . intense anxiety is one of the most tormenting affects we can have. Patients who have gone through an intense fit of anxiety will tell you that they would rather die than have a recurrence of that experience."[1]

Mental illness in the depression-based family, suffered by 17.4 million Americans or 9.5 percent of the population, is a worthy rival of the intense physical pain and the anxiety of which Horney wrote. Many people who have lived through the suicidal obsessions, compulsions, depressions or manic-depressions of such persons before they finally do themselves in will find it incredible that any form of human suffering can "rival" these at their worst. Moreover, feelings of depression are frequently accompanied by rages, incoherent explanations and inconsecutive reasonings. The severely depressed person may have the power to do as he or she chooses, but she seems (to herself) absolutely incapable of controlling her wants and choices themselves. Her will seems, even to her, both perverse and all-powerful. She does not want to want to die; she does not want to choose to die; but in the end her real wants and choices get swept along with her illness. She knows she will lose control in the end; that she will come to *want* all-powerfully to choose death, and of course she will choose it. This impotence in the face of an irresistible avalanche of affect is almost universally a part of the testimony of depressives who have been rescued.

AN ALTERNATIVE APPROACH TO THE RELATIVITY PROBLEMS

Conventionalist positions in value theory define some evaluative term ("good" and "bad") in terms of what some person or group of persons (subjects) believe, what customs they have, or what rules they have adopted. Then it will follow that that thing is good, in their theory, because those persons act or believe as they do. Good things are good, and right acts are right, precisely because of what that person or group of persons thinks about these things or acts in respect to them. All value judgments, according to a subjectivist theory, are elliptical. When we assert that "X is good," our understanding is that we have left unspoken something that we expect to be understood: "X is good" means "X is approved or put in practice by some Ys or is *good for* those Ys or *good according* to those Ys, or good *in that group*."

The general name for positions opposed to subjectivism or conventionalism is "ethical objectivism," or "ethical absolutism." According to this view, no such elliptical qualifications are called for. The rightness of conduct and the goodness of some states of mind are properties of objects themselves, quite independently of the opinions and actions of human beings. In that respect value judgments are like statements of natural laws.

Let us consider for a moment judgments that are clearly as the conventionalist says all value judgments are. The two most prominent classes of such judgments and rules are rules of etiquette and the judgments of good or bad manners that apply them, on the one hand, and legal statutes like traffic and criminal codes, on the other.

This kind of relativity also includes much statute law, as is well understood by international travelers. In some countries it is illegal to have an abortion, or to gamble in a casino, or to drive on the right side of the road; in others, it is not. While we may argue rationally over which customs and laws are wiser, more useful, better or worse than others, we do not say that the better customs of etiquette, simply by virtue of being better customs of etiquette, really apply everywhere. One must specify the group or the country when one states that a practice is good manners or legal, otherwise one's statement is elliptical, waiting to be filled in for full sense. "Good manners," we might ask, "according to whom?" or "relative to which norms?" or "legal in which political jurisdiction?"

The ethical relativist is likely to claim that the same is true of moral rules (or *some* moral rules). If one tribe holds that it is virtuous to go wild with drink periodically or to dispatch one's elderly grandparents, then those things are morally right in that tribe, though they may be wrong elsewhere. The absolutistic view, on the other hand, is that these things are morally wrong everywhere, regardless of local beliefs, though we may moderate or withdraw our blame when it is pointed out to us that a given wrongdoer was merely doing what was widely believed to be morally right in his community.

Philosophers of medicine often begin their works by formulating definitions of health and sickness. Some of these definitions "reduce" statements about health and sickness to statements of an ordinary nonmedical kind. Others will reduce some or all health-sickness statements (diagnostic and therapeutic) to value judgments, arguing along the way for the impossibility of value-free medical statements. Some of these value judgments are moral judgments proper; others are mere "normative" judgments with the more specific type under consideration not spelled out.

Examples of the sorts of judgment that are the subjects of these controversies are those just discussed. Consider the role of health judgments in societies with values of a very different kind from our own. All are devoted to lives of calm, quiet, detached, dispassionate "contemplation." A person who successfully "trains" for life in a society of that unphysical kind might be called, because of this successful adaptation to his social environment, a healthy human specimen. But in a society like our own, which seems dedicated to struggle and labor and the bodily vitality that promotes it, the drooping, languid, unenergetic visitor from Mysticland will be a figure of mockery. It simply evokes derisive laughter in the active athletic world to call the drowsy visitor "a model of good health." Well, maybe we should say that the mystic would be healthy in Mysticland and the athlete in Athleticland, but neither could be considered healthy if he were a permanent resident in a land to which his suffering body could not adapt. The next step is to compromise and say that people are not simply healthy or sick *tout court*. They are healthy relative to the structure and governing laws of their society or relative to the requirement of a job, or relative to their talents, and their preferred activities, and so on.

There are some standard borderline judgments of health or sickness that generate disputes among theorists. Is baldness (in a man) a disease? Is baldness (in a woman) a disease? Is aging a disease? Is menopause? Is extreme ugliness? Is a moderately weak big toe a defect? An injury? For a place kicker on a professional football team? Is an inability to digest cellulose (when 90 percent of the human race, let us suppose, has acquired that ability) a disease? Are the answers to these questions "purely factual" or medical judgments? Which, if any, of them express implicit value judgments? Of those that express value judgments, which express moral judgments (one species of value judgments)? Insofar as the judgments of health and illness are involved somehow with values, to what kind of independent analysis are value statements themselves properly subject? Those writers who reject the possibility of "value-free" judgments of health and sickness have been impressed by examples of this sort. At least some of the times when we make health-sickness judgments, we are making some sort of judgment about comparative *value, service,* to continuing *interest, importance, worthiness.*

NORMATIVISM AND RELATIVISM OF HEALTH JUDGMENTS

Some puzzlement over the concepts of health and sickness is produced by the fact that physicians are sometimes asked to formulate criteria of sickness and health and/or to apply criteria to difficult factual situations. Medical people are not accustomed to being asked such questions. Often the answers they are requested to produce require decision-making rather than discovery. On other occasions, the answer to what appears at first to be a medical question must be answered simply: "that depends on what you mean." If the question then is "what *should* we mean by 'sick'?" the physician complains that he is being asked to reply in his capacity as a medical person to an essentially nonmedical question. The physician then may be tempted to generalize. Questions about the meaning of "health" and "sickness" are essentially and irreducibly normative. Physicians are not accustomed to dealing professionally with normative questions like those asked above.

Normally, say many physicians, we are asked questions that draw on our special expertise, and we answer by doing laboratory tests of blood and urine samples, or by reading gauges or turning dials, or seeking biopsies of tumors. We are not called upon to evaluate mysticism and athleticism as ways of life, or to appraise a given face's degree of ugliness, or to rule on whether baldness can impair a person's proper functioning, or whether a condition such as a fever that indirectly benefits or pleases a person by preventing him from honoring what would otherwise be an obligation can still be called a "sickness." Questions like these, their physician says, are not mere factual questions subject to special medical techniques of investigation. They are value questions over which reasonable persons differ, and answers to which are relative to one's community.

How shall we respond to this argument? Are questions about health and sickness always at bottom questions about values and behavioral norms? If so, is the value judgment they call for itself subject to relativistic (unscientific) analysis, as the normativists[2] claim, or are medical judgments value-free and confirmable, in the manner of ordinary factual statements? It seems clear to me that:

1. It is false that *all* medical judgments are disguised normative statements or "value judgments" beyond the special competence of the physician. When the manager of a football team asks a doctor to examine his star player to determine whether he is healthy or sick, injured, or likely to be injured, he is asking a purely medical "factual" question. He may, in his next breath, ask the doctor for moral advice: "Should I call on the star player to play in this game or would that be too dangerous a risk to him?" That is a moral question about what it would be right to do. Clearly the two questions are intertwined, and the answer to one is even found to be dependent on the answer to the other. But they are not the same question; nor are they the same *kind* of question.

2. It is false that no medical judgments are at bottom normative. The following are basically normative: "Homosexuality is a disease." "Homosexuality is not a disease." "Baldness is a disease." "Abortion is (is not) a properly medical treatment." "Jones's occasionally aching big toe is not a genuine injury or sickness, but the very same symptom in a professional football kicker is an injury or illness."

3. Therefore it is true that some medical judgments are disguised normative judgments, and that some medical judgments are irreducibly and distinctively factual statements: "The tumor in your left breast is malignant" (or "benign") is factual. Of course, "health" and "sickness" are more abstract and more difficult to define than "malignant" and "benign," but apart from that, they are words of similar function. The normativist contention is that all health judgments are value judgments. Put another way, all judgments of health include value judgments as part of their meaning.[3] To call a condition "sick" is to judge it adversely, since adverse evaluation and favorable evaluation are characteristic functions of normative terms. The final move of the normativist, then, is to interpret the normative terms he cannot avoid in the relativist fashion. Vitality really is the essence of health in one society; physical inactivity in another. Homosexuality is a sickness in some societies, a functionally normal genetic variation in others.

In summary, medical normativism, which is meant to apply to all judgments of health and sickness, claims too much. Some such judgments seem to be value-free, factual ones.

But medical factualism also claims too much when it asserts that all health and sickness judgments are value-free. There are contexts, then, though perhaps not many, in which moral and medical judgments are interinvolved, and are so in virtue of their conceptual linkages prior to complications contributed by the confrontation of psychiatry and crime.

RELATIVITY PROBLEMS AND PRESUPPOSED VALUE JUDGMENTS IN MEDICINE

By and large, theorists of medicine have been dissatisfied with analyses of such terms as "healthy" and "sick" that fail to mark off the domain of the medical from other kinds of scientific judgments. It is distinctive of the medical judgments, they insist, that they are not merely statements of fact confirmed or disconfirmed once and for all by simple observations. Rather they are more controversial. Reasonable persons differ about them and search more widely for the types of consideration that are relevant to their testing. Medical judgments, they soon discover, are rarely value-free, but in many cases they are even value-saturated. Often, then, a disagreement over medical judgments is a consequence of the invasion of value considerations into the medical domain. At this some point with pride and others with alarm—those who think of themselves as bringing good news and those who fear that their own news is bad news.

There is no way to interpret and appraise the value-acknowledgers except by looking at the examples commonly used by them of how medical judgments can be said to incorporate value judgments and how that in turn can lead to a kind of vicious relativism that will be said to discredit the premises that generated it. A number of years ago I wrote an article about the incorporation of value in medical judgments. I shall go back to 1967 and try to remember just what I had in mind, before turning to various other examples from other writers. I seem to have begun, as I would still begin, with a functionalist account of illness. Then I proceeded directly to the point:

> there is in fact very little disagreement among us over what constitutes the proper working order of the human *body*. We all would agree that a body with paralyzed limbs is no more in a "good working order" than a car with flat tires; and in general our culture identifies bodily health with vigor and vitality. But we can imagine a society of mystics or ascetics who find vitality a kind of nervous distraction (much as we regard hyperthyroid activity)—a frustrating barrier to contemplation and mystic experience, and a source of material needs that make constant and unreasonable demands for gratification. Such a group might regard bodily vitality as a sickness and certain kinds of vapidity as exemplarily health. Our disagreement with these people would not be a purely medical matter.[4]

This is not a bad argument exactly, but I am no longer terribly impressed by it. A stubborn medical philosopher on the other side will not be silenced so quickly. He can admit that there are two ways of interpreting my old example, one "value-free" and the other value-based (or even "suffused"). But having admitted that much, he wonders now what advantage either interpretation might have the other. The value-free approach would describe the "vapid mystic" as a person in excellent health; the value-based writer could describe that person as "excellent," insightful, creative, magnanimous, but he would hesitate to ascribe "good health" or "healthy mindedness" to him as well. Instead he might point out that the mystic has a constant cough, that he trips and stumbles frequently when he tries to move or change his position, and he groans with headache. Nevertheless, just to be polite, he compliments the ascetic visitor by admiring his "robust and energetic bodily vigor."

A third party listens with astonishment and cannot suppress his spontaneous laughter. In general, people from Mysticland get lots of admiring compliments for their quiet way of life. Healthiness is simple not one of them. Would most of us not say that they are unhealthy and vapid, that they mistreat their bodies and are doomed to early deaths even though they have many virtues distinct from health, both of a moral and an intellectual kind? It is open to us to praise our way of life by calling it excellent, happy, virtuous, fulfilling, holy and good. Or we can be linguistically eccentric and express our general praise for it through the use of one word—"healthy"—at the cost of confusion and surprise.

I borrowed another example from my friend and former student, Stephanie Lewis, who commented in a seminar that if 90 percent of humanity came, through evolution, to be able to digest cellulose and if, further, this capacity became importantly useful (perhaps through critical shortages of other foods), the remaining 10 percent (who are physiologically exactly the same as us, their ancestors) would quite properly be said to be deformed, or sick, or lacking in "basic" human equipment. What is "healthy" then, is relative to our resources, technical capacities and purposes.

Similarly, in my own example of the mystic society, what is healthy is "relative" to the comparative values ascribed to altered states of consciousness, on the one hand, and athletic vigor, on the other. Actually, in the "mystic versus athlete" example, we can say that what is healthy is independent and various, and thus "relative" to neither alternative lifestyle, or we can say that relative to the mystic life, the one group is healthier; whereas relative to the athletic lifestyle, the other mode of living is healthier. Psychiatric writers have long defended a kind of cultural relativism marked by a refusal to make bold ethical judgments. So we should be cautious of using the phrase "relative to" too frequently. In summary of our discussion of the mystic and cellulose examples, which way of life is healthier—the mystic's or the athlete's—depends upon which set of values is the more appealing. So says the value-based theory. I am no longer so sure. We could say (and I see no strong reason against it), that (say) the mystic's life is superior all told, even though the athlete's is healthier, since health is not everything but just one value among many.

The cellulose example is typical of a class of examples that employ the concept of *adaptation* as basic. Health, they say, just is harmonious adaptation to the environment. That conception makes Mrs. Lewis's example possible in a variety of forms. Can I be healthy now, one asks, and change not a bit in, say, the next ten years, and nonetheless, at that time be sick not because I changed, but because the world external to me changed? If health is determined by one's adaptation to the environment, then it can be affected for better or worse in either of two ways—either through the person's body changing or the environment changing. Quite clearly, if all the changes in this example take place external to the person, and all the changes needed to bring back the initial adaptation are changes in the external circumstances (absolutely none of them through surgery, medication or hypnosis on the "sick person" but only via environmental changes (such as the destruction of trees to which many persons are allergic), it would seem odd to say that the person has been "cured." The paradox all writers seek to avoid is that in which a sickness to one party can be cured by treatment of another. If the only cure for an allergy is the destruction of a whole species of tree, we would have the delightful situation in which many human beings could describe how their human sickness was cured by a tree surgeon!

Many of these examples have a common form. In these stories, whether or not some standard of health is correct is said to *depend upon* (or be *relative to*) whether some "value judgment" is true. The "that depends" clause in the next example is not a physical contingency, nor is it the usual sort of value judgment. Rather it is a judgment of physical attractiveness. There are value judgments galore, however, in examples of these kinds. Whether or not one holds baldness to be a genetic disease depends on one's judgment of the importance to a proper human form of a full head of hair. Is a different analysis required for a woman? Should we add "cosmetic" goals to ordinary therapeutic ones? Or do we already? People in this category include those who are plain ugly, by our local cultural standards of attractiveness, of course. Is an ugly man or woman *per se* unable to function properly? Must he or she suffer pain, deformity or functional impairment because of his or her ugliness? Is one answer to that question a *medical* judgment, or a "purely factual judgment"? The closest this question comes to being a purely factual one is when we interpret it as asking a medical authority whether the condition in question amounts to an impairment of a vital human function, for example, walking, lifting, breathing, digesting, talking, remembering, calculating, seeing, hearing, lovemaking and so on. Most of the examples on this list are noncontroversial, but perhaps some would be controversial if we could ask, say, whether baldness impairs one's capacity to walk, to see, to make love, or whether it is a fact that a bald person cannot make love, digest protein or hear sounds. These are not exactly open questions.

CATEGORIZING PSYCHOPATHY

While philosophers have been grappling with such concepts as function and abnormalcy and such distinctions as that between physical and mental, psychiatrists, too, have been wrestling with terminology in the regular revisions of their *Diagnostic and Statistical Manual of Mental Disorders (DSM-IV)*. Their efforts are a good illustration of the intermingling of factual and evaluative judgments. I interpret their classification principles as follows.

The term "disorder" is apparently the most generic category. Disorders can be divided into various subsystems depending on our diagnostic purposes. There are some minor exceptions to this usage, as when the *Manual* speaks of "conditions" as a basic category, and also where a particular term has been placed in certain categories by the law for forensic purposes. The legally assigned basic categories include mental "defect," "illness," "syndrome" and "incapacity." For any biological or psychological function, the human organism may be in "proper working order" (functional language for "healthy") or "out of order" (that is to say, suffering a "disorder"). The disorders can be divided according to a number of principles, but it is clear that the primary divisions are those specifying the range of the organic functions found to be disordered, though etiological distinctions are also used, for example, "substance-related," or disorders first appearing in a particular stage of life such as infancy or old age.

I counted 17 basic categories of disorder described in the most recent edition of the *Manual*. All but a few of these form the basic system of classification, namely in terms of the function that is impaired by the disorder. The disorders classified in this manner are: schizophrenia and other psychotic disorders, other cognitive disorders, mood disorders, anxiety disorder, somatoform disorders, factitious disorders, sexual and gender identity disorders, eating disorders, sleep disorders, impulse-control disorders, adjustment disorders, personality disorders and other conditions.

Each of these judgments does its own distinctive job (function) and each finds as it begins that its job is already partially done by the other. In some cases, the psychiatric task of diagnosis depends on a moralistic judgment about *rights* (a moral concept if ever there was one). For example, the definition of antisocial personality disorder rests partially on judgments about what other people's actual rights really are. This is an interesting contrast with earlier language that evades moral judgments and speaks instead of "behavior that deviates markedly from expectation of the individual's culture." That final passage might very well have been composed by the kind of social scientist who is *embarrassed* to use a moralistic term or to acknowledge that there are such things as moral judgments. The disorder which for many years has been called "psychopathy" has been renamed and classified as one of the "personality disorders." A "personality disorder" is defined in turn as an enduring pattern of inner experience and behavior that deviates markedly from the expectations of the individual's culture, is pervasive and inflexible, has an onset in adolescence or early adulthood, is stable over time and leads to distress or impairment. If the impairment is appropriately severe, the disorder can also be called a mental illness, though my impression is that psychiatrists are more comfortable with the "disorder" vocabulary.

There are ten basic Personality Disorders recognized in the *Manual:* paranoid personality disorder, schizotypal disorder, borderline personality disorder, histrionic personality disorder, narcissistic personality disorder, avoidant personality disorder, dependent personality disorder, obsessive-compulsive personality disorder and personality disorder not otherwise specified. The classification no longer includes psychopathic personality disorder, which has been replaced by antisocial personality disorder and defined as a pattern of disregard for and violation of the rights of others. Once more we encounter a kind of definitional blending of the psychiatric and the moral, the psychiatric disorder being defined in moral terms ("others' rights").

For all the merits these new definitions have, there are various ways in which they can confuse a moral philosopher. The philosopher will find it easy to distinguish "personality disorder" from "character flaw," but he may not understand how he is to interpret a "personality defect." In ordinary language, we usually assess the personalities of our friends not by applying to their dispositions basic moral terms such as honest-dishonest, cruel-kind, generous-mean and so on, but rather such terms as "nice guy," "bore," "lively," "dull," "witty," "dour," "pleasant," "feisty," "sweet." We could then loan those personality-appraised terms that are negative to the psychiatric classifiers. They are clear and familiar. The only trouble is that they are probably not what psychiatric classifiers have in mind.

Their intentions would be better fulfilled, I suspect, if they used the word "personal" where they now use the word "personality." Personal disorder could be understood to be a disorder of one's person—one's whole person, that is, and not just his arm or leg, or his eating or sleeping. A personal disorder involves the person, probably by impairing her capacity to act or have feelings of a desired and appropriate kind in the appropriately matching circumstances.

Some definitions of "personality disorder" listed in the *Manual* employ terms of moral condemnation—flaws of character (formerly called "vices") instead of defects of personality. In ordinary language we would reserve such phrases as "defective personality" for people otherwise decent but obnoxious, unpleasant, humorless, boring and the like. It might be taken as an interesting suggestion that psychiatrists should help people improve their sense of humor and call that "therapy." The descriptions in the *Manual* that seem to be morally condemnatory include "detachment from social relationships," "disregard for and violation of the rights of others," instability in interpersonal relationships, excessive emotionality and attention-seeking, grandiosity, need for admiration, lack of empathy, "hypersensitivity to negative evaluation" and compulsive preoccupation with orderliness, perfectionism and control.

Some of these traits are clearly character flaws, and some of the character flaws are clearly moral faults. Some others are clearly just personality defects—ways of being unpleasant, though without necessarily leading to harm or doing anything immoral. Consider, for example, from among the traits already mentioned, suspiciousness, emotional inexpressiveness, eccentricities of behavior, excessive emotionality, need for admiration, feelings of inadequacy, hypersensitivity to negative evaluation, excessive need to be taken care of, clinging and preoccupation with orderliness, perfectionism and control.

In fact, the defects of feeling and behavior that define the ten basic personality disorders are almost all personality defects as opposed to character flaws; those that are character flaws are almost all nonmoral flaws. A mentally disordered person who is preoccupied with orderliness and who suffers from feelings of inadequacy or an excessive need to be admired can be a "pain in the neck" to those who must frequently be in his company; that makes him a bore, not a brute. Almost all the personality disorders are compatible with honorable behavior, the keeping of promises and repayment of debts, and the abstention from violence. The one big exception among the *DSM-IV* personality disorders is the one called antisocial personality disorder. That is a new name for one class of disordered persons. They used to be called psychopaths, and they continue to be defined in moral terms.

NOTES

[1]Karen Horney. *The Neurotic Personality of Our Time.* New York: W. W. Norton, 1937, 46.

[2]This term is assigned to these writers by Christopher Boorse, "On the Distinction between Disease and Illness," *Philosophy and Public Affairs* 5: 44–68 (1975).

[3]Ibid.

[4]Joel Feinberg, "Crime Clutchability and *Mens Rea*," in *Doing and Deserving*. Princeton, NJ: Princeton University Press, 1970, 245–255.

Mental Disabilities, Equal Opportunity and the ADA

NORMAN DANIELS

Mental and physical disabilities achieve parity in the legal protections afforded them through the Americans with Disabilities Act (ADA), at least on paper if not in practice. No such parity in health care benefits was recognized in President Clinton's Health Security Act or in any of the alternatives, even though members of the Benefits and Ethics Working Groups advising the White House Health Care Task Force urged parity. Instead the plan only promised that "future savings" in the system would be used to establish parity of benefits early in the next millennium (and the check is in the mail). Strong arguments for parity in both contexts derive from a commitment to protecting fair equality of opportunity. In both settings, it is the impairment of opportunity that matters, not whether its etiology lies in mental rather than physical disease or disability (Daniels 1985).

In what follows, I shall explore in more detail whether other key features of the ADA, especially as it is applied to mental disabilities, are adequately explained or justified by a principle assuring fair equality of opportunity. I will argue that the ADA is a reasonably good legislative approximation to what is required to implement such a principle. My interest in the issue is in part theoretical: showing that a general principle can provide a unified view of our commitments in two areas of public policy strengthens support for it. But the issue is also of practical interest, because the rationale for legislation affects its application and interpretation. Specifically, I shall focus on three issues.

The first concerns the strength of our commitment to provide work opportunities to the mentally (and physically) disabled, even where there are significant costs involved in reasonable accommodation. In some cases, employers may be obliged to ignore modest decrements in relevant talents and skills, decrements that would have been grounds for replacing a nondisabled employee. Can this strong commitment to allowing the mentally disabled to work be explained by a commitment to fair equality of opportunity? Or do we need to posit a "right to work" (see Kavka, this volume pp. 174–192)? Is the obligation to assure access to work to people with disabilities a general social obligation or one that specifically falls on employers? Does the scope of the obligation match the distribution of its burdens?

The second issue concerns the relationship between our commitments to provide protection of employment opportunities for the mentally disabled and our commitments to provide them with income support. Does the strong commitment embodied in the ADA to protecting the opportunities to work of those with disabilities imply some special responsibility on their part to work? What is the relationship between entitlements to work opportunities and entitlements to income support for those with disabilities? How should

Editors' note: This essay is a slightly abridged version of Norman Daniels, "Mental Disabilities, Equal Opportunity, and the ADA," pp. 281–297 in *Mental Disorder, Work Disability, and the Law*, ed. Richard J. Bonnie and John Monahan, Chicago: University of Chicago Press (1997), reprinted here with permission. Omitted material is indicated by * * *.

we mesh our commitments to protecting opportunity and to providing income support, given that these commitments may derive from different principles of distributive justice?

The third issue concerns the difficulty of drawing boundaries, especially in many cases of mental disabilities. Talents and skills are "normally" distributed across a population, and ordinarily we think employers are free to make decisions about hiring and promotion based on their judgments about how different employees manifest the relevant talents and skills. But some mental disorders adversely affect talents and skills, for example, interpersonal social skills that might be important in many jobs. If a "normal" person simply has trouble "relating" to others, it is the employer's prerogative to make appropriate hiring and firing decisions. But if difficulty in interacting with others is the result of some mental disorder (e.g., something given an appropriate place in *DSM-IV* or subsequent revisions), then the ADA requires judgments about whether the employee is "disabled" yet "otherwise qualified" and about what reasonable accommodation involves. Similarly, in health care contexts, the diagnostic category can place a deficit in social skills in a special category. Insurers may then be obliged to provide assistance (for instance, treatment for shyness) that would not be available to the "normally" shy person. How similar, however, are these contexts in which third parties are obligated to take special steps on behalf of those with mental disorders? Should the same set of conditions trigger health care and employment protection obligations?

FAIR EQUALITY OF OPPORTUNITY AND DISABILITY RIGHTS

The standard account of disability rights rests, quite plausibly, on a commitment to assuring everyone equality of opportunity. Historically, protection for people with disabilities against workplace and educational discrimination followed and was modeled on equal opportunity legislation aimed at racist and sexist practices at work and in schools. The historical analogy seemed obvious and appropriate. Race and sex were widely used to determine access to jobs and educational opportunities in ways that have no relationship to the "morally relevant" grounds for distributing those goods. Talents and skills, including personality and character traits, are relevant grounds for awarding employment and educational opportunities because they have a reasonable relationship to being able to perform well, that is, effectively or productively. But race and sex have no relationship to being able to perform well at the required educational or employment tasks. . . . Legislation aimed at sex and race discrimination had to sweep away the many rationales and excuses that had been developed to justify discriminatory practices.

Disability legislation was aimed at a similar historical problem and rested on a similar underlying philosophical analysis. Because of discriminatory stereotypes, those with disabilities were kept out of jobs they could perform as well as those who were not disabled. In many cases, the disability was just as "morally irrelevant" to job or educational placement as race or sex, but it was being used to justify exclusion or reduced access. These employment and educational practices were supported by widely held stereotypes that ascribed a broad range of reduced capabilities to those whose disabilities were quite narrow and specific. The parallel to racist and sexist stereotypes is widely recognized.

To some extent, antidiscrimination legislation of all kinds looks backwards. It aims to correct for the historical effects on current practices of past attitudes and practices. It is a legacy of past attitudes that keeps us from being color-, gender- or disability-neutral now. Still, there is some difference between the case of disabilities and that of race and sex. Unlike race, which never has, and sex, which almost never has any real (as opposed to imagined) effects on capabilities to perform a job, mental and physical disabilities have some real effects. We can imagine (if only imagine) a more perfect world in which the legacies of past discrimination are eliminated and in which issues about race and gender bias disappear. But issues about placement of people with disabilities would remain to the extent that there were measurable effects on job- or education-related capabilities.

To that extent, legislation protecting the job rights of those with disabilities also looks forward: it addresses a residual problem we will always face. The legislation says we must make "reasonable accommodation," at some social cost, to provide employment opportunities to people with disabilities who are "otherwise qualified" to perform "the essential tasks" involved in jobs or educational slots. We cannot be disability-neutral but must instead wear corrective lenses that keep us from perceiving those social costs as an excuse to ignore or perpetuate barriers against people with disabilities. Of course, once we have invested in making the workplace more accessible to people with disabilities, the incremental cost of employing them will be reduced, at least for many disabilities.

The ADA forces us to accept the costs of reasonable accommodation. Focusing on this point and these costs should not mislead us into thinking that all accommodation is costly—some is not at all (Blanck, this volume, pp. 209–220). Furthermore, except in many rigidly defined assembly-line or service jobs, employers generally make some accommodation to the needs and preferences of workers, and they do not generally look at these adjustments as costs. Nor should it mislead us into ignoring some important benefits, such as the benefits to others that come from increasing diversity in the workplace. * * *

The burden of "reasonable accommodation" may lead some people to think that disability rights in the ADA take us beyond the scope of a principle assuring equality of opportunity. Reasonable accommodation asks us—actually, it *requires* employers, who pass these costs along to consumers—to ignore some inequalities in capabilities, including some effects on talents and skills, even though ignoring them actually affects productivity or otherwise increases costs. The cost increases may result from modifications in the workplace, in job structures, or from most (acceptable) decrements in performance. Truly neutral consideration of abilities would require no such reasonable accommodation for the effects of disabilities. If equality of opportunity simply required us to consider only relevant characteristics, then it might seem not to carry us as far as the ADA and earlier legislation do toward reasonable accommodation.

A suitable appeal to a plausible interpretation of equality of opportunity can, however, justify the reasonable accommodation requirement. Consider first, the "reasonable accommodation" we must make in the case of race and sex. If sexist or racist practices have distorted the development of the talents and skills of women or minorities, then some accommodation must be made. We would not be protecting equality of opportunity if we simply ignored the impact of unfair social practices and formally made point-by-point comparison of existing talents and skills. We are obliged to commit social resources to rectifying the distortions caused by these practices; we are obliged to seek fair and not merely formal equality of opportunity (Rawls 1971). Suddenly becoming color- or gender-neutral without considering the varied effects of unjust practices on real opportunity is insufficient. The costs we must bear do not only take the form of compensatory training programs aimed at restoring talents and skills to the levels that would have existed in a nonsexist, nonracist environment. We must also ignore the costs that derive from altering expectations of employers and coworkers, as well as clients and customers. Simply calculating whether a female or minority employee is as productive "at the margin" as a competing white male hides existing biases behind the formally "neutral" calculation.

Many of the incremental costs of adding disabled workers to a workplace that is acclimatized to bias against the handicapped are strictly analogous to the costs of rectifying sex and race bias in the workplace. This is more obvious in the case of physical than mental disabilities. Modifying a workplace to make it accessible to a physically handicapped worker is much more costly than building an accessible workplace from the start. Counting the costs of modification as part of the "inefficiency" of hiring the handicapped understates what protecting equality of opportunity requires. So, too, altering job descriptions so that they reflect essential functions, or reassigning tasks so that job structures are more accessible to people with disabilities—modifications that may be necessary for the mentally disabled—may involve transition costs that should not count as true inefficiencies. We calculate the costs of protecting equality of opportunity not simply from the perspective of present structures and present costs, but from the perspective of what a fairer work context would have involved, had we been concerned with equal opportunity from the start.

There may be a significant residue of cases, especially when we consider the effects of mental disabilities, where the costs of making reasonable accommodation cannot simply be accounted for by appeal to what a fair "baseline" would have involved, had the workplace adequately assured equality of opportunity from the start. A person with mental disabilities may require modest concessions on the job—more frequent breaks, release time for counseling, or shifting job responsibilities—that involve extra costs even from the perspective of a workplace that already was structured to protect equality of opportunity. Hiring or retaining the mentally disabled worker under these conditions—as opposed to hiring or retaining the slightly more efficient nonhandicapped worker—might be a reasonable accommodation, but it would seem to involve "more than equal" opportunity. Or can this case, regardless of whether it is hypothetical or rare, be accommodated within concern about equality of opportunity?

To see why I believe it can be accounted for, we should back away from workplace contexts for a moment and think about how a commitment to equality of opportunity operates in the context of health care (Daniels 1985, 1988). Disease and disability both impair the range of opportunities open to individuals. To characterize the scope of this impairment, consider the array of plans for their lives that reasonable people in a given society might choose, given their talents and skills. This broad array of opportunities is the "normal opportunity range" for a given society. A given individual with a particular set of talents and skills occupies a subspace of the normal opportunity range. Each person has a fair share of the normal opportunity range, determined by her talents and skills. When people are diseased or disabled, their opportunities shrink to occupy only a part of this fair share. A commitment to equality of opportunity, however, is a commitment to keeping people functioning as closely as possible to normal, so that their shares of the normal range are as close to their fair share as possible given reasonable resource constraints. Health care systems and institutions should be designed with that goal in mind. The principle of distributive justice governing their design should be the principle of fair equality of opportunity, construed in this way as a principle protecting the range of opportunities open to people.

A commitment to equality of opportunity leads us to accept somewhat greater costs to protect the range of opportunities of those who are most impaired as compared to those who already enjoy more of their fair shares of opportunity. Though we are not committed to pouring all of our resources into the most impaired cases—we do not "maximin"—we also do not simply calculate the most efficient allocation of medical resources (Daniels 1993). We give some but not full priority to treating sicker or more disabled patients—or that is what a commitment to protecting equality of opportunity seems to require. (It does not tell us, however, just how much priority to give; see Daniels 1993.) The loss of efficiency here—we do not allocate resources so that they maximize medical benefits at the margin—is a reasonable accommodation to the demand of equality of opportunity. We go an extra distance to bring those whose opportunities are most impaired or threatened as close to normal functioning as we can. Of course, health care settings are not competitive in the same way job competition is, even where we must make resource-allocation decisions among different categories of patients competing for scarce medical services or dollars. Still, it is instructive to see that a commitment to equality of opportunity in the health care setting has an analogue to reasonable accommodation in the employment setting.

The interpretation of equality of opportunity appropriate to health care contexts has the goal of keeping people functioning as normally as possible (Daniels 1985, 1988; Rawls 1993). This conception . . . has some bearing on how we should think about the residual problem of reasonable accommodation for people with disabilities in workplace settings. Keeping people with disabilities functioning as close to normally as possible in the workplace setting may require that we take modest extra steps to open employment doors. We go beyond strict or formal comparison of the mentally handicapped to equally capable nonhandicapped workers, even if doing so involves a trade-off between protecting their opportunities and efficiency that is somewhat steeper than the one we must otherwise make. (The argument here suggests there should also be special vocational rehabilitation or other services to fill in the gap between the limits of health care and reasonable accommodation on the job. I shall not discuss this issue here.)

I believe there is no deep compromise with principle in making this extra concession. One way to think about it is that we make up in the employment sphere for what we cannot quite accomplish in the health care sector. To see this point, we need to think about how concerns about equality of opportunity fit together with other concerns about distributive justice. The account I have sketched of equal opportunity (Rawls 1971; Daniels 1985) accepts the existing distribution of talents and skills, corrected for unjust social practices, as an inevitable source of inequality. Economic redistribution should (following Rawls) aim at making those whose life prospects are worst end up as well-off as possible. But this only mimics the effects of the distribution of talents and skills on equality; it does not eliminate them. (Others argue that the demands of equality or equality of opportunity require more forceful or direct efforts to equalize capabilities and eliminate the disadvantage that would otherwise come from the natural distribution of talents and skills; see Sen 1990, 1992; Cohen 1989.)

Accepting the existing distribution of talents and skills and its effects, combined with appropriate redistribution, thus puts that distribution of talents and skills to work in a way that tends to maximize the benefit of those worst off in marketable talents and skills. There is nothing sacred, however, about the existing distribution of talents and skills. The modest compromise with efficiency involved in reasonable accommodation thus is equivalent to slightly redistributing the talents and skills, or altering their market value, albeit at some cost. We put those with disabilities closer to where they would have been had they had no disability. Since we cannot make this correction in the sphere of health care, we do the next best thing in employment. Of course, this is only rough justice, but it recognizes the special importance of work opportunities in our lives.

Although I have argued that we can explain the reasonable-accommodation requirement by appealing to an appropriate account of equal opportunity, some may think we should look elsewhere for such a justification. I want briefly to consider one alternative, Kavka's (this volume, pp. 174–192) valuable discussion of a "strong right to work," which he claims gives an account of the employment rights of people with disabilities. Kavka argues that people with disabilities have a right to work with these five features:

1. They (but not other workers) have a right to employment rather than just an income stream (call this the special right).
2. They have a right to nondiscrimination.
3. They have a right to compensatory training and education.
4. They have a right to reasonable accommodation, where that involves some societal investment to make the workplace more disability-friendly.
5. They have a right to tiebreaking uses of preferential treatment in placement practices.

Taken by itself, the special right of those with disabilities (but not others) to employment, as opposed to an income stream, is at once too strong and too weak. It is too weak because, by itself, it would assure access of people with disabilities only to some job or other, perhaps a quite minimal job commensurate with the abilities of the handicapped worker. To make the right to work resemble the much more robust requirements of the ADA, features 2 to 4, and possibly 5, must be added to the special right. But these additional features of the right to work do not depend on the special right. They cannot be derived from it, nor can they be derived from the appeal Kavka makes to the importance of self-respect in trying to establish the special right. Some of the additional features, including reasonable accommodation, can, however, be given plausible foundations by appealing to a developed account of fair equality of opportunity, or so I have argued.

The special right Kavka claims for those with disabilities is also too strong. By this I mean two things. First, it goes beyond the scope of the disability rights we recognize in the ADA. The ADA carries no implication that it is more important to provide work to people with disabilities than it is to people without disabilities; its primary concern is to level the playing field. (Of course, this does not show that Kavka is wrong and the ADA right. It only shows how what he argues for is much stronger than what is needed to justify features of the ADA.) Second, and more important, Kavka's special right goes beyond the employment rights we ought to claim for the handicapped and can reasonably justify. To see this, consider Kavka's central argument.

Kavka's argument for this strong right to work, especially the special right, turns crucially on the relationship between working and self-respect. Kavka argues, correctly I believe, that working has a fundamental impact on self-esteem, especially in cultures like ours that attach so many other awards to work. Following Rawls (1971), he views the social bases of self-respect as a primary or basic good, and argues that contractors (whether Rawlsian, acting from behind a veil of ignorance, or Hobbesian, acting without a veil) would insist on securing that good for themselves through the design of social institutions. Taken so generally, the argument might provide some basis for explaining the importance of keeping people at work, including those with disabilities, rather than simply providing them with income streams. It supplements, in other words, the argument I offered earlier for accepting the costs of reasonable accommodation.

But Kavka argues more specifically that work is more important to the self-respect of people with disabilities than it is to people without them. It is more important, he speculates, because those with disabilities have fewer other ways to sustain self-esteem. Consequently, he argues, as social contractors we would give priority to putting our disabled future or possible selves to work over our nondisabled future selves. Here I believe Kavka draws on speculative psychological claims that cannot support his conclusion. Is self-respect sustained better when preferential treatment in access to jobs is our policy than when equal opportunity is assured? This very matter is the focus of sociological debate in the context of affirmative action programs regarding race and sex. Critics of preferential treatment argue that it undermines self-respect because it raises doubts about the ability of those who obtain jobs or educational opportunities.

The more secure inference from this argument about self-respect is that keeping people with disabilities at work is just as important as providing work to others. Consequently, equal opportunity requires reasonable accommodation. Abandoning Kavka's special right to work thus still leaves us with a strong defense of the features of disability rights provided by the ADA.

One qualification is needed to the argument so far. The obligation to guarantee equality of opportunity is a social obligation, and translating this social obligation into obligations that fall on different individuals or groups is complex. In the health care context, this implies an obligation to assure access to appropriate health care regardless of ability to pay, and the fairest way to distribute the burden of that obligation would be through progressive tax-based financing. In employment and education settings, the social obligation imposes a duty on employers and educational institutions not to discriminate against people with disabilities. The ADA also, however, imposes a duty to provide "reasonable accommodation," which implies that some costs will be borne by employers. Assuming these costs are passed on to consumers, there is a dispersion of the burden; if all employers bear some burdens, we may suppose the dispersion of the burdens to consumers will be widespread, though it is less likely to be as progressive as it would be if it were subsidized by taxes. A subsidy to employers who make more expensive accommodations to the handicapped would be a way to create further incentives to keep the mentally disabled at work, but the administrative burden of such a program, plus its visibility in public budgets, may constitute reasons why the strategy was not adopted when the ADA was passed.

INCOME SUPPORT AND DISABILITY RIGHTS

What relationships hold between our obligations to support those who cannot work by providing them with income support and our obligations to assure people with disabilities access to work? When there are significant barriers to work for the disabled because of discrimination or because reasonable accommodation is lacking, then there is clearly more need for income support for those with disabilities. Presumably, if more people with disabilities work, then there is less need for income support. Very generous income support for those who do not work would also have some negative impact on the willingness of people with disabilities to work, especially those whose prospects are for lower wages.

These interactions between support for disability rights and income support are not particularly interesting, however important they are from the point of view of institutional design. Two quite different moral principles underlie our commitment to disability rights and income support. Whereas disability rights rest on a commitment to a principle protecting fair equality of opportunity, or so I have argued, income-support policies rest on other principles of distributive justice. Minimally, they can be thought of as social insurance protecting us against short-term disruptions of income (for example, for temporary disabilities or other short-term unemployment). But they also reflect a concern to constrain the lifetime inequalities in income and wealth that can emerge in a society because some people are unable to work for protracted periods. Equal opportunity and income-support principles are not completely independent: lack of income support undermines equal opportunity, and lack of equal opportunity leads to unfair income inequalities.

Clearly, we need both principles at work and institutions to embody them. We cannot say that because we are protecting equal opportunity, we need not provide income support, or vice versa. * * *

Some people believe that a more interesting relationship between disability rights and income support surfaces when we meet our social obligations to improve work prospects for those with disabilities. They ask: Don't the disabled have a responsibility to work now that discriminatory barriers are lowered? Can we reduce access to income support or make it contingent on serious efforts to secure work? We should be leery of the presuppositions behind these questions. The fact that we failed in the past to provide equal opportunity for people with disabilities did not make our obligation to provide income support greater: it only made the *need* for it greater. Similarly, providing generous income support does not relieve us of the obligation to protect equality of opportunity, though it may lower the demand of those with disabilities (or malingerers) to work. So too, protecting the work rights of people with disabilities does not make our obligation to provide income support less, though it may reduce the need for it. Similarly, I do not think people with disabilities "owe" us something more, in the form of a greater responsibility to work, simply because we now aim to protect opportunity in ways that we always should have. Their responsibility to work is neither greater nor less than the responsibility of anyone else.

The serious danger in thinking that the responsibility of people with disabilities to work increases as society meets its responsibility to protect opportunity is that we will overestimate the success of our efforts to protect opportunity. If we overestimate the improvement in access to work, we will underestimate the need for income support. In our eagerness to cut back on income support, we will then hold people with disabilities responsible for failing to meet their obligation to work. This is blaming the victim. We must avoid it. At the same time we cannot ignore whatever real work disincentives are created by income support and whatever real abuse occurs because of malingering and fraud. * * *

MENTAL DISABILITIES AND BOUNDARY ISSUES

I want to consider two objections to my claim that a principle providing for fair equality of opportunity gives a unified account of rights to health care and disability rights. The first objection is that the conditions that trigger treatment and employment protection differ significantly. How can they then be encompassed by the same principle? The second objection is that by treating disease and protecting people with disabilities, we in fact draw arbitrary distinctions that ignore other ways in which equal opportunity is ignored in health care and employment contexts. I conclude with a comment on the difficulty of establishing parity in the protections afforded to mental and physical disabilities.

Although I have appealed to a fair-equality-of-opportunity principle in both health care and work disability contexts, eligibility for treatment or protection is triggered by different criteria in these domains. A departure from normal functioning that makes someone eligible for medical treatment may not count as a disability for purposes of the ADA. Many illnesses have an impact on normal functioning, and thus on the range of opportunities open to an individual, without, for example, impairing a "major life function." . . . Many treatable mental illnesses or disorders will not constitute ADA-protected disabilities because of their limited effect on functioning, especially in the workplace. Similarly, a condition might trigger disability rights but not access to medical treatment, for example, because no effective medical treatment is available for it. * * *

These differences in the eligibility requirements for medical treatment and ADA protection do not undercut the claim that both share the same general function of protecting equality of opportunity. Rather, the difference reflects differences in the means and context in which this function can be carried out in health care and employment settings. Once we think about it, identical eligibility requirements or triggers for treatment and employment entitlements would be totally inappropriate given these differences.

The issue of perceived disabilities aside, we might suppose that a more fully developed medical technology would eliminate the need for many of the protections afforded by the ADA. Suppose we could cure all mental illness, restore normal functioning to quadriplegics, grow new limbs for amputees, or replace enzymes that enhanced the intelligence of the mildly retarded. In this fantasy, much of what we consider disability would be eliminated, and we could narrow the scope of the ADA dramatically. This suggests that much of what we do through the ADA for mental and physical disabilities corrects for what we cannot do through health care. Where we cannot cure, we must compensate for loss of functioning and keep people functioning as close to the levels they would enjoy if we could do more medically. Though there is some divergence between the conditions that trigger medical entitlements and those that trigger employment protections, both sets of protections serve the same general purpose: keeping functioning as close to normal as they can. Employment protections are invoked where our limited capabilities mean we could not eliminate the need for them through health care interventions.

The second objection is that certain "hard cases," or boundary problems, confound the appeal to equal opportunity in employment contexts. These hard cases can arise for both physical and mental disabilities, but the latter seem particularly difficult to resolve. Consider first a hard case involving a physical disability: a disabled worker with reduced motor capability may be somewhat slower than a nondisabled worker at certain tasks. In the absence of the disability, the employer might have preferred to replace a worker who was so slow at those tasks. Nevertheless, reasonable accommodation might require retaining the disabled worker. In effect, the protection keeps the disabled worker in place at some cost in order to keep her functioning in life as close as possible to the level she would have enjoyed had she not been disabled. Here the protection is compensatory. We do not accommodate the "normal" worker who is just plain slow.

More complex cases arise for mental disabilities. A "normal" but irascible worker, or a very shy, withdrawn or lethargic but otherwise "normal" worker, might be replaced by an employer for lack of social skills in certain jobs. If equally irascible, shy or lethargic workers have mental diseases or disorders that qualify them as "mentally disabled," however, their employers may have to provide them with "reasonable accommodation." Is there some inequity here? Why should a compromise of performance be excused and compensated for in one case and not the other?

This problem may seem particularly hard at the extremes. Suppose two workers are seriously lacking in certain social skills. One has a mental disorder that triggers ADA eligibility—his shyness (or irascibility) is the result of a bipolar condition, for example. The other, however, is just as shy (or irascible), but we find no mental disease or disorder. He is just at the extreme of the normal distribution for shyness (or irascibility). Since the lack of skill is seriously disadvantaging in exactly the same way, then it seems troublesome that one is protected but the other not.

The very same problem arises in health care contexts. If a bipolar patient was extremely shy, we might provide insurance coverage for group therapy to address the shyness, even though we might not provide such coverage for an otherwise normal but equally shy person. The rationale would be that we were treating an effect of the disease. Similarly, very short children with diagnosable growth hormone deficiency are eligible for reimbursement for growth hormone treatment; this counts as "treatment." But shortness that results from just being at the extreme end of the normal distribution for height would not be reimbursable; this counts as mere "enhancement." In these cases, we are particularly troubled because the suffering or disadvantage in each case is similar for those eligible for treatment and those not. It seems arbitrary to treat in one way those people who have a biologically based condition we call "disease" and in another way those whose biologically based condition is "normal" even though they suffer or are disadvantaged identically. Despite the challenge of such hard cases, the treatment/enhancement distinction should play a role in deciding what obligations we have to provide medical services, and I think an analogous distinction can be defended in the case of employment rights for people with disabilities. To show that this distinction is not arbitrary from the point of view of justice, despite the hard cases, I shall argue that it fits better than alternatives with the approach I have taken toward fair equality of opportunity. This approach (call it the *standard model*) helps to specify a reasonable limit on the central task of health care, and its analogue does the same for disability rights.

I have argued that health care services aim to restore people to the range of capabilities they would have had without disease or disability, given their allotment of talents and skills. The *standard model* for thinking about equality of opportunity thus takes as a given the fact that talents and skills and other capabilities are not distributed equally among people. Some people are better at some things than others. Accordingly, we assure people *fair* equality of opportunity if we judge them by their capabilities while ignoring "morally irrelevant" traits like sex or race when we place people in schools, jobs, and offices. Often, however, we must correct for cases in which capabilities have been misdeveloped through racist, sexist or other discriminatory practices. Similarly, by preventing or treating disease and disability, we can correct for impairment of the capabilities people would otherwise have. Reasonable accommodation for people with disabilities further corrects for the impairment of capabilities that we cannot correct through medical treatment. The standard model does not call for us to eliminate all differences in capabilities through medical enhancement, but only those that result from disease and disability (Daniels 1990; Sabin and Daniels 1994, Daniels 1996). Similarly, it does not call for "reasonable accommodation" of all differences in capabilities among unequally skilled workers; we provide reasonable accommodation only for the decrements that can be attributed to the disability for "otherwise qualified" workers.

This limitation of the standard model can appear arbitrary. Our capabilities are themselves the result of a natural and social lottery, and we do not "deserve" them; we are just fortunate or unfortunate in having them. We can mitigate this underlying arbitrariness *somewhat* as follows. Those who are better endowed with marketable capabilities are likely to enjoy more goods such as income, wealth and power. If we constrain inequalities in these goods so that those who are worst-off do as well as possible, considering alternatives, then social cooperation will work to the benefit of all (Rawls 1971). Still, this constraint does not eliminate all inequalities in the capabilities people have and thus in the opportunities they enjoy, especially since we are enjoined to judge people in light of their capabilities. If our egalitarian concerns require that we strive to give people equal capabilities wherever technologically feasible, then we should not settle for mitigating the effects of relying on equality of opportunity as standardly understood (Sen 1990, 1992; Cohen

1989). Rejecting the standard model pushes us toward leveling all differences in capabilities; from that perspective, the distinction between treatment and enhancement has no point.

From the perspective of the standard model of fair equality of opportunity, however, it is reasonable to limit the task of medical services to restoring people to normal functioning and thus to the range of opportunities they would have had absent disease or disability. In the standard model, the treatment/enhancement distinction retains its point. For purposes of justice, it is enough that the line between disease or disability and its absence is *uncontroversial* and *ascertainable through publicly acceptable methods,* such as those of the biomedical sciences, for the general run of cases. Being able to draw a line in this way allows us to refer counterfactually in a relatively clear and objective way to the range of opportunities a person would have had in the absence of disease and disability; it facilitates public agreement. * * * Abandoning the treatment/enhancement distinction would push us toward a much more radical form of egalitarianism. * * * It begins a cascade of changes in the scope of medicine that would forever change its face and might threaten the social consensus that gives medicine the strong moral grip it has on us and our resources.

It might be thought that we do not need to adopt such an extreme position if we abandon the notion of disease or disability. If extreme shortness or shyness could be considered a handicapping condition, then we might still be able to appeal to the standard model of equality of opportunity (Allen and Fost 1990). Growth hormone therapy would simply move people into the range of capabilities they would have had were they not handicapped. This compromise approach does not seek full equality in capabilities, only the end of handicapping disadvantages.

There are serious objections to dropping the reference to disease or disability in drawing this version of the treatment/enhancement distinction. First, we need a clear notion of "handicap." Specifying the shortest 1 percent as handicapped will itself seem arbitrary after the first cycle of therapies creates a new group of shortest people. Not treating the newest group would then seem arbitrary in light of a new set of hard cases. Second, it will now be medicine's task to eliminate all comparable handicapping conditions. In our racist society, this means black, brown or red skin. Should we eliminate melanin or oppose discrimination? Although the compromise approach does not seek quality of capabilities, it vastly expands the function of medicine and, by medicalizing social problems, it risks losing whatever consensus exists on the moral importance of meeting health care needs.

The problem raised for the treatment/enhancement distinction by our hard cases is similar to the kind of problem all rules face when their justification derives from the fact that general conformity to them is on the whole either better or fairer. We can almost always describe hard cases in which the very reasons that lead us to adopt a rule to cover the general case also lead us to think the rule is nonoptimal or unfair when applied to them. Though troubling, hard cases do not always count as counterexamples that force us to reject the rule. Sometimes we must swallow the discrepancy between the particular case and the general run of things if we want a generally better or fairer distributive scheme.

Employment rights as specified in the ADA similarly rest on an appeal to the standard model of equal opportunity. Reasonable accommodation is given only for those with disabilities, not for those whose capabilities—whose talents and skills—put them at a market disadvantage. Hard cases in employment contexts retain a residual arbitrariness, just as they do in medical contexts, but the alternative is a radical egalitarianism aimed at leveling all differences in capabilities, with radical consequences for productivity. The leveling approach is no more plausible or feasible in employment than in medical contexts.

I shall conclude by returning to my starting point, the issue of parity—on paper, in law—between the treatment of mental and physical disabilities. Mental disabilities pose more difficult problems than physical ones. They force us to steer a narrow course between the Scylla of "otherwise qualified" and the Charybdis of "disabled." To show that a mental disorder constitutes a disability, we must show that it impairs a major life function. For many mental disorders, the impact on social skills has its primary effect on work. It is not possible to point to its effects on mobility, hearing or seeing, the major life functions affected by physical disabilities. But showing that the disability has an impact on work makes it more difficult to show that someone with mental disabilities is "otherwise qualified" to work. Distinguishing essential and nonessential tasks may be harder when the job requires some level of social skills or some degree of "reliability."

For similar reasons, what constitutes reasonable accommodation may be more difficult to determine for mental than physical disabilities. Reasonable accommodation may require, for example, more extensive restructuring of job requirements or provision of breaks and other supports than for many physical disabilities. Here social prejudice against mental disabilities—strong biases and degrading stereotypes—is particularly difficult to guard against. It is much easier to moralize about mental disability than physical disability—easier to blame the victim. It is easier, for example, to imagine that if someone were more cooperative or tried harder, his performance would improve, and he would need less accommodation. These features of mental disabilities and the strength of social prejudice concerning them give us strong reason to demand objective assessment of performance, essential tasks and costs of accommodation. The point of the comparison is the suggestion that real parity between mental and physical disabilities exists only on paper, despite the best intentions behind the ADA. The fair equality of opportunity account nevertheless provides a basis for diligent insistence on reasonable accommodation and the attempt to achieve real parity.

REFERENCES

Allen, David B., and Norman C. Fost. "Growth Hormone Therapy for Short Stature: Panacea or Pandora's Box?" *Journal of Pediatrics* 117 (1990): 16–21.

Cohen, G. A. "On the Currency of Egalitarian Justice." *Ethics* 99 (1989): 906–944.

Daniels, Norman. *Just Health Care.* New York: Cambridge University Press, 1985.

Daniels, Norman. *Am I My Parents' Keeper? An Essay On Justice between the Young and the Old.* New York: Oxford, 1988.

Daniels, Norman. "Equality of What: Welfare, Resources, or Capabilities?" *Philosophy and Phenomenological Research* 50 (Supp.) (1990): 273–296.

Daniels, Norman. "Rationing Fairly: Programmatic Considerations." *Bioethics* 7(2,3) (1993): 224–233.

Daniels, Norman. *Justice and Justification: Reflective Equilibrium in Theory and Practice.* New York: Cambridge University Press, 1996.

Kavka, Gregory S. "Disability and the Right to Work," this volume, pp. 174–192.

Rawls, John. *A Theory of Justice.* Cambridge, MA: Harvard University Press, 1971.

Rawls, John. *Political Liberalism.* New York: Columbia University Press, 1993.

Sabin, James, and Norman Daniels. "Determining 'Medical Necessity' in Mental Health Practice: A Study of Clinical Reasoning and a Proposal for Insurance Policy." Hasting Center Report 24(6) (1994): 5–13.

Sen, Amartya. "Justice: Means vs. Freedoms." *Philosophy and Public Affairs* 19 (1990): 111–121.

Sen, Amartya. *Inequality Reexamined.* Cambridge, MA: Harvard University Press, 1992.

Congress and the Courts

Disputing the Doctrine of Benign Neglect
A Challenge to the Disparate Treatment
of Americans with Disabilities

HARLAN HAHN

One of the major obstacles to the effort to gain equal rights for Americans with disabilities has been the failure of judges and legal commentators to apply a consistent understanding to cases of discrimination occasioned by disability and by other human characteristics such as gender and race or ethnicity. While the courts have long recognized the harmful effects of the separation of white and African-American children in public schools, for example, the prevalent influence of the medical model—and of assumptions concerning biological inferiority—has prevented them from adopting a similar approach to disparities between disabled and nondisabled citizens. The impact of paternalism and the concept of benign neglect has not only spawned inconsistent constitutional interpretations but has also deprived disabled people of the benefits that might otherwise be expected to flow from the minority-group paradigm for the study of disability. This essay, therefore, seeks to explore improvements in judicial decisions that could result from increased acceptance of the view that citizens with disabilities comprise a minority group comparable to other disadvantaged segments of the population.

RACIAL AND DISABILITY DISCRIMINATION

In 1954, a unanimous Supreme Court outlawed racial segregation in public schools.[1] This historic ruling was founded on a declaration that was compelling in its simplicity and straightforwardness: "Separate educational facilities are inherently unequal."[2] Significantly, the justices did not make exceptions to the doctrine. They did not cite any physical attribute that would make it constitutionally permissible to require that a youngster be separated from the mainstream of children in order to receive an education. Nor did they insert qualifications that designate certain types of inequality as being tolerable in the schools.

Moreover, the *Brown* decision relied on social science research that demonstrated the psychological damage imposed on African-American children as a result of attitudes reflected by the segregation of education.[3] Not only were they damaged in respect to identity and self-esteem, but their separation from the mainstream of American children induced the latter to view them with suspicion and contempt. Ample evidence from comparable studies shows that isolation based on disability exposes disabled children to analogous antipathy.[4] Yet from the date of *Brown,* seventeen years would elapse before the courts finally ruled that young people with disabilities must be afforded at least some access to the schools,[5] and another four more years went by before the initial implementation of this policy would occur.[6] The lag in time between the initiation of desegregated education for African-American children and the guarantee that disabled children would have any access

269

to education at all is especially remarkable because most Americans take as an article of faith that there is no animus against people in virtue of their being disabled. In fact, at the time, the prospect of placing Americans of different colors in close proximity to each other aroused much more heated controversy and much more obstinate opposition than proposals for inclusiveness for Americans with disabilities. That the overtly expressed antagonism toward people with disabilities does not usually rise to the level suffered by people of color has helped to obscure the similarities between racial and disability discrimination.

THE INFLUENCE OF THE MEDICAL MODEL

Perhaps the principal difference between racial and disability discrimination, and the conception that must be altered to facilitate the elimination of discrimination, is the idea that disability is largely a medical condition. Most nondisabled people regard disability primarily as a physiological deficit rooted in the living organism—that is, in the organic individual—that interferes with ordinary human functioning. Medicalizing disability may result from confusing the notion of impairment, which refers to limitations attributable solely to deficits of body or mind, with the notion of disability, which refers to restrictions imposed on the individual by an environment that places the individual at a social or economic disadvantage.

The domination of the medical model in analyzing disability has impeded the ambition of disabled people to achieve what appears to be a basic prerequisite for their recognition as citizens entitled to equal rights, namely, putting to rest the mistaken belief that their disadvantage results from biological inferiority. During the nineteenth century, most Americans believed that women and racial minorities were biologically inferior to nondisabled white males. The struggle of members of both groups to gain equal standing in the courts required enormous efforts both of scholarship, in order to refute the charges of their biological failings, and of political organization, in order to embed the findings of this research in the culture.

The difficulty of achieving a comparable advance today is magnified because equating disability with impairment, and defining disability by reference to the functional limitations impairment occasions, obscures a crucial component of discrimination: the stigmatization of disability and the negative attitudes directed at people so stigmatized. Many impairments have visible attributes that are disconcerting to those who observe them. So-called "hidden" impairments—for instance, learning disabilities or bipolar disorder—are designated in a way that attracts unfavorable attention to those so labeled. Visible and labeled differences that are imagined to be deficits have a decisive and usually detrimental effect on how disabled people, including disabled children, are judged. Yet the courts have been reluctant to recognize and rely upon the vast literature concerning prejudicial attitudes aroused by signs that a person has a disability and to respect first-person testimony as to the harm of stigma. As a leading commentator on the concept of stigma observed: "By definition, of course, we believe the person with a stigma is not quite human."[7]

PATERNALISM AND CONSTITUTIONAL INTERPRETATION

The tendency to accept the assumption that people with disabilities are biologically inferior and therefore to neglect the negative impact of stigmatizing attitudes has resulted in a climate permeated with paternalism. The belief that nondisabled persons do not harbor feelings of hostility or animus toward people with disabilities has contributed to the formation of a relatively weak constitutional standard for assessing discrimination against disabled citizens. From a paternalistic perspective which regards public attitudes about disability as favorable rather than unfavorable, the inequality that results from factors such as architectural barriers and employment discrimination is frequently ascribed to happenstance or coincidence rather than intentional conduct. This doctrine has been invoked to hold that a disparate impact, instead of overt bigotry, is an appropriate basis for determining discrimination on the basis of disability. In *Alexander v. Choate* (1985), Justice Thurgood Marshall, delivering the opinion of the Supreme Court, found that discrimination against the handicapped was perceived by Congress to be most often the product not of invidious animus but rather of thoughtlessness and indifference—of benign neglect.[8] Yet the assumption that the interests of disabled people are actually served by inattention to the issue of discrimination has seemed to undermine judicial decisions about this subject. In the same year, in the case of *Cleburne v. Cleburne Living Center,*[9] arguably one of the most important Supreme Court decisions regarding the constitutional status of people with mental retardation, Justice Byron White addressed the question of whether the class of people with this diagnosis should be regarded as a constitutionally protected suspect class. White's discussion is indicative in its confusion. It shows how problematically the courts think about citizens with disabilities.

First, White acknowledges that, like traditional protected classes, mentally retarded citizens have been subjected to a long history of discrimination and oppression. Second, he admits that they do not themselves constitute a political group powerful enough to alter their status through the political process. Given these premises, the Court's conclusion seems to be nothing other than a *non sequitur*. White concludes, for the majority, that: "the distinctive legislative response, both national and state, to the plight of those who are mentally retarded demonstrates not only that they have unique problems, but also that the lawmakers have been addressing their difficulties in a manner that belies a continuing antipathy or prejudice . . . the legislative response . . . negates any claim that the mentally retarded are politically powerless in the sense that they have no ability to attract the attention of the lawmakers."[10] Thus the Court's 1985 doctrine about the status of people with disabilities appears to be that, while neglect is benign for them, legislative attention is to be understood as even more benign. The evidence that segregation and isolation intend them no harm is to be found in both the neglect and the attention to which they are subjected.

Justice White describes citizens with mental retardation as having "a reduced ability to cope with and function in the everyday world."[11] The discrepancy between the assertion that members of this group have decreased capacities to function and the assertion that they have power over legislators is striking. Of course, the legislative favor to which White refers consists in the establishment of programs sought by nondisabled professionals and family members rather than by mentally retarded citizens themselves. Having to rely on others to secure one's social needs is, of course, characteristic of being subjected to paternalism. Dependence on such political alliances not only prevents members of a disadvantaged group from achieving self-determination but also places them at risk of being abandoned or harmed when the dominant partner in a paternalistic coalition finds it convenient to act contrary to their interests.

This danger apparently did not trouble White, who wrote: "because both State and Federal Governments have recently committed themselves to assisting the retarded, we will not presume that any given legislative action, even one that disadvantages retarded individuals, is rooted in considerations that the Constitution will not tolerate."[12] Thus the Court's reasoning suggests that, contrary to the experience of other historically oppressed minorities, policies admitted to be harmful to disabled people should nevertheless be understood as the product of benign neglect rather than the result of intentionally unequal treatment.

THE MINORITY GROUP PERSPECTIVE

Yet a well-documented literature supporting the similarity between the situation of people with disabilities and other marginalized minorities was available to the 1985 Court. In 1953, a year before *Brown,* the Social Sciences Research Council endorsed "the very general assumption that in American culture physically disabled persons, like Negroes and children, for instance, have the position of an underprivileged minority."[13] This view was reaffirmed in 1970 by a sociological analysis which concluded that: "the concept of the minority group can be applied in the case of the disabled despite minor differences."[14] A decade later, the first major attempt to analyze disability through the exclusive use of the minority-group paradigm was sponsored by the Carnegie Council on Children.[15] In 1986, a Harris survey found that 45 percent of Americans with disabilities believed "that disabled persons are a minority group in the same sense as are blacks and Hispanics," and 74 percent indicated that they experienced "a sense of common identity with other disabled people."[16] Further, the Harris survey found: "For all disabled persons, however, the ultimate goal is the freedom to choose, to belong, to participate, to have dignity and freedom to achieve. It is the end of the caste of the handicapped and the stereotypes and prejudices that persons with disabilities lack essential human attributes necessary to be considered a part of organized society."[17] In the last quarter-century, perhaps the principal change in the understanding of disability has begun to affect the doctrine of benign neglect. This has meant provoking a radical alteration of paradigms. Increasingly, the medical model, which supported the functional-limitation analysis of disability and influenced health care and social welfare policies accordingly, has been challenged by adherents of the minority-group model. This approach identifies stigmatization, and the prejudicially disparate treatment of disabled individuals that results from it, as the most important impediment for disabled people. The minority-group perspective analyzes disability as a sociopolitical construction occasioned by the impact on physically and mentally disabled people of an environment shaped by and for the dominant majority.[18] Thus the minority-group model became the theoretical foundation for the Americans with Disabilities Act.

IMPLICATIONS OF THE NEW PARADIGM

Embedding the minority-group model of disability into American political and cultural thought has sweeping implications for people for disabilities, especially for young children whose self-concepts have not yet been mutilated by experiences of stigmatization. First, the awareness that their problems, including some degree of their incapacities, are created by defects of their social environment rather than of themselves relieves them from the enormous burden of psychological distress imposed by guilt and shame. Second, raising their consciousness in this regard is vital to promoting disabled people's sense of personal and political identity and empowerment.

This new perspective may facilitate the transmission of strategies for coping with socially imposed obstacles. Consequently, the minority-group model has the potential to elicit intergenerational interaction that fashions and preserves a cultural legacy—a disability tradition—able to sustain an extended struggle for equality and justice. Finally, these analyses revise the agenda for actions aimed at improving the lives of people with disabilities. An expanded recognition of the environmental causes of disability not only enhances self-esteem but is also an essential organizing tool for political activism by people with disabilities. The understanding elicited by the analogy between disabled and other minority groups makes it clear that integrating people with disabilities into society is not a matter of making psychological adjustments so as to accept the limitations society imposes on them. The sociopolitical perspective postulates that: (a) public policy shapes the social environment, (b) public policy reflects the attitudes—in a sense, the will—of the majority; and (c) it is from the stigmatizing social attitudes of the majority that the basic problems confronting the disabled minority flow.[19] It follows from these premises that collective action will be needed to purge public policy of the effects of stigmatizing attitudes.

Hence there is a crucial role for antidiscrimination law, which allows individuals to challenge being disadvantaged by practices permitted or even promoted by existing public policy. In the "Findings" of the 1990 Americans with Disabilities Act, Congress addresses the doctrine of benign neglect promulgated by the 1985 Supreme Court in *Alexander* and in *Cleburne*. Finding 5 declares: "individuals with disabilities continually encounter various forms of discrimination, including outright intentional exclusion. . . ." Finding 7 affirms: "individuals with disabilities are a discrete and insular minority who have been faced with restrictions and limitations, subjected to a history of purposeful unequal treatment, and relegated to a position of political powerlessness in our society."

However, subsequent judiciaries may be as impervious to the evidence of disparate treatment of disabled people as was the 1985 Court. As Jacobus tenBroek wrote in the *California Law Review* in 1966, "jurors are almost entirely able-bodied, . . . and the judge has sound . . . limbs, fair enough eyesight, and, according to counsel, can hear everything but a good argument. The judge or juror . . . provide . . . a standard of reasonableness . . . including some often quite erroneous imaginings about the nature of . . . disability."[20] To combat this unfortunate tendency to imagine that the lives of disabled persons are buoyed by the benignity with which others treat them, it is desirable to supplement social science research with narrative accounts contributed by people who are living with disabilities. Doing so would reveal the malignity of life in environments hostile to disability and the ways in which practices can be altered to remedy this effect. Without judicial recognition of the importance of weighing the effects of a barrier-ridden physical environment and a stigmatizing social environment in deciding whether equality between the disabled and nondisabled portions of the population has been achieved, the aptness of the minority-group model for the effective political conceptualization of disability may remain an unrealized opportunity.

ACKNOWLEDGMENTS

The author wishes to acknowledge support from the Southern California Study Center and the James Irvine Foundation.

NOTES

[1] *Brown v. Board of Education,* 347 U.S. 483 (1954).

[2] Ibid., 495.

[3] Kenneth B. Clark and M. P. Clark, "Racial Identification and Preference in Negro Children," in Guy E. Swenson, Theodore M. Hartley and E. L. Hartley, eds., *Readings in Social Psychology.* New York: Holt, 1952, 551–560.

[4]Harlan Hahn, "Antidiscrimination Laws and Social Research on Disability: The Minority Group Perspective," *Behavioral Sciences and the Law* 14: 41–59 (1996).

[5]*Pennsylvania Association of Retarded Children (PARC) v. Commonwealth of Pennsylvania,* 334 F. Supp. 1257 (E.D. Penn., 1971); *Mills v. Board of Education,* 348 F. Supp. 866 (D.D.C., 1972).

[6]For a study of the passage and implementation of the 1975 law, see Erwin L. Levine and Elizabeth M. Wexler, *P.L. 94–142: An Act of Congress.* New York: Macmillan, 1981.

[7]Erving Goffman, *Stigma Notes on Management of Spoiled Identity.* Englewood Cliffs, NJ: Prentice-Hall, 1963, 5.

[8]469 U.S. 287 (1985) at 296. Justice Marshall may have invoked the phrase "benign neglect," which was first used in a sardonic sense by Daniel Patrick Moynihan when he was President Nixon's advisor on domestic policy to justify the lack of new civil rights initiatives. Supreme Court Justices often write opinions to attract the support of other members of the Court. This concept also might have been a persuasive argument for choosing disparate impact rather than "prejudicial intent" as a standard for determining discrimination on the basis of disability. In any event, if Justice Marshall intended to use the phrase sardonically, the other justices did not appear to recognize it.

[9]473 U.S. 432 (1985).

[10]Ibid., 442.

[11]Ibid.

[12]Ibid., 446.

[13]Roger G. Barker, Beatrice A. Wright, Lee Meyerson and Mollie R. Gonick, *Adjustment to Physical Handicap and Illness: A Survey of the Social Psychology of Physique and Disability.* New York: Social Sciences Research Council, 1953, 102.

[14]Constantina Safilios-Rothschild, *The Sociology and Social Psychology of Disability and Rehabilitation.* New York: Random House, 1970.

[15]John Gliedman and William Roth, *The Unexpected Minority: Handicapped Children in America.* New York: Harcourt Brace Jovanovich, 1980.

[16]"The ICD Survey of Disabled Americans." New York: Louis Harris and Associates, 1986.

[17]Ibid.

[18]Harlan Hahn, "Toward a Politics of Disability: Definitions, Disciplines, and Policies," *The Social Journal* 22: 87–105 (1985).

[19]Harlan Hahn, "Disability and the Urban Environment: A Perspective on Los Angeles," *Society and Space* 4: 273–288 (1986).

[20]Jacobus tenBroek, "The Right to Live in the World: The Disabled in the Law of Torts," *California Law Review* 54: 841–919 (1966).

Making Change
The ADA as an Instrument of Social Reform

RICHARD K. SCOTCH

The Americans with Disabilities Act was passed by a large bipartisan majority and signed into law by President Bush on July 26, 1990, with great fanfare. While the immediate objective of the ADA was to bar discrimination on the basis of disability in private employment, public accommodation, telecommunications and other institutions of public life, disability advocates hoped that the larger impact of the ADA would be to further full social participation for tens of millions of Americans with disabilities.

In many people's minds, these two goals were clearly linked. The explicit rationale for the ADA was that many of the problems associated with having a disability were the result of a socially constructed environment which arbitrarily and perniciously excluded or limited the social participation of people with physical or mental impairments. The cultural assumption that having a disability inevitably meant that someone was unable to live independently or participate in everyday economic, political or social life became a self-fulfilling prophecy embedded in employment practices, the design and operation of public accommodations and incentives in public benefit systems. Disability community advocates hoped that the ADA would be an important step in redefining how disability is constructed in public policy and ultimately in public life.

The conception of disability as a social construction is typically linked to a social model of disability that conceptualizes disability as a social construction that is the result of interaction between physical or mental impairment and the social environment. The nature of the social environment determines the extent to which an impairment results in incapacity and/or exclusion from mainstream social processes, rather than this being determined by merely the impairment itself. Technology, architecture and spatial organization all reflect concepts of what is "normal" and how "normal" people function, as do cultural attitudes and institutional processes (Higgins, 1992). By characterizing the social isolation and enforced dependency of people with disabilities as the result of social and political choices rather than as inevitable results of impairment, the social model suggests analogies between the social status of people with disabilities and other marginalized groups such as racial and ethnic minorities, women, or gays and lesbians.

People with disabilities clearly share many of the experiences and characteristics of other groups commonly recognized as minorities. They are subject to prejudiced attitudes, discriminatory behavior and institutional and legal constraints that parallel those experienced by African-Americans and other disadvantaged and excluded groups. People with disabilities are victimized by negative stereotypes of dependence and incapacity which lead to discriminatory attitudes and practices resulting in exclusion and social isolation. They may lack access to employment, public facilities, voting and other forms of civic involvement due to barriers of stigma, fear and disabling assumptions. Thus people with disabilities are denied the opportunity fully to participate in society. Within this political framework, disputes over civil rights have become central in disability policy and politics (Scotch, 1984, 1988, 1989).

The ADA explicitly built upon this minority-group analogy by taking as its model previous federal statutes such as the Civil Rights Act of 1964, which prohibited discrimination on the basis of race, religion and gender. (Other models were Title IX of the Education Amendments of 1972 and Section 504 of the Rehabilitation Act of 1973.) Using the Civil Rights Act of 1964 as a legislative template, the ADA seeks to eliminate the marginalization of people with disabilities through established civil rights remedies to discrimination. Paul Higgins (1992) writes of the ADA:

> Rather than (primarily) looking to individual characteristics to understand the difficulties experienced by people with disabilities, rights encourage us, even require us, to evaluate our practices that may limit people with disabilities. Rights empower people with disabilities. With rights, people with disabilities may legitimately contest what they perceive to be illegitimate treatment of them. . . . No longer must they endure arrangements that disadvantage them to the advantage of nondisabled citizens. (199–200)

The ADA can be seen as more than a specific protection from discrimination—it is also a policy commitment to the social inclusion of people with disabilities. In 1986, the National Council on the Handicapped, a presidentially appointed advisory body, issued a report titled *Toward Independence* that was a major step toward the ADA. The report built upon the results of a survey conducted by Louis Harris Associates along with the anecdotal experience of many people with disabilities in asserting that discrimination was a major barrier to social participation and in particular employment for disabled Americans. The report stated that preceding "handicap discrimination laws fail to serve the purpose of any human rights law—providing a strong statement of a societal imperative. An adequate equal opportunity law for persons with disabilities will seek to obtain the voluntary compliance of the great majority of law-abiding citizens by notifying them that discrimination against people with disabilities will no longer be tolerated by our society" (1986, 18).

Similarly, Jane West (1991) wrote, shortly after the act's passage: "The ADA is a law that sends a clear message about what our society's attitudes should be toward people with disabilities. The ADA is an orienting framework that can be used to construct a comprehensive service delivery system. . . . The ADA is intended to open the doors of society and keep them open" (22).

Despite the ten years since its enactment, the direct impact of the ADA on discriminatory practices remains unclear. In one recent discussion of the ADA, Collignon (1997) addressed the difficulties in assessing the act's impact, including the dearth of available information about the population of Americans living with disabilities and the problem of operationalizing objectives found in the act such as economic self-sufficiency, full participation or equal opportunity.

Further, implementation has been slow, and many employers and providers of public accommodation have been slow to respond. In part, this delayed response is due to the perceived ambiguity of several statutory provisions and the desire for judicial clarification of how and to whom the law would specifically apply. Many affected entities have taken a wait-and-see approach or have responded to individual situations on an *ad hoc* basis, while others appear to have resisted change unless forced by enforcement agencies or the courts.

It is difficult to measure the extent of voluntary actions taken in response to the law, since compliance requires a responsiveness to individual situations rather than simply physical alterations or procedural adaptations. Certainly many employers and public accommodation providers have made their facilities more accessible, and public commitment to ensuring access appears to be high. However, one cannot easily attribute such changes to the ADA as opposed to general social trends toward greater inclusion of people with disabilities. Technological changes, activism by the disability rights and independent living movements, and the effects of prior federal statutes such as the Rehabilitation Acts of 1973 and 1978 and the Individuals with Disabilities Education Act have all helped to give people with disabilities more public visibility and (perhaps) stimulated greater public understanding of the experience of disability.

In terms of the full panoply of federal disability policies, the ADA appears to be a modest effort, albeit a self-consciously ambitious one. One analysis, by Monroe Berkowitz, compiled the costs of all federal programs in the 1995 federal fiscal year, categorized by their broad purposes (Berkowitz, 1996). Of nearly $184 billion for all programs, more than 90 percent went for health care ($91 billion) or income maintenance ($78 billion). Thirty-eight million dollars, a mere 0.02 percent, went for civil rights, of which $1.6 million was directly related to the Americans with Disabilities Act (1996, 50). Nevertheless, the Americans with Disabilities Act has been seen as very important and a potential catalyst for social change by the disability community that advocated for it, the business community and others that are subject to its requirements, and many policy-makers and their observers in the mass media.

THE CIVIL RIGHTS ACT OF 1964 AND CIVIL RIGHTS FOR AFRICAN-AMERICANS

One way of thinking about the impact of the Americans with Disabilities Act and its capacity to serve as an engine of social change is to examine the role of comparable civil rights laws on the social position of other minority groups. Of such laws, perhaps closest to the ADA in breadth and focus of coverage is the Civil Rights Act of 1964. The experience of African-Americans since the passage of the civil rights legislation of the 1960s may have implications for the potential of disability civil rights statutes as vehicles for overcoming social disadvantage. While Jim Crow laws and legal segregation have been abolished, and many well-educated African-Americans have unprecedented access to employment and middle-class status, poorly educated African-Americans as a group are relatively worse-off in terms of earnings or employment than they were thirty years ago, and the state of intergroup relations remains far short of the goals of the civil rights movement of the 1960s. In fact, one of the most contentious issues in the current debate over race relations is affirmative action, a concept in some ways analogous to the accommodations needed to make employment, education, public accommodations and other institutional spheres truly accessible to Americans with disabilities.

One prominent study of employment discrimination legislation is the 1985 book *Discrimination, Jobs, and Politics* by the sociologist Paul Burstein. One of Burstein's objectives was to determine whether Title VII of the Civil Rights Act of 1964, the model for the ADA's Title I, had improved employment opportunities for African-Americans. He addresses what he refers to as "structural looseness," the gap between the intentions of legislation and its formulation and actual impact (1985, 190–191). He notes a finding common to the sociology of social protest movements, that the success of a movement "depends upon changes in the social and political context over which it has little or no control" (188).

Nevertheless, Burstein contends that equal employment opportunity legislation (EEO) did have a significant economic and political impact, substantially raising the income of nonwhite men and women (149–150). He acknowledges but criticizes several technical analyses of earnings that, he argues, minimize the impact of EEO by ignoring the broad social and political consequences of the Civil Rights Act (182). He concludes:

> Finally, and perhaps most important, analysis of the consequences of the struggle for EEO can be improved by examining the struggle as a whole—that is, as a conflict over access to resources waged in many ways, including, but not limited to, the enforcement of legislation. Work that focuses solely on the enforcement of EEO legislation . . . simply misses much of what is important about the struggle—the role of social protest, changes in the social context, and the implications of the decision to work through the democratic political process. Only an approach that considers how social change and political organization impinge upon economic outcomes can hope to lead to an understanding of the struggle for EEO and where it is taking us. (154)

A different point about the Civil Rights Act of 1964 is made by William Julius Wilson in his study of urban poverty among African-Americans, *The Truly Disadvantaged*. Citing the hope that the act's passage would lead to racial progress and the end of racial discrimination, Wilson notes that antidiscrimination laws are, even where successful, inadequate "to deal with the complex problems of race in America because they are not designed to address the substantive inequality that exists at the time discrimination is eliminated" (1987, 146). He continues that the "problems of the truly disadvantaged [racial minority group members] may require *nonracial* solutions such as full employment, balanced economic growth, and manpower training and education . . ." (147). Wilson makes a similar point in *When Work Disappears* (1996), where he writes that: "less advantaged blacks are extremely vulnerable to changes in modern industrial society, leading to problems that are difficult to combat by means of race-based strategies alone—either those that embody equality of individual opportunity, such as the Civil Rights Act of 1964, or those that represent affirmative action. Now more than ever, we need broader solutions" (1996, 199). Examples of such broader policy solutions include employment and training programs, national health care, expanded child care and improved public education (1996, 205–206).

IMPACT OF THE ADA

I would contend that, at least in its first ten years, the ADA appears to have fallen short of its more optimistic goal of fundamentally changing the lives of most Americans with disabilities. In the aggregate, people with disabilities are still disproportionately unemployed and underemployed, and their incomes are below those of people without disabilities. While survey data suggest that most Americans are supportive of the ADA's goal of inclusion and nondiscrimination, stigma that constrains individuals with disabilities persists in individual attitudes and institutional processes.

Further, the ability to participate of Americans with disabilities is constrained by many indirect factors. People with disabilities tend to have lower levels of education and training due to historical exclusion from schooling, making them more vulnerable to trends in our increasingly postindustrial labor market. Many people with disabilities are also disadvantaged in the labor market by work disincentives built into benefit and insurance programs and by inadequate systems of social support. Inadequate health insurance coverage for chronic conditions creates barriers to employment, as do difficulties with transportation. Further, disability interacts with class, race, gender and age in complex ways that compound isolation and inequity. While these disadvantages can be attributed to a legacy of stigmatization and isolation, they may not be overcome solely by framing the problem in terms of discrimination.

People with disabilities are also affected by rapidly changing economic conditions, including global competition, deregulation and the growth of the service sector, which have led to considerable turbulence in work relationships, job longevity and the organizational, geographic and spatial settings in which work is done. Some of these trends increase access to jobs, while others may make work less accessible to the many disabled people seeking employment.

Just as the economic and social challenges facing many African-Americans are not likely to be resolved by civil rights laws alone, the social exclusion of people with disabilities will not be resolved by the ADA on its own. Access to good jobs, health insurance, personal assistance, community-based services and accessible technologies may be enhanced but is not guaranteed by laws such as the ADA. Antidiscrimination laws may be necessary but not sufficient for major institutional change.

Of course, we may disregard the optimistic aspirations of disability advocates for the ADA and focus more concretely on its narrow impact, examining administrative records of complaints and on judicial rulings. Based on her review of these sources with regard to Title I, Nancy Mudrick reports that: "there is no clear assessment of whether court decisions have affected the employment experiences of people with disabilities" (1997, 66). She notes that those most likely to seek redress are individuals already employed and those whose disabilities are acquired from chronic diseases that may begin with mid-life (66–67), and that the ADA may be less effective at increasing the employment opportunities and options of people seeking to enter the workforce with a disability (69). Similarly, Jane West noted in 1994 that: "the ADA does not appear to be making a difference for people who are not currently working, and may make it even harder for those with significant disabilities to find employment" (cited in Baldwin 1997, 51). Mudrick concludes that while the cost of providing accommodation under the ADA's requirements have been modest, its impact may be modest as well. She writes that: "It may be the case that . . . people with disabilities have overestimated the ability of a civil rights act to significantly alter employment rates and circumstances" (70).

Further, the record of recent court rulings suggests that the ADA may be available to a far smaller number of people with disabilities than was intended by its framers. In an exhaustive analysis of ADA decisions in 1997, Robert Burgdorf, the author of the original 1988 bill that would become the ADA, discusses how many decisions have perpetuated the incorrect concept that people with disabilities are some special group of individuals who are "drastically different from others and, therefore, should be treated differently and given special protection" rather than as "regular Janes and Joes" who despite their impairments are not essentially different from other people (1997, 534). He concludes that: "in the name of restricting this special treatment to the supposed truly deserving beneficiaries, obstacles have been erected that have kept many of the supposed core group along with many other citizens from the protection these laws were enacted to provide" (585).

More recent Supreme Court rulings in 1999 have excluded individuals from the ADA's protection from discrimination if their impairments can be corrected with medication or devices. The impact of these rulings is that while correctable impairments may lead to discrimination, that discrimination is permissible even if the correction means that the person is capable of performing a job. Another person involved in drafting the ADA, Chai Feldblum, responded by pointing out that the decisions "create the absurd result of a person being disabled enough to be fired from a job, but not disabled enough to challenge the firing" (quoted in Greenhouse 1999, A16).

However, the ADA may have led to considerable reconsideration of exclusionary and prejudicial practices across American society independent of how its legal remedies have been applied. Marjorie Baldwin notes that: "The fact that the ADA exists at all may be a sufficient condition to reduce some labor market discrimination based on employer prejudice," due to changing, less stigmatizing conceptions of disability (1997, 48). However, she continues: "It is likely that it will require more than a change in public awareness generated by the passage of the law to allay employer concerns" about the employability of persons with disabilities (50).

DISABILITY AND SOCIAL CHANGE

The ADA might be seen as having both narrow direct effects and broader indirect ones. I would suggest that the latter are far more important but are also quite difficult to disentangle from changes in the economy, the overall society and the ways in which disability fits into larger social institutions and processes. Ultimately, however, the ADA needs to be examined contextually to understand its full significance. It may be more useful to see the law as representative of social trends rather than as a major change agent in itself. Such an interpretation is quite consistent with the social model of disability, which suggests that disability may be defined as an interaction between an impairment and the social environment. While the law may prompt some changes in behavior, its impact is likely to be modest in the face of the commonly held assumption that having a disability is inextricably linked with incapacity and dependence. The judges and regulatory officials who enforce the law are unlikely to get very far ahead of popular notions about what disability is and what it means. On the other hand, if a less stigmatizing view of disability is prominent in the culture, then an antidiscrimination law may become more efficacious but less necessary.

The facileness of the analogy between racial discrimination and discrimination on the basis of disability masks the potentially radical nature of the ADA's mandates and the fundamental institutional changes required for it to attain its promise. Although contention perseveres about the duration needed for race-conscious remedies to persist, the ADA requires a permanent transformation of workplaces, public facilities and the infrastructures that support them. Disability is diverse, dynamic and idiosyncratic. While there are occasionally individual difficulties to be worked out, race and gender discrimination can typically be eliminated through wholesale changes in policy and practice. Because of the diversity of disabling conditions and the variety of coping strategies of individuals who have them, many accommodations under the ADA must be tailored to the individual involved and may require periodic alterations to reflect changes in the individual's impairment or the environment in and outside the workplace. Truly accommodating people with disabilities may require a constant willingness to change, the periodic restructuring of expectations, tasks and techniques, and a constructive communication between persons with disabilities and those responsible for their environments, such as employers.

Can a law such as the ADA accomplish such a humane, responsive and individuated environment in work and public life? If social institutions were already inclined to accommodate the range of individual needs, it would be no great leap to be sure to accommodate those individuals who had disabilities. Some social trends, such as the decentralization of computer technology and the disaggregation of much work, enhance the capacity to accommodate individual situations. But there are countervailing trends which make the capacity to accommodate problematic by imposing standardization and routinization on many common tasks. These trends can be overcome, but an antidiscrimination law may be a blunt instrument to accomplish such change.

The Americans with Disabilities Act is a crucial protection for people with disabilities. The ADA's mandates have led to significant expansion of access to the social, economic and political mainstream, independent of the workings of the courts and regulatory bodies. However, whatever legal standing for protection from discrimination has been gained, it would be very difficult to argue that people with disabilities have achieved social or economic parity as the result of ADA, or that having a disability is no longer a relevant factor in the life chances of many individuals.

But that might be far too much to expect from a civil rights law. People with disabilities face a variety of barriers to social participation, including limited human capital, social isolation and cultural stereotypes. While many of these can be directly or indirectly linked to discrimination, none of them will be easily changed by an act of Congress. Fundamental and far-reaching social change will be necessary for people with disabilities to enjoy full access to American society.

Might we then expect that the ADA can at least end overt discrimination on the basis of disability? If the social model of disability is correct, even this may be too great a burden to place on the legal system. The stigma associated with disability is so embedded and reinforced within our culture and social structure that it will take tremendous efforts to root out. As Donald L. Horowitz (1977) points out, the courts have a built-in emphasis on formal relationships and may lack the capacity to alter informal patterns of behavior. Such an effort may be a task more appropriate for a broadly based social and political disability movement than for a law dependent on judicial and regulatory enforcement. People-to-people contacts may help to break down pernicious stereotypes and arbitrary limitations on people with disabilities. Grassroots advocates may be better able to educate communities about the nature of the barriers faced by people with disabilities and how the participation of people with disabilities can be achieved with beneficial results.

Legal protections from discriminatory practice are probably indispensable, but such guarantees cannot be the only strategy toward ending the discrimination and social exclusion faced by Americans with disabilities. What may be needed as well is a broad-based political mobilization of people with disabilities to educate the public and policy-makers about the actual experience and consequences of disability and to advocate for laws and programs that promote integration, full participation and nondiscrimination, the goals established in the Americans with Disabilities Act.

REFERENCES

Baldwin, Marjorie L. "Can the ADA Achieve Its Employment Goals?" *Annals of the American Academy of Political and Social Science* 549 (1997): 37–52.

Berkowitz, Monroe. "Federal Programs for Persons with Disabilities." Presented at Conference on Employment and Return to Work for People with Disabilities, Social Security Administration and National Institute on Disability and Rehabilitation Research, Washington, DC, 1996.

Burgdorf, Jr. Robert L. "'Substantially Limited' Protection from Disability Discrimination: The Special Treatment Model and Misconstructions of the Definition of Disability." *Vill. L. R.* 42:2 (1997) 409–585.

Burstein, Paul. *Discrimination, Jobs, and Politics: The Struggle for Equal Employment Opportunity in the United States since the New Deal.* Chicago: University of Chicago Press, 1985.

Collignon, Frederick C. "Is the ADA Successful? Indicators for Tracking Gains." *Annals of the American Academy of Political and Social Science* 549 (1997): 129–147.

Greenhouse, Linda. "High Court Limits Who is Protected by Disability Law." *New York Times,* June 23, 1999, A1, A16.

Hahn, Harlan. "Disability Policy and the Problem of Discrimination." *American Behavioral Scientist* 28:3 (1985): 293–318.

Higgins, Paul C. *Making Disability: Exploring the Social Transformation of Human Variation.* Springfield, IL: Charles C. Thomas, 1992.

Horowitz, Donald L. *The Courts and Social Policy.* Washington, DC: Brookings Institution, 1977.

Mudrick, Nancy R. "Employment Discrimination Laws for Disability: Utilization and Outcome." *Annals of the American Academy of Political and Social Science* 549 (1997): 53–70.

National Council on the Handicapped. *Toward Independence: An Assessment of Federal Laws and Programs Affecting People with Disabilities With Legislative Recommendations.* Washington, DC: U.S. Government Printing Office, 1986.

Scotch, Richard K. *From Good Will to Civil Rights: Transforming Federal Disability Policy.* Philadelphia: Temple University Press, 1984.

Scotch, Richard K. "Disability as the Basis for a Social Movement: Advocacy and the Politics of Definition." *Journal of Social Issues* 44:1 (1988): 159–172.

Scotch, Richard K. "Politics and Policy in the History of the Disability Rights Movement." *Milbank Quarterly* 67:(Supp. 2 Pt 2) (1989): 380–400.

West, Jane. "The Social and Policy Context of the Act," in Jane West, ed., *The Americans with Disabilities Act: From Policy to Practice.* New York: Milbank Memorial Fund, 1991.

Wilson, William Julius. *The Truly Disadvantaged: The Inner City, the Underclass, and Public Policy.* Chicago: University of Chicago Press, 1987.

Wilson, William Julius. *When Work Disappears: The World of the New Urban Poor.* New York: Knopf, 1996.

Ten Years Later
The ADA and the Future of Disability Policy

ANDREW I. BATAVIA

The Americans with Disabilities Act (ADA)[1] has improved the life circumstances of most people with disabilities. However, there continue to be wide gaps between people with and without disabilities in almost all major social indicators, and the number of people with disabilities who are employed, educated and socially active has not improved substantially in the past decade. The inability of the ADA in its first ten years significantly to increase these numbers and narrow the gaps was predictable. The policy assumptions of other components of our nation's disability policy, such as Social Security Disability Insurance (SSDI) and Supplemental Security Income (SSI) programs, are still not consistent with those underlying the ADA. Moreover, the ADA was not designed to resolve all problems experienced by people with disabilities. There has also been little progress in addressing those policy issues that cannot be resolved fully by the ADA, such as access to health care coverage, personal assistance services, smoke-free environments and full employment. Additional efforts will be needed to conform existing disability policy to the premises and goals of the ADA and to further empower people with disabilities in resolving those issues that the ADA was not designed to address fully.

Ten years after the enactment of the ADA, the effects on people with disabilities have varied.[2] There have been some significant improvements in the lives of many individuals with disabilities. In that brief period of time, our society has become much more physically accessible, particularly for people with mobility impairments.[3] Access to higher education for many individuals with disabilities has also improved. However, as a group, people with disabilities remain among the most socially deprived Americans, with about 70 percent unemployed, 33 percent living in households with incomes of less than $15,000 and 20 percent not completing high school.[4] Over the past 15 years, these key social indicators for people with disabilities have not improved significantly,[5] and there continue to be large discrepancies between individuals with and without disabilities.[6]

Many of us who supported the ADA from the outset are not surprised that it did not achieve dramatic improvements across the entire disability population, particularly by the end of its first decade.[7–9] The ADA is only one of many disability laws in this country, albeit the most far-reaching and arguably the most important one. Shortly after the enactment of the law, Gerben DeJong and I pointed out the philosophical and practical inconsistency between disability-based civil rights laws such as the ADA and the other two components of disability policy in this country: (1) income and in-kind assistance programs, and (2) skill-enhancement programs such as vocational rehabilitation.[10] These programs were established years before the ADA, often with assumptions that were never true (for example, that people are either totally disabled or not disabled) or that became obsolete over time as people with disabilities became more independent and employable (for example, that people with the most "severe" disabilities cannot work). We argued that the goals of the ADA are not likely to be achieved until these other programs become more consistent with the premises and goals of the ADA.[11]

For example, the SSDI and SSI programs, which provide cash benefits to people who are not capable of gainful employment, were based fundamentally on an assumption that people with significant disabilities are basically unemployable. This assumption has been disproven by the many people with significant disabilities, such as quadriplegia, who are now working and living independently in their communities.

Moreover, even if all existing disability policy in this country were to be consistent with the ADA, there are some inherent limits to the extent to which a civil rights law such as the ADA, or any law for that matter, can achieve fundamental social change. Notwithstanding some of the rhetoric of the independent living movement, some people with disabilities (such as many people with severe brain injuries) are simply too functionally limited to pursue education and employment in the community. However, this should not be overstated, because most people with disabilities are capable of some functional activity, and many are capable of full-time gainful employment.

The majority of people with disabilities who are capable of employment attempt to enter markets for unskilled and semiskilled laborers with high levels of unemployment.[12] Many of them must compete in these markets despite educational deficits that occurred years prior to the enactment of the ADA. Those who have been excluded from the job market as a result of discrimination have been placed at a substantial disadvantage because they do not have a record of employment. This is particularly problematic in a youth-oriented labor market.

The ADA has an extremely broad scope, but it was not designed to resolve all social problems of people with disabilities. It cannot, by itself, fully address problems of access to health insurance, personal assistance services, and environments that are free of tobacco smoke and other chemical irritants that have a profound impact on individuals who are particularly sensitive to these stimuli. Additional laws or other approaches to achieving significant social change will be needed to address these issues.

This essay examines the extent to which, ten years after the enactment of the ADA, our disability programs have changed to be more compatible with the goals of the ADA. It further considers the extent to which the ADA is likely to achieve its goals even if all disability policy in this country became compatible with the goals of employment and independence, and what further policies or other interventions will be necessary to achieve these goals more fully.

INCOME AND IN-KIND BENEFITS PROGRAMS

The SSDI program provides cash assistance to people with disabilities who have worked previously and who have contributed payroll taxes to the Social Security System for a requisite number of quarters. The SSI program provides cash assistance to people with disabilities who have extremely limited incomes. Both are significant beyond their direct budgetary impact, because their eligibility criteria also determine an individual's eligibility for Medicare and Medicaid respectively. This link between income and in-kind health care programs has enormous implications for the prospects of people with disabilities to become gainfully employed.[13]

Specifically, the prospect of eventually losing access to health care coverage as a result of leaving the programs through gainful employment creates a strong disincentive to work.[14] In fact, despite several amendments to the programs during the 1980s, including the ability to retain health benefits for a certain period of time after becoming employed, very few people with disabilities have left the SSDI or SSI programs over the years.[15] The message that should have been learned from this experience is that tinkering with systems that are based on fundamentally erroneous premises will not be sufficient to cause substantial increases in the number of employable people with disabilities who choose to become employed.[16]

Several proposals for significant social security disability reform have been advanced. One approach developed would time-limit benefits for the large majority of people with disabilities who are capable of gainful employment but not for those who are truly "too disabled" to work, such as most people with severe brain damage.[17] Substantial resources for accommodations, including access to health care coverage, would be provided to ensure the individual would have the capacity to maintain employment and that the individual would be better-off financially by working.

This and other proposals for substantial structural reform of the programs have not been considered seriously by the Congress. Instead, Congress recently enacted the Ticket to Work and Work Incentives Improvement Act of 1999, P.L. 106–170, which adopts a more incremental approach that retains the basic assumptions of the program and attempts to affect its incentive structure. Among its reforms are:

1. Creating a "ticket" that will enable SSI or SSDI beneficiaries to choose among a range of public or private providers of vocational rehabilitation, rewarding providers that assist beneficiaries to become employed with a portion of the benefits saved.
2. Expanding the ability of states to provide Medicaid buy-ins to people with disabilities who return to work.
3. Extending Medicare coverage for people with disabilities who return to work.
4. Creating a new Medicaid buy-in demonstration to help working people with impairments that are not severe enough to qualify for health assistance but that are likely to lead to significant disabilities in the absence of medical treatment.
5. Providing for appropriate protection and advocacy services to beneficiaries who attempt a return to work.
6. Creating a work incentive grant program to provide community-based benefits planning and assistance, facilitate access to information about work incentives, and better integrate services to people with disabilities who are working or returning to work.
7. Establishing a corps of trained, accessible SSA work-incentive specialists.
8. Authorizing a mandatory demonstration project on the effectiveness of reducing SSI cash assistance to beneficiaries on a sliding scale of one dollar of cash assistance for every two dollars of earned income as an incentive to employment.
9. Providing for an expedited reentry process so that people with disabilities know that supports are there should they fail in their first attempts at work.
10. Adding a provision to ensure that work is not used as evidence of medical improvement, prohibiting work activity from triggering a medical improvement review.
11. Ensuring that a work incentive advisory panel strongly reflects the views of consumers but fairly addresses the views of all the stakeholders.

I supported this bill from the outset, despite the fact that it does not fundamentally alter the premises of the programs, because the provisions discussed above are clearly a significant step in the right direction. Moreover, more fundamental reform is likely to be politically infeasible, particularly in the Senate, where any such fundamental reform is likely to be subject to filibuster either by liberal Democrats influenced by elements of the disability community or by conservative Republicans, depending upon the specific nature of the fundamental reform.

While I worked with the Social Security Task Force of the National Council of Independent Living to secure the new law's passage, I am under no illusions that it will result in a mass exodus from the programs to payrolls. The most that can reasonably be expected, I believe, is that those beneficiaries with marketable employment skills who are currently on the disability rolls because it is not currently in their economic self-interest to work may now be induced to seek employment. A certain percentage of these individuals will be successful in that endeavor and will become full-time employees throughout the remainder of their working lives.

To achieve significant reductions in the disability rolls will require a substantial push rather than a gentle pull. For many people with disabilities who have been on the programs for a long time and who have grown accustomed to the feeling of security under them, a substantial push may be the best thing that ever happened to them. I would advise them that the security they are feeling is "the security of the zoo"; although they will probably never starve as program beneficiaries, they will also probably never experience the freedom to achieve their highest potentials. Whatever reform is ultimately adopted should ideally provide sufficient push to encourage the beneficiary to escape the zoo permanently, but also should not place the beneficiary in the jeopardy of the jungle. Supports and safeguards are necessary to ensure that the beneficiary has a real chance to obtain employment and, if the effort fails, to ensure that the beneficiary will still have the resources to survive.

Some might argue that freedom involves risk, and the state has no obligation to provide opportunity if individuals are not willing to assume risk. I would generally agree with this proposition. However, in the case of the Social Security disability programs, the state has actually created the incentive structure that disempowers people with disabilities. Therefore, the state has some obligation to assist people with disabilities to escape the programs. Whether this means that the disabled individual must not be subject to risk, or that the risk should be significantly reduced to assist the individual, is a matter for policy debate. I would encourage people with disabilities to work, but would provide an adequate safety net in the event of failure.

It is important to note that the SSDI and SSI programs together cover only approximately 6 million people with disabilities; the majority of the approximately 54 million Americans with disabilities have no involvement in these systems. Consequently, while social security disability reform is an important piece of the empowerment puzzle, and these programs should be made consistent with the ADA as soon as possible, such reform will not resolve the problems of the many people with disabilities who are not beneficiaries of these programs and who are also not adequately achieving their employment and independent-living potentials.

TRAINING AND EDUCATION PROGRAMS

Programs to enhance the skills and employability of people with disabilities have adapted more rapidly in conforming to the assumptions and goals of the ADA. This is, in part, because many of these programs are administered by state agencies that are subject to the requirements of Title II of the ADA. Failure to comply with these requirements could result in costly litigation as well as adverse political effects. Moreover, the financial consequences to the federal and state governments and the political consequences to government officials of modifying these skill-enhancement programs are not nearly as dramatic as the corresponding potential consequences of fundamentally altering the Social Security disability programs. The stakes, both financially and politically, are much smaller. Increasing efforts have been made for vocational rehabilitation programs to address the needs of people with substantial disabilities. Still, there have not been any dramatic innovations to enhance significantly the employment and independent-living objectives of people with disabilities.

CAN THE ADA ACHIEVE ITS OBJECTIVES?

The ADA assumes that people with disabilities should be allowed to pursue their potential and should not be discriminated against or discouraged from achieving their objectives. Even if all of our disability policies were entirely consistent with the premises and goals of the ADA, it is unlikely that the enormous gaps between people would close entirely. They probably would be reduced to some extent. But they are not all attributable to discrimination. They are also a result of a broad array of factors that range from societal attitudes and practices to the specific circumstances of the individual. Societal factors include governmental and institutional policies that disempower people with disabilities. Individual factors include functional limitations, family support, personal responsibility and personal motivations. The latter two, of course, may be influenced by socialization patterns.[18]

Moreover, the ADA does not prohibit every form of disparate treatment of people with disabilities. For example, certain practices and policies by insurance plans and health maintenance organizations that have discriminatory and adverse effects on people with disabilities are not invalidated by the ADA.[19, 20] Although the ADA specifically prohibits discrimination in employee compensation and discrimination by places of public accommodation (including insurance offices and health maintenance organizations), it protects these organizations in underwriting risks, classifying risks or administering risks in a manner that is consistent with state law, unless they are doing so as a subterfuge to discriminate against people with disabilities.[21] This confusing set of provisions in the ADA has been clarified by Department of Justice regulations stating that insurers may no longer treat people differently on the basis of disability unless their differential treatment is justified by sound actuarial principles or reasonably anticipated experience.

Similarly, problems in gaining access to personal assistance services are not necessarily resolved by the ADA.[22] For example, there is nothing in the ADA that requires that a hotel or restaurant provide assistance in bathing or eating to an individual with a disability who requires such assistance. There may be some circumstances in which employers may be required under Title I of the ADA to provide or pay for personal assistance services, such as when an employee with a disability is required by the job to travel overnight, but this is the exception rather than the rule. Also, the recent decision of the U.S. Supreme Court in the *Olmstead* case suggests strongly that some states may be required under Title II of the ADA to provide personal assistance services in the community as an alternative to institutionalization.[23]

Places of public accommodation generally are not required to offer completely smoke-free environments to accommodate the needs of people with respiratory problems, although at least one court has found such an obligation.[24] Similarly, they are not required to provide environments that are free of other chemicals irritants to meet the needs of people with multiple chemical sensitivity, otherwise known as environmental disease.

In the employment context, in particular, the ADA does not ensure people with disabilities of a job.[25-27] The employment provisions of Title I do not include affirmative-action obligations. Employers are not required to hire a certain number of people with disabilities, nor are they required to hire any individual, disabled or not disabled, who is not the most qualified applicant for the particular job. They are required to provide reasonable accommodations to those people with disabilities whom they hire and to consider the ability of job applicants to do the job with the reasonable accommodations provided.

Therefore, if an employer does do not wish to hire a person with a disability, the employer can always claim that the applicant was not the most qualified, even after claiming to take into consideration the individual's ability to do the job with necessary reasonable accommodations, or the employer can claim that the candidate was not a good fit for the job. In fact, many people with disabilities are not the most qualified for the job, because our primary and secondary education systems continue to provide less-adequate education for people with disabilities than for those without disabilities despite years of implementation of the Individuals with Disabilities Education Act (IDEA).[28] Even if all people with disabilities on the programs were the most qualified for the jobs they would like to have, our economy typically is not adequate to provide all the job opportunities desired.

Moreover, the ADA is likely to suffer diminishing marginal returns over time. In other words, those who are amenable to complying with the ADA voluntarily or with limited reluctance have probably already complied. Those who are most resistant to compliance and who have been clever enough to evade their responsibilities under the law so far are likely to remain noncompliant. Therefore, the ADA's capacity to achieve its goals is likely to diminish relatively. Of course, our society will continue to become more and more accessible over time directly as a result of the ADA. The point is that the rate at which such accessibility will increase will slow down. The ADA will always be necessary, because without it there is likely to be a reversal in the trend toward greater accessibility. However, the ADA will never achieve the level of accessibility that is optimal for people with disabilities.

WHAT FURTHER POLICY TOOLS ARE NEEDED?

In the coming century, a two-pronged approach will be needed. First, all disability policy should be made consistent with the premises and goals of the ADA. Second, to the extent that the ADA itself cannot achieve its laudatory objectives, additional policy intervention will be needed. The question is: What should be the nature of this intervention? The answer will depend in large part on the specific aspects of the problem that remain to be remedied. Some problems are likely to be amenable to further legislation.

For example, to the extent that the ADA does not adequately address the problem of people with disabilities being excluded from health insurance by virtue of preexisting-conditions clauses and lifetime maximum benefits in insurance policies, legislation is feasible. The number of people who are excluded from coverage for preexisting conditions could potentially increase dramatically as science allows us better to identify genetic predispositions. The U.S. Supreme Court's recent decision in *Sutton* indicates that such "potential disabilities" are not protected under the ADA. For this reason, additional legislation will be necessary to protect such individuals from discrimination based upon genetic predisposition.

On the other hand, to the extent that people with disabilities continue to be unemployed, there are real limits to the extent that additional legislation will be fruitful. As indicated earlier, an employer who is intent upon rejecting an applicant with a disability is likely to find ways in which to do so without being subjected to the substantial risk of a lawsuit. It is difficult to conceive of a law that would be politically feasible and would induce an otherwise recalcitrant employer to hire such an applicant. By increasing the penalties of the ADA, the reaction may even be counterproductive, in that employers know that current employees are more likely than potential employees to sue under the ADA, and therefore it may be preferable from their business perspective not to hire the person with a disability in the first place.

Some disability rights advocates will demand extremely aggressive social policy, such as requiring that a certain percentage of each employer's workforce consist of people with disabilities. There are several reasons why this approach would not be productive. First, from a political point of view, it would never be enacted in this country. The current backlash against affirmative action in this country makes clear that such legislation would be rejected. Americans are particularly resistant to numerical quotas and would be extremely concerned that employers would be required to hire people who were not qualified for the job.

Second, even if such legislation were politically feasible, it would not be technically feasible. We would first have to define precisely what we mean by a numerical quota of people with disabilities. Is a person with quadriplegia equivalent to a person with diabetes? Does a person with back pain qualify as a person with a disability for purposes of such employment protection? How much back pain would be necessary to qualify? Even if such questions could be answered theoretically, in practice they would lead to an enormous amount of conflict and potentially litigation. The databases on people with disabilities, particularly at the local level, are simply not adequate to support such an implementation effort.

In the area of employment, our best hope for people with disabilities is to affect positively the attitudes of employers and managers about people with disabilities. This may prove to be the most enduring legacy of the ADA. Over time, as people with disabilities are brought into the mainstream of our society, primarily through the mandates of Title II on state and local government and of Title III on places of public accommodation, attitudes are changing and will continue to change. Appropriate public policy in the area of employment may, therefore, entail efforts to supplement this positive effect on attitudes through public service announcements and other public relations campaigns.

WHAT IS THE FUTURE OF DISABILITY POLICY?

The success of future disability policy will depend upon the extent to which it continues to empower individuals to achieve their goals. The ADA has provided an essential first step in this regard. It empowers the individual against discriminatory treatment. However, for reasons discussed above, it will never achieve the full level of empowerment that will allow people with disabilities to achieve their goals. Other approaches will be needed to supplement the ADA.

One key issue will be how the various disability programs should be structured or restructured best to empower people with disabilities.[29] Under any program, benefits can potentially be provided in-kind (i.e., direct provision of services), in cash or in some form of cash equivalent, such as a voucher, a tax credit or a medical savings account. Theoretically, providing benefits in cash offers the greatest empowerment of the beneficiary, because it offers that individual the greatest flexibility in meeting his or her needs. However, for a variety of reasons relating to distrust of program beneficiaries by public officials and taxpayers, and beneficiary concerns that the cash payments will be reduced in response to budgetary pressures, many programs such as Medicare and Medicaid provide benefits in-kind.

Increasingly, we should attempt to achieve the goals of fiscal responsibility, taxpayer confidence and beneficiary control and flexibility through an intermediate approach between pure cash and in-kind benefits. A cash-equivalent approach, in which the beneficiary receives something with a cash value that can be spent on a variety of specifically delineated services and providers, is likely to achieve this balance. For example, in lieu of traditional Medicare and Medicaid in-kind services, beneficiaries with disabilities could receive "medical savings accounts" (MSAs) with a catastrophic coverage policy to provide protection in the event of a significant illness or injury, and a savings account that could be spent on any qualified service (including many services that are not covered under Medicare or Medicaid).

This essay has demonstrated the inadequacy of the ADA in addressing access to health care for people with disabilities. The problem is that, although the ADA prohibits discriminatory treatment of people with disabilities that is not "justified" by sound actuarial data or reasonably anticipated experience, many people with disabilities are high-cost users of health care services.[30] These individuals are not adequately protected by the ADA against insurance mechanisms that have an adverse impact on them. To protect them, we will need mechanisms to "adjust risks" such that greater resources are allocated to people with disabilities who have high health care costs, thereby offering providers a greater incentive to treat them.[31]

With respect to personal assistance services, we need a national program or at least a national policy to subsidize the needs of people with disabilities in a manner in which both the individual and the program have significant responsibilities. A national approach is needed both to ensure coordination of services and to avoid the so-called "race to the bottom," in which the various states attempt to reduce the personal assistance services they cover in order to discourage people with disabilities and expensive related expenses from moving to their jurisdictions.

With respect to the social security disability area, we need program modifications which provide individuals with disabilities a greater incentive to leave the programs. Ideally, the revised programs should make it easier for beneficiaries to enter and leave the programs. Perhaps most important, the revised programs must include a strong component of individual responsibility. This essential component is largely lacking in the current programs, which have a strong historical and philosophical basis of social paternalism (i.e., to provide for individuals who are incapable of providing for themselves). In the context of such a paternalistically based system, notwithstanding several efforts to make the programs more empowering, it is not realistic to assume that large numbers of beneficiaries with disabilities will be able to assert their independence. Perhaps the most disturbing aspect of the current system is that it convinces many people, including many younger people, that they are too disabled ever to work or to live independently.

The ADA is the cornerstone of disability policy in this country. It offers a sound foundation for building our future disability policy based on goals of equality of opportunity, full participation, independent living, and economic self-sufficiency. However, a cornerstone is not adequate alone to provide the support needed by people with disabilities. It is only a major component of one of the three legs of disability policy—antidiscrimination policy. The two other existing legs—income and in-kind support programs, and training and education programs—must also be structurally sound. To the extent that some of their building blocks are defective conceptually or in their implementation, whether they have always been defective or they lost their effectiveness over time, they must be replaced.

Finally, a fourth leg—which we may refer to as empowerment policy—must be constructed to fill in the gaps of the other three legs, and to ensure that societal circumstances are such that the individual is able to succeed. If we wish to achieve the laudable goals of the ADA, we must build from its foundation the full structure necessary to support the aspirations of people with disabilities.

NOTES

[1]P.L. 101–336, 104 Stat. 327 (July 26, 1990), codified at 42 USC §§ 12101 et seq.

[2]West, J. "Introduction" in *Implementing the Americans with Disabilities Act,* West, J. ed., Cambridge, MA: Milbank Memorial Fund and Blackwell Publishers, Inc., 1996.

[3]Batavia, A. I. "Public Accommodations" in *Implementing the Americans with Disabilities Act,* West, J., ed., Cambridge, MA: Milbank Memorial Fund and Blackwell Publishers, Inc., 1996.

[4]"NOD/Harris Survey of Americans with Disabilities." Washington, DC: Louis Harris and Associates, 1998.

[5]Louis Harris and Associates. "The ICD Survey of Disabled Americans: Bringing Disabled Americans into the Mainstream." New York: International Center for the Disabled, 1986.

[6]Compared with the 30 percent of working-age adults with disabilities, 80 percent of adults without disabilities are employed full or part-time; the employment of people with disabilities has not improved significantly in the past decade (Louis Harris and Associates, 1986). Compared with the 33 percent of adults with disabilities who live in households with incomes of less than $15,000, only 12 percent of adults without disabilities live in such households. Some 20 percent of people with disabilities do not complete high school, compared with 10 percent of those without disabilities (Louis Harris and Associates, 1998).

[7]Batavia, A. I., and Schriner, K. "The ADA as Engine of Social Change: The Strengths and Limitations of a Civil Rights Approach to Meeting the Needs of People with Disabilities," *Policy Studies Journal,* forthcoming.

[8]Daly, M. C. "Who Is Protected by the ADA: Evidence from the German Experience." *Annals of the American Academy of Political and Social Science* 549 (January 1997): 101–116.

[9]Mudrick, N. R. "Employment Discrimination Laws for Disability: Utilization and Outcome" *Annals of the American Academy of Political and Social Science* 549 (January 1997): 53–70.

[10]DeJong, G., and Batavia, A. I. "The Americans With Disabilities Act and the Current State of Disability Policy," *Journal of Disability Policy Studies* 1(3) (Fall 1990): 65–75.

[11]The ADA states, "The Nation's proper goals regarding individuals with disabilities are to assure equality of opportunity, full participation, independent living, and economic self-sufficiency for such individuals." Section 2 (a) (8) of the ADA (29 U.S.C. 12101 (a) (8)).

[12]Yelin, E. H. "The Employment of People With and Without Disabilities in an Age of Insecurity." *Annals of the American Academy of Political and Social Science* 549 (January 1997): 117–128.

[13]Mashaw, J. L. et al., eds., *Disability, Cash Benefits and Work,* Kalamazoo, MI: W. E. Upjohn Institute for Employment Research, 1996.

[14]Berkowitz, E. D. "Implications for Income Maintenance Policy," in *Implementing the Americans with Disabilities Act,* West, J., ed. Cambridge, MA: Milbank Memorial Fund and Blackwell Publishers, 1996.

[15]Rupp, K., and Stapleton, D., eds. *Growth in Disability Benefits: Explanations and Policy Implications,* Kalamazoo, MI: W. E. Upjohn Institute for Employment Research, 1998.

[16]Batavia, A. I. 1998. "Unsustainable Growth: Preserving Disability Programs for Americans with Disabilities," in *Growth in Disability Benefits: Explanations and Policy Implications,* K. Rupp and D. Stapleton, eds. Kalamazoo, MI: W. E. Upjohn Institute for Employment Research, 1998, 325–336.

[17]Batavia, A. I., and Parker, S. "From Disability Rolls to Payrolls: A Proposal for Social Security Program Reform." *Journal of Disability Policy Studies* 6(1) (August 1995): 73–86.

[18]Some disability rights advocates and researchers would argue that by focusing on individual factors, we are in fact "blaming the victims." Although I agree that the primary focus should not be on the

individual, individual factors cannot be ignored in identifying and addressing the problems that are keeping people with disabilities from achieving their objectives. The fact is that some individuals with disabilities, like some members of any population, either generally or on occasion act in an irresponsible manner, and this personal behavior can have negative effects on them and others. For example, a large percentage of people with disabilities who use government-sponsored paratransit services neglect to inform the service when they need to cancel a trip, thereby causing a waste of valuable resources and inconvenience for other passengers and drivers. Although it is fashionable in some circles to blame such behavior on society, based on the premise that these are socially oppressed individuals, ultimately they (just like nondisabled individuals) must be held accountable for their own behavior.

[19]Batavia, A. I. "Health Care Reform and People with Disabilities," *Health Affairs* 12(1) (Spring 1993): 40–57.

[20]Feldblum, C. "The Employment Sector: Medical Inquiries, Reasonable Accommodation, and Health Insurance" in *Implementing the Americans with Disabilities Act,* West, J., ed. Cambridge, MA: Milbank Memorial Fund and Blackwell Publishers, 1996.

[21]Section 501 (c) (1) and (2) state that the ADA "shall not be construed to prohibit or restrict [insurers, HMOs and other entities that administer benefit plans] from underwriting risks, classifying risks, or administering" such risks that are based on or not inconsistent with state law. On the other hand, Section 501(c) also states that these sections "shall not be used as a subterfuge to evade the purposes of title I and III."

[22]Batavia, A. I., DeJong, G. and McKnew, L. "Toward a National Personal Assistance Program: The Independent Living Model of Long-Term Care for Persons with Disabilities." *Journal of Health Politics, Policy and Law* 16(3) (1991): 525–547.

[23]*Tommy Olmstead, Commissioner, Georgia Department of Human Resources, et al. v. L.C.,* 98–536, 119 S. Ct. 617 (cert. granted, December 14, 1998).

[24]Recently, the U.S. Court of Appeals for the Second Circuit ruled in *Staron v. MacDonald's Corp.,* 51 F.3d 353 (April 4, 1995), that the ADA can be used to protect people who are particularly vulnerable to cigarette smoke.

[25]Burkhauser, R. V. "Post-ADA: Are People with Disabilities Expected to Work?" *Annals of the American Academy of Political and Social Science,* 549 (January 1997): 71–83.

[26]Burkhauser, R. V., and Daly, M. C. "The Potential Impact on the Employment of People with Disabilities," in *Implementing the Americans with Disabilities Act,* West, J., ed. Cambridge, MA: Milbank Memorial Fund and Blackwell Publishers, 1996.

[27]Baldwin, Marjorie L. "Can the ADA Achieve its Employment Goals." *Annals of the American Academy of Political and Social Science* 549 (January 1997): 37–52.

[28]Moreover, many people with disabilities who were of working age prior to the enactment of the ADA do not have competitive work records.

[29]Batavia, A. I. "Health Care, Personal Assistance, and Assistive Technology: Are In-Kind Benefits Key to Independence or Dependence for People with Disabilities?" in *Disability, Cash Benefits and Work,* J. L. Mashaw, et al., eds., Kalamazoo, MI: W. E. Upjohn Institute for Employment Research, 1996.

[30]DeJong, G., Batavia, A. I., and Griss, R. "America's Neglected Health Minority: Working-Age Persons with Disabilities." *Milbank Quarterly* 67 (Suppl. 2, Part 2) (1989): 311–351.

[31]Kronick, R. Dreyfus, T., Lee, L., and Zhou, Z. "Diagnostic Risk Adjustment for Medicaid: The Disability Payment System." *Health Care Financing Review* 17(3)(Spring 1996): 7–33.

ADA Title III
A Fragile Compromise

RUTH COLKER

Title III of the Americans with Disabilities Act[1] (ADA Title III) protects individuals with disabilities from discrimination at places of public accommodation.[2] Such discrimination takes the form of outright exclusion, policies and eligibility criteria that have a disparate impact against individuals with disabilities, and physical barriers that impede accessibility.[3]

Although the employment title of the ADA (Title I)[4] has received the most public attention, ADA Title III is equally important, because it applies to all individuals with disabilities—irrespective of whether they are sufficiently qualified to engage in employment.[5] Because the definition of "public accommodation" under ADA Title III is broad,[6] this title provides accessibility and nondiscrimination at entities that individuals visit on a frequent basis in order to obtain the basic essentials such as food, lodging and health care, as well as at entities that individuals visit to enhance the quality of their lives, such as restaurants, hotels and places of amusement and recreation. ADA Title III therefore plays an enormously important role in the integration of individuals with disabilities into society in general.

However, the broad coverage of ADA Title III came at a price—as part of a "fragile compromise."[7] In return for a broad list of covered entities, civil rights advocates agreed to a limited set of remedies under ADA Title III. When private parties bring suit under ADA Title III, they are able to obtain only injunctive relief and are *not* able to obtain monetary damages.[8] This compromise was modeled after an agreement reached in 1964 when Title II of the Civil Rights Act of 1964[9] (CRA Title II) was enacted to prohibit racial discrimination at places of public accommodation. CRA Title II, like ADA Title III, permits private individuals to seek only injunctive relief.[10] CRA Title II, however, unlike ADA Title III, covers only a few categories of public accommodations.[11] Proponents of the ADA were therefore able to obtain broader coverage than previous civil rights activists had been able to obtain under CRA Title II, but they were not able to move beyond the limited set of remedies enacted under CRA Title II.

In order to seek broader remedies under ADA Title III than under CRA Title II, disability rights advocates argued for Congress to consider a different legislative model—the Fair Housing Act (FHA)—which prohibits discrimination in the sale or rental of housing to any buyer or renter. Enacted in 1968 to prohibit housing discrimination on the basis of race, the FHA has always contained compensatory and punitive damages as a potential source for relief. In 1988, when the act was amended to provide protection against discrimination for individuals with disabilities,[12] it was also amended to remove the cap on punitive damages[13] and to provide for *mandatory* enforcement by the Attorney General (AG) when the Secretary of Housing and Urban Development (HUD) "determines that

A longer version of this essay appeared in the *Berkeley Journal of Employment and Labor Law.*

reasonable cause exists to believe that a discriminatory housing practice has occurred or is about to occur,"[14] and a complainant chooses judicial rather than administrative relief. Senator Harkin argued that the FHA compensatory and punitive damages remedial scheme rather than the CRA Title II injunctive remedial scheme was appropriate for ADA Title III.[15] In the end, however, the limited relief available under CRA Title II prevailed in a spirit of compromise.[16]

When legislation is being considered by Congress, compromises are an essential ingredient of enactment. In this context, ADA proponents traded expanded coverage for limited relief. This compromise, however, was reached as part of a "one step at a time" approach, leaving to another day the question of whether this limited scheme of relief would be effective. Because CRA Title II has been relatively effective in vindicating the rights of racial minorities who are denied access to public accommodations, this compromise seemed a reasonable one in 1990 when the ADA was enacted. Proponents of ADA Title III could claim victory because they obtained broader coverage than exists under CRA Title II with equivalent remedies.

This time—ten years after the enactment of ADA Title III—is a good moment to assess the success of this compromise. I will argue that ADA Title III has been less successful than was originally hoped. Due in part to the limited avenue for relief,[17] ADA Title III has spawned few lawsuits. In addition, courts have rendered exceedingly narrow interpretations of their already-limited authority to grant injunctive relief. The second problem feeds into the first problem. By narrowly interpreting an already-limited remedy, the courts have further reduced plaintiffs' incentives to bring a lawsuit under ADA Title III. Although state law can sometimes serve as a remedial gap-filler in such situations, that result has not occurred under ADA Title III. Many states passed their own civil rights laws subsequent to the passage of CRA Title II with broader remedial provisions,[18] but few states have used the passage of ADA Title III as impetus for broadening their state antidiscrimination remedies in the area of disability discrimination. It has only been ten years since the passage of the ADA, and further state legislative action may be forthcoming, but there is little reason to believe that further "filling the gap" will occur under ADA Title III. State law remedies in this area are very limited and are sometimes contained in antiquated statutes which are in serious need of updating, yet little legislative activity is occurring in this area of the law on the state level.[19]

The lack of success under ADA Title III has been hidden by the seeming success of the plaintiff in the first major ADA Title III case—Sidney Abbott.[20] Sidney Abbott brought suit under ADA Title III when Dr. Randon Bragdon refused to fill her cavity in his office in September 1994. Four and a half years later, the courts have concluded that Abbott is an individual with a disability and that she is entitled to injunctive relief under ADA Title III.[21]

Sidney Abbott is one of only a few plaintiffs who have been able to obtain effective relief for a violation of ADA Title III.[22] Her ability to obtain relief, however, can be attributed more to the fact that both of the parties were ideologically committed to having a court resolve this matter than to the design of the statute. Dr. Randon Bragdon had made his views on not treating patients with HIV publicly known and apparently welcomed a legal challenge to his position. Abbott was a "test" plaintiff who visited Dr. Bragdon's office knowing that he would refuse to fill her cavity in his office. Abbott needed no financial incentive to file suit and, in truth, could have readily obtained dental treatment elsewhere. Abbott was entitled to $10,000 in damages under Maine law,[23] but she decided not to pursue that relief because "the lawsuit was filed on principle."[24] Although Dr. Bragdon could have challenged her standing to bring suit on justiciability grounds, he never made that claim, most likely because he desired a decision on the merits.[25] Both parties therefore actually sought—and received—a decision on the merits. Because the case was primarily one of principle, injunctive relief was satisfactory to Abbott.

The little academic discussion that has occurred on ADA Title III has criticized the Justice Department for preferring education to litigation and for not vigorously enforcing the title.[26] Although I agree that Title III poses enforcement problems, it is wrong to blame the Justice Department for the enforcement problems. Enforcement problems with Title III exist because of the limited relief available under the statute coupled with courts' narrow interpretations of that relief provision. Rather than criticizing the Department of Justice for a lack of enforcement, a review of the settlements that Justice Department attorneys have entered suggests that the department should be applauded for settlements that often go beyond the requirements of the statutory language.

In the first section of this essay, I will discuss the relief available under ADA Title III, CRA Title II and the FHA. In the second section, I will examine the existing evidence of the effectiveness of ADA Title III and in particular, judicial outcomes, verdict outcomes and settlement outcomes. I will argue that this evidence indicates that Title III suffers from underenforcement due to the limited range of remedies that courts have construed are available. In the third section, I will discuss the limited remedies currently available under state law to show that state law is not currently "filling the gaps" in remedies under ADA Title III as has historically occurred under CRA Title II. In the final section, I will conclude that the current trend of underenforcement of ADA Title III should cause us to consider enhancing remedies at the state and federal level.

LEGISLATIVE HISTORY

The First Bill

The Americans with Disabilities Act was first introduced as H.R. 4498[27] by Representative Coelho and as S. 2345 [28] by Senator Weicker in 1988. These bills were the outgrowth of the work on the National Council on the Handicapped, an independent federal agency whose 15 members were appointed by President Reagan and confirmed by the Senate.[29]

These two initial bills contained much broader antidiscrimination coverage than the bill that was eventually enacted as the Americans with Disabilities Act.[30] The original bill was not divided into titles as was the final bill. Instead, it had sections banning different types of discriminatory activities. Section 4 prohibited discrimination in employment. Section 5 prohibited discrimination in access to services or programs, prohibited architectural and other barriers, and made it unlawful to: (1) refuse to grant reasonable accommodations, (2) impose disqualifying selection criteria, and (3) engage in associational discrimination because of someone's relationship to an individual with a disability.[31]

The original bill contained much stronger language than the ultimately enacted ADA.[32] Most importantly for the purposes of the present discussion, the enforcement section of the original bill was much stronger than the enforcement provision in the finally enacted ADA because it provided for monetary relief.[33] The exhaustion of administrative enforcement procedures was required only for actions involving employment discrimination. Claims of discrimination involving barriers to access at public accommodations could be brought by private citizens for monetary damages. In contrast, the bill that was finally enacted permitted private parties to obtain only injunctive relief[34]—a weaker remedy.

Weakening of Legislation

Even on the day when the ADA was first introduced, Senator Dole, a key sponsor of the ADA, spoke in favor of the need for such a bill but also stated that compromises were needed which would weaken the bill.[35]

Subcommittees of the United States Senate held hearings nearly a year later on S. 933, a modified version of the ADA which was introduced in the next Congress by Senator Harkin. Senator Harkin, who was the key sponsor of the ADA in the Senate, did not immediately acquiesce to Senator Dole's views about the need to limit the provision on relief. Senate Bill 933, which Senator Harkin introduced in the Senate on May 9, 1989, provided that the enforcement scheme for the FHA (which included both compensatory and punitive damages) should be available to redress discrimination at places of public accommodation.[36]

Attorney General Thornburgh spoke in favor of the new bill, but made it clear that ADA Title III needed serious revision to limit its scope and protection. His objections were threefold: (1) that businesses could not make accurate predictions of the types of modifications required because the "readily achievable" compliance standard was not well defined and did not preexist under Section 504; (2) the remedies for violations of ADA Title III should parallel the remedies already existing under CRA Title II rather than the broader remedies existing in the FHA; and (3) the scope of businesses covered by ADA Title III should be narrowed so as not to impose undue hardship on small businesses.[37] Most of these suggested amendments were adopted before enactment of the final bill. The term "readily achievable" was retained but was defined as meaning "easily accomplishable and able to be carried out without much difficulty or expense."[38] Explicit factors, such as the size and financial resources of the covered entity were added as factors to be considered when determining whether an accommodation was readily achievable, to make clear that the burden on small businesses would be minimal.[39]

Despite his recognition of the need for strong remedies, Senator Harkin capitulated on the remedies issue five months later, making it clear that this compromise was necessary to attain a bipartisan bill with a broad scope of coverage:

> Senator Kennedy and I are committed to this compromise. We will oppose all weakening amendments. We will also oppose any amendments that are intended to strengthen the substitute, if these amendments do not have the support of the administration and Senator Dole. We are pleased that the administration and Senator Dole share this commitment. We hope that other Senators will understand how fragile this compromise is and will support it. *The major component of the compromise was the agreement by the chief Senate sponsors to cutback the remedies included in the original bill in exchange for a broad scope of coverage under the public accommodations title of the bill; in other words to extend protections to most commercial establishments large and small and open to the public.* We would thus consider any amendment that pertains to either of these two aspects of the legislation an amendment designed to destroy this fragile compromise.[40]

In the name of a "fragile compromise," the remedies underlying ADA Title III were limited in exchange for an expansive list of commercial entities covered by the statute. The compromises accepted during passage of the ADA are not unusual. Enforcement was traded for scope of coverage. The participants in this compromise recognized, however, that the ADA would need to be reevaluated over time to see if it was effective. Attorney General Thornburgh recommended a "cautious" approach, with continuing discussion and dialogue over time to see if a purely injunctive strategy would work.[41] This chapter therefore next examines the effectiveness of the ADA Title III remedies in light of our first decade of enforcement experience.

Thus the scope of coverage and strength of enforcement of ADA Title III were limited during the legislative process. The argument advanced for weakening the remedial scheme was that injunctive relief had proven effective under CRA Title II. Therefore there was no need for other relief, such as monetary relief. Nonetheless, proponents of the ADA were concerned whether injunctive relief would be effective.

Limitations of Civil Rights Act Analogies

A fuller understanding of our experience under the civil rights laws should cause us to question the assumption that injunctive relief serves the objectives of ADA Title III. The scope of CRA Title II is narrower than the scope of ADA Title III. In addition, there is a broader array of state law remedies to supplement CRA Title II remedies than there are state law remedies to supplement ADA Title III remedies. Even assuming the effectiveness of the remedial scheme of CRA Title II, there are many reasons to doubt that a similar remedial scheme would be effective under ADA Title III. A better analogy for ADA Title III is found by looking at the FHA. With the passage of time, Congress concluded that broad compensatory and punitive damages are required to provide effective remedies under the FHA (along with an ambitious government enforcement scheme). The limited remedies passed under CRA Title II were part of a fragile compromise in order to enhance passage of the statute in a bipartisan atmosphere. To date, these remedies have not proven effective under ADA Title III.

Title II of the Civil Rights Act of 1964. Although CRA Title VII has received the most legal attention in the past several decades, it was the need for CRA Title II that was most vividly in the public's imagination at the time the Civil Rights Act was passed. Four black students who were refused cups of coffee in a Woolworth's store in Greensboro, North Carolina on February 1, 1960, began a series of sit-ins and civil disobedience that formed the backdrop for the passage of the Civil Rights Act.[42]

Senator Weicker emphasized the analogy to those four black students in his opening remarks as sponsor of the ADA. Senator Weicker could also have described the analogy to CRA Title II in another way—that ADA Title III, like its counterpart in the Civil Rights Act of 1964, was watered down during the legislative process to enhance its potential for enactment.

In the original civil rights bill proposed to Congress by President John F. Kennedy, the scope of protection under CRA Title II was somewhat broader than what was ultimately enacted. The original bill prohibited discrimination in public accommodations, including all places of lodging, eating, and amusement and other retail or service establishments.[43] That bill was modified many times before ultimate passage. Most importantly, as a result of the McCulloch Justice Department compromise,[44] it specifically exempted private clubs and failed explicitly to cover "any retail shop, department store, market, drugstore, gasoline station, or other public places which keep goods for sale."[45] Like ADA Title III, the final CRA Title II listed specific entities that are covered, such as hotels, restaurants and places of entertainment, rather than including a more expansive generic definition of places open to the public. Although the rationale for limiting CRA Title II to those entities was never fully explained in the legislative history, one comment by Representative "Judge" Smith may have captured some of the sentiment at the time. Referring to the fact that a chiropodist whose office was in a hotel would be covered by CRA Title, he is reported to have made a "shrill outburst": "If I were cutting corns," he cried, "I would want to know whose feet I would have to be monkeying around with. I would want to know whether they smelled good or bad."[46]

Civil rights proponents, by contrast, saw no reason to exempt retail or service establishments from CRA Title II. For example, Representative Robert W. Kastenmeier criticized the limited scope of CRA Title II in his additional views that he filed as part of the House Judiciary Committee Report.[47]

Similarly, in a stinging concurrence in one of the few constitutional cases to discuss the right of a property owner to have the state enforce his desire to exclude blacks from a restaurant, Justice Douglas argued in *Bell v. Maryland*[48] that the Constitution permits no discrimination of this sort in any place of public accommodation.[49]

Ironically, the day that Justice Douglas issued the concurring opinion in *Bell v. Maryland* was also the day that the Civil Rights Act of 1964 returned to the Senate for deliberation. By then, it was far too late to consider any amendments to expand the act's coverage to encompass the reach of what Justice Douglas considered constitutional. The bill was able to become law two weeks later only as a result of extraordinary political maneuvering.[50] Political rather than constitutional concerns resulted in the limited scope of CRA Title II. Without the McCulloch Justice Department compromise, the Civil Rights Act of 1964 would never have become law.

Not only did CRA Title II, as enacted in 1964, not cover retail and personal service establishments, but the act has never been amended to provide broader protection. Although state law prohibits discrimination in retail stores in most states, seven states (Alabama, Florida, Georgia, Mississippi, North Carolina, South Carolina and Texas) have no such statute.[51]

Another issue that had to be confronted when the CRA was considered was the question of what kinds of remedies should be enacted. Civil rights activists had examined possible enforcement schemes. In a book published in 1959, civil rights activist Jack Greenberg observed that three enforcement schemes are generally possible: "criminal prosecution, private civil suit for damages or injunction by an aggrieved person, and administrative or injunctive implementation by public officials."[52] He considered criminal enforcement to be problematic because of the high burden of proof and the fact that "[t]rial has to be by jury, which may very likely be as prejudiced as the defendant."[53] Civil suits for damages, he argued, are similarly problematic because of the problems of jury trials and the costs of engaging counsel. His preferred mechanism was use of an administrative agency or attorney general which would vigorously enforce antidiscrimination laws at public expense and without jury trials.[54] Other commentators argued that the token amounts that are awarded in actions for civil damages may not act as an effective deterrent;[55] whereas injunctive relief might be effective insofar as it would have a continuing effect, thereby permitting punishment for contempt if the injunctive order was violated.[56] Based on the experience with states that used criminal penalties and private civil actions for damages, some commentators argued "that neither criminal prosecutions nor private civil actions for damages appreciably decrease the incidence of discrimination or give its victims an adequate legal remedy."[57] They emphasized the importance of injunctive relief with possible enforcement by an administrative agency,[58] although some commentators suggested that there could be an option for a private civil action for damages.[59]

The Civil Rights Act generally reflected the approach recommended by Greenberg and other commentators, although each title of the Civil Rights Act utilized somewhat different enforcement schemes. CRA Title VII (the employment discrimination title) created a private right of action for make-whole relief and a modest administrative enforcement mechanism.[60] These remedies were enhanced in 1972 to create a stronger administrative enforcement structure,[61] and in 1991 to create the possibility of compensatory or punitive damages.[62] CRA Title II (the public accommodation title) created a private right of action for preventive or injunctive relief with the possibility of intervention by the attorney general if a complaining party could certify to the court that the case was of general public importance.[63] However, even when the attorney general intervened, CRA Title II did not provide for any kind of monetary damages.[64] Moreover, unlike CRA Title VII, the remedies have not been enhanced since 1964. And unlike the FHA, the intervention on the part of the attorney general is entirely discretionary.

Nevertheless, CRA Title II has proven to be a relatively effective tool in eliminating discrimination in places of public accommodation. Its effect has been twofold. First, the availability of structural injunctions has led to large-scale changes in the way public accommodations conduct business.[65] Second, state law has filled the remedial gap by providing compensatory damages and more expansive statutory coverage than CRA Title II.[66] Thus an ability to effectively enforce an antidiscrimination principle in the area of public accommodations may be attributable to the partnership of state antidiscrimination laws and CRA Title II rather than attributable to CRA Title II alone.

The effectiveness of banning race discrimination at places of public accommodation may have also occurred through another important statutory vehicle—Section 1981.[67] Several courts have concluded that private plaintiffs can sue for infringement of contract under Section 1981 to obtain monetary damages when they are denied access to or discriminated against by public accommodations.[68] That cause of action is not available in the disability area, however, because Section 1981 applies only to race discrimination.[69]

In assessing the performance of ADA Title III, one needs to ask whether structural injunctions and supplemental state or federal law remedies are likely in this area. Given the narrow way that many courts have interpreted their remedial powers under ADA Title III, structural injunctions appear unlikely. Moreover, the ten-year record of limited state law amendments suggests that enhanced relief at the state law level is unlikely. It may be that an amendment to the ADA is the only possible way to improve the enforcement of ADA Title III, since Section 1981 is not available to enhance the penalties in the disability area.

Fair Housing Act Amendments of 1988. Another analogy was also available when ADA Title III was being debated—the Fair Housing Act (FHA). As enacted in 1968, the FHA provided that plaintiffs could recover "actual damages and not more than $1,000 punitive damages, together with court costs and reasonable attorney fees in the case of a prevailing plaintiff"[70] to remedy race discrimination in the rental or sale of housing. The act was amended in 1988 to prohibit disability-based discrimination and to eliminate the cap on punitive damages.[71] As noted in the House Judiciary Committee Report section-by-section analysis, the limitation on punitive damages was eliminated because the committee concluded "that the limit on punitive damages served as a major impediment to imposing an effective deterrent on violators and a disincentive for private persons to bring suits under existing law."[72] Thus, although the FHA always contained a more ambitious range of remedies than ADA Title III, these remedies were broadened even further when disability discrimination in housing became unlawful.

During the debate over the ADA, Senator Harkin questioned why the FHA was not the appropriate analogy for ADA Title III, rather than CRA Title II.[73] The FHA contains important parallels to ADA Title III. Whereas the FHA covers the rental of apartments to individuals with disabilities, ADA Title III covers the rental of hotel rooms to people with disabilities.[74] Yet under current law, if a rental agent refuses to rent a house to an individual with a disability, he or she is subject to the full set of remedies provided under the FHA, while if a motel owner refused to rent a motel room to that same individual, the individual would be able to obtain only injunctive relief.

It is arguable that housing discrimination has longer-term consequences for individual tenants than does discrimination at a place of temporary lodging, and thus stiffer penalties are appropriate for the former rather than the latter. But the lack of accessibility at places of public accommodation serves to impede the mobility of many individuals with disabilities. Given the nature of our highly mobile society, such impediments have daily effects on the basic requirements of living (e.g., grocery stores), and broader effects on the ability of an individual to work and travel (e.g., hotels and restaurants). Being confined to one's home due to the inaccessibility of the outside community can be as significant as having difficulty obtaining housing itself. Moreover, even if housing discrimination is somewhat more significant than discrimination at places of public accommodation, it is questionable whether the degree of difference is sufficiently significant to justify such widely divergent relief.

In deciding which analogy makes more sense—CRA Title II or the FHA—we must consider the change in social consensus since the passage of the Civil Rights Act in 1964. The Civil Rights Act was passed after what has been termed the "longest debate" due to a lengthy filibuster in the United States Senate. CRA Title II was also passed at a time when civil rights advocates had serious reservations about jury trials for victims of race discrimination. Those fears are largely unfounded today and, in any event, are not particularly relevant to the law of disability discrimination.[75] Jury trials are now commonplace under the Civil Rights Act of 1964 and state antidiscrimination laws.

By contrast, the Fair Housing Act Amendments of 1988 were passed by a bipartisan Congress. The remedies provided reflected the strong political and social commitment to making affordable housing available without discrimination on the basis of disability. The ADA was passed only two years later, again by a strongly bipartisan Congress. Although the scope of entities covered was narrowed during the legislative debate—as the scope was narrowed during the legislative debate of CRA Title II—the list of entities ultimately covered under the ADA was much more comprehensive than the list covered by CRA Title II. Our emerging social consensus about the inappropriateness of discrimination is strong enough to justify a more stringent set of remedies for both race and disability discrimination than in 1964.

Nonetheless, the proponents of the ADA were never able to move the discussion of remedies beyond that of injunctive relief. They were stuck with the limited remedies that had been negotiated at another time—1964—and in another context—race discrimination—where the fear of jury trials was particularly strong. Senator Harkin understood the importance of ensuring that the Fair Housing Act remedies rather than the CRA Title II remedies would be available under the ADA. The bill introduced by Senator Harkin in the Senate Committee on Labor and Human Resources contained the FHA remedies for violations of the ADA's public accommodation section (which was eventually enacted as ADA Title III).

But Senator Harkin compromised in order to attain bipartisan support of the ADA. He nonetheless forecast that the limited remedial scheme of ADA Title III would lead to few lawsuits and underenforcement of the statute's mandate. Attorney General Thornburgh

seemingly agreed that there may be few lawsuits but predicted that there would be sufficient voluntary compliance to enforce the statute's mandate. The experience under the
FHA, however, was that even a remedial scheme providing actual damages and limited
punitive damages was insufficient to enforce the mandate of the act. Limited remedial
schemes therefore need to be periodically revisited to see if they are effective.[76]

Effectiveness of Remedies

Despite the limited scope of relief available under CRA Title II, there is far less discrimination on the basis of race at public accommodations today than there was in 1964. One no
longer finds "Whites Only" signs on the doors of restaurants. The problems today are what
we might call "second-order" problems of discrimination—lesser service rather than a
denial of entrance. Thus, in one of the most well publicized public accommodation cases
in recent years, a Denny's Restaurant in Maryland allegedly failed to serve six African-
American Secret Service agents while the white agents were served second and third help-
ings. Two class action lawsuits were filed on behalf of 294,537 plaintiffs under federal and
state law, with a reported settlement two years later of $46 million and the discharge of
more than a hundred employees for discriminatory behavior.[77] Denny's relatively prompt
attempt to settle this lawsuit reflects the changing moral climate that has occurred since
1964. It is no longer good business, especially for a restaurant chain, to have the image of
excluding African-American customers.

The second-order problems in the area of race discrimination are being redressed
through a combination of state and federal law. Federal law gave the plaintiffs authority to
seek a structural injunction against Denny's, while state law provided plaintiffs the opportunity to seek compensatory relief. The $46 million price tag in the Denny's case was the
result of broader protection available under state than federal antidiscrimination law. In
addition, Section 1981 can be used to enhance the penalty when individuals are denied
service because of race.[78]

By contrast, the injunctive relief remedial scheme of ADA Title III has not been sufficiently effective in eliminating barriers to access for individuals with disabilities. Physical
barriers such as steps—which preclude entrance by people who use wheelchairs—and the
lack of Telecommunication Devices for the Deaf (TDD)[79] services at hotels—which impede the traveling opportunities of people who have hearing impairments—are only two
commonplace examples of exclusion on the basis of disability by many places of public
accommodation. Remedying violations of ADA Title III is different from remedying violations of CRA Title II. An apt analogy would be a case in which a restaurant refuses service
because of the physical appearance of an individual with a disability. In the more typical
case, however, the restaurant has effectively denied service by having a step at the front
door. The step may have predated passage of the ADA, and was probably not constructed
with the intention of excluding a category of potential customers. In order to comply with
the ADA, the restaurant must take the proactive step of removing the barrier which, in
turn, entails a cost for the restaurant. Under CRA Title II, it arguably makes economic
sense to ban discrimination, because a restaurant, for example, would ultimately incur
more business if it began to serve African-Americans.[80] That fact may also be true under
ADA Title III. A restaurant that can serve customers who use wheelchairs will also attain
increased business, not only from individuals with disabilities, but also from the friends
and family of the individuals with disabilities. But the increased service will not result until
after an initial expenditure of money on the part of the restaurant owner. The threat of
injunctive relief is not sufficient to create compliance, because compliance requires a more

proactive step than merely removing a "Whites Only" sign and may entail what is perceived to be a significant expense.[81]

Further, injunctive relief has been ineffective under ADA Title III because of courts' narrow interpretations of their power to issue such relief. Courts have repeatedly concluded that they lacked jurisdiction to hear ADA Title III cases because the plaintiffs' individual instances of discrimination did not create standing to seek injunctive relief.[82] Many of the ADA Title III cases have involved a failure to provide medical services to individuals with disabilities, particularly individuals with AIDS. In such a situation, the plaintiff is likely to file suit against the doctor who provided treatment while also seeking treatment from another physician. Because the plaintiff obtained treatment from another physician, the courts reason that the case is moot since the injury is unlikely to recur and compensatory relief is not available. Thus the courts have concluded that they are powerless to order any relief even though a flagrant violation of the ADA may have occurred. When a court can issue no relief, it often cannot maintain jurisdiction over the case; it must dismiss the case or, if there is a supplemental state action, remand the case to state court.[83]

Courts that have applied mootness doctrine to ADA Title III cases have applied the doctrine too stringently and have arguably misconstrued the nature of these Title III actions. ADA Title III cases do not involve extreme situations in which only a plaintiff's criminal conduct could cause future discrimination to occur. Instead, these are cases in which plaintiffs represent a class of litigants who repeatedly face instances of discrimination as a result of their own voluntary and lawful conduct. Although Bragdon and other ADA plaintiffs may not be at risk of physical harm as a result of defendants' conduct, they have the ability to put themselves in the position of having to face unlawful conduct in the future. Sidney Abbott *could* seek medical services from Dr. Bragdon in the future.[84] And it is unlikely that Dr. Bragdon's refusal to treat patients with HIV infection in his office would change absent a court-ordered injunction, especially since he had taken a strong public position concerning his right not to treat patients with HIV. The choice of service provider belongs to Abbott; the right to choose is reinforced in the ADA. The choice of service provider is hers under the ADA; an injunction would maintain the right to lawful choice. To preserve that right, an injunction is absolutely essential as a remedy.

ADA TITLE III RESULTS

The most significant impact of ADA Title III's limited scope of relief is probably the small number of cases that have been filed under that title. In an earlier article,[85] I concluded that the courts of appeals had issued decisions in 475 cases under ADA Title I (the employment title) from June 1992 to July 1998. By contrast, I have been able to locate only 25 ADA Title III appellate decisions for the same time period. (Only 5 percent of the reported appellate cases are, therefore, ADA Title III cases.)

Twenty-five appellate decisions are too few to provide a clear sense of how effective ADA Title III has been in remedying discrimination problems. I have therefore tried to supplement these results with other kinds of results—verdicts and settlements. The verdict data is discussed below; the settlement data is discussed after the verdict data. The verdict and settlement data suggest that Title III may be effective, particularly when supplemental state actions are available. It also may be effective when the federal government brings suit and seeks broad relief. But the verdict and settlement data still reflect small sample sizes, suggesting that ADA Title III's effectiveness may be largely dependent on voluntary compliance rather than litigation. Attorney General Thornburgh may have been correct to suggest that incentives to pursue litigation would be diminished through a limited remedial scheme, but it is hard to imagine that voluntary enforcement is effective when private parties can calculate that it is highly unlikely that any enforcement action for noncompliance would be brought against them. Twenty-five appellate decisions is quite disproportionate to the 475 cases decided under ADA Title I. While 475 cases may be considered excessive, 25 would appear to be too few.

Appellate Litigation Results

I was able to find only 25 appellate decisions under ADA Title III that were reported on Westlaw. Of those 25 decisions, defendants prevailed in the lower court through dismissal or summary judgment in 18 cases (72 percent). After the appellate process was completed, defendants still prevailed in 18 of 25 cases (although the mix of cases changed through six reversals). Although this result is a prodefendant outcome, it is less prodefendant in its orientation than the comparable results I have found under ADA Title I. Under ADA Title I, defendants prevail in 94 percent of the cases from which appeals were taken (448 of 475). After the appeal process was completed, defendants continued to prevail in 82 percent of the cases from which appeals were taken (389 of 475). In the Title I area, the appeals courts appear to have played a modestly corrective role, lessening the defendant-win rate from 94 percent to 82 percent. Apparently, plaintiffs have a somewhat easier time prevailing under ADA Title III than under ADA Title I but are not very inclined even to attempt litigation under ADA Title III.

Verdict Data. The verdict data confirms that plaintiffs are unlikely to sue under ADA Title III. Verdicts are rarely reported in published decisions, so they are not a part of the set of cases discussed above. Although not all verdicts are readily available, there are verdict services in various regions of the country which report verdict data. Westlaw and Lexis report the results from many of these services.

I used these verdict services to locate all ADA cases reported by September 28, 1998. I was able to locate 109 verdicts in ADA cases heard in either state or federal court. Of these 109 cases, there were only 16 ADA Title III cases. (ADA Title III cases were therefore about 16 percent of all ADA verdicts.) Seven of these cases were brought in federal court and nine were brought in state court. Plaintiffs were successful in four of seven federal court actions and four of nine state court actions, with an overall success rate of eight of 16. The success rates for Title I and III actions were comparable. In Title I actions, plaintiffs were successful in 27 of 51 actions, and in Title III actions, plaintiffs were successful in 17 of 39 actions. These figures are consistent with what the judicial expectations model would suggest. Cases are most likely to go to trial when both parties estimate that they have about a 50 percent chance of prevailing. Very strong and very weak cases should settle, since the losing party should calculate that it is not economical to take the case to trial.

It is interesting to note the discrepancy between cases which go to a jury trial and are not appealed, and cases decided by the judge or jury which are appealed. Jury trials rarely occurred in the cases in my appellate sample. Most of the cases ended at a pretrial stage through the entry of summary judgment. In the cases which did *not* go to a jury, plaintiffs had a much lower chance of prevailing than in cases which did go to the jury. In an earlier article, I have hypothesized in the Title I context that judges are misusing the summary judgment device to avoid having potentially meritorious cases go to the jury.[86] These Title III statistics, although not as extreme as the Title I statistics, provide further confirmation for this hypothesis.

The Title III data also suggest that we need not be concerned about excessive jury awards if compensatory and punitive damages were available under ADA Title III. All of these ADA Title III cases also included a supplemental state law action in which compensatory or punitive damages were available, such as a negligence *per se* theory. The typical plaintiff suffered a serious injury as a result of faulty accessibility standards and therefore was eligible for damages under a negligence *per se* theory for a violation of a substantive standard (ADA) which led to an injury. Such plaintiffs typically received an award of about $10,000, although one plaintiff attained an award of $512,000 against a physician and a hospital for the failure to admit him to the hospital in violation of the ADA and other laws.[87] These awards reflected compensation for actual physical injury due to a failure to meet ADA Title III standards.

Very few of these cases involved what might be considered stigmatic harm due to a lack of accessibility. The only exception to this pattern was a case against Sunnyvale Town Center for failing to provide crosswalks and parking for individuals with disabilities at its mall.[88] The jury awarded a verdict for the plaintiff of $74,097 in economic damages and $160,000 in noneconomic damages. The case was then settled for $145,000 including costs.

These verdicts suggest that where plaintiffs have only a stigmatic claim of injury due to lack of accessibility but no physical injury, juries will tend to calculate their injury as relatively minor. If the ADA were amended to include a right to relief for compensatory damages, it is reasonable to conclude that this trend would continue.[89]

It is also important to recognize that the jury verdict cases almost always involve situations where the plaintiff suffered a physical injury as a result of the failure to comply with ADA standards. Few of these cases involved solely a lack of access. The purpose of ADA Title III, however, was to remedy the lack of access to places of public accommodation by individuals with disabilities. State tort law already provides relief where an individual becomes injured due to a negligent design feature. With the unavailability of compensatory damages, the pure lack-of-access cases are not going to juries. They are being decided exclusively by judges. And, unfortunately, the reported decision data suggest that judges are not as sympathetic to ADA Title III cases as are juries.

The lack of availability of compensatory damages therefore causes two results: (1) a limited availability for relief, and (2) judge rather than jury decisions. Not only do plaintiffs fail to obtain compensatory damages, but they often fail to prevail altogether before an unsympathetic judiciary. When CRA Title II was passed, the thinking about the judge/jury distinction was quite different. Civil rights proponents feared that white Southern juries might be unsympathetic to CRA Title II claims, so that the decision to permit only injunctive relief had the additional advantage of having the case not eligible for jury determination. The choice of permitting only injunctive relief under the law of race was considered by some civil rights advocates to be the best choice because of the problem of prejudiced juries.[90] By contrast, injunctive relief was considered to be more effective because "the expenses involved are borne by the government, a trial by a prejudiced jury is never necessary, and the remedy is of continuing effect, permitting punishment for contempt when the injunctive order to violated."[91]

Under ADA Title III, however, we usually have reason to come to the opposite conclusion, since the existing data show that juries are more likely to rule in favor of plaintiffs than are judges in bench trials.[92] The limitation to purely injunctive relief not only precludes plaintiffs from obtaining compensatory damages but also causes them to have their cases heard before judges rather than juries.

Settlements

One might argue that reported decision and verdict data offer an incomplete picture of ADA compliance because they do not include settlements. Settlement data are probably the hardest to acquire, since settlements are often not made public. Nonetheless, the Department of Justice (DOJ) reports its settlements on its Web site. The Web site indicates that the DOJ has attained settlements in 46 ADA Title III cases as of September 1998.

When the DOJ settles an ADA Title III case, it has leverage that is not available to private plaintiffs—it has the statutory authority to seek civil damages if it brings suit.[93] Private parties can also intervene in their cases to seek damages under state law. Despite this financial leverage, the DOJ obtained a significant civil fine only in one case of $50,000. Of the other 16 cases in which the DOJ obtained monetary settlements, the amounts ranged from $250 to $10,000. Two of the fines were in the form of gift certificates of $500 and $900.

A typical settlement involved claimants with mobility impairments who alleged that an existing facility was not accessible although accessibility was "readily achievable."[94] Often the case was coupled with a claim that the entity failed to provide an auxiliary aid. Twelve cases involved the "readily achievable" standard; only two cases involved the more lenient standard for new construction.[95]

The remedies obtained by the DOJ under the "readily achievable" standard for existing entities were often quite significant. For example, Comfort Inn agreed to remove barriers relating to parking, ramps and walkways; to replace emergency lights; to create accessible rest rooms; to lower restaurant cash registers; to provide a lift to the swimming pools; to create accessible drinking fountains; and to create accessible rooms and doorways at their motels throughout the country. Similarly, Friendly Ice Cream (which was also assessed a $50,000 fine) agreed to remove steps; widen doors; redesign vestibules and dining areas for wheelchairs; provide accessible parking, rest rooms and routes; install curb cuts; relocate telephones; and read menus to people with visual impairments at their stores throughout the country. There were also many cases with effective but inexpensive compliance, such as changing policies to permit service animals into an entity or changing policies about use of a driver's license as an exclusive form of identification.

While the DOJ settlements appear to be effective, they are few in number. Forty-six settlements in approximately six years of statutory enforcement reflects less than one settlement a month by an agency charged with national enforcement. Although it may be the case that DOJ can attain effective enforcement in the cases it prosecutes, it is unrealistic to expect that such efforts will have much impact on the pattern of denial of accommodation that may exist in the larger society. It is hard to believe that the kinds of general problems that DOJ found—inaccessible hotels and restaurants, improper service animal policies, and inappropriate photo identification policies—are isolated to those 46 entities.

Under the existing statutory scheme, DOJ enforcement is a theoretically important part of statutory compliance because the DOJ is settling the pure access cases that ADA Title III was designed to remedy. With the limited financial incentives to file suit for this kind of violation (when a physical injury has not occurred), it is unrealistic to expect the private bar to take many of these cases. Yet the DOJ has only a few attorneys assigned to national enforcement under ADA Title III. In considering the ineffectiveness of DOJ ADA Title III enforcement, it is helpful to make a comparison with the FHA. Under the FHA, if the Secretary of Housing determines that reasonable cause exists to believe that a discriminatory housing practice has occurred or is about to occur, the secretary is required to issue a charge on behalf of the aggrieved person for further enforcement proceedings by the attorney general. If the aggrieved individual elects a judicial remedy, then "the

Secretary shall authorize, and not later than 30 days after the election is made the Attorney General shall commence and maintain, a civil action on behalf of the aggrieved person in a United States district court seeking relief under this subsection."[96] By contrast, the aggrieved individual has the right to intervene in that lawsuit, thereby pursuing both a public and private cause of action at little expense to the aggrieved individual. Thus when Congress so desires, it knows how to make enforcement by the DOJ effective for the aggrieved individual.[97] The public enforcement opportunities under ADA Title III, by contrast, are quite limited, in part due to Congress's limited allocation of resources to DOJ enforcement.

It is important to remember that when CRA II was passed, individuals who were familiar with state enforcement efforts under state civil rights statutes noted the importance of an administrative enforcement scheme for civil rights laws to be effective.[98] Congress was not willing in 1964 to develop such an enforcement scheme for CRA II, but demonstrated its ability to create such an enforcement scheme for FHA in 1998. It is therefore disappointing to see Congress backpedal in 1990 and enact an administrative enforcement scheme that was obviously inadequate.

FILLING THE REMEDIAL GAP

It is arguable that despite the limited relief under ADA Title III, the ADA might spur states to pass or amend their own antidiscrimination laws to provide effective remedies. Some states do have broader remedial provisions under their racial nondiscrimination laws than Congress provided under CRA Title II, which have served as an impetus for lawsuits such as the case against Denny's.

Even states with a strong commitment to antidiscrimination in the disability arena have not amended their state statutes to provide more effective relief than is available under ADA Title III. For example, Maine amended its disability antidiscrimination statute in 1995 to parallel the scope of coverage under the federal ADA. It repealed and replaced the section defining "places of public accommodation" so that its scope of coverage was identical to the coverage under federal law.[99] But it left intact the relief provision already existing under Maine law for cases of discrimination brought against places of public accommodation. This provision caps relief at $10,000 for first-time offenders, $25,000 for second-time offenders, and $50,000 for third-time offenders.[100] While this relief is more generous than the relief available under the ADA, because the civil damages can be awarded directly to the victim of discrimination and are available without the intervention of the state attorney general, this relief is not a product of a deliberate attempt by the state to fill the enforcement gap under ADA Title III. The relief provisions found in the Maine antidiscrimination law *preceded* the enactment of the ADA. Thus the passage of the ADA had an impact on the substantive law of Maine—the scope of coverage—but no impact on the relief available to victims of discrimination at places of public accommodation.

State disability law on discrimination at places of public accommodation can be divided into three categories: (1) states which do not have a state law banning discrimination at places of public accommodation on the basis of disability; (2) states which have a statute which prohibits such discrimination, but provide narrow remedies such as purely injunctive relief or a modest fine under the criminal code; and (3) states which provide broader remedies than the ADA.

The following table summarizes the overall results:

TABLE 1: State Public Accommodation Statutes Prohibiting Disability Discrimination

Category One *(No prohibition)*	*Category Two* *(Narrow remedies)*	*Category Three* *(Broad remedies) (date adopted)*[106]
Oklahoma[101]	Alabama+(M)	**Arizona (1992)**
South Carolina [102]	Alaska($500 cap)	California (1976)
Tennessee[103]	Arkansas(M)	**Delaware (1996)**
Texas[104]	Colorado+($10–300)(M)	**Florida +(1992)**
Washington[105]	Connecticut($25–100)(M)	Hawaii (1988)
	District of Columbia	**Idaho + (compensatory:**
	Georgia+($100)(M)	**1990, punitive: 1997)**
	Iowa+(M)	Illinois (1989)
	Kansas+ ($2000 cap)(M)	Indiana (1978)
	Maryland($500–2500)	Kentucky (1974)
	Massachusetts++ ($2500 cap)(M)	Louisiana (1980)
	Mississippi +(M)($100)	Maine($10,000—$50,000 in
	Montana+(M)	penal damages)(1989)[107]
	Nebraska+(M)	Michigan(1980)
	New Hampshire(M)	Minnesota (1969)
	New Mexico+(M)	Missouri(1986)
	New York($100–$500) (M)	Nevada(1965)
	North Carolina	**New Jersey(1990)**
	North Dakota	Ohio(1987)
	Oregon($1,000 cap)	**South Dakota(1991)**
	Pennsylvania($500 cap) (M)	Vermont(1987)
	Rhode Island	Virginia(1985)
	Utah+(M)	Wisconsin(1975)
	West Virginia ($5000 cap)	
	Wyoming+ ($750 cap) (M)	

+Definition of disability includes individuals who have visual or auditory impairments or are otherwise physically disabled.
++Definition of disability includes individuals who are deaf, blind or have any physical or mental disability.
(M) Misdemeanor statute.
States in boldface amended their statutes in or after 1990 to include compensatory damages.

The 5 states in category one do not generally offer the protections of nondiscrimination at places of public accommodation except to provide the right to use a service animal at a place of public accommodation.[108] The 25 states in category two prohibit discrimination at public accommodations but provide narrow remedies. The most typical remedy provided in these states is a misdemeanor remedy; 17 of 25 states provide that violating their law against public accommodation is a misdemeanor. These misdemeanor statutes provide virtually no relief at all. As indicated in parenthesis after the statutes, the misdemeanor penalties range from $10 to $5,000. Many of these states also have very antiquated statutes which cover only a subcategory of individuals with disabilities. I have marked the states that limit their coverage to individuals with visual, hearing or other physical disabilities; 12 of the 25 states in category two fit this description.

The states with the most effective remedies are listed in category three. Twenty-one states provide some form of compensatory relief. Twenty-one of 51 states (including the District of Columbia) therefore provide for reasonably effective relief beyond what ADA Title III requires.

However, to the extent that gap-filling exists under state law, it does not appear that the passage of the ADA has been a major factor. I have marked the states that have statutes that were amended in or after 1990 to include compensatory damages with boldface type. Only six states fit that description. California, for example, has the most generous relief provision, making it possible for plaintiffs to obtain "up to three times the amount of actual damages but in no case less than one thousand dollars ($1,000) and attorney's fees."[109] Although California has increased the minimum penalty several times, the provision for relief has existed since 1976. Similarly, Vermont enacted its disability discrimination statute in 1987 and provided for injunctive relief and compensatory and punitive damages.[110] States' decisions to offer broader relief than the ADA generally seem to be independent of the passage of the ADA. Although many states amended their statutes after the passage of the ADA to make their definition of "public accommodation" more consistent with the ADA's definition, only six of those states broadened the relief available in their state statute at that time. There is therefore no current groundswell for state law to serve a "gap-filling" function under the law of public accommodations.

By contrast, significant gap-filling at the state level has occurred in the area of racial nondiscrimination statutes since the passage of CRA Title II. Four states have no statute banning race discrimination at places of public accommodation. Fifteen states have statutes which go no further than CRA Title II. Thirty-one states provide at least compensatory relief. Of these 31 states, 18 took more than a decade to include compensatory damages. Table 2 on page 309 summarizes these results:

The issue of relief, however, has a unique quality in the area of race nondiscrimination legislation that may not translate into the area of disability nondiscrimination legislation. The choice of permitting only injunctive relief under the law of race was considered by some civil rights advocates to be the best choice because of the problem of prejudiced juries, as discussed above. Thus state legislatures may have always been willing to create compensatory damages under their race nondiscrimination statutes; they were not asked to do so until the jury climate became more favorably disposed to claims of race discrimination. There is little or no evidence that state legislatures which enacted legislation forbidding disability-based discrimination but which limited the remedies to injunctive relief were willing to consider compensatory damages at the time of enactment.

Nearly every state has a statute prohibiting disability discrimination at places of public accommodation. The question is whether legislatures can be mobilized to conclude that legislative action is necessary to improve the existing statutory law. One rationale for legislative action in the disability area may be that many states have quite antiquated disability statutes, such as "white cane laws" which provide for a very limited prohibition against discrimination.[111] If states perceive a need to update these antiquated statutes, there is the possibility that they also may be persuaded to improve their remedial scheme more generally.

A final difficulty that may exist for the law of disability discrimination is the public perception that this is now an area that is primarily the subject of federal, not state, regulation.[112] When states have amended their disability statutes, they have frequently used the federal government as a "benchmark" or limit for what are the proper contours of a statute in this area. In the racial civil rights area, we may have once thought of the states as a labo-

TABLE 2: State Statutes Prohibiting Race Discrimination at Places of Public Accommodation

Category One (No prohibition against discrimination)	No Compensatory or Punitive Damages (Date enforcement scheme established)	Compensatory or Punitive Damages (Original date compensatory damages adopted)
Alabama	Arizona (1965)	Alaska (1970)
Georgia	Colorado (1979)	**Arkansas (1993)**
Mississippi	Connecticut (1980)	California (1905)
North Carolina	Idaho (1961)	**District of Columbia (1977)**
Texas	Illinois (1989)	**Florida (1992)**
	Kansas (1961)	**Delaware (1996)**
	Maine (1971)	**Hawaii (1989)**
	Maryland (1963)	**Indiana (1978)**
	Massachusetts (1933)	Iowa (1965)
	Nebraska (1969)	**Kentucky (1974)**
	North Dakota (1983)	**Louisiana (1988)**
	Rhode Island (1991)	**Michigan (1976)**
	Virginia (1987)	Minnesota (1969)
	West Virginia (1967)	**Missouri (1986)**
	Wyoming (1982)	Montana (1895)
		Nevada (1965)
		New Hampshire (1992)
		New Jersey (1990)
		New Mexico (1969)
		New York (1965)
		Ohio (1987)
		Oklahoma (1968)
		Oregon (1973)
		Pennsylvania (1955)
		South Carolina (1990)
		South Dakota (1991)
		Tennessee (1978)
		Utah (1965)
		Vermont (1987)
		Washington (1973)
		Wisconsin (1980)

States in boldface took a decade or longer after the passage of the Civil Rights Act to enact a remedial scheme that included compensatory damages.

ratory for innovative legal developments, but in the disability discrimination area, we may now be expecting the federal government to be the leading laboratory. If so, the only way to spur significant change would be for the federal government to take a significant step rather than to expect the states to do so.

CONCLUSION

ADA Title III was modeled on CRA Title II, specifically borrowing its limited remedial scheme. Plaintiffs who have litigated under ADA Title III have had a reasonable chance of prevailing, but litigation also appears to be a seldom-used tool due to the limited remedies available. Settlements have occurred and their remedies have been effective, but there is little incentive for private individuals to seek settlements unless the Department of Justice initiates an enforcement proceeding. Voluntary compliance is difficult to measure, but any casual observation of the accessibility of places of public accommodation reveals that there is much work to be done in order to attain compliance.[113]

The tenth anniversary of the ADA provides a good opportunity to assess the effectiveness of the ADA's remedies. Nearly all of the ADA Title III verdicts involved cases with a state law claim for compensatory damages under a negligence *per se* theory. Plaintiffs were able to attain verdicts only if they had actual physical injuries, for instance, from a fall due to negligent construction. The ADA Title III cases which resulted in reported opinions or DOJ settlements did involve pure right to access issues—without the requirement of an actual physical injury—but those cases were very few in number. The DOJ's enforcement authority enhanced the relief available in those cases, but the DOJ is able to bring very few cases despite its national enforcement authority. Its enforcement authority is much more limited under ADA Title III than it is under the FHA. At a minimum, Congress should enhance DOJ enforcement authority to increase compliance with ADA Title III.

State law is also in serious need of expansion. While 21 states provide for greater relief than ADA Title III, and six of those states have enhanced their remedial scheme since 1990, not only do states need to enhance the relief available under their state statutes, but they need to revisit the scope of protection generally provided under state law in the area of disability discrimination. Many state statutes are woefully antiquated and in serious need of updating.

Revision of state law, however, is not an adequate ultimate solution to the remedy problem. The purpose of national legislation like the ADA is to provide a uniform and national set of antidiscrimination standards. Yet that reality has not been realized. Plaintiffs who suffer physical injuries as a result of inaccessibility may have a viable state law claim for negligence with the possibility of compensatory relief. Plaintiffs in 16 states can sue to challenge inaccessibility problems and recover more than injunctive relief under state law. And a handful of plaintiffs each year can benefit from the DOJ's enforcement efforts on their behalf. But the remaining victims of discrimination under ADA Title III have little, if any, recourse if their accessibility problems have not caused physical injury. If Congress is serious about providing access to public accommodations for all Americans, such regional differences are unacceptable.

To attain uniform enforcement, we should move toward a compensatory damage scheme under ADA Title III, borrowing from the damages scheme available under the FHA. Experience at the state level suggests that there is little reason to fear runaway juries if damages were to be expanded under ADA Title III. The very fact that we need not fear runaway juries, however, also gives pause to wonder whether we should not be even more ambitious for seeking effective remedies under ADA Title III. By permitting injunctive relief and limited compensatory relief, we still may not be giving businesses sufficient incentives to comply with ADA Title III. Businesses might calculate that it is cheaper not to comply, since statutory enforcement is unlikely to be as expensive as compliance from the date of enactment of the ADA. In other words, a business that is sued in the year 2000 for failing to comply with ADA Title III may have benefited for ten years by saving money on an auxiliary service or device. Offering that device prospectively and paying a modest compensatory award to an individual victim of discrimination as a result of enforcement activity may be cost-effective. But if the remedial scheme required a business to pay a fine for all the years in which it did not comply with the ADA, then the failure of the business to comply with the statute might not be cost-effective. The DOJ's civil fine authority provides that incentive structure but, given the DOJ's limited enforcement resources, it cannot act as a serious deterrent against unlawful conduct under ADA Title III. The FHA's mandatory enforcement scheme by the attorney general would create a significant improvement in ADA compliance.

ADA Title III was a significant and important step in improving the lives of individuals with disabilities. It is now time to ask, however, whether we can do a better job in creating an effective enforcement scheme to achieve those aspirations. Our experience under the FHA and state disability antidiscrimination law should provide models for more effective enforcement.

ACKNOWLEDGMENTS

I would like to thank the USX Foundation for supporting the research which underlies this chapter. I also would like to think my many excellent research assistants: Amanda Dine-Gamble, Leslie Kerns, Beth Paxton and Theodore Wern. I would like to thank the following people who offered feedback on an earlier draft: Samuel Bagenstos, Jim Brudney, Chai Feldblum, Joseph William Singer and Bonnie Poitras Tucker. Finally, I would like to thank the participants at a Berkeley symposium who were a wonderful and helpful audience for an earlier draft.

NOTES

[1] 42 U.S.C. § 12181–12189 (1994 & Supp. 1997).

[2] "No individual shall be discriminated against on the basis of disability in the full and equal enjoyment of the goods, services, facilities, privileges, advantages or accommodations of any place of public accommodation by any person who owns, leases (or leases to), or operates a place of public accommodation." 42 U.S.C. § 12182(a).

[3] See 42 U.S.C. § 12182(b)(2) (defining "discrimination").

[4] See 42 U.S.C. § 12101–12117 (1994) (prohibiting employment discrimination).

[5] See 42 U.S.C. § 12111(8) (defining "qualified individual with a disability" as "an individual with a disability who, with or without reasonable accommodation, can perform the essential functions of the employment position that such individual holds or desires.")

[6] The definition of "public accommodation" covers 12 categories of covered entities, ranging from laundromats to bowling alleys. See 42 U.S.C. § 12181(7) (defining "public accommodations). In addition, the term "commercial facilities" is defined as "facilities (a) that are intended for nonresidential use; and (b) whose operations will affect commerce." See 42 U.S.C. § 12181(2). Although the prohibitions against discrimination do not generally apply to all commercial facilities, see 42 U.S.C. § 12182 (prohibition of discrimination by public accommodations), the accessibility requirements for new construction and alterations do apply to commercial facilities as well as public accommodations. See 42 U.S.C. § 12183. The definition of disability is also arguably broad. See 42 U.S.C. § 12102 (2) ("The term 'disability' means, with respect to an individual—(a) a physical or mental impairment that substantially limits one or more of the major life activities of such individual; (b) a record of such an impairment; or (c) being regarded as having such an impairment.")

[7] See note 40 (remarks of Senator Harkin).

[8] See 42 U.S.C. § 12188(a)(2) (providing for injunctive relief in private suits by affected parties). See also 42 U.S.C. § 12188(b) (providing for enforcement by the attorney general with potential civil penalties ranging from $50,000 to $100,000).

[9] 42 U.S.C. § 2000a (1994).

[10] 42 U.S.C. §2000a-3 (1994) (providing for civil action for preventive relief by a private party and intervention by the attorney general "if he certifies that the case is of general public importance.")

[11]CRA Title II covers places which provide lodging to transient guests, facilities principally engaged in selling food for consumption, gasoline stations, and places of exhibition or entertainment. 42 U.S.C. §2000a(b).

[12]See Fair Housing Amendments Act of 1988, Pub. L. 100–430, sec. 5(b), § 802(h), 102 Stat. 1619, 1619–20 (1988) (codified as amended at 42 U.S.C. § 3602(h) (1994)) (amending the definition section to include "handicap"); Pub. L. 100–430, sec. 6 (a), § 804, 102 Stat. 1619, 1620–22 (1988) (codified as amended at 42 U.S.C. § 3604 (1994)) (amending this section to include at the end a prohibition against discrimination on the basis of handicap in the sale or rental of housing to any buyer or renter).

[13]When originally enacted, the Fair Housing Act provided the following provision for relief:

> The court may grant as relief, as it deems appropriate, any permanent or temporary injunction, temporary restraining order, or other order, and may award to the plaintiff actual damages and not more than $1,000 punitive damages, together with court costs and reasonable attorney fees in the case of a prevailing plaintiff: *Provided,* That the said plaintiff in the opinion of the court is not financially able to assume said attorney's fees.

Fair Housing Act, Pub. L. No. 90–284, § 812, 82 Stat. 73, 88 (1968) (codified at 42 U.S.C. § 3612(c) (Supp. 1965–1969)) (amended 1988).

In 1988, the Fair Housing Act was amended. The relief provision for private parties who sought civil actions was moved to section 3613. The amended and renumbered provision provided:

> (1) In a civil action under subsection (a), if the court finds that a discriminatory housing practice has occurred or is about to occur, the court may award to the plaintiff actual and punitive damages, and subject to subsection (d) of this section, may grant as relief, as the court deems appropriate, any permanent or temporary injunction, temporary restraining order, or other order (including an order enjoining the defendant from engaging in such practice or ordering such affirmative action as may be appropriate).

> (2) In a civil action under subsection (a) of this section, the court, in its discretion, may allow the prevailing party, other than the United States, a reasonable attorney's fee and costs. The United States shall be liable for such fees and costs to the same extent as a private person.

Fair Housing Amendments Act of 1988, Pub. L. 100–430, sec. 8(2), § 813(c), 102 Stat. 1619, 1633–34 (1988) (codified as amended at 42 U.S.C. § 3613(c) (1994)).

[14]See Fair Housing Amendments Act of 1988, Pub. L. 100–430, sec. 8(2), § 810(g)(2)(A), 102 Stat. 1619, 1628 (1988) (codified as amended at 42 U.S.C. § 3610(g)(2)(A) (1994)).

[15]See note 40. No one, however, suggested that the regime of mandatory enforcement by the Department of Justice when a reasonable cause determination has been made by another federal agency should be imported into ADA Title III from the Fair Housing Amendments Act of 1988.

[16]Nonetheless, because of the availability of civil damages in an action brought by the attorney general under ADA Title III, this title has a somewhat broader relief provision than CRA Title II. CRA Title II has never been amended to provide for civil damages when the attorney general brings suit.

[17]Although this article deals with the relief problems under ADA Title III, as causing few lawsuits to be filed, that is not the only explanation for this pattern. Another plausible explanation is that it is difficult to file class action remedies under this Title.

[18]*Cf. infra* Tables 1 and 2.

[19]See *infra* Table 1.

[20]*Bragdon v. Abbott,* 118 S. Ct. 2196 (1998). Abbott was denied dental treatment at her dentist's office because she is HIV-positive. She prevailed on a motion for summary judgment at the trial court level on the issues of whether she was an individual with a disability (yes) and whether she posed a direct threat to the dentist (no). *Abbott v. Bragdon,* 912 F. Supp. 580 (D. Maine 1995). Her case was affirmed by the First Circuit, 107 F.3d 934 (1st Cir. 1997), and affirmed and remanded by the United States Supreme Court on the direct threat issue, 118 S.Ct. 2196. On remand, the First Circuit again affirmed the grant of summary judgment. 163 F.3d 87 (1st Cir. 1998). Bragdon's request for certiorari to the United States Supreme Court was denied, *Bragdon v. Abbott,* 119 S.Ct. 185 (1999).

[21]Dr. Bragdon is legally obligated to fill her cavity in his office, because his services are covered under ADA Title III and such dental treatment would not pose a significant risk to the health or safety of himself or others. See *Abbott v. Bragdon,* 163 F.3d 87 (1st Cir. 1998), cert. denied, 119 S.Ct. 185 (1999).

[22]See section on ADA Title III Results.

[23]See ME Rev. Stat. Ann. tit. 5, § 4613(2)(B)(7) (West Supp. 1998) (providing for "civil penal damages [to the victim of unlawful discrimination] not in excess of $10,000 in the case of the first order under this Act against the respondent, not in excess of $25,000 in the case of a 2nd order against the respondent arising under the same subchapter of this Act and not in excess of $50,000 in the case of a 3rd or subsequent order against the respondent arising under the same subchapter of this Act, except that the total amount of civil penal damages awarded in any action filed under this Act may not exceed the limits contained in this subparagraph").

[24]John Ripley, "Ruling Upheld on HIV Dental Patient Treatment," *Bangor Daily News,* April 13, 1996, available in LEXIS, NEWS Library, BGRDLY File.

[25]A court, of course, could have raised the jurisdiction issue *sua sponte* but none of the courts of record raised the issue.

[26]See Paul V. Sullivan, Note, "The Americans with Disabilities Act of 1990: An Analysis of Title III and Applicable Case Law," 29 *Suffolk U. L. Rev.* 1117, 1141 (1995) ("Settlement agreements with the Department of Justice have resulted in many of the accomplishments of Title III. Commentators reason that initial litigation has been sparse because the government has placed a greater emphasis on education. Commentators, however, have noted that litigation should increase as the Department of Justice shifts from ADA education to ADA enforcement. Currently, many disability advocates are dismayed because some entities are not voluntarily complying with Title III, and compliance comes only after threats of litigation or actual litigation. In addition, the disabled and their advocates are concerned that political eagerness to shrink government might undermine the effectiveness of the ADA.") The only significant discussion of ADA Title III was written by Professor Robert L. Burgdorf who himself was a leading advocate for the passage of the ADA. See Robert L. Burgdorf, "'Equal Members of the Community': The Public Accommodations Provisions of the Americans with Disabilities Act," 64 *Temp. L. Rev.* 551 (1991). The article does an excellent job of describing the requirements of ADA Title III but has little discussion of its legislative history or subsequent case development. (It was written before the ADA had become effective.)

[27]It was referred jointly to the Committees on Education and Labor, the Judiciary, Energy and Commerce, and Public Works and Transportation Committees. See H.R. 4498, 100th Cong. (1988).

[28]See 134 *Cong. Rec.* 9357 (1988).

[29]See 134 *Cong. Rec.* 9357 (1988) (statement of Senator Weicker in introducing S. 2345). See also 134 *Cong. Rec.* 9382 (statement of Senator Harkin as chairman of the Subcommittee on the Handicapped).

[30]Most notably, the definition of "disability" (which was then termed "on the basis of handicap") was much broader. An individual need only demonstrate that he or she was treated differently "because of a physical or mental impairment, perceived impairment, or record of impairment." H.R. 4498, Sec. 3(1). The term "physical or mental impairment" was also much broader, requiring only proof of a "physiological disorder or condition, cosmetic disfigurement, or anatomical loss affecting one or more systems of the body" or "any mental or psychological disorder, such as mental retardation, organic brain syndrome, emotional or mental illness, and specific learning disabilities." H.R. 4498, § 3(2).

[31]Each of these sections was stronger than the ultimately enacted bill.

[32]The barriers section makes no distinction between new, altered or existing structures. It also specifically mentions transportation barriers which were not listed in the finally enacted ADA. The defenses that are provided for this section are minimal. This early version of the ADA also included considerably stronger language with respect to the removal of communication barriers than the final bill. Ultimately, the only of these requirements to survive passage was the telephone relay services requirement.

Whereas the ultimately enacted statute requires only the removal of barriers for existing entities that meet the narrow definition of public accommodation, the original bill covered all commercial entities. Senator Weicker explained that "simple justice argues strongly for requiring the removal of barriers that exclude or limit the participation of people with disabilities." 134 *Cong. Rec.* at 9378.

[33]H.R. 4498, Sec. 9(b).

[34]42 U.S.C. § 12188 (1994).

[35]134 *Cong. Rec.* at 9386.

[36]S. 933, 101st Cong., § 405 (1989) (enforcement section incorporating Fair Housing Act remedies with "reference to a practice that is discriminatory under this title concerning a public accommodation or public transportation service operated by a private entity").

[37]See generally "Hearings Before the Committee on Labor and Human Resources and the Subcommittee of the Handicapped on S. 933," 101st Cong. (May 9, 10, 16, and June 22, 1989).

[38]42 U.S.C. §12181(9) (1994).

[39]42 U.S.C. § 12181(9)(a)-(d).

[40]135 *Cong. Rec.* 19,803 (1989) (emphasis added).

[41]"Hearings," note 37, 210.

[42]For further discussion of the impact of CRA Title II on ADA Title III, see Burgdorf, note 26, at 552–553.

[43]Charles Whalen and Barbara Whalen. *The Longest Debate: A Legislative History of the 1964 Civil Rights Act.* 1, 1985.

[44]William McCulloch (R-Ohio) was the ranking Republican member of the subcommittee of the House Judiciary Committee when the Civil Rights Act was introduced in the House in 1963 and assigned to his subcommittee. He agreed to provide seven Republican votes for support of the Civil Rights Act in exchange for various compromises which weakened the bill but also enhanced its likelihood of ultimate passage. See Whalen and Whalen, *The Longest Debate,* 10–14, 59–64.

[45]Whalen and Whalen, *The Longest Debate,* 239. See Staff of the House of Representatives Comm. on the Judiciary, 88th Cong., H.R. 7152 43 (Committee Print No. 2 1963) (compare previous language on page 14 with new language on page 43 of Committee Print of bill).

[46]Whalen and Whalen, *The Longest Debate,* 110. (Smith supposedly removed the sentences from the official transcript of the proceedings in the *Congressional Record.*)

[47]"Additional Majority Views of Hon. Robert W. Kastenmeier," *House Judiciary Committee Report* No. 88–914 (1963), reprinted in United States Equal Employment Opportunity Commission, *Legislative History of Titles VII and XI of Civil Rights Act of 1964* 2040–2041 (undated).

[48]378 U.S. 226 (1964).

[49]*Bell v. Maryland,* 378 U.S. 226, 252–253, 254–255 (1964).

[50]See generally Whalen and Whalen, *The Longest Debate,* 218–229.

[51]Joseph William Singer, "No Right to Exclude: Public Accommodations and Private Property," 90 *Nw. U. L. Rev.* 1283, 1290 (1996).

[52]Jack Greenberg, *Race Relations and American Law* 15 (1959).

[53]Id., 15.

[54]"Here, injunctive suits or administrative implementation by the federal government would seem to be the most efficient way to proceed," Id., 17.

[55]See Arthur Earl Bonfield, "State Civil Rights Statutes: Some Proposals," 49 *Iowa L. Rev.* 1067, 1114 (1964).

[56]See Dennis L. Wright, Note, "State Legislative Response to the Federal Civil Rights Act: A Proposal," 9 *Utah L. Rev.* 434, 449 (1964–65).

[57]See Bonfield, "State Civil Rights," 1114.

[58]See Wright, note, "State Legislative Response," 449.

[59]See Bonfield, "State Civil Rights," 1119.

[60]See Civil Rights Act of 1964, Pub. L. 88–352, § 706, July 2, 1964, 78 Stat. 241, 259 (1964) (codified at 42 U.S.C. § 2000e-5 (Supp. 1964–1969)) (amended 1972).

[61]The administrative enforcement mechanism under Title VII was enhanced considerably in 1972 when the Equal Employment Opportunity Commission was given the power to bring a civil action against any respondent not a government, governmental agency, or political subdivision where the commission has determined that there is reasonable cause to believe that the charge is true. When the respondent is a governmental entity, the commission is required to refer the charge to the attorney general who may bring a civil action against the respondent in a federal court. See Equal Employment Opportunity Act of 1972, Pub. L. 92–261, sec. 4(a), § 706, 86 Stat. 103, 104–05 (1972) (codified as amended at 42 U.S.C. § 2000e-5 (1988)) (amended 1991).

[62]The private cause of action was enhanced in 1991 when compensatory and punitive damages became available. See Civil Rights Act of 1991, Pub. L. 102–166, sec. 102, § 1977A(b), 105 Stat. 1071, 1073 (1991) (codified at 42 U.S.C. § 1981a(b) (1994)).

[63]42 U.S.C. § 2000a-3(a) (1994).

[64]42 U.S.C. § 2000a-3(b).

[65]See section on Effectiveness of Remedies.

[66]See Table 2.

[67]Civil Rights Act of 1866, 42 U.S.C. §1981 (1994).

[68]See, e.g., *Perry v. Command Performance*, 913 F.2d 99 (3rd Cir. 1990) (Section 1981 action based on a beauty salon's refusal to provide services to an African-American woman); *Watson v. Fraternal Order of Eagles*, 915 F.2d 235 (6th Cir. 1990) (allegations of refusal to sell soft drinks to guests at club violated Section 1981); *Perry v. Burger King Corp.*, 924 F. Supp. 548 (S.D. N.Y. 1996) (refusal to allow plaintiff to use bathroom was sufficient to state a cause of action under Section 1981); *McCaleb v. Pizza Hut of America, Inc.*, 28 F. Supp.2d 1043 (N.D. Ill. 1998) (cause of action under Section 1981 for failing to provide plaintiffs with range of services while eating their meals); *Harrison v. Denny's Restaurant*, No. C-96-0343 (PJH), 1997 WL 227963 (N.D. Calif. Apr. 24, 1997) (denial of service at restaurant can violate Section 1981 although mere slow service does not violate Section 1981); *Franceschi v. Hyatt Corp.*, 782 F. Supp. 712 (D. Puerto Rico 1992) (denial of access to hotel can state a cause of action under Section 1981).

[69]Section 1981, by its wording, limits itself to issues of race discrimination. See 42 U.S.C. § 1981.

[70]Pub. L. 90–284, title VIII, § 812(c), 82 Stat. 73, 88 (codified at 42 U.S.C. § 3612(c) (Supp. 1964–1969)) (amended 1988).

[71]Pub. L. 100–430, sec. 8(2), § 813(c), 102 Stat. 1619, 1633–34 (1988) (codified as amended at 42 U.S.C. § 3613(c) (1994)). See note 13 (quoting text of section).

[72]H.R. Rep. No. 100–711, at 40 (1988), reprinted in 1988 U.S.C.C.A.N. 2173, 2201.

[73]See note 40.

[74]See 42 U.S.C. § 12181(2)(defining ADA Title III as only covering facilities for nonresidential use).

[75]My own research, in fact, suggests that victims of disability discrimination should be wary of bench trials because of the strong propensity of trial court judges to grant motions for summary judgment on behalf of defendants. See Ruth Colker, "The Americans with Disabilities Act: A Windfall for Defendants," 34 *Harv. C. R.-C.L. L. Rev.* 99 (1999). When civil rights activists expressed concern about jury trials in the race area, they were assuming all-white juries. That assumption is no longer appropriate. See *Batson v. Kentucky*, 476 U.S. 79 (1986) (invalidating the use of race-based peremptory challenges).

[76]Some people might argue that the FHA is ineffective even with an enhanced remedial scheme. The merit of that argument is beyond the scope of this essay.

[77]Betsy Pisik, "Denny's Mails Checks to Suit's Black Diners," *Washington Times*, Dec. 12, 1995, B10.

[78]See Civil Rights Act of 1866, 42 U.S.C. §1981 (1994).

[79]A TDD is a telecommunication device attached to a telephone that permits individuals to communicate by typing their messages back and forth. Both parties must have a TDD for the system to operate properly. A TDD is a relatively inexpensive device (around $200), yet most businesses do not own a TDD or, if they do own one, do not use it when telephoned by a person on a TDD. (The TDD emits a signal to let a hearing listener know to switch his or her telephone to the TDD device.)

[80]In the short term, some white customers might fail to patronize the restaurant, however, in the long term, the overall customer population would surely rise. Justice Douglas made this assertion through anecdotal data. See *Bell v. Maryland*, 378 U.S. 226, 265 n.2 (1964).

[81]Even if the expense is fairly minimal, there may be no entity proactively taking responsibility for the barrier removal. For example, in a landlord-tenant situation, neither entity may consider himself or herself to be responsible for the design or construction of the entrance. Inertia may therefore act as a deterrent to action.

[82]See, e.g., *Jairath v. Dyer*, 154 F.3d 1280 (11th Cir. 1998) (filed suit under ADA Title III and state law after doctor refused to perform a Gore-Tex implant procedure on plaintiff; district court granted defendant's motion for summary judgment and refused to remand state law claim to state court; court of appeals reversed and remanded case with instruction to remand it to state court for consideration of the state law issue). See also *Hoepfl v. Barlow*, 906 F. Supp. 317 (E.D. Va. 1995) (no standing to sue for injunctive relief under ADA, absent showing that realistic possibility existed that defendant's future discriminatory conduct would cause harm to plaintiff); *Delil v. El Torito Restaurants*, No. C 94–3900–CAL., 1997 WL 714866 (N.D. Cal. 1997) (no standing to sue for injunctive relief because there is no "'real and imminent threat' of future injury"); *Atakpa v. Perimeter Ob-Gyn Associates*, P.C., 912 F. Supp.

1566 (N.D. Ga. 1994) (patient did not have standing to seek injunctive relief under the ADA because she failed to allege that she will ever seek services from defendants in the future).

[83]See generally 28 U.S.C. § 1367 (c)(3) (1994) (governing supplementary jurisdiction of related state law claims).

[84]I understand that Abbott did state in an interrogatory that she had not had the cavity filled prior to filing suit and would use Dr. Bragdon to fill her cavity if she obtained injunctive relief.

[85]See id.

[86]See Colker, *The Americans,* 126.

[87]See *Howe v. Hull,* No. 3:92CV7658 (Ohio) (June 14, 1994), available in LEXIS, VERDCT Library.

[88]See *Gladys Haney v. Sunnyvale Town Center et al.,* No. CV 762408 (Santa Clara County Superior Court, California) (August 11, 1997), available in LEXIS, VERDCT Library.

[89]In private conversations with attorneys I have learned that they had found it very difficult even to get judges to consider their client's right to relief for stigmatic injury. It may be that society's lack of recognition of the importance of accessibility to individuals with disabilities has contributed to my findings of relatively low jury awards. Those results may change someday, but, at present, there appears to be little evidence suggesting that juries would award substantial claims for lack of accessibility cases.

[90]Wright, note, "State Legislative Response," 449.

[91]Id.

[92]Abbott's lawyers, however, were concerned about the possibility of a prejudiced jury in the HIV context. Even if compensatory damages became available, some plaintiffs might choose to forgo that possibility and seek only injunctive relief in order to avoid the possibility of a prejudiced jury.

[93]See 42 U.S.C. § 12188 (b)(2)(C)(I)-(iii) (1994) (providing for a civil penalty of $50,000 for a first violation and $100,000 for any subsequent violation).

[94]See 42 U.S.C. § 12182(b)(2)(A)(iv) (1994) (providing that unlawful discrimination includes "a failure to remove architectural barriers, and communication barriers that are structural in nature, in existing facilities . . . where such removal is readily achievable"). The term "readily achievable" is defined as meaning "easily accomplishable and able to be carried out without much difficulty or expense." 42 U.S.C. § 12181(9).

[95]Cf. ADA Title III, 42 U.S.C. § 12183(a)(1) (1994) (new construction) with § 12182(b)(2)(A)(iv) (existing construction). For new construction, the ADA provides that an entity must be "readily accessible to and usable by individuals with disabilities, except where an entity can demonstrate that it is structurally impracticable to meet the requirements of such subsection." 42 U.S.C. § 12183(a)(1).

[96]See Fair Housing Amendments Act, Pub. L. 100–430, sec. 8(2), § 812(o), 102 Stat. 1619, 1632 (1988) (codified at 42 U.S.C. § 3612(o)(1) (1994)).

[97]From March 12, 1989, to December 6, 1993, the Department of Justice handled 293 "judicial election" cases—reasonable cause determinations from HUD in which the aggrieved party chose a judicial rather than administrative remedy. A consent decree or settlement was achieved in 171 of those cases; 12 went to trial and 86 were pending when these statistics were collected. United States Commission on Civil Rights, *The Fair Housing Amendments Act of 1988: The Enforcement Report* 212, Table 11.4 (1994). These statistics would appear to reflect a vigorous and effective enforcement mechanism, but this enforcement scheme has its critics. (Of these 292 cases, charges were filed on the basis of race (49 cases), family status (180 cases), disability (40 cases), sex (6 cases), national origin (3 cases), religion (2 cases), and combined basis (13 cases). Thus, there were virtually as many disability cases as race cases, suggesting that disability discrimination is an area of law requiring as much enforcement activity as race discrimination. Id.)

Despite the evidence of significant enforcement activity on the part of DOJ, the DOJ's exercise of its enforcement authority has received some criticism. For example, the United States Commission on Civil Rights found:

> Although the FHAA required DOJ to file a claim in every election, DOJ has returned a few election charges for further investigation by HUD. Although FHAA regulations provide that DOJ may consult with the General Counsel if new court decisions or new evidence affect HUD's initial reasonable cause determination, OGC finds it troubling that DOJ refuses to proceed in some cases. OGC asserts that DOJ returns elected charges

when DOJ does not agree with the substantive issues involved in HUD's reasonable cause determination. However, DOJ maintains that it only returns an elected HUD charge when new information makes filing a claim inappropriate or frivolous. While DOJ acknowledges that it must support the Secretary's reasonable cause determination, DOJ argues that it must also fulfill its obligations to the Federal courts to file only sound claims.

—Commission on Civil Rights, *The Enforcement Report* 213–214 (1994).

[98]See Bonfield, "State Civil Rights," 1117–1118.

[99]1995 Me. Laws 393, §7 (codified as ME Rev. Stat. Ann. tit. 5, § 4553(8))(West Supp. 1998).

[100]ME Rev. Stat. Ann. tit. 5, § 4613(2)(B)(7) (West Supp.1998).

[101]Oklahoma law provides that "a blind, physically handicapped, deaf or hard-of-hearing person and his or her guide, signal, or service dog or a dog trainer . . . shall not be denied admittance [to public facilities or public accommodations] because of such dog." Okla. Stat. Ann. tit. 7, § 19.1(B)(West Supp. 1999).

[102]South Carolina law does appear to make conduct unlawful that is already made unlawful by the ADA. See S.C. Code 1976 §§ 1–13–20; 1–13–100. But there appears to be little or no enforcement authority to remedy violations of any nonemployment complaints. See S.C. Code Ann. § 1–13–90(e)(West Supp. 1998)(providing solely for voluntary conciliation with the Human Rights Commission).

[103]Tennessee law prohibits discrimination on the basis of race, creed, color, religion, sex, age or national origin, but not disability. See Tenn. Code Ann. § 4–21–501 (1998).

[104]Texas law provides "persons with disabilities" with "the same right as the able-bodied to the full use and enjoyment of any public facility in the state" and provides for nondiscrimination in the rent or leasing of housing. See Tex. Hum. Res. Code Ann. § 121.003(a) (West Supp. 1999).

[105]Washington state has a public policy concerning the right of "the blind, the visually handicapped, the hearing impaired, and the otherwise physical disabled" to place of public accommodation; see Wash. Rev. Code Ann. § 70.84.010(3)(1992), but provides no remedy other than in the "white cane law" context; see Wash. Rev. Code Ann. § 70.84.040 (West Supp. 1999); Wash. Rev. Code Ann. § 70.84.050 (West Supp. 1999); and Wash Rev. Code Ann. § 70.84.070 (1992).

[106]Boldfaced type indicates statute amended after 1990 to create compensatory damages.

[107]Civil penal damages were first created in the Maine statute in 1971. The damages remedy has been raised over time from an original range of $100–$1,000 to the current $10,000–$50,000 cap. See ME Rev. Stat. Ann. tit. 5, §4613. (West 1989 and West Supp. 1998).

[108]I placed South Carolina in category one, although it appears to provide a right of access to public accommodations but no remedy other than voluntary conciliation. See note 126.

[109]Cal. Civ. Code §54.3 (West Supp. 1999).

[110]VT Stat. Ann. tit. 9, § 4506 (1993).

[111]White cane laws abrogate the common law contributory negligence *per se* rules when an individual who is blind is injured when not using a cane or a dog. See generally Adam A. Milani, "Living in the World: A New Look at the Disabled in the Law of Torts," 48 *Cath. U. L. Rev.* 323, 350–53 (1999). These laws do enhance the ability of individuals who are blind to travel safely, but are not a sufficient mechanism for providing the right to nondiscrimination at places of public accommodation for individuals in general who have disabilities. In some states, the only protection against discrimination at places of public accommodation is the white cane law. In such cases, the state needs to update its law of nondiscrimination.

[112]By contrast, when the Civil Rights Act of 1964 was passed, the federal government was careful to recognize the importance of existing state laws in this area. See Wright, note 57, at 434 (concluding that Title II of the Civil Rights Act actually encouraged state action).

[113]Each year, I have my students in my disability discrimination course conduct an accessibility study of an entity covered by ADA Title III. I do not limit their choice, except by geography. Each student, every year, finds accessibility violations at the site that he or she studies. In my own personal travels, I virtually always find accessibility problems at a site that I visit.

Courts and Wrongful Birth
Can Disability Itself Be Viewed as a Legal Wrong?

LORI B. ANDREWS AND MICHELLE HIBBERT

In 1990, the U.S. Congress launched a $3 billion scientific endeavor to uncover the specific links between genes and disease. The Human Genome Project was designed to map (that is, determine the location of) and sequence (or analyze the constituent parts of) each of the 50,000 to 100,000 genes in each human cell. Described by proponents as "biology's moon shot" and by opponents as "the Manhattan Project of science," the Human Genome Project's ultimate goal is to facilitate the development of genetic diagnostic tests and genetic treatment modalities for the nearly 5,000 diseases that have a genetic basis.

The Human Genome Project is producing an explosion of information. The genetic tests that are being developed determine the presence of genes signaling current and future diseases that may affect a person. People are able to learn of their risks of developing a particular genetic disease or of the possibility that they may develop a particular illness after exposure to certain environmental stimuli. They can also learn about the genetic makeup of their fetus, thus providing information that the couple can use to decide whether to continue or terminate the pregnancy.

As the volume of genetic information increases, prospective parents are beginning to expect health care professionals to inform them of genetic risks to their potential children due to their age, ethnic group and family history. Many couples seek genetic testing of themselves and their fetuses. They expect doctors to be able to predict genetic risk, to undertake genetic tests in a careful manner, and to convey the results accurately. When potential parents' expectations are not met—and they give birth to a child with a genetic disorder—they may sue the health professionals for "wrongful birth." In some cases, the child himself or herself might sue the health care provider for "wrongful life"; in such cases, the child's attorney claims the child would rather not have been born than have been born with the genetic-based disability.

The very notion of wrongful birth and wrongful life—conveying the idea that having a child with a disability that could have been "prevented" through abortion is a legal wrong—seems vastly at odds with the ideas about disability that serve as the foundation for the Americans with Disabilities Act. At the same time, however, some disability rights activists are strongly pro-choice and feel uncomfortable restricting women's rights to terminate a pregnancy. Moreover, because of altercations that people with disabilities have had with the medical system, they are sometimes troubled by taking the side of negligent doctors in these legal actions.

How, then, are we to reconcile the genetic tort actions with our goals in enacting and enforcing the Americans with Disabilities Act? To begin to answer that question, we need to analyze closely the social and legal context in which prenatal screening occurs and the perceptions of disability that undergird the wrongful birth and wrongful life cases.

318

DISABILITY AND CHANGING CONCEPTS OF NORMALITY

In large measure, the history of eugenics is a history of brutality against the disabled. People who were mentally disabled were involuntarily sterilized in the United States by the thousands at the turn of the century. In Nazi Germany, people with disabilities were systematically exterminated. Even today, much of the writing about genetic discoveries includes economic analyses about the cost of care for people with a particular genetic mutation, implying that society would be better off had they not been born.[1]

Genetic technologies have a major impact on people with disabilities. Indeed, genetic testing changes the very categories of "disabled." As bioethicist Paul Ramsey pointed out when amniocentesis was first introduced, "the concept of 'normality' sufficient to make life worth living is bound to be 'upgraded'"[2] as testing is increasingly offered for less and less serious disorders. Currently, some parents choose to abort for reasons that seem trivial or inappropriate to other people. Some parents abort fetuses with an XYY chromosomal complement, for example, even though research has disproven the hypothesis that this is a "criminal" gene. People with dwarfism "are incensed that by the idea that a woman or couple would choose to abort simply because the fetus would become a dwarf."[3] As time passes, an increasing number of women abort based on particular types of genetic information, which also changes the boundaries of normality. The percentage of women in Scotland who aborted fetuses with spina bifida rose from 21 percent in 1976 to 74 percent in 1985.[4]

Newer genetic technologies provide the opportunity for users to choose to avoid very minor deviations from some perceived normality. Consider the use of preimplantation screening, which Marsha Saxton refers to as "admission standards" for fetuses.[5] A couple undergoes *in vitro* fertilization, produces multiple embryos, and each one is genetically tested. If a couple has ten embryos in petri dishes, they might use different criteria to determine the "genetic worth" of the embryos to be implanted than they would in determining whether a single *in utero* fetus at four months of development should be aborted. While a couple may not be likely to abort a fetus based on its sex or based on being an unaffected carrier of a recessive disorder, they may, when faced with a high volume of embryos, only a few of which can be safely implanted in the woman, decide to implant only noncarrier embryos or embryos of a particular sex. With ten embryos, the couple must refuse implantation of some of the embryos for the safety of the woman and any resulting fetuses. If a couple chooses to move from randomly selecting the embryos to be implanted to doing so on genetic grounds, this may seem less morally problematic to them than aborting a particular fetus. The decision may be viewed differently for several reasons. The woman is not physically pregnant, so there has not been attachment to a particular fetus. She has not felt the fetus move or begun to bond with it. In addition, the process may be viewed less as choosing *against* a particular individual (the developing fetus) than choosing *for* a set of individuals (the embryos to be implanted).

Some genetic testing programs go even further than reporting known conditions; they also report any unusual genetic pattern, even where there is no clear indication about whether the genetic deviation has *any* health implications whatsoever. Thus couples may choose not to implant embryos and not to carry to term fetuses that do not meet some gold standard of normality, even in instances where the fetus would face absolutely no health risk.

In addition to possibly making even less-serious departures from the model genome seem like a disability, genetic predispositional testing is creating a new form of disability in which currently "able" individuals are being treated by insurers, employers and others as "disabled" because of a potentially increased future propensity to illness.

Genetic tests are also stigmatizing existing people with disabilities as having slipped through the net of prenatal screening. The mere existence—and marketing—of genetic testing may seem like an affront to many people with disabilities, given the numerous ways in which "genetic" information was used in oppressive ways in the past, as with the mandatory sterilization laws at the turn of the century in this country, and the way in which disabled individuals continue to be discriminated against today.[6] The fact that the birth of children with certain disabilities can be "prevented" can aggravate the stigmatization of such children.

There is much in common between women who undergo genetic testing on themselves or their fetuses and people with disabilities. Both groups may suffer from medical manipulation. A woman whose genetic test results indicate that her fetus is affected with a genetic disorder—or that she herself is likely to develop a genetic disorder later in life—may be discriminated against by various social institutions such as insurers or employers. Yet despite certain commonalities, these two groups may appear to be at odds with each other. This is because some women's use of prenatal diagnosis to identify fetuses with particular disorders and abort them may be seen as devaluing existing people with those same disorders. In some—perhaps many—instances, the decision may be based on ignorance or even misinformation about what life with that disability is like, or even whether people with that condition consider it a disability at all.

PRESSURE TO USE GENETIC SERVICES TO ELIMINATE DISABILITY

"Prenatal screening seems to give women more power," says disability rights activist Laura Hershey, "but is it actually asking women to ratify social prejudice through their reproductive 'choice'?"[7]

Genetic testing creates an environment in which people believe that if a test is offered they should take it and act upon the information. "Women are increasingly pressured to use prenatal testing by claims that undergoing these tests is the 'responsible thing to do.' Strangers in the supermarket, even characters in TV sit-coms, readily ask a woman with a pregnant belly, 'Did you get your amnio?'" notes Martha Saxton.[8] Even a government agency, the Office of Technology Assessment of the U.S. Congress, exemplified this approach. After describing new genetic tests, an Office of Technology Assessment report stated "individuals have a paramount right to be born with a normal, adequate hereditary endowment."[9]

The way in which physicians describe a genetic condition may make it seem much more grim than it seems to a person with that condition. "Medical descriptions of Down's syndrome—rather than revealing the variability of the condition—selectively represent the condition in uniform, distancing, negative, ungendered, and static teams," notes Diane Beeson.[10] In the prenatal setting, as an increasing number of tests are being developed for less-serious disorders, parents may be pressured into feeling that something is "wrong" or "unfit" with their baby if there is the slightest departure from a socially conditioned perfection. Prenatal diagnosis, asserts McGill University epidemiology professor Abby Lippman, is "an assembly line approach to the products of conception, separating out those we wish to develop from those we wish to discontinue. . . ."[11]

Genetic testing may also "privatize" disability. Once prenatal diagnosis and testing are made available for a particular disorder, there may be a tendency not to continue to provide funds for research to help combat the medical problems for existing people with that disorder and not to continue social services for such individuals. Once genetic disease is no longer seen as a random characteristic, this may reduce our communal commitment to people with genetic disabilities.[12] This may be especially true in the coming years as wealthier women get access to prenatal diagnosis and abortion and poorer women do not.[13] If a disproportionate number of disadvantaged women have children with disabilities, their lack of clout in state legislatures may make it less likely that legal protections such as educational opportunities for people with disabilities will be continued.

Couples may be made to feel guilty by relatives, health care providers, insurers and other social institutions if they give birth to a child whose departure from "normality" could have been determined prenatally. This is particularly true in the case of mothers who already have children with a genetic disorder and who give birth to additional children with the same disorder.[14] Couples may be the subject of hostility for carrying a child with even a slight disability to term, as occurred with broadcaster Bree Walker-Lampley's decision to give birth to a child with ectrodactyly, a mild genetic condition which fuses the bones in the hands.[15]

Testing is being offered for such a wide range of conditions and disorders that the women being offered prenatal testing—and even some of the obstetricians ordering the tests—have no idea what the life of a child with such a genetic makeup would be like. They must increasingly depend on the people marketing the tests, such as biotechnology companies, for information about how serious the disorder being tested for might be. In the context of breast cancer genetic testing, a biotechnology company exaggerated the risk of cancer that women with the genetic mutation faced. Such tactics can push people into undergoing testing who otherwise would not have. Moreover, decisions may be made about terminating fetuses based on certain stereotypes about disability. Adrienne Asch, a disability rights activist and professor at Wellesley College, points to research studies which show that "whites and middle-class people in general showed more discomfort with Down syndrome and retardation, whereas people of color and those of lower socioeconomic status expressed more fear of physical vulnerability."[16]

Relying on physicians' assessments of disability can be problematic. Even those physicians who treat people with disabilities may have inaccurate impressions of the lives of such people if the physicians interact with such individuals only in a medical setting.

Physicians have very different views of particular disabilities from those of people with those disabilities. When asked to evaluate the quality of their lives, 80 percent of doctors said pretty good,[17] but 82 percent indicated that their life quality would be pretty low if they had quadriplegia. In contrast, 80 percent of people with quadriplegia rated the quality of their lives as pretty good. Consequently, as Adrienne Asch indicates, "those wishing to use the [genetic] technology should receive substantially more information about life with disability than they now do. . . ."

Laura Hershey is a poet and newspaper columnist. "I have a rare neuromuscular condition," she says. "I rely on a motorized wheelchair for mobility, a voice-activated computer for my writing, and the assistance of Medicaid-funded attendants for daily needs—dressing, bathing, eating, going to the bathroom."[18]

"My life of disability has not been easy or carefree," she continues. "But in measuring the quality of my life, other factors—education, friends, and meaningful work, for example—have been decisive. If I were asked for an opinion on whether to bring a child into the world, knowing she would have the same limitations and opportunities I have had, I would not hesitate to say, 'Yes.'"[19]

In 1999, a British philanthropic organization, RADAR (Royal Association for Disability and Rehabilitation) surveyed people with disabilities and genetic predispositions to a disability. Thirty-seven percent would ban abortion for Down syndrome, 53 percent for blindness and 72 percent for a correctable genetic condition such as cleft palate.[20]

Other people note the strange contradiction that just at the political moment when laws such as the Americans with Disabilities Act have been enacted to protect people with disabilities, genetic technologies are aimed at preventing their birth. "It is ironic," says Marsha Saxton, "that just when disabled citizens have achieved so much, the new reproductive and genetic technologies are promising to eliminate their kind—people with Down Syndrome, spina bifida, muscular dystrophy, sickle cell anemia and hundreds of other conditions."[21]

WRONGFUL BIRTH

Courts initially resisted recognizing a cause of action for wrongful birth.[22] The early cases befuddled the courts because, unlike traditional malpractice cases, nothing that the health care provider could have done would have prevented harm to the child.[23] The logic behind these early suits was that if the parents of the affected child had received proper counseling or diagnosis, they could have decided not to conceive or to seek an abortion. Early case law dealing with wrongful birth actions rejected the notion that the failure to warn the parents of a fetus's risk of an apparently serious genetic disease was actionable because the physician was not the proximate cause of the defect.[24] Seven states—Idaho, Minnesota, Missouri, North Carolina, Pennsylvania, South Dakota and Utah—currently statutorily bar wrongful birth claims.

However, wrongful birth cases are now recognized in 22 states and the District of Columbia.[25] In those states, the law creates a duty on the part of physicians to offer genetic services to high-risk patients. Physicians, genetic counselors or genetic testing laboratories may be found liable in a wrongful birth claim for negligent actions or negligent inactions. Since women have a constitutional right to reproductive choice, they are viewed as having a right to know about their increased genetic risks and the availability of genetic testing so they can either avoid conceiving a child with a particular genetic disorder or terminate a pregnancy with an affected fetus. Recognizing wrongful birth actions is also seen as an important way to deter physician negligence.

A variety of actions and inactions can give rise to a wrongful birth claim. Such a suit may be brought when a reasonable health care provider should have known of the risk because the couple's previous child had a genetic disorder. Or the negligence may consist of a health care provider's failing to offer certain tests, such as amniocentesis, to alert that the fetus has Down syndrome even though the health care provider should have known of the risk because of the woman's advanced age.[26] Other plaintiff parents have successfully brought wrongful birth claims against health care providers who actively discouraged use of genetic testing,[27] and against health care providers who failed to advise prospective parents of the risk that their fetus may suffer from a genetic disorder by virtue of one or both parents belonging to a particular ethnic or racial group.[28]

Wrongful birth claims have also successfully been brought against laboratories that performed a test negligently and against physicians who misinterpreted test results,[29] and such suits are likely to increase in the future. For instance, a recent study showed that one third of physicians misinterpreted genetic tests for colorectal cancer.[30] Thus, a test's predictability may depend not only on the actual ability of the test to identify the disease gene, but also on who is reading the results of the tests.

However, because hundreds or even thousands of genetic risks may become predictable, it may be unreasonable to assume that physicians will be able to warn each patient of all the potential risks and tests available to determine those risks. Thus courts have already begun to limit the types of genetic risks that physicians must disclose. Most states recognize wrongful birth cases only if the disorder is "serious." One court indicated, for example, that deafness was not sufficiently serious. However, parents have won cases in which the resulting child had Down syndrome, cystic fibrosis and polycystic kidney disease (which, to most people, would certainly not be considered so serious as to make life not worth living).

WRONGFUL LIFE

Courts have been much less willing to recognize wrongful life suits on behalf of the child, rather than on behalf of the parents. The claim of the child in a wrongful life case is that he or she would rather not have been born than be born with a particular disorder—and most courts have believed that was a matter for philosophers, rather than judges, to decide.[31]

Only three states—California, New Jersey and Washington—currently recognize wrongful life claims, and nine states statutorily bar such claims.[32] Jurisdictions that have refused to recognize the validity of wrongful life actions justify the decision by simply stating that they refuse to grapple with the philosophical and ethical implications of such an allegation. In a wrongful life action, "the child does not allege that the physician's negligence caused the child's deformity. Rather, the claim is that the physician's negligence—his failure to adequately inform the parents of the risk—has caused the birth of the deformed child. The child argues that but for the inadequate advice, it would not have been born to experience the pain and suffering attributable to the deformity."[33]

Courts *have* recognized a wrongful life cause of action in a few states when doctors failed to advise prospective parents of genetic risks[34] or provided erroneous information.[35] In such cases, the child may even be allowed to recover damages for "diminished childhood." In 1984, in *Procanik v. Cillo,* the New Jersey Supreme Court let the child recover damages for "diminished childhood" where the child sued her doctor for negligently denying her parents information regarding her health *in utero.* This court found wrongful life damages appropriate because it assumed that a child would rather not have been born than to have been born disabled and born to parents whose ability to care for her would be negatively impacted because of her disability.[36]

At least one court *in dicta* suggested that children may bring wrongful life actions against their parents in addition to, or instead of, against the negligent health care provider. A California court stated: "If a case arose where, despite due care by the medical profession in transmitting the necessary warnings, parents made a conscious choice to proceed with a pregnancy, with full knowledge that a seriously impaired infant would be born . . . we see no sound policy which should protect those parents from being answerable for the pain, suffering and misery which they have wrought upon their offspring."[37]

Thus far, no court has recognized a wrongful life suit by a child against a parent. Indeed, after the California decision, that state's legislature passed a law stating: "No cause of action arises against a parent of the child based upon the claim that the child should not have been conceived or, if conceived, should not have been allowed to have been born alive."[38]

The courts recognizing wrongful life claims have done so mainly because they find that the focus should not be on whether an impaired life is better than no life at all—which has been historically cited as justification for refusing to recognize wrongful life causes of action; instead these courts have focused on awarding damages for the child with the disability. In *Curlender v. Bio-Science Laboratories,* the court allowed a child born with Tay-Sachs disease to bring a wrongful life suit against a medical testing facility and a physician for negligently telling the child's parents that they were not carriers of the Tay-Sachs gene. The court stated: "the reality of the 'wrongful life' concept is that such a plaintiff both exists and suffers, due to the negligence of others. . . . The certainty of genetic impairment is no longer a mystery."[39] Similarly, a New Jersey court allowed a child to bring a claim of wrongful life and stated that a wrongful life claim "is not premised on the concept that non-life is preferable to an impaired life, but it's predicated on the needs of the living."[40]

Damages recoverable under causes of action for wrongful birth and wrongful life claims differ between jurisdictions. As a general rule, either the parents or the child—but not both—may recover the extraordinary costs associated with the child's illnesses. Furthermore, some jurisdictions allow the recovery of emotional-distress damages in wrongful birth or wrongful life cases and may award damages for "diminished parental capacity" or "diminished childhood."

The New Jersey supreme court allows damages for "diminished parental capacity" based on the theory that "[p]arents can suffer diminished parental capacity as a result of . . . being excluded from perhaps the most important decision in their lives—whether to give birth to a congenitally defective child. . . . Thus, parents victimized by negligent genetic counseling bear a multiple burden."[41] Another court allowed parents to recover for wrongful birth under the theory that such a holding would enhance, rather than disparage, the emotional well-being of the entire family.[42]

The legal cases view a child with a disability as a tragedy for the whole family. In some jurisdictions, siblings of a child with a disability may bring wrongful birth claims against a negligent doctor and may also be permitted to recover damages for "loss of parental services." In 1994, in *Batson v. U.S.,* the court held that the sister of a child born with neural tube defects could recover for loss of parental services. The court believed that the extra financial and emotional burden placed on parents by virtue of having a child whose doctor negligently failed to prenatally diagnose the disorder would cause the "healthy" sibling necessarily to lose out on "care, counsel, and training and education which a child might . . . have reasonably received otherwise."[43] An earlier court, however, refused to recognize a wrongful birth claim brought by parents and a child's siblings in part because the court felt the life of their sister did not constitute an actionable injury.[44]

In the first suit of its kind, a New Jersey appellate court held that a grandfather cannot bring a wrongful birth suit on his behalf to recover emotional distress arising from the birth of his grandson. The grandfather alleged that a grandparent is a "filament of family life" and that the birth of the child affected the entire family. Thus, he argued, he should also be entitled to recover damages for the emotional distress he suffered when the defendants failed to inform the mother of his grandson of fetal abnormalities.[45] The appellate court held that only the parents of the child may recover for pain and suffering resulting from the birth of the child.[46]

HOW DO JUDGES VIEW DISABILITY?

"There is reason for us to fear wrongful birth suits and oppose suits for wrongful life," says Adrienne Asch: "it is the message they send to the children themselves, disabled people, and society about the worth of life with impairments."[47]

An analysis of judges' opinions does give cause for concern about the social messages being sent about disability. Today's courts' willingness to recognize wrongful birth suits contrasts greatly with decisions in the 1960s when courts did not allow such suits, in part because it would devalue people with disabilities. In *Gleitman v. Cosgrove,*[48] a 1967 case, for example, the court stated:

> The right to life is inalienable in our society. A court cannot say what defects should prevent an embryo from being allowed life such that denial of the opportunity to terminate the existence of a defective child in embryo can support a cause for action. Examples of famous persons who have had great achievement despite physical defects come readily to mind, and many of us can think of examples close to home. A child need not be perfect to have a worthwhile life. We are not faced here with the necessity of balancing the mother's life against that of her child. The sanctity of the single human life is the decisive factor in this suit in tort. Eugenic considerations are not controlling. We are not talking here about the breeding of prize cattle. It may have been easier for the mother and less expensive for the father to have terminated the life of the child while he was an embryo, but these alleged detriments cannot stand against the preciousness of the single human life to support a remedy in tort.

The court even went so far as to cite Jonathan Swift's "A Modest Proposal"[49] to support the last point.

A 1979 case similarly ruled:

> [One] of the most deeply held beliefs of our society is that life—whether experienced with or without a major physical handicap—is more precious than non-life . . . [the child] by virtue of her birth, will be able to love and be loved and to experience happiness and pleasure—emotions which are truly the essence of life and which are far more valuable than the suffering she may endure. To rule otherwise would require us to disavow the basic assumption upon which our society is based. This we cannot do.[50]

The way the judges today talk about people with disabilities has moved from a right-to-life analysis to the right of parents to use their best judgment about their future children. However, a discussion of the affected child's abilities is almost never discussed in the cases allowing some form of damages. Instead, the courts have focused on the child's disabilities and the degree to which this caused his or her parents, as well as the entire family, to suffer. The impact on the parents is seen as virtually unbearable. "The psychological trauma is much deeper and the impairment more pernicious than a seeming lack of love. . . . such parents 'are consumed with an awful sorrow. Not the surgical sorrow of death, but an hourly, daily, yearly sorrow—an agonizing shattering, tearing sorrow.'"[51] Another judge said: "No one can fail to deplore the anguish experienced by these unfortunate parents. A pecuniary award, regardless of its size, cannot compensate them for their sorrow."[52]

The diseases at issue are painted in gloomy terms. Cystic fibrosis is described as an "insidious and incurable disease. . . . The prospects for one suffering from cystic fibrosis . . .

are grim."[53] A child with a disability is seen as having "to bear the frightful weight of his abnormality throughout life."[54]

WHAT WOULD BE A DISABILITY-CENTERED APPROACH TO WRONGFUL BIRTH AND WRONGFUL LIFE SUITS?

What might an ADA-type approach to wrongful birth and wrongful life cases look like? One approach might be to eliminate such causes of action entirely. Courts recognize, for example, that a child cannot sue his father for being born illegitimate.[55] The California Court of Appeals, in the wrongful life suit, *Curlender v. Bio-Science,* said "it cannot be disputed that in present society such a circumstance [illegitimacy], both socially and legally, no longer need present an overwhelming obstacle."[56] It could be argued that, similarly, being born with a disability should no longer be actionable since the ADA and related laws remove many social and legal obstacles previously encountered by people with disabilities.

Even if wrongful birth and wrongful life cases were not eliminated entirely, people concerned about disability rights could try to ensure that they are not applied to less serious disabilities. Drawing such a line is obviously a sensitive and troubling matter. Perhaps it is hubris even to try. But there may be some disorders—painful, serious, causing early death, such as Tay-Sachs disease—where there may be fairly widespread support for parents' uncoerced and private decisions to undergo testing and abort to avert their child's pain and suffering. In all other instances, then, such legal actions could be forbidden.

There is at least some legal precedent for this second approach of line-drawing. Some early courts that entertained wrongful birth or wrongful life causes of action presumed that only children "born with gross deficiencies"[57] or "invidious and incurable" diseases would bring such suits.[58] For example, in *Turpin v. Sortini,* a wrongful birth case, the California Supreme Court asserted: "[i]n this case, in which the plaintiff's only affliction is deafness, it seems quite unlikely that a jury would ever conclude that life with such a condition is worse than not being born at all."[59]

Such line-drawing is appropriate if we do not want to require children to come with a genetic warranty. It seems totally inappropriate, for example, to screen a fetus for late-onset disorders, such as Huntington's disease or Alzheimer's.

The push to test—even for trivial or treatable conditions—is strong, in part because there is a financial benefit to the companies, patent holders and physicians who offer testing for less serious disorders. Yet certain tests should not be offered—because the condition is so trivial or is treatable after birth, or because the existence of the test seems to demean already-existing individuals with that condition. We discourage prenatal sex selection, because it is assumed that fetuses should not be aborted just because the individual will be discriminated against later in life. As we are flooded with new genetic tests, we need a societywide assessment about where to draw the line on the use of genetic services.

A third approach would focus not on limiting the legal claims but on trying to better inform potential parents about the nature of various disabilities so that they will not equate the birth of a child with a legal wrong. Disability rights activist Lisa Blumberg notes: "[t]oo often counselors do little more than provide future parents with a dreary laundry list of problems their child could have and express sympathy."[60] Before testing, an individual should be told about the genetic conditions for which he or she or the fetus is being tested, whether they are treatable, and about whether, in the prenatal context, the parents will be faced with a decision about whether to abort the fetus. He or she should have the opportunity to meet people with the disability for which testing is being done. Much thought should be given to the type of information that should be presented; this is an area in which disability activists can provide considerable aid to physicians and counselors.

Providing more accurate information about an individual's life with disabilities, and assuring that people in general have more contact with such individuals in the course of their daily lives,[61] may help prevent some couples from being coerced into testing and abortion and may deter lawsuits. Personal knowledge of a particular disorder can lessen the tendency of people unthinkingly to seek a "genetic fix." Some genetic counselors, for example, find that after working with patients with cystic fibrosis, they are no longer willing to participate in counseling for prenatal tests (since they personally do not feel that such a child should be aborted).

CONCLUSION

Preventing the birth of an individual with a disease is morally different from preventing a disease. "It suggests that the lives of some persons with a disability or illness are not worth living, that such persons are to be understood only as social or economic drains and never as sources of either independent value or enrichment for the lives of others," says Ruth Faden, director of the Program in Law, Ethics, and Health at Johns Hopkins University.[62] To the extent that judges deciding wrongful birth and wrongful life convey the message that disability itself is a legal wrong, it is time to take action to address these misperceptions forcefully.

NOTES

[1]This problem is exacerbated by the fact that few people have contact with individuals with a disability and consequently may overestimate their cost to society and underestimate their contribution to society.

[2]Paul Ramsey, "Screening: An Ethicist's View," in B. Hilton, D. Callahan, M. Harris, P Condliffe, and B. Berkley, eds. *Ethical Issues in Human Genetics: Genetic Counseling and the Use of Genetic Knowledge.* 163 Fogarty International Proceedings No. 13, 1973: 147, 159.

[3]Marsha Saxton, "Disability Rights and Selective Abortion," in Ricki Solinger, ed. *The Fifty Years War: Abortion Politics, 1950 to 2000.* Berkeley, CA: University of California Press, in press.

[4]Dorothy C. Wertz and John C. Fletcher, "A Critique of Some Feminist Challenges to Prenatal Diagnosis," 2 *J. Women's Health* 173–188, 181 (1993).

[5]Saxton, "Disability Rights."

[6]Adrienne Asch, for example, points out that blind parents are sometimes denied custody and visitation rights based on their disability. Adrienne Asch, "Reproductive Technology and Disability," in Sherrill Cohen and Nadine Taub, eds. *Reproductive Laws in the 1990s* Clifton, NJ: Humana Press, 1989 (citations omitted), 69–123, 79.

[7]Laura Hershey, "Choosing Disability," *Ms.,* July/August 1994, 26–32, 29.

[8]Saxton, "Disability Rights."

[9]Office of Technology Assessment, U.S. Congress, *Mapping Our Genes* 84 (1988).

[10]Diane Beeson, "Social and Ethical Issues in the Prenatal Diagnosis of Fetal Disorders," in Benedict M. Ashley and Kevin D. O'Rourke, eds. *Health Care Ethics: A Theological Analysis,* 3d ed., St. Louis, MO: Catholic Health Association of the United States, 1989, 76–86, 81.

[11]Abby Lippman, "The Genetic Construction of Prenatal Testing, Choice, Consent, or Conformity for Women?" in Karen H. Rothenberg and Elizabeth Thomson, eds. *Women and Prenatal Testing: Facing the Challenges of Genetic Technology.* Columbus, OH: Ohio University Press, 1994, 9–34, 15.

[12]Adrienne Asch and Gail Geller, "Feminism, Bioethics, and Genetics," in Susan M. Wolf, ed. *Feminism and Bioethics: Beyond Reproduction.* London: Oxford University Press, 1996 (footnote omitted), 318–350, 330.

[13]In one study, "60% of urban white women over age 40 in Georgia, but only 0.5% of African women over 40 in rural areas used prenatal diagnosis." Wertz and Fletcher, note 4 at 178, citing D. C. Sokol, J. R. Byrd, A.T.L. Chen, M. F. Goldberg and G. P. Oakley, "Prenatal Chromosome Diagnosis: Racial and Geographical Variation for Older Women in Georgia," 244 *JAMA* 1355–1357 (1980).

[14]Id.

[15]See Lori B. Andrews, "Body Science," 83 *American Bar Association Journal* 44 (1997).

[16]Asch, "Reproductive Technology," 87.

[17]Hugh Gregory Gallagher, "Can We Afford Disabled People?" 14th Annual James C. Hemphill Lecture, September 7, 1995, Rehabilitation Institute of Chicago, 21.

[18]Hershey, "Choosing Disability," 28.

[19]Id., 30.

[20]"Disabled People Mixed Over Genetic Future," BBC News, September 28, 1999, available at http://news.bbc.co.uk/hi/english/health/newsid_459000/459330.htm.

[21]Saxton, "Disability Rights."

[22]See, eg., *Gildiner v. Thomas Jefferson Univer. Hosp.* 451 F.Supp. 692, 695 (E.D. Pa. 1978); *Lininger v. Eisenbaum,* 764 P.2d 1202, 1212 (Colo. 1988); *Blake v. Cruz,* 698 P.2d 315, 332 (Idaho 1984); *Dorlin v. Providence Hosp.,* 325 N.W.2d 600, 601 (Mich. Ct. App. 1982); *Eisbrennery v. Stanley,* 308 N.W. 2d 2O9,213 (Mich. Ct. App. 1–981); *Azzolino v. Dingfelder,* 337 S.E.2d 528, 532033 (N.C. 1985), cert. denied, 479 U.S. 835 (1986); *Schroeder v. Perkel,* 432 A.2d 834, 840 (N.J. 1981); *Berman v. Allen,* 404 A.2d 8, 12 (N.J. 1972); *Gleitman v. Cosgrove,* 227 A.2d 689, 692 (N.J. 1967); *Alquijay v. St. Luke's-Roosevelt Hosp. Ctr.,* 473 N.E.2d 244, 245 (N.Y. 1984); *Becker v. Schwartz,* 386 N.E.2d 807, 812 (N.Y. 1978); *Ellis v. Sherman,* 478 A.2d 1339, 1342 (Pa. Sup. Ct. 1984), aff'd, 515 A.2d 1327 (Pa. 1986); *Nelson v. Krusen,* 678 S.W.2d 918 (Tex. 1984); *James G. v. Caserta,* 332 S.E.2d 872, 881 (W.Va. 1985); *Dumer v. St. Michael's Hosp.,* 233 N.W.2d 372, 377 (Wis. 1975); *Beardsley v. Wierdsman,* 650 P.2d 288 289–90 (Wyo. 1982).

[23]See, eg., *Procanik v. Cillo,* 478 A.2d 755, 760 (N.J. 1984) (plaintiffs could not assert that the physician's negligence caused the child's congenital rubella syndrome or that the child ever had a chance to live a normal life).

[24]See *Gleitman v. Cosgrove,* 227 A.2d 689, 692–93 (N.J. 1967) (holding that no casual link existed between a fetus's injury resulting from its mother's exposure to German measles and the doctor's failure to warn the parents of the risk of such an injury).

[25]See *Keel v. Banach,* 624 So.2d 1022 (Ala 1993); *University of Arizona Health Services Center v. Superior Court,* 136 Ariz. 579, 667 P.2d 1294 (1983); *Turpin v. Sortini,* 31 Cal. 3d 220, 182 Cal. Rptr. 337, 643 P.2d 954 (1982); *Lininger v. Eisenbaum,* 764 P.2d 1202 (Colo. 1988); *Haymon v. Wilkerson,* 535 A.2d 880 (D.C. 1987); *Garrison v. Medical Center of Delaware, Inc.,* 581 A.2d 288 (Del. 1989); *Kush v. Lloyd,* 616 So.2d 415 (Fla. 1992); *Arche v. United States Dep't of AM,* 247 Kan. 276, 798 P.2d 477 (1990); *Reed v. Campagnolo,* 332 Md. 226, 630 A.2d 1145(1993); *Viccaro v. Milun* 406 Mass. 777, 551 N.E.2d 8 (1990); *Greco v. United States,* III Nev. 405, 893 P.2d 345 (1995); *Smith v. Cote* 128 N.H. 231, 513 A.2d 341 (1986); *Schroeder v Perkel,* 87 N.J. 53, 432 A.2d 834 (1981); *Becker v. Schwartz,* 46 N.Y.2d 401, 413 N.Y.S.2d 895, 386 N.E.2d 807 (1978); *Owens v. Foote,* 773 S.W.2d 911 (Tenn. 1989); *Jacobs v. Theimer,* 519 S.W.2d 846 (Tex. 1975); *Naccash v. Burge* 223 Va. 406, 290 S.E.2d 825 (1982); *Harbeson v. Parke-Davis, Inc.,* 98 Wash.2d 460, 656 P.2d 483 (1983); *James G. v. Caserta,* 175 W.Va. 406, 332 S.E.2d 872 (1985); *Dumer v. St. Michael's Hospital,* 69 Wis.2d 766, 233 N.W.2d 372 (1975); *Goldberg v. Ruskin,* 128 111. App. 3d 1029, 84 111. Dec. 1, 471 N.E.2d 530 (1984); *Eisbrenner v. Stanley,* 106 Mich. App. 357, 308 N.W.2d 209 (1981); *Flanagan v. Williams,* 87 Ohio App. 3d 768, 623 N.E.2d 185 (1993). Georgia and North Carolina bar wrongful birth causes of action by judicial decision. See *Atlanta Obstetrics & Gynecology Group v. Abelson* 260 Ga. 711, 398 S.E.2d 557 (1990); see also *Azzolino v. Dingfelder,* 315 N.C. 103, 337 S.E.2d 528 (1985).

[26]See, eg., *Becker v. Schwartz,* 386 N.E.2d 807, 814 (N.Y. 1978) (noting the effect of a mother's age on the development of a fetus).

[27]See *Haymon v. Wilkerson,* 535 Acted 880, 881 (D.C. 1987) (finding liability when a couple followed a physician's advice discouraging genetic testing of their fetus and the fetus was subsequently diagnosed as having Down syndrome).

[28]See *Naccash v. Burg,* 290 S.E.2d 825, 837 (Va. 1982) (allowing recovery for a physician's failure to use a blood test to determine the risk that an Eastern-European Jewish couple had of passing Tay-Sachs disease to their children).

[29]See, eg., *Gallagher v. Duke University,* 822 F.2d 793 (4th Cir. 1988).

[30]See F. Giardiello, J. Brensinger, G. Peterson, M. Luce, L. Hyland, J. Bacon, S. Booker, R. Parker, and S. Hamilton, "The Use and Interpretation of Commercial APC Gene Testing for Familial Adenomatous Polyposis," 336 *N. Eng. J. Med.* 823–27 (1997).

[31]See, eg., *Gleitman v. Cosgrove,* 227 A.2d 689 (N.J. 1967); *Becker v. Schwartz,* 386 N.E.2d 807 (N.Y. 1978).

[32]See Idaho Code § 5–334 (1995) (statutorily barring both wrongful life and wrongful birth claim); Ind. Code Ann. § 34–1–1–11 (1996) (barring wrongful life causes of action); Minn. Stat. § 145.424(l), (2) (1993) (barring wrongful life and wrongful birth claims, respectively); Mo. Rev. Stat. § 188.130 (1995) (barring both wrongful life and wrongful birth claims); N.C. Gen. Stat. § 14.45. 1 (e) (1996) (conscience clause used by courts to bar both claims); N.D. Cent. Code § 32 03–43 (1995) (barring wrongful life causes of action); 42 Pa. Cons. Stat. § 8305 (1993) (barring both wrongful life and wrongful birth claims); S.D. Codified Laws Ann. §§ 21–55–1 & 21–55–2 (1987) (wrongful life, birth and conception claims explicitly barred); Utah Code Ann. § 78–11–24 (1993) (barring wrongful life and wrongful birth claims).

[33]See Thomas D. Rogers, "Wrongful Life and Wrongful Birth: Medical Malpractice in Genetic Counseling and Prenatal Testing," 33 *S.C. L. Rev.* 713 (1982).

[34]See, eg., *Turpin v. Sortini,* 643 P.2d 954, 965 (Cal. 1982) (bringing a claim against a health care provider for failure to advise parent of a hereditary hearing defect).

[35]See *Curlender v. Bio-Science Lab.,* 165 Cal. Rptr. 477, 479–80 (Ct. App. 1980) (bringing suit against a laboratory for negligently conducting genetic tests).

[36]See 478 A.2d 755, 764–66.

[37]See *Curlender v. Bio-Science Lab.,* 165 Cal. Rptr. 477, 488 (Ct. App. 1980).

[38]See Cal. Civ. Code § 43.6 (West 1998).

[39]See 165 Cal. Rptr. 477, 488 (App. Ct. 1980).

[40]See *Procanik v. Cillo,* 478 A.2d 755, 763 (N.J. 1984).

[41]See *Procanik v. Cillo,* 478 A.2d 755, 766–67 (N.J. 1984) (Handler, J., concurring in part and dissenting in part).

[42]See *Marciniak v. Lundborg,* 450 N.W.2d 243, 246 (Wisc. 1990).

[43]See 848 F.Supp. 962, 973 (U.S. Dist. Ct. 1994).

[44]See *Azzolino v. Dingfelder,* 337 S.E.2d–528, 537 (N.C. 1985).

[45]See Molly J. Liskow, "Grandfather of Tay-Sachs Baby Cannot Sue for Wrongful Birth," *New Jersey Lawyer,* May 11, 1998, 46 (citing *Michelman v. Erlich,* N.J. Appellate Division, A-3846–96TI, May 6, 1998).

[46]Id.

[47]Asch, "Reproductive Technology," 94.

[48]44 N.J. 22, 227 A.2d 689 (1967).

[49]Jonathan Swift, "A Modest Proposal" in *Gulliver's Travels and Other Writings.* New York: Modern Library, 1958, 488–496.

[50]*Berman v. Allan,* 404 A.2d 8, 12–13 (1979).

[51]*Procanik v. Cillo,* 97 N.J. 339, 363 (Handler, J., dissenting) (quoting G. Stigen, *Heartaches and Handicaps* 6 (1976)).

[52]*Naccash v. Burger,* 223 Va. 406,420 (1982) (dissent).

[53]*Schroeder,* 87 N.J. at 58–59.

[54]*Gleitman v. Cosgrove,* 227 A.2d 689, 704 (1967) (Jacobs, J., dissenting).

[55]*Zepeda v. Zepeda,* 190 N.E.2d 849 (111. App. Ct. 1963).

[56]*Curlender,* 106 Cal. App. 3d 811, 825 (1980).

[57]See *Becker,* 386 N.E.2d 812 (consolidated case where children suffered from Down syndrome and polycystic kidney disease).

[58]See *Shroeder v. Perkel,* 432 A.2d 834, 836 (N.J. 1981) (child suffered from cystic fibrosis).

[59]See 643 P.2d 954, 962 (Cal. 1982).

[60]Lisa Blumberg, "Eugenics vs. Reproductive Choice," *The Disability Rag and ReSource,* January/February 1994, 5.

[61]This could be a benefit of the Americans with Disabilities Act, which provides legal protections to assure that individuals with disabilities are better integrated into society.

[62]Ruth Faden, "Reproductive Genetic Testing, Prevention, and the Ethics of Mothering," in Karen H. Rothenberg and Elizabeth Thomson, eds. *Women and Prenatal Testing: Facing the Challenges of Genetic Technology.* Columbus, OH: Ohio University Press, 1994, 92.

Go to the Margins of the Class
Hate Crimes and Disability

LENNARD J. DAVIS

With great ceremony, the press reported the February 1999 conviction of white-supremacist John William King for the kidnapping and murder of James Byrd Jr., who had been chained to a truck in Jasper, Texas, dragged two miles, and dismembered. Likewise, the conviction of coconspirator Lawrence Russell Brewer in September 1999 seemed to imply that justice had been done. If justice in a broader sense is to be served, however, another fact of the case deserves attention. Byrd was not only black and the victim of race hatred; he was also disabled. The press has so casually noted this that few people realize it; those who do, including myself, found out that Byrd was severely arthritic and subject to seizures. This information was ferreted out only after extensive searches of news reports.

Indeed, I myself was uncertain that Byrd was a person with disabilities. I recalled reading, on the day the crime was first reported, that a disabled African-American had been brutally murdered. Since I was interested in disability, the article caught my eye. Yet when the story reappeared days, weeks and months later, Byrd was simply referred to as African-American. Almost all the news stories contained this simplification. Indeed, when I decided to write a piece on the subject for *The Nation,* I at first thought I might have made an error in thinking that Byrd was a person with disabilities. When I went to the library to look up the articles on microfilm, I found that the *New York Times* mentioned only twice, in the first two reports, that Byrd was a person with disabilities. Any newspaper story I checked tended to follow that pattern.

I decided that in order to write this piece, I had to find out what Byrd's disability was. When I called the sheriff's office, the local newspaper, the district attorney's office, Byrd's family and lawyers, no one could or would tell me. Finally, fact-checkers at *The Nation* managed to discover that Byrd was severely arthritic. When I wrote the article for *The Nation,* the war in Kosovo was beginning. Because of the journalistic space taken up by the war, my article kept being delayed and then further delayed. Finally, the story was no longer current, so the editors and I decided we would aim to publish it when the second defendant went on trial. By the time that happened, the immediacy of the issue had faded. Perhaps the rather complex notion of identity made the piece seem less of a priority, and *The Nation* decided in the end to cancel the story. The reason I am telling this tale, no anomaly in the annals of journalism, is that it signals the difficulty of talking about the issue of disability in the face of race.

At the risk of being overly anecdotal, let me add another bit in the biography of this article. Initially, I wanted to write this story as an op-ed piece for the *New York Times.* An acquaintance who is on the editorial board of the paper read my initial article and responded in a somewhat condescending and negative way. He asked me if I seriously thought that race could be equated with disability, whether the history of lynching and slavery could be meaningfully equated with occasional violence against people with disabilities. The

331

responses of editors for both of these progressive journals was to see race as the primary category and disability as a poor third cousin of race. Their assumption was that violence toward a person of color with disabilities is primarily the result of the color and much less the result of the disability.

But disability is hardly a minor category. Approximately 16 percent of Americans have a disability and, as such, they comprise a significant minority group with an inordinately high rate of abuse.[1] According to the Center for Women's Policy Studies, disabled women are raped and abused at a rate more than twice that of nondisabled women.[2] The risk of physical assault, robbery and rape, according to researcher Dick Sobsey, is at least four times as great for adults with disabilities as for the general population.[3] In February 1999, for example, a mentally retarded man in Keansburg, New Jersey, was abducted by a group of young people who tortured, humiliated and assaulted him.[4] In March 1999, advocates for another mentally retarded man filed a lawsuit against a group of Nassau Country, New York, police officers who beat him while he was in custody.[5]

People with disabilities and deaf people report that they are routinely harassed verbally, physically and sexually in public places. In private institutions or group homes, they are often the prime victims of violence and sexual abuse; in their own homes, they are subjected to sexual abuse, domestic violence and incest, preyed upon by family members, family "friends" and "caretakers."[6] So the question remains, why is American society largely unaware of or indifferent to the plight of people with disabilities? Is it because as an ableist society, we do not really believe that disability constitutes a serious category of oppression? Whenever race and disability come together, as in the King case, ethnicity tends to be considered so much the "stronger" category that disability disappears altogether.

As a society, we have long been confronted by the existence of discrimination against people of color. Students pour over the subject of race in their textbooks and read the work of multicultural writers in high school and college. Martin Luther King Day and Kwanzaa raise our consciousness, and the heroic tales of people like Rosa Parks inspire us.

But while we may acknowledge we are racist, we barely know we are ableist. Our schools, our textbooks, our media utterly ignore the history of disability. The dominant culture renders invisible the works of disabled and deaf poets, writers and performance artists. The closest we have come to a national media engagement is the 1998 six-part NPR radio series *Beyond Affliction* and a few references to deafness in the TV series *ER*. Motion pictures still largely romanticize or pathologize disability. There is not much else to make the experience of 16 percent of the population come alive realistically and politically.

Yet 72 percent of people with disabilities are unemployed, and their income is half the national average.[7] Among working-age adults with disabilities, the poverty rate is three times that of those without impairments. One third of all disabled children live in poverty.[8] And despite the Americans with Disabilities Act, a judicial backlash has been underway ever since its passage in 1990. From 90 to 98 percent of discrimination cases brought under the ADA by people with disabilities have been lost in court. Immigration policy with respect to the disabled emulates the restrictive 1920s naturalization policies aimed at other "undesirable" groups.[9]

With the aging of the war-baby generation, there will be a disability boomlet in the near future. But children constitute the fastest growing segment of the disabled population. From 1990 to 1994 the number of children and young adults with disabilities rocketed by 1.5 million and 1.9 million, respectively—largely due to rising rates of asthma, mental disorders, mental retardation, learning disabilities and spinal cord injuries.[10] The last of these result mostly from sports and automobile accidents among whites and from gunshot wounds among African-Americans.

Legal theorists have a term for the way that race eclipses disability—intersectionality. Kimberle Crenshaw, writing about the way that color obliterates gender, notes that antidiscrimination law rotates around "a single-axis framework."[11] Thus people are marginalized who do not fit clearly into a recognized minority status. Crenshaw makes this case for African-American women who are, according to her analysis, edited out of civil rights and employment decisions which tend to focus more on the issue of race than the combination of race and gender. For example, in *DeGraffenreid v. General Motors,* five African-American women brought a suit against General Motors claiming that the seniority system perpetuated the effects of past discrimination against African-American women. Although evidence adduced at trial revealed that General Motors engaged in discriminatory activities against such women, the district court granted summary judgment for the defendant, stating: "[P]laintiffs have failed to cite any decisions which have stated that Black women are a special class to be protected from discrimination."[12] Because GM had hired women, no sex discrimination was found; the court thought the issue should have been pursued on the basis of race alone. The idea that race and gender could create a special category or have negative synergistic effects seems to have eluded the court entirely.

Anita Silvers notes this fact when she writes: "the courts tend to implement prohibitions against discrimination so as to favor paradigmatic members of the protected class. In doing so, they propel individuals whose experiences diverge from those of the class's prototypes, but who are equally at risk, to the class's margins."[13] Thus when disability meets race, disability is propelled to the margins of the class.

From a legal perspective, one wants to make sure that members of an historically unprotected class receive proper justice and consideration under the law. Thus in America, women and minorities have been the focus of antidiscrimination law. There has been much cultural work done to make it acceptable at the end of the millennium that such groups have public respect and sympathy. Countless novels, movies and plays have accomplished this goal over the course of the twentieth century. It is unimaginable that a film could be made now that would present African-Americans, Native Americans or women as members of a deservedly subordinate, disenfranchised group. Thus the courts will, in the most obvious cases, uphold the right of members of such groups to redress wrongs in housing, employment, discrimination and so on.

However, disability occupies a different place in the culture at this moment. Although considerable effort has been expended on the part of activists, legislators and scholars, disability is still a largely ignored and marginalized area. Every week, films and television programs are made containing the most egregious stereotypes of people with disabilities, and hardly anyone notices. Legal decisions filled with ableist language and attitudes are handed down without anyone batting an eye. It is telling that a professor who is perceived to take an openly antidisability stance was hired in 1999 by Princeton University to fill a prestigious chair over the protests of leaders of the disability community.[14] Such a hire would have been impossible for someone who harbored racist or sexist views. Newspapers and magazines barely notice the existence of disability and largely use ableist language and metaphors in their articles. In other words, disability may still be the last significant area of discrimination that has not been resolved, at least on the judicial, cultural and ethical level, in this century. Likewise, there are no nationally known advocates of disability rights or scholars of disability studies who have anything remotely like the visibility of scholars who deal with race, gender and postcoloniality.

This lack of visibility and of widespread legitimation through cultural and pedagogical institutions has left disability the weaker term. Further, the way that disability has been constructed as an identity category in the popular imagination leads to a lessened status in a pecking order of abuses. Tobin Seibers has written about the way that people with disabilities will necessarily be regarded as narcissists, and I have taken his insight and written about the way that legal cases tend to view people with disabilities.[15]

Because of the nature of disability discrimination, plaintiffs will often protest rather large claims based on rather small infractions. That is, if a particular stairway is not ramped or an employer provides an accessible sink for drinking water in a bathroom but not in the kitchen, a plaintiff can claim violations of the ADA. However, the issue around lack of access can often seen to be minor and trivial, and at the same time, the plaintiff will appear overly concerned about such details, petty, narcissistic and not a good sport or a team player.

The issue of the water fountain, which is one of the violations cited in *Vande Zande v. State of Wisconsin Dept. of Admin.*, seems incredibly trivial. Lori Vande Zande, a paraplegic who uses a wheelchair, worked for the State of Wisconsin, and complained about a pattern of discrimination, one aspect of which involved the state's agreeing to make a bathroom accessible but not a kitchen. Vande Zande would have to fill her drinking cup, clean her dishes, and so on in the bathroom while her coworkers would use the kitchen. Vande Zande claimed that being forced to use the bathroom sink "stigmatized her as different and inferior."[16] Such a claim appears narcissistic in the setting of the office when the category of disability is considered. However, when placed in a setting concerning race, the nature of the claim changes. An African-American who had to use a separate, although equal, water fountain in public accommodations because of his or her identity would more clearly be an obvious violation of civil rights. From the point of view of a white Southerner in the 1960s the person using the fountain was still able to drink the same water and only the location of the fountain was at issue. But from the point of view of the late twentieth century, such segregated drinking fountains are unjust—unless the person is one with disabilities and the employer, not the state, has to provide the accommodation.

Since so much substance in legal cases is based on the state of mind of the plaintiff and the defendant rather than on any major egregious wrong done, these cases seem all the more ephemeral and trivial. If an obese woman claims that she was not hired because the manager thought she was too fat,[17] the case rises or falls on one's assessment of various internal states of mind. Often, to a judge or jury unfamiliar with disability, the claimant can seem paranoid, self-centered, whiny or overly dramatic. Such ideological obstructions stood in the way of earlier cases in which race or gender were considered, but now these categories are so well established that the claimants will not seem petty in asserting discrimination based on these issues.

So when it comes to violence against people with disabilities, several factors intervene. Although many states have statutes that describe disability in a list of categories that are protected under hate crime legislation, the actual enforcement of such policies may be muted by the intersectionality I have been describing. The Violent Crime Control and Law Enforcement Act of 1994 defines a hate crime as one: "in which the defendant intentionally selects a victim, or in the case of a property crime, the property that is the object of the crime, because of the actual or perceived race, color, religion, national origin, ethnicity, gender, disability or sexual orientation of any person."[18] The following states include disability in their hate crime law although not all of these states have actually passed this legislation: Alaska, Arkansas, Arizona, California, the District of Columbia, Delaware, Illinois,

Iowa, Louisiana, Maine, Minnesota, Nebraska, Nevada, New Hampshire, New Jersey, New York, Oklahoma, Rhode Island, Vermont, Washington and Wisconsin.

Tellingly, though, a distinction is often made in this legislation. For example, previously under California's hate crime law, a murder committed because of the victim's race, color, religion, ancestry or national origin could bring the death penalty or life in prison without parole. However, the maximum penalty for a murder based on gender, sexual orientation or disability was 25 years to life in prison. A new bill signed in September 1999 increases the maximum in those latter categories to life in prison without parole. Federal efforts to prevent hate crimes, however, are now restricted to race, color, religion and national origin.

Several United States senators have sponsored legislation to extend efforts to gender, disability and sexual orientation. But at this writing it seems unlikely that this idea will pass into law and, even if it did, that hate crimes based on disability will carry as stringent a penalty as crimes based on hate for race, color, religion or national origin. In September 1999, the National Organization for Women (NOW) and other advocacy groups met with key senators to urge that prohibitions against sex-based and disability-based hate crimes be retained in the Hate Crimes Prevention Act (S. 622, HCPA). But senators opposed to including the new categories prevailed, and the extension of the act's protection to disability, as well as to sex, was defeated in October 1999.

The hierarchy of hate in such legislation is telling. The general idea behind hate crime legislation, ratified in *Wisconsin v. Mitchell*[19] and up to this point without significant appellate action, is that a crime is committed whenever the defendant, in the words of the Wisconsin statute: "[i]ntentionally selects the person against whom the crime . . . is committed . . . because of the race, religion, color, disability, sexual orientation, national origin or ancestry of that person."[20] Although the Wisconsin statute includes disability on a par with other identity categories, California and other states consider that to be a victim because of one's race or religion is substantially more troubling than being a victim because of one's gender, disability status or sexual preference.

But how do we determine, in any philosophical sense, that one kind of identity is more important than another? Historically, although the United States was founded on a separation of church and state, religion has been seen as a "holy" category certainly higher in status than, for example, one's sexual preference; race, so embroiled in the nation's history, must be more important than something like disability; and so on—the arguments are based more on *ad hoc* judgments about the viciousness of different kinds of prejudice than on any principle one can articulate. This seems to be the same unreflective influence that gives priority of race over gender or disability in the intersectionality argument.

We can see this contradiction in another arena. The FBI is required to keep track of hate crimes. It has produced a report that found of the 8,049 incidents of hate crime reported to police in 1997, 12 were motivated by bias based on disability; of these, nine were based on the victim's physical condition and three were based on the victim's mental condition. These numbers seem shockingly low when compared to other studies such as Dick Sobsey's tabulations,[21] which I mentioned earlier. Sobsey also notes that when a crime occurs to a person with disabilities, the crime tends to be a violent crime rather than a property crime.

With women who are disabled, according to the Center for Women's Policy Studies, the fact of disability raises the chances that a woman will be the victim of a crime, and women of color even more so. The Colorado Department of Health estimates that at least 85 percent of women with disabilities are victims of domestic violence, compared with 25 to 50 percent of nondisabled women.[22] Most crimes against women with disabilities go unreported and are substantially higher than the mere 20 per cent of rapes of nondisabled women that are reported. Given these special considerations, is it any wonder that the FBI has such low statistics? The answer must be that when confronted with hate crimes, the FBI, like the journalists reporting on Byrd's case, will often tend to look for the bigger category. Indeed, I am sure that when it comes time for the FBI to list the report on Byrd, they will file it under racial hate crime rather than a disability-related crime. Also, many of the crimes against people with disabilities will simply be seen as ordinary rather than hate crimes. So the rape or murder of a mentally ill resident of a sheltered facility will be seen as a rape or murder, not as one motivated by the status of the person involved. Indeed, one of the arguments used by opponents of hate crime legislation, particularly as it applies to gender or disability, is that crimes such as rapes will have to be investigated by the FBI, putting an undue burden on that organization. Since such crimes are daily occurrences, and since it could be argued that rape itself is a hate crime against women, the FBI will be taxed to the utmost in trying to detail all of these acts of violence.

Intersectionality argues that individuals who fall into the intersect of two catagories of oppression will, because of their membership in the weaker class, be sent to the margins of the stronger class. What these statistics suggest is that the category of disability, while a weak one to judges or legislators, is a powerful one to those who seek to victimize. Rather than minimizing an identity, victimizers are drawn to the double or triple categories of race, gender and disability. Each of these categories enhances the opportunity for hate and the likelihood that the crime will go unnoticed, unreported, disbelieved. For example, the Center for Women's Policy Studies reports that virtually half of the perpetrators of sexual abuse against women with disabilities gained access to their victims through disability services, and that caregivers commit at least 25 percent of all crimes against women with disabilities.[23] In other words, the dependency of such women, escalated by their lower economic status, ethnicity and diminished mobility or ability to communicate to authorities is an enticement to victimizers.

Not only do authorities pay less heed to people with disabilities with diminished capacities who are dependent, they do so because they are unaware, for the most part, of the way that ableism is built into the social, physical and ideological environment. It has only been through the work of disability scholars in the recent past that this situation has come to be articulated in a public and widespread way. As Harlan Hahn observes in "Disputing the Doctrine of Benign Neglect: A Challenge to the Disparate Treatment of Americans with Disabilities," in this volume, the public paternalistically imagines that people with disabilities are usually treated with kindness. This rationalization then is used to invoke happenstance to explain practices that harm people with disabilities. For example, a recent lawsuit by students and the California Faculty Association against San Francisco State University was prompted by such conditions as the university's disregard of the safety of blind people and mobility-impaired people during a period when campus paths of travel were disrupted by construction. Although the student newspaper ran a front-page story and students with disabilities petitioned the university president, the university did not respond. This public university exacted bodily injury as the price students with disabilities had to pay for their education, but deflected its responsibility by construing the dangerous conditions as accidental.[24]

Hahn criticizes the tendency of the justice system to fail to come to grips with the fact that much injurious conduct toward people with disabilities is knowingly imposed. The doctrine of benign neglect which suffuses judicial interpretation of disability discrimination law denies that overt bigotry is the cause of inequities in the protection of people with disabilities. Instead, as Justice Thurgood Marshall insisted in 1985: "discrimination against the handicapped [is] . . . most often the product, not of invidious animus, but rather of thoughtlessness and indifference—of benign neglect." As Hahn comments in a footnote, Justice Marshall may have invoked the phrase "benign neglect" ironically, but the other justices did not appear to recognize it.[25]

The point here is that the general climate of ableism makes it comfortable for us to regard systematic violence against people with disabilities as accidental. Could one claim that the university's policy of negligence toward students with disabilities, especially after being forewarned, is a willed act of violence? The consciousness of the general public and the legal system would have to undergo a dramatic change for the truth of such a claim to be obvious.

Likewise, the definition of "hate" has to change as well. One of the reasons that attacks against people with disabilities are resisted as "hate" crimes is because the general ideology toward people with disabilities rules out hate as a viable emotion. In our culture, it is permissible to "pity" or even "resent" people with disabilities. It is sometimes loosely permitted to make fun of some disabilities (stutters, mental retardation, age-associated deafness, myopia, etc.), but one is generally not supposed to "hate" disabled people. Thus the idea that crimes against people with disabilities might be a result of "hate" seems to most people somehow wrong. Who would act violently toward a person using a wheelchair merely because they could not walk? But the "hate" against people with disabilities is a much more subtle and ingrained hatred. It is a hatred of difference, of the fact that someone cannot see a clearly posted sign, cannot walk up unblocked stairs, need special assistance above what other "normal" citizens need. This kind of hatred is one that abhors the possibility that all bodies are not configured the same, that weakness and impairment are the legacy of a cult of perfection and able embodiment. When the law begins to catch on to this level of hatred, then justice will be served.

Considering that we are entering a new millennium when people with disabilities may make up 20 percent or more of the population, as a society we ought seriously to set about educating ourselves just as we have on issues of race, gender and sexual preference. Let us never forget that the deaf, the feeble-minded and other "defectives" were rounded up first by the Nazis to be sent to the death camps. Only when the camps had consumed people with disabilities did the Nazis begin bringing in the racial undesirables. Disability is not a category that should be obliterated by race or gender. Rather, all these forms of oppression should walk, or wheel, side by side.

NOTES

[1]H. Stephen Kaye, *Disability Watch: The Status of People with Disabilities in the United States.* Oakland, CA: Disability Rights Advocates, 1997, 11.

[2]Barbara Waxman, "Fact Sheet: Violence Against Disabled Women," Center for Women's Policy Studies, e-mail document.

[3]Private communication.

[4]"9th Is Charged in Torture Case as Prosecutors Look for Bias," *New York Times*, February 18, 1999, B5.

[5]David M. Halbfinger, "Man Says Union Chief Beat Him in Jail," *New York Times*, February 24, 1999, B5.

[6]Waxman, "Fact Sheet."

[7]Kaye, *Disability Watch*, 31.

[8]Ibid., 18.

[9] *New York Times,* February 18, 1999, B1.

[10] Kaye, *Disability Watch,* 16.

[11] Kimberly Crenshaw, "Demarginalizing the Intersection of Race and Sex: A Black Feminist Critique of Antidiscrimination Doctrine, Feminist Theory, and Antiracist Politics," in *Living With Contradiction: Controversies in Feminist Social Ethics,* ed. Allison Jagger, Boulder, CO: Westview, 1994, 40.

[12] *De Graffenreid,* 413 F Supp at 143.

[13] Anita Silvers, "The Unprotected: Constructing Disability in the Context of Antidiscrimination Law," this volume.

[14] Katha Pollit, "Peter Singer Comes to Princeton," *The Nation* 268; 16 (May 3, 1999), 10.

[15] Tobin Siebers, "Tender Organs, Narcissism and Identity Politics," in *Disturbing Discourses: A Disability Studies Sourcebook,* Brenda Jo Brueggemann et al., eds., forthcoming; Lennard J. Davis, "Bending Over Backwards: Disability, Narcissism, and the Law," *Berkeley Journal of Labor and Employment Law,* forthcoming.

[16] *Vande Zande v. State of Wisconsin Dept. of Admin.* 44 F. 3d 538, 545 (7th cir. 1995).

[17] *Cassista v. Community Foods,* 5 Cal. 4th 1050 (1993).

[18] Pub. L. No. 103–322, 108 Stat. 1815 (Sept. 13, 1994).

[19] 508 U.S. 476 (1993).

[20] Wisc. Stat. § 939.645.

[21] Dick Sobsey, *Violence and Abuse in the Lives of People With Disabilities.* Baltimore, MD: Paul Brookes Press, 1997.

[22] Waxman, "Fact Sheet."

[23] Waxman, "Fact Sheet."

[24] Thompson, Carolyn. "Special Report, Disabled Students Settle Lawsuit Against San Francisco State University", KGO-TV (ABC affiliate). Eleven O'Clock News, November 5, 1999.

[25] *Alexander v. Choate,* 469 U.S. 287 (1985) at 296.

Viewing U.S. Law from Elsewhere

Canada, the United Kingdom and Australia

Disability rights are an issue worldwide, within and beyond advanced industrialized societies. (Some writers in this volume, such as Gregory Kavka, explicitly limit their remarks to relatively wealthy societies, but others do not.) The United Nations General Assembly first addressed disability in a "Declaration of the Rights of Disabled Persons" in 1975 and subsequently, in 1993, issued the "Standard Rules of the Equalization of Opportunities for People with Disabilities." In its 1994 White Paper on Social Policy, the European Commission of the European Union included a section on "Promoting the Social Integration of Disabled People," which set forth policies aimed at building equal opportunities for the disabled. These and other efforts have elicited heightened attention to disability rights in many nations.

From Birmingham to Bangkok, international, national and local governmental and nongovernmental organizations are exploring ways to create "nonhandicapping" social and physical environments for people with disabilities and elder people. Both the conceptualization and the implementation of disability rights vary from nation to nation. For instance, the 1987 Philippines constitution explicitly lists rights of people with disabilities, including the right to vote without assistance, while Nepal adopts the approach of the United Nations' International Covenant of Economic, Social, and Cultural Rights by making special provisions to protect disabled persons' welfare so they can be active citizens. Germany enforces a requirement that employers ensure the representation of disabled people in their workforces, but a similar British provision, adopted just after World War II, was never enforced and has been superseded recently by a new disability discrimination statute. Other variations of emphasis and enforcement characterize the approaches different nations take to disability rights.

This final section of the volume, presents three views from elsewhere: Canada, the United Kingdom and Australia. Together with the United States, these societies are four of the principal common law and anglophone (at least outside of Quebec) legal systems in the world. Yet they evidence importantly different approaches to disability law within quite different constitutional and civil rights traditions.

In 1985, Canada was the first country in the world to include disability explicitly in a full equality test in its constitution. As Jerome Bickenbach relates, the Charter of Rights and Freedoms includes physical and mental disability along with race, sex and other characteristics singled out for the equal protection of the laws. Thus Canada, unlike the United States, gives explicit constitutional recognition to the right to equality for people with disabilities.

Like disability law in the United States, however, the Canadian approach exemplifies what Bickenbach calls the "human rights approach" to disability policy. Seeking to analogize disability rights to other civil rights, this approach relies in turn on the social conception of disability, rather than the understanding of disability in individualized, medicalized terms. Bickenbach offers a careful characterization of the human rights approach, with disability understood socially, and praises its undoubted achievements. He believes, however, that the analogy between race and disability as characterizing "minority groups" is forced at best; people with disabilities represent a wide range of characteristics and only in limited cases (such as the deaf) are there well-defined communities among them. (However, see the essays by Amundson, Silvers and Hahn in this volume for differing assessments of the aptness of this analogy.) Further, reliance on labeling as a group bears its own risks of adverse stereotyping. Perhaps of deepest theoretical importance, the characterization of "disability," at least in the American ADA as understood in the courts, has reverted back to the medical model of disability in order to limit the numbers who can claim the protection of the civil rights model. The irony, in Bickenbach's judgment, is that the civil rights paradigm thus threatens to undermine the social model of disability that it requires. Bickenbach concludes with praise for the Canadian constitutional approach, because it opens the possibility of understanding the rights of people with disabilities in the broader context of equality rather than in the narrow context of nondiscrimination.

Mairian Corker both describes and criticizes the British counterpart to the ADA, which is called the Disability Discrimination Act, or DDA. In 1995, the DDA was enacted by Parliament as a compromise after successive failures to pass a stronger alternative, the Civil Rights (Disabled Persons) Bill. The DDA protects only a relatively narrow class; people with impairments that have substantial and long-term adverse effects on normal day-to-day activities. The DDA prohibits treating individuals with disabilities less favorably than others are or would be treated, unless the treatment in question can be shown to be justified. There is no theoretical constraint on the various values that may be invoked to justify unfavorable treatment of individuals who are disabled. Corker finds that the DDA—and in some respects the ADA as well—relies on a set of individualistic assumptions which are deeply problematic. Problematic as well are the separation between mind and body represented in the statutory definitions of disability. Finally, the way language constructs our understanding of disability deepens oppression. The DDA does not provide adequate protection for people with disabilities, nor does it insure that they will even be included in the public debates about disability policy.

Finally, Melinda Jones and Lee Ann Marks offer an analysis of the new Australian disabilities law. Australia, unlike the U.S., does not have a significant civil rights tradition. Unlike in both Canada and in the U.S., in Australia there is no tradition of protection of constitutional rights. There are, however, several statutes protecting the civil and political rights of people with disabilities, including the recently enacted Disability Discrimination Act (DDA), modeled in part on the American ADA. Disability law in Australia has developed against the background of a work-based social safety net that relies on improving employment, wages and working conditions, rather than a social security system. One central difference is that the Australian DDA incorporates a very broad definition of disability—going so far as to include physical malformation or disfigurement explicitly—it shifts attention from the status of the complainant to whether he or she has suffered from discriminatory treatment. An implication of the Australian approach is that it does not assign rights which others in the community do not have to a narrowly defined class of disabled people. An important feature of the Australian DDA is its incorporation of strategies for ending discrimination that function as alternatives to individual complaints. These strategies are based on the insight that much discrimination against people with disabilities is structural.

These comparative discussions illustrate a variety of efforts to come to terms with the civil rights of people with disabilities, the rights Jacobus tenBroek pursued over 30 years ago. The authors in Part D are not entirely satisfied with the success of the efforts in their own countries and they are insightful in regard to the lessons, some positive and some not, to be learned from the United States' experience with the ADA. Nevertheless, it is significant that within the past 15 years, each of the four countries, with similar heritages and shared traditions of law, has enacted a major statute protecting the rights of people with disabilities. Today, in each of these countries, Jacobus tenBroek would have an explicit claim to legal protection against the instances of social exclusion he cites in his plea for the right to be in the world. What remains is the continued struggle to understand and bring to fruition this commitment to the achievement of justice, good lives and good communities.

The ADA v. the Canadian Charter of Rights

Disability Rights and the Social Model of Disability

The Americans with Disabilities Act (ADA) has, in its decade of operation, become the model for disability antidiscrimination legislation around the world.[1] To be sure, there are other legal mechanisms for responding to discrimination: Canada, Poland and the Netherlands have constitutional guarantees of equality for persons with disabilities;[2] France, Germany and several other European countries have strict affirmative-action provisions, primarily in the employment sector;[3] and Japan and China, among other countries, have strongly worded though not legally binding or enforceable "prohibitions" of discrimination against persons with mental or physical disabilities[4] which are founded on the equally nonbinding United Nations declarations.[5]

The contrast with the Canadian constitutional approach to disability rights provides an interesting comparison with the ADA. The Canadian Charter of Rights and Freedoms provides in Section 15(1) for a general, and on the face of it very broad, guarantee of equality: "Every individual is equal before and under the law and has the right to the equal protection and equal benefit of the law without discrimination and, in particular, without discrimination based on race, national or ethnic origin, colour, religion, sex, age or mental or physical disability." The Canadian Supreme Court has been cautious in its interpretation of the scope of this provision as it affects persons with disabilities.[6] Inasmuch as successful adjudication using the Charter has constitutional force, all levels of government are bound to act in accordance with the decision. Although individuals can initiate constitutional legal challenges, the federal government of Canada, as well as certain provinces, have found it in their interests to initiate constitutional reviews of their own acts or policies so as to avoid future litigation.

In addition to the constitutional recognition and protection of equality, each Canadian province and the federal government have enacted explicit antidiscrimination legislation (or human rights acts, as they are called), that provide protection against discrimination on the basis of disability. These acts apply to the private sector, unlike the Charter protection, which binds only the various levels of government and its agencies. Their focus, however, is on arbitration and conciliation, and only a few cases make their way (and with extreme slowness) up through the court system. There have been, however, interesting and creative results. For example, a child with cerebral palsy who wished to compete in a bowling tournament won the right to do so, even though that required a change in the rules of the game, inasmuch as she needed to use a ramp to deliver the ball.[7] Unfortunately, in recent years, human rights agencies have been dramatically underfunded, with the result that what was once a slow process is now a glacially slow process.

Ultimately, when human rights are guaranteed, constitutionally or otherwise, enforcement becomes a judicial matter and is not restricted to providing compensation to one individual whose rights have been violated. Indeed, on occasion courts in Canada have creatively devised techniques for altering offensive legislative provisions, up to the point of excising certain wordings and substituting others. The bluntest tool available to a Canadian court is a declaration that a law (and so state action taken in accordance with the law) is *ultra vires;* but in practice, Canadian courts have taken to issuing far more subtle and effective orders in order to ensure that equality for persons with disabilities is enhanced and protected. Relying on the Charter's internal logic, courts have held that forms of discriminatory treatment, though arguably justified by a background pressing and substantial state objective (for example, highway safety), nonetheless violated equality because the means in which that objective was sought to be achieved were not rationally connected to the objective.[8] In another high profile case a deaf individual who had argued that hospitals in British Columbia which fail to provide sign language interpreters discriminate against people who are deaf was successful. The Supreme Court of Canada had little difficulty demanding that legislative changes be implemented forthwith to ensure that the province's health sector functioned in line with the constitutional protection of equality.[9]

At the same time, "judicial legislation" of this sort certainly has its critics and is highly dependent on the membership of the court and their political views.

The Canadian approach to the constitutional enforcement of disability human rights is not without its problems. The discourse of human rights becomes specialized and removed from common understanding. An individual or group who wants to bring a case against a law or policy has the onerous task of bringing before the courts complex constitutional argumentation. The process can take years, is extremely expensive, and can be dismissed without comment by a court that judges the issues of insignificant constitutional importance. Courts, finally, as rule are understandably reluctant to move too quickly or too far when interpreting the highest law of the land.

Although there are many procedural and substantive differences between the Canadian constitutional approach and that adopted in the U.S. and elsewhere, all examples of legal protections against discrimination are a manifestation of what might be called "the human rights approach" to disability social policy. Undoubtedly the single most important social event in international disability advocacy in the past couple of decades, the human rights approach was the product of political action and lobbying in the U.S. and elsewhere from the early 1960s on.[10] The disability rights movement followed and adhered to the strategies and inspiration of civil rights movements responding to racial discrimination, which, certainly in the U.S. context, accounts for the reliance on antidiscrimination protection as the primary expression of disability rights and the mode of their protection.

Early on, disability advocates realized that an essential theoretical presupposition of the human rights approach was a very different conception of disability from that standardly used in the medical community. Relying on decades of work by sociologists and sociopsychologists,[11] advocates gravitated towards the "social model" of disability, in which disability is seen as the outcome of an interaction between intrinsic features of the individual's body or mind (impairments) and the complete social and physical context or environment in which that the person carries out his or her life.[12]

Hints of the social model can be discerned in the definition of "handicapped individual" found in the original version of the Rehabilitation Act of 1973 (mirroring the language of Title VI of the Civil Rights Act of 1964), which created a parallel between the disadvantageous social reception of disability and that of race.[13] A more explicit and considerably more radical expression of the social model came in 1976 from a group of disabled individuals in the U.K. calling themselves the Union of the Physically Impaired Against Segregation (UPIAS), who defined "disability" as "the loss or limitation of opportunities to take part in the normal life of the community on an equal level with others due to physical and social barriers."[14]

More moderate and defensible versions of the social model of disability argue that while having a disability means being limited in the range of activities one can perform, what accounts for this limitation is often if not always a matter of the environmental context in which human actions occur.[15] In particular, physical and socially created or tolerated barriers limit when they do not prevent the performance of human activities, roles or behaviors which, in composite, account for the sum total of human life in all its social dimensions. The physical and social world creates barriers for people with impairments: stigmatizing attitudes and presumptions of incompetence, failures to accommodate impairment needs, and a general neglect that makes possible the design of products and the built environment that are not fully useable for people with mobility, communication or intellectual impairments. The social world that produces barriers or fails to remove them creates much of the disadvantage of having a disability.

Other recent attempts to describe the social model of disability have sought to describe more carefully the relationship between the intrinsic features of human bodies and minds that account for impairments and the extrinsic features of the physical and social world that, in interaction, yield the experience of disability. Moreover, the relationship between impairments and limitations in the performance of activities is more complex than usually believed. The disabilities that people experience can be linked to a wide range of background impairments, and it is rare to be able to infer from impairment to disability, or vice versa. For example, a person may have limitations in his or her ability to move around in an open public area because of impairments that interfere with walking, or with seeing obstacles or with being able psychologically to deal with strangers. On the other hand, we should be wary of predictions about what people who have visual impairments can or cannot do: some of these predictions merely reflect stigmatizing preconceptions.

The social model of disability, in brief, can be characterized by adherence to the following propositions:

1. Disability is a complex phenomenon that results from interactions between intrinsic features of human minds and bodies and features of the physical and social environment in which people live and act.
2. Disability cannot be reduced to or be predicted from underlying physical or mental states of the person.
3. Disability is not a dichotomous state that people either have or do not have, but is rather "fluid and continuous,"[16] existing in various forms and degrees; moreover, disability is a universal human experience.
4. Disability cannot be understood independently of the complete context—that is, features of the physical and social environment—of the person's life.

THE ADA AND THE DISABILITY RIGHTS APPROACH

In the U.S. and other industrialized countries, the disability rights movement—underpinned by one or another version of the social model of disability—played itself out against a background of specific social entitlements and related provisions, primarily in the areas of health, rehabilitation, transportation, education and employment. Historically, these provisions were overtly political responses to the demands of disabled veterans, with the result that disability programming, despite the rights revolution, tends to be reactive and piecemeal.[17] Often, too, disability policies have seemed to be more responsive to the professional needs of service providers and bureaucrats than to people with disabilities themselves.

As an essentially consumer protest, the disability rights movement was fueled by a rejection of this manner of meeting disabled people's needs. Initially at least, what was demanded was not more social programming or even specific entitlements, but a reorientation of the very foundation of disability law and policy. What was needed was an explicit recognition of the human rights of persons with disabilities. All change for the better would flow once it was acknowledged that people with disabilities are not given their rights as a matter of charity or the goodwill of others, but are entitled to them as equal members of society.

The human rights approach, in other words, was at bottom a demand for equality for persons with disabilities. Following the pattern of other civil rights movements, that demand was, so to speak, legally operationalized as antidiscrimination enforcement. The legal mechanism for securing equality thus became enforceable protections against discrimination on the grounds of disability. While the human rights approach put full participation and equality foremost on its agenda, it also reacted against the stereotypes of infirmity and childlike dependency and set its sights on the goals of independence and self-sufficiency. Especially in the U.S., disability advocates adopted and made their own the culture of individualism and a rejection of a paternalistic state. Rather than entitlement programming, which fosters dependence, the goal should be economic self-sufficiency, usually in the form of remunerative employment. Equality, advocates believed, could be best served by enabling people with disabilities to be competitive in the open labor market, giving them a fair and equal opportunity to get and keep a job. The strategy of encouraging people with disabilities to make demands for full inclusion into existing economic structures was motivated by the fundamental faith that full employment for persons with disability was bound to have long-range economic advantages for the society at large. This suggested that what prevented fully inclusive employment could not be the labor market itself but, rather, economically irrational stigma and prejudice of the sort that antidiscrimination legislation is perfectly designed to remedy.

In retrospect, the disability rights approach can be credited with nearly every change in attitude and treatment of people with disabilities in the last two decades, from curb cuts and accessible bathrooms to programs to integrate developmentally disabled children into the public schools. As it has matured, the approach has adopted some of the theoretical developments introduced by feminists and black theorists. More recently, the approach has taken on some of the flavor of identity politics. Yet through it all, faith has been retained in the legal representation of disability rights in antidiscrimination legislation in general and the ADA in particular.

In the face of proven success, it might seem churlish to raise objections to theory and practice of antidiscrimination law or to question whether equality-seeking is always and only a matter of preventing discrimination. Nonetheless, cautious critique is justified if, as I believe, in the contemporary social and economic climate legislation like the ADA yields doctrine and results that are in conflict with the underlying political and ideological components of the disability rights movement, namely the social model of disability and the goal of political equality. This conflict manifests itself when the ADA is viewed either as an appropriate and adequate legal remedy for rights violations or, more broadly, as a constructive social response to the inequality that people with disabilities experience.

THE ADA AS A REMEDY FOR RIGHTS VIOLATIONS

The ADA sets out detailed legal and administrative mechanisms for determining, adjudicating and remedying complaints of discrimination on the basis of disability as explicitly defined by its provisions. This role is accomplished by means of provisions that provide adjudicators with the legal tools for distinguishing discriminatory from nondiscriminatory treatment within protected sectors represented by the four primary titles of the act: Employment, Public Services, Public Accommodations, and Telecommunications. And the purposes of the act are clear—namely, to provide "clear, strong, consistent, enforceable standards" that address discrimination against individuals with disabilities, such as will establish a clear and comprehensive mandate for the elimination of that discrimination.[18]

The governing assumptions of the act are nowhere better expressed than in the "finding" that individuals with disabilities are a: "discrete and insular minority who have been faced with restrictions and limitations, subjected to a history of purposeful unequal treatment, and relegated to a position of political powerlessness in our society, based on characteristics that are beyond the control of such individuals and resulting from stereotypic assumptions not truly indicative of the individual ability of such individuals to participate in, and contribute to, society. . . ."[19] The cause of discrimination is here portrayed as "purposeful unequal treatment" founded on "stereotypic assumptions" directed at a "discrete and insular minority." These salient phrases, adopted directly from the developed law on racial discrimination, firmly root the ADA in a conception of discrimination that informs not only the substantive provisions that follow but also the jurisprudence that has developed.

The ADA presumes that people with disabilities see themselves and are seen by others as a minority group analogous to a racial minority who have historically suffered discriminatory treatment that is fundamentally irrational and prejudicial. Unfortunately, the analogy between disability and race is forced and awkward. The social stigma and stereotyping that undoubtedly exist in the case of disability vary widely between mental and physical impairments. People with disabilities do not have common experiences, nor, the Deaf community notwithstanding, is there a unifying culture or language that people with disabilities can point to in order to establish transdisability solidarity. One does not have to be an anthropologist to observe that the leaders of the disability movement have tended to be highly educated, white, middle-class males with late onset physical disabilities and minimal medical needs, a group that is hardly representative of the population of people with disabilities around the world.

But even if the minority model fitted the facts, and people with disabilities did constitute a "discrete and insular minority," there is a fundamental dilemma in relying on this characterization. Unlike race and gender, in the case of disability adverse labeling is a justifiable concern on its own. Yet in order to benefit from the protections of the ADA, one is required to embrace a label and a minority group status which is explicitly described to be socially discredited.

But surely, it might be argued, the ADA and its operation over the years have helped to destigmatize the label of "person with disability," perhaps even infusing it with new and invigorated positive value. There is little evidence that this has occurred, nor is it clear how it could happen since the purpose of the ADA is explicitly negative, namely to eliminate discrimination against persons with disabilities. Given that purpose, the essence of the ADA as a legal tool rests on its conception not of the minority group nor of an individual with a disability but on discriminatory treatment based on disability.

The key to the ADA's characterization of discriminatory treatment flows from a legal protocol that has gained wide acceptance across jurisdictions that adopted antidiscrimination legislation in the last decade.[20] The protocol, most clearly applied in the employment sector, envisages an individual who is "otherwise qualified" to perform a job, but who is prevented from doing so—or denied some other opportunity or benefit—solely because of a disability (or perceptions that others have of the individual's disability or presumed disability). Such treatment is discriminatory, subject to the conditional defence that no reasonable way exists of accommodating the disability, that is of providing an accommodation, modification, or other alteration that would enable the individual to perform the essential functions of the job. Accommodations are "reasonable" only if their provision would not constitute an "undue hardship" for those charged with providing them.

Inevitably, legislation such as the ADA will lead to proactive or anticipatory responses by individuals and agencies to avoid potential ADA complaints. This is undoubtedly a good thing, but this social response depends entirely on the primary function of the ADA to deal *post hoc* with instances of putatively discriminatory treatment. In short, the ADA is designed to be reactive and complaint-driven. It is legislation that seeks to protect human rights by giving people a legal tool to use when they feel that their rights to equal participation and equal respect are being infringed. Antidiscrimination is, in the first instance, "individualistic" legislation, inasmuch as the onus is on the individual to take the initiative to use the power it provides.

The ADA envisages a situation in which an individual is prevented from achieving goals that he or she could plausibly achieve solely because of artificial barriers founded on irrational beliefs, stereotypes or prejudice about disability. Each individual is presumed to have the motivational and other merit-creating abilities required for full participation in a protected area of social life, so as to plausibly argue that he or she would succeed but for these artificial and irrational obstacles. If nothing else, this presumption in practice clearly favors intelligent people with late-onset mobility or sensory or mild psychiatric impairments that have not affected either their motivation or their general capacity to work. The largest class of complainants under the ADA employment provisions have been from people with lower-back pain—a classic late-onset debilitating condition—and the upper range of compensation awards involve damages such as those awarded against a law firm that failed to accommodate an attorney with depression.

Arguably, the paradigm instance of disability discrimination presumed by the ADA is not representative of the condition of social inequality faced by persons with disabilities. But even if it were, the process of determining whether an individual qualifies for ADA protection has become entangled in complex and subtle legal argumentation and distinction-drawing as the intentionally vague components of the protocol just described are applied to concrete cases. The growing complexity and legal subtlety of ADA case law are clearly seen in the voluminous detail of the Equal Employment Opportunity Commission's (EEOC) ADA Compliance Manual and related interpretative guidelines.[21]

THE ADA AND THE DEFINITION OF DISABILITY

One might suggest that ever-increasing complexity and subtlety are a common characteristic of the maturation of legal concepts and rules as they are modified by application in particular cases. The cynic might suggest that this trend is just a by-product of the legal profession creating work for itself. What is ironic, however, is the message this growing complexity seems to embody. It is as if the moral clarity expressed in the opening sections of the ADA needs to be reconsidered: we thought that it was obvious that people with disabilities "continually encounter" discrimination and are "severely disadvantaged," but now we cannot be so sure. This message is, of course, considerably reinforced by recent Supreme Court cases such as *Sutton v. United Airlines, Inc.,* in which the scope of ADA coverage has been significantly restricted, in part on the basis of the claim, reinforced by the ADA itself, that disability can affect only "a discrete and insular minority."[22]

Indeed, the practical value of the ADA as a response to rights violation is cast into doubt by the clear direction that the legal interpretation of disability has taken. It is understandable that the ADA should define the term "disability" consistent with its purpose of eliminating discrimination and so, perhaps, very differently from legislation that, for example, determines eligibility for disability pensions or workers' compensation. Yet the ADA's statutory definition of "disability" and subsequent interpretations are arguably inconsistent with the social model of disability that underwrote the disability rights movement and generated the political will to enact the ADA in the first place.

There are two components of the statutory definition of "disability" in the ADA—the first from the act itself, and the second from the regulations:

> sec. 3 (2) Disability.—The term "disability" means, with respect to an individual
>> a physical or mental impairment that substantially limits one or more of the major life activities of such individual:[23]
>> (A) a record of such an impairment; or
>> (B) being regarded as having such an impairment.

> sec. 1630. 2(h) A physical or mental impairment means:
>> any physiological disorder, or condition, cosmetic disfigurement, or anatomical loss affecting one or more of the following body systems: neurological, musculoskeletal, special sense organs, respiratory (including speech organs), cardiovascular, reproductive, digestive, genito-urinary, hemic and lymphatic, skin, and endocrine; or any mental or psychological disorder, such as mental retardation, organic brain syndrome, emotional or mental illness, and specific learning disabilities.[24]

There is as well a third component, namely a list of exceptions to what qualifies as a disability or an impairment:

> sec. 510. Illegal Use of Drugs.
>> In General.—For purposes of this Act, the term "individual with a disability" does not include an individual who is currently engaging in the illegal use of drugs. . . .

> sec. 511 Definitions.
>> Homosexuality and bisexuality.—For purposes of the definition of "disability" in section 3(2), homosexuality and bisexuality are not impairments and as such are not disabilities under this Act.
>> Certain Conditions.—Under this Act, the term "disability" shall not include—
>>> transvestitism, transsexualism, pedophilia, exhibitionism, voyeurism, gender identity disorders not resulting from physical impairments, or other sexual behavior disorders;

compulsive gambling, kleptomania, or pyromania; or psychoactive substance use disorders resulting from current illegal use of drugs.

Setting aside the exclusions for the moment, the primary definition of "disability" accords well with the antidiscrimination mandate of the act. In particular, it is perfectly appropriate that there be three prongs to the definition of disability—namely, having a disability, having a record of a disability, and being regarded as having a disability. Since prejudice, stigma and other adverse and discriminatory attitudes are based on perception rather than reality, it is perfectly sensible to define the protected class of people both in terms of physical conditions that they have as well as those they no longer have or never had. Discrimination on the basis of the perception of a disability is as much a social ill as discrimination on the basis of an actual disability. As well, it is surely defensible to separate the determination of disability from that of eligibility to bring a complaint, that is, the determination that one is a "qualified individual with a disability." That said, these statutory definitions reveal a conception of disability that is surprisingly at odds with the social model, as characterized by the four basic principles noted above.

ADA disabilities and impairments exist on a continuum, in the sense that a disability is defined as an impairment that meets a threshold of severity. Since impairments are viewed as exclusively biomedical phenomena—disorders, conditions, losses or diseases—on this definition, so too are disabilities. In practical terms, this means that, where it is not obvious, some form of medical documentation of impairment is essential to qualify as a person with a disability. But this is to fall back on the medical model of disability that was explicitly rejected by disability rights advocates. And it was rejected for a good reason, since disability is not a personal trait but an outcome of an interaction between an impairment and the physical and social environment in which the individual lives. Disabilities are not severe instances of impairment; they are categorically different entities.

Does this matter for the aims of the ADA? There is, of course, the blatant inconsistency between the first and the third prongs of the definition. Why demand medical evidence that one has a severe enough impairment to qualify for protection against stigma, stereotyping and prejudice, when no such evidence is needed to qualify as being "regarded as having a disability"? If the social issue is discrimination, that is a matter of how other people treat a person with disabilities, and that treatment is not directly correlated with the medical status of a person or the range and extent of that individual's functional capabilities in real-life situations. Making a determination of whether a person's rights have been violated by others in terms of that individual's medical condition seems perverse and utterly beside the point.

This is precisely why disability theorists and activists rejected the medical model of disability. On the social model, disability is entirely context- or environment-dependent, in the sense that the existence of a disability or its quality as a limitation on a person's range of social roles and activities is as much a function of features of the world as of his or her physical or mental condition. This fact has been recently recognized by the World Health Organization and embodied in its revised international classification of disability, the ICIDH-2.[25] Although traditionally viewed as an international organization devoted to the provision of medical assistance and advice, the WHO has, consistent with its own very broad definition of "health," stated that health is not merely a matter of the absence of disease but also the extent and range of an individual's functioning. In the ICIDH-2, disability is modeled as a limitation in the range or extent of a person's activity performance. Yet, as activities are always performed in the context of a world shaped by features of the physical and human-made environment, the ICIDH-2 recognizes that the outcome of extent of participation will typically be the product of an interaction between the individual, his or her health status, and the physical and social world. Thus two people may have the same impairment with the same severity, but because of different occupational demands, social supports or climatic conditions, one may have a disability and the other may not. Disabilities are rarely directly inferable from impairments precisely because disabilities are context-dependent and impairments are medical abstractions from context.

There are many reasons why the ADA, contrary to the intentions of its advocates, seems always to be belabored by a medicalized version of disability. But prominent among these reasons is the fact that the ADA is an evolutionary development from the Rehabilitation Act of 1973, an act which deals primarily with provision for and access to medical and rehabilitation services. Medically based services presumed genuine medically determined needs, so a medical qualification for eligibility is appropriate. As mentioned, the ADA is also influenced by the Civil Rights Act of 1964, in which membership in a "discrete and insular minority" is the rationale for protection. In order to qualify for membership in a minority group, some objective determination is required and, for well-known reasons,[26] medical determination has always been the administrative approach taken in matters involving disability.

The result has been an inordinate expenditure of judicial time and energy on ever more precise rules for determining the medically based qualifications for disability. And this has invariably been at the expense of illuminating the genuine issue of whether a person has been treated in a discriminatory fashion. Perhaps the more notorious examples of misplaced energy and injustice have been in ADA complaints founded on obesity.

On the social model, obesity is understood as a common impairment that is amenable to a relatively uncontentious medical definition—namely, a state of weighing more than a statistically defined normal range for height and sex.[27] Whether or not obesity can lead to disabilities is entirely a matter of whether a person's weight limits the performance of activities, which in turn is a question of what activities a person wants or needs to do, and, more importantly, the environmental context in which those activities are to be performed. If activities are limited, these are the disabilities, not the obesity, which is the underlying impairment. Except in very extreme cases, it would be impossible to predict, without knowing details about the physical and social environment of an obese individual, what disabilities he or she experiences, if any. One thing is sure: if a person is ridiculed for being overweight, assumed to be slothful, gluttonous or unintelligent, or denied employment or other opportunities, then these reactions are *prima facie* discriminatory. And we can be sure of this whether or not the person involved is obese (rather than merely at the upper bounds of normal weight) and without having to be concerned about *why* he or she is overweight or obese.

The treatment of obesity under the ADA is quite different. Obesity is conceptualized as a "disability" rather than an impairment, and counts as a disability only if (a) the condition is truly one of obesity rather than merely high but normal weight; and (b) there are underlying medical causes for it (often termed "morbid obesity").[28] In short, the etiology of the obesity is the crucial issue. If obesity is a "physiological disorder," it qualifies as a disability; otherwise, not. This issue dominates the judicial scrutiny.[29] The question of what activities were limited by the excess weight, if any, and the issue of how employers, coworkers or others treated the complainant are pushed into the background. Despite constant academic criticism, it is unlikely that courts will move away from this approach.[30] Canadian human rights tribunals mirror this approach.[31]

To be sure, in some cases, courts have been sympathetic to the argument that, though not disabled, the obese individual who was denied employment or presumed to be unintelligent qualifies under the third prong of the definition and was "regarded as having a disability." Though effective in the result, this ploy is not a satisfactory solution to the core problem: the "regarded as" prong of the definition is appropriate when either the complainant has no impairment or his or her impairment does not in fact substantially limit his or her activities. So argued, the complainant cannot point to a failure to make reasonable accommodations at the workplace, since the complaint is founded on the premise that there are no actual activity limitations caused by the impairment. Although reliance on the third prong can save the day for a few, it does not address the central problem that obesity may lead to disabilities, irrespective of its causes or medical etiology.

At bottom, the problem represented by the obesity cases—involving not only the ADA but many other state antidiscrimination acts—is a failure to adhere to the social model of disability. Disabilities are not simply severe impairments; to identify a disability, it is essential to contextualize the discussion and to understand how environmental factors contribute to the disadvantage at the core of the complaint. The compulsive line-drawing that invariably medicalizes the discussion ignores the fact that disability is not a categorical or "bipolar" phenomenon, but context-dependent and continuous.[32] Moreover, the concern with disability ought to be discriminatory disadvantage associated with disability, and this issue (which ought to be the core of antidiscrimination law) has nothing to do with the etiology of the disability.

The obesity cases are emblematic of yet another current of ADA jurisprudence: that discrimination is not legally possible for individuals whose disabilities were "voluntarily induced." Despite a clear rejection of this proposition in the EEOC Compliance Manual,[33] judicial remarks in a variety of contexts make it clear that part of the reason courts insist on an underlying medical cause of obesity is to ensure that the condition was not the product of voluntary overeating.[34] Similarly, the consistent refusal to recognize as impairments adverse personality traits such as poor judgment, irresponsible behavior and poor impulse control—unless the result of a psychological disease or disorder—can be traced to the assumption that these conditions are voluntary.[35] Finally, and most blatantly, the ADA's treatment of illegal drug and alcohol use indicates a presumption that, however much these practices may contribute to disability (as they plainly do), they will not be so considered because these conditions are voluntary. The Supreme Court has made this last point abundantly clear in a Veterans' Administration case in which two honorably discharged veterans were denied educational assistance benefits because, as alcoholics, they had "engaged with some degree of wilfulness in the conduct that caused them to become disabled."[36] By contrast, there is law in Canada to the effect that alcohol dependency is itself a disability, whether wilful or not.[37]

The twin motivations of moralism and paternalism at work here may also be responsible for the explicit legislative exclusions listed above. Being a transvestite, voyeur or compulsive gambler does not mean that all adverse treatment that one experiences is discriminatory or not. It all depends. Although there is more than enough judicial affirmation of the principle that ADA discrimination must be determined on a individual basis, in full apprisal of the particular circumstances involved, these exclusions simply rule out an individualized, context-sensitive determination.

It would be naïve to ignore the fact that antidiscrimination legislation is invariably the product of a political compromise in which irrelevant ideological positions can leave their imprint. In the cases of the ADA this has yielded the peculiar result that some classes of persons with disabilities are excluded, not because they do not have medically ascertained impairments, or are believed to have, but because their conditions are perceived to be indicative of moral fault or weakness of character. There are also instances where this attitude has spilled over to conditions that are not excluded. There are, for example, several cases of the denial of ADA protection to students with learning disabilities on the grounds that their proposed accommodation of more time and a quiet room for exam-taking is compatible with lack of motivation or weakness of the will to overcome stress and nervousness.[38]

All of these features of the statutory definition of "disability" distance the ADA from the social model of disability; if anything, judicial interpretations, especially in recent years, have further emphasized this conceptual gap. This can only limit the effectiveness, or indeed relevance, of antidiscrimination law as a remedy to the violation of basic rights inherent in the unequal treatment that people with disabilities experience in all sectors of social life. Viewing disability as a severe form of an impairment, determined by etiology and categorical, is a persistent and perhaps inevitable flaw in the legal definition used in the ADA and most other antidiscrimination legislation. More troubling is the failure to acknowledge the essential role that the environmental context plays in creating or worsening disability. The ADA appears to undermine the very model of disability that created its rationale.

THE ADA AS A RESPONSE TO INEQUALITY

There remains a deeper concern.[39] Even if the ADA and antidiscrimination law in general could be made to work effectively and without these drawbacks, the advocacy strategy that sets its sights entirely on responding to discrimination may be of limited value to people with disabilities. Although undoubtedly there is discrimination against people with disabilities, and this should be corrected, the condition of inequality that people with disabilities face cannot always fit into the conceptual mold or legal test of discrimination. People with disabilities internationally face nonaccommodating physical and organizational environments; lack of educational or training programming; impoverished or nonexistent employment prospects; inadequate income-support programs founded on insulting eligibility requirements; limited access to assistive technologies; a general lack of resources to meet impairment-related needs; neglect; and minimal political influence. These are all social ills brought about by a maldistribution of power and resources. But they are not forms of discrimination.

But why not discrimination? Because that is not what is going on. Discrimination is a wrongful limitation of someone's freedom; it is the creation of an obstacle or barrier to full participation or benefit, to which the wronged party has a claim, based on a feature of that individual that is, in the context of the treatment, irrelevant. A discriminatory action is offensive because it is disrespectful and assaults the dignity of an individual or a group.[40] Because discrimination is an indignity, compensation to the victim of the insult is meaningful and appropriate. But first the complainant needs to show that he or she has been denied a benefit or opportunity available to others and that the disadvantage followed from perceptions about disability that are irrational and unjustifiable. But for reasons already mentioned, this is a difficult case to make out, even in clear cases.

In practice, of course, antidiscrimination law has moved considerably beyond this core meaning. It is common in this jurisprudence to speak of derivative forms of discrimination—"indirect," "adverse effect," or "constructive"—which often serves the important legal function of applying legislative remedies where there is no clear evidence of a discriminatory intent or even a discriminator. In the hands of rights advocates, the term "discrimination" has often been extended to encompass any social injustice whatsoever. The term has become elastic and threatens to be stripped of concrete meaning. Judicial backlash was inevitable. In order to sustain the distinction between those disadvantages that are and those that are not discriminatory, judges will, since they have little option, rely on the core notion of "discrimination" in order to recenter their intuitions about when and why discriminatory distinction-drawing violates antidiscrimination law.

But why pursue the dubious tactic of stretching the meaning of discrimination beyond its natural bounds? Unemployment undoubtedly makes life harder for people with disabilities; but why assign the responsibility for these complex, multifactorial and systemic phenomena to some discriminator? Undoubtedly people with disabilities do face discrimination in this central sense; and for that reason, antidiscrimination legislation is justifiable and important. But that is not all there is to a recognition of human rights. Especially when economic factors create real disadvantages for persons with disabilities, there is no insult, because there is no insulter. There is a social evil; there is injustice and inequality. But it is an evil of a different sort.

The characteristic feature of the inequality and denial of human rights suffered by people with disabilities around the world is the unjust limitation of their equal right to participate in the full range of social roles and ways of living. This may be the consequence of neglect, lack of political clout or a systemic social failure to provide the resources and opportunities needed to make participation feasible. Inequality is exemplified in concrete and practical terms by the absence of resources and opportunities that make it realistically possible for a person to achieve what he or she wishes to achieve.

The denial of opportunities and resources is an issue not of discrimination but of distributive injustice—an unfair distribution of society's resources and opportunities that results in limitations of participation in all areas of social life. Opportunities and resources respond to needs, and a key disadvantage linked to disability is an inequality in the satisfaction of human needs. Impairment-related needs, variable across the population, are met for some people but not others. Some needs are catered to, while others are ignored. Resources are allocated to satisfy the repertoire of functional capacities of some people, but not others. These allocations create a distributive imbalance unfairly disadvantaging some people. This accounts for the fact that the most accurate indicator of the social status of being a person with disabilities is poverty. The social construction of disability creates inequality of access to social resources.

Distributive injustice persists because of the variation in impairment-related needs and disability accommodations. Statistically, the higher the level of impairment need, the smaller the population cohort, with the result that more trivial and more common impairment needs (such as glasses for mild visual impairment) tend to be catered to, while more complex and less common needs (say those for spina bifida) are more likely to be underserved. Overlying this is the arbitrary allocation of socially constructed disadvantages distributed across the population of impairments. Generally speaking, there are far more disadvantages associated with mental and psychiatric impairments than the actual needs linked to those impairments would predict. Many of the complaints against managed care as a mode of distribution of health care reflect these same injustices. In the end, distributional injustice is the product of structural and impersonal economic forces, forces that cannot be explained in terms of discrimination in any of its many senses.

CONCLUSION

Antidiscrimination laws such as the ADA are shaped by social and legal forces that, perhaps inevitably, turn their attention away from distributional issues. In the abstract, this is not a criticism; indeed, the corrective focus of the ADA is the primary source of its strength and relevance to people with disabilities. Yet there are reasons to think that, both in conception and in operation, the ADA conflicts with the fundamental ideological components of the disability rights movement: the social model of disability and the goal of political equality. The conflict is theoretical, to be sure, but there are many concrete instances where the theoretical disequilibrium has produced inexplicable or unjust results. The Canadian approach, with its twin reliance on a fundamental, constitutional guarantee of equality and flexible and conciliation-based antidiscrimination legislation, provides a contrast to the ADA regime. In principle, the Canadian approach offers a stronger protection, since, grounded in constitutional law, the changes a successful complaint could engender would be far-reaching in scope. But precisely because of this, Canadian courts are cautious and, although far less so now than previously, deferential to the objectives of the legislature.

To be sure, none of this provides grounds for moving away from antidiscrimination legislation, either in the ADA model or by means of the more complex Canadian approach. On the contrary, it should be the motivation for supplementing antidiscrimination law with a more vigorous and multisectorial pursuit of equality of participation for persons with disabilities. In the end, perhaps, what is needed is a rethinking not so much of what disability is or who qualifies as a *bona fide* person with a disability with a valid and enforceable complaint of discrimination, but rather of our social and political commitment to equality.

NOTES

[1]Some examples of legislation closely modeled on the ADA are the Disability Discrimination Act, 1992 (Australia), Disability Discrimination Act, 1995, c 50 (U.K.), Human Rights Act, 1993, No. 82 (New Zealand), Disabled Persons Act (India), and Israel's Disabled Persons Act, 1998. As noted in the text, Canadian human rights acts, at the federal and provincial levels, also follow the pattern set by the ADA and the Vocational Rehabilitation Act 1973, but they must be seen in the context of the constitutional protections found in the Canadian Charter of Rights and Freedoms (enacted as the Canada Act, 1982 (U.K.), c. 11, Schedule B, part I).

[2]Canadian Charter of Rights and Freedoms, section 15(1) and Antidiscrimination Act (Poland).

[3]Severely Disabled Persons Act (Germany), and Israel's Employment (equal opportunities) Law, 5574 (1988).

[4]Disabled Person's Fundamental Law (Japan); Disability Discrimination Ordinance, 1996 (Hong Kong); and Disabled Persons Act (China).

[5]In particular, Standard Rules on the Equalization of Opportunities for Persons with Disabilities, adopted by the United Nations General Assembly, resolution 48/96 (UN 48th session, 2012.93).

[6]See, for example, *Eaton v. Brant County Board of Education* (1997) 1 S.C.R. 241, in which a 12-year-old child with cerebral palsy was denied mainstreamed education in part on the ground that the ground of disability differed from those of race and sex, since disability admitted of individual variation, and hence the need on the part of courts to determine what government measures best served the interests of equality in the accommodation of difference. The court felt that specialized but segregated education services met that test in this case.

[7] *Youth Bowling Council of Ontario v. McLeod* (1990) 14 C.H.R.R. D/120 (Ont. Div. Ct.).

[8] *Hines v. Nova Scotia* (1990) 73 D.L.R. (4th) 491 (N.S.S.C.), in which the court struck down a provision of the Motor Vehicle Act of Nova Scotia that prevented diabetic truck drivers from getting a license on the ground that there were other ways of securing the objective of highway safety that were less offensive to the values of equality. And see a similar result for flying a plane: *Bahlsen v. Canada* (1996) 141 D.L.R. (4th) 712 (Fed. C.A.)

[9] *Eldridge v. British Columbia* (1997) 151 D.L.R. (4th) 577 (S.C.C.).

[10] Scotch, R. *From Goodwill to Civil Rights.* Philadelphia, PA: Temple University Press, 1984; and "Politics and Policy in the History of the Disability Rights Movement" (1989) 67 [Suppl. 2] *Milbank Quarterly* 380; Driedger, D. *The Last Civil Rights Movement.* London: Hurst and Co., 1989; Anspach, Renee R. "From Stigma to Identity Politics: Political Activism among the Physically Disabled and Former Mental Patients" (1979) 13 *Social Science and Medicine* 765.

[11] E.g., Safilos-Rothschild, C. *The Sociology and Social Psychology of Disability and Rehabilitation.* New York: Random House, 1970; Wright, B. *Physical Disability—A Psychosocial Approach,* 2nd ed. New York: Harper & Row, 1983; Sagarin, E., ed. *The Other Minorities: Nonethnic Collectivies Conceptualized as Minority Groups.* Toronto: Ginn, 1971; and Bury, M. "Social Aspects of Rehabilitation" (1987) 10 [Suppl. 5] *International Journal of Rehabilitation Research* 25.

[12] See, e.g., Imrie, R. *Disability and the City: International Perspectives.* London: Paul Chapman, 1996; Bickenbach, J. *Physical Disability and Social Policy.* Toronto: University of Toronto Press, 1993; and Barnes, C., and G. Mercer, eds. *Exploring the Divide: Illness and Disability.* Leeds: Disability Press, 1996. And compare the construct of disability used in the revised *International Classification of Functioning and Disability (ICIDH-2).* Geneva: World Health Organization, 1999.

[13] For a review of the history and development of this definition, see J. Wegner "The Antidiscrimination Model Reconsidered: Ensuring Equal Opportunity without Respect to Handicap under Section 504 of the Rehabilitation Act of 1973" (1983) 69 *Cornell Law Review* 401.

[14] UPIAS *Fundamental Principles of Disability.* London: Union of the Physically Impaired Against Segregation, 1976.

[15] The "social model" and "social-political perspective" are examples of social constructivist theories, sometimes called "interactive" or "environmental" approaches; see Imrie, R. "Rethinking the Relationships between Disability, Rehabilitation, and Society" (1997) 19 *Disability and Rehabilitation* 263, for the former, and Amundson, R. "Disability, Handicap, and the Environment" (1992) 9 *Journal of Social Philosophy* 105, for the latter. The sociopolitical perspective on disability has a complex history in sociology, tracing its origins both to Parson's notion of the "sick role," Parson, T. "Definitions of Health and Illness in the Light of American Values and Social Structure" in E. Jaco, ed. *Patients, Physicians, and Illness.* New York: Free Press, 1979; and the work of E. Goffman, in particular *Asylums.* New York: Doubleday, 1961 and *Stigma: Notes on the Management of Spoiled Identity.* Englewood Cliffs, NJ: Prentice Hall, 1963, on the process of stigmatizing and the creation of "deviance." In Britain, sociologists sought their explanations outside the more individualistic, American approach, adopting more overtly political theoretical accounts. For a description of some of the history of the sociopolitical perspective (or "paradigm," as it is sometimes called), see Bickenbach, *Physical Disability,* 135–181, and for the contrasting U.K. history, see Barnes, C. "Theories of Disability and the Origins of the Oppression of Disabled People in Western Society" in Len Barton, ed. *Disability and Society.* London: Longman, 1996.

[16] The phrase is I. Zola's, in "Toward the Necessary Universalizing of a Disability Policy" (1989) 67 *The Milbank Quarterly* 401.

[17] Stone, D. *The Disabled State.* Philadelphia, PA: Temple University Press, 1984; and Liachowitz, C. *Disability as a Social Construct: Legislative Roots.* Philadelphia, PA: University of Pennsylvania Press, 1988.

[18] PL. 101–336 Sec. 2 (b) (1), (2).

[19] PL. 101–336 Sec. 2 (a) (7).

[20] Cf. sec. 16 Ontario Human Rights Act, S.O. 181, c. 53; sec. 22 Human Rights Act, 1993, No. 82 (New Zealand); secs. 5,6 Disability Discrimination Act, 1995, c. 50 (U.K.); secs. 8–12 Disability Discrimination Act, 1992 (Australia).

[21] E.g., the comments and analysis on section 1630 of the EEOC's regulations on the implementation of Title I of the ADA run to several hundred pages and are expanding yearly.

[22] *Sutton v. United Airlines, Inc.,* 130 F.3d 893 (1999).

[23]Like many aspects of the ADA, this definition is closely followed in other jurisdictions In the U.K.'s Disability Discrimination Act, 1995, for example, "disability" is defined as "a physical or mental impairment which has a substantial and long-term adverse effect on his ability to carry out normal day-to-day activities."

[24]29 C.F.R. sec. 1630.2(h).

[25]*ICIDH-2.*

[26]Stone, *The Disabled State.*

[27]"Obesity" is defined by the World Health Organization as being more than 5 percent above the upper range of the "normal" category measured by the body mass index (BMI).

[28]See *Underwood v. Trans World Airlines,* 710 F. Supp. 78, 83–84 (S.D.N.Y. 1989) (dealing with obesity under the Rehabilitation Act, 1973) and *Cook v. Rhode Island Department of Mental Health,* 10 F.3d 17 (1st Cir. 1993).

[29]E.g. *Francis v. City of Merriden,* 7 AD Cases 955 (1997). And cf. under state antidiscrimination laws: *Cassita v. Community Foods,* 2 AD Cases 1188 (Calif. Sup. Ct. 1993); *Civil Services Commission v. Penn. Human Relations Commission,* 2 AD Cases 1345 (PA Sup. Ct. 1991).

[30]See Peterson, S. "Discrimination against Overweight People: Can Society Still Get Away with It?" (1994–1995) 30 *Gonzola Law Review* 105; Kramer, K., and A. Magerson. "Obesity, Discrimination in the Workplace: Protection through a Perceived Disability Claim under the Rehabilitation Act and the Americans with Disability Act" (1994) 31 *California Western Law Review* 41; Taussig, W. "Weighing in against Obesity Discrimination" (1994) 35 *California Law Review* 927; and Hartnett, P. "Nature or Nurturing Lifestyle or Fate: Employment Discrimination against Obese Workers" (1993) 24 *Rutgers Law Journal* 807.

[31]E.g. *Horton v. Niagara* (1987) 9 C.H.R.R. D/4611 (Ont. Bd. of Inquiry) and *Ontario v. Vogue Shoes* (1991) 14 C.H.R.R. D/425 (Ont. Bd. of Inquiry).

[32]For a similar critique of the ADA's treatment of disability, see R. Colker *Hybrid—Bisexuals, Multiracials, and Other Misfits under American Law.* New York: New York University Press, 1996.

[33]"Voluntariness is irrelevant when determining whether a condition constitutes an impairment" EEOC Compliance Manual, sec. 902.2(e).

[34]This line of argument can be found arising in earlier Rehabilitation Act, 1973 cases: *Greene v. Union Pacific Railroad Co.,* 548 F. Supp. 3 (1981); and *State Division of Human Rights v. Xerox Corp.,* 480 N.E. (2d.) 695 (1985).

[35]See *Daley v. Koch,* 892 F.2d 212 (2nd Cir. 1989).

[36]*Traynor v. Turnage,* 485 U.S. 535.

[37]*Entrop v. Imperial Oil Ltd.* (1995) 95 C.L.L.C. 230–022 (Ont. Bd. of Inquiry).

[38]See *Argen v. N.Y. State Board of Law Examiners,* 860 F. Supp. 84 (W.D.N.Y. 1994).

[39]The concern in what follows—that inequality in the case of disability is best conceptualized as a matter of distributive rather than corrective justice—is a large issue that can only be touched on here. See the recent extensive debate on this issue in Silvers, A., Wasserman, D. and Mahowald, M.. *Disability, Difference, Discrimination.* New York: Rowman & Littlefield Publishers, Inc., 1998.

[40]See David Wasserman, "The Concept of Discrimination," in R. Chadwick, ed. *Encyclopaedia of Applied Ethics.* San Diego, CA: Academic Press, 1997.

The U.K. Disability Discrimination Act
disabling language, justifying inequitable social participation

MAIRIAN CORKER

When I failed basic English on the first attempt, *they* said that
was what was to be expected of the deaf. When I passed it on
the second attempt, *they* were silent. When I passed it at
advanced level, *they* said it was a fluke. Funny how most of the
other things they said never got through. Now when I read or
write anything, it's my way of continuing to defy them. And now
they say I've got it wrong and that I don't understand my own
history.   —*Notes from a diary, 1974*

To be injured by speech is to suffer a loss of context, that is,
not to know where you are. Indeed, it may be that what is unanticipated about the injurious speech act is what constitutes its
injury, the sense of putting its addressee out of control. To be
addressed injuriously is not only to be open to an unknown
future, but not to know the time and place of injury, and to suffer the disorientation of one's situation as the effect of such
speech. Exposed at the moment of such a shattering is precisely
the volatility of one's "place" within the community of speakers;
one can be "put in one's place" by such speech, but such a
place may be no place.   —*Butler 1997, 4*

INTRODUCTION

The claim of disabled people to social or civil rights has been high on the agenda of the
U.K. disabled people's movement since the publication of the document *Fundamental
Principles of Disability* by the Union of Physically Impaired Against Segregation (UPIAS
1976), although individual disabled people, who drew inspiration from grassroots organizations of disabled people, were writing from a "rights" perspective a decade before (Hunt
1966). Disability rights discourse has traditionally "advocated policies based upon according disabled people full citizenship rights through anti-discrimination legislation." (Oliver
1996b, 123). The pursuit of this goal at the level of national policy has seen no less than
thirteen Private Members' Bills pass through the British Parliament, most of which have
fallen foul of outdated mechanisms of parliamentary procedure.

   This period of intense political mobilization in the U.K. also saw the generation of an
increasing body of knowledge and practice which has come to be known as "the social
model of disability" (Barnes, Mercer and Shakespeare 1999, 2). There is not the space here
to document these developments in detail.[1] For the purposes of this essay, it is important to

357

note, however, that the social model of disability rests on a sharp, often rigorously applied, conceptual distinction between *disability* and *impairment*. Disability is seen as a form of social oppression that is institutionalized in Western society, whereas impairment is nothing more than a description of physical, sensory or mental difference. Indeed, the importance of this distinction is underscored by the resistance amongst many U.K. disability theorists to considering impairment in its interpenetrative, interdependent relation to disability, and the insistence of some that impairment should be examined separately (Oliver 1996a).

Barnes, Mercer and Shakespeare (1999) have suggested that the adoption of this conceptual model marks an important difference between U.S. and U.K. approaches to understanding and theorizing disability. The other main distinction is that U.K. approaches are heavily influenced by the discipline of sociology and social policy, whereas U.S. approaches have sought to explore disability within a broad humanities context. Citing Linton (1998a, 1998b), Barnes and colleagues suggest that the latter "have been linked to the denial of civil rights to a minority group rather than a specific theoretical explanation of disability and the exclusion of disabled people from the mainstream of economic and social activity" (1999, 4). There are nevertheless important exceptions to this rule, most notably in the campaigns of Deaf[2] people in both the U.S. and the U.K. for linguistic minority rights and status and their pursuit of a political agenda that is in many ways disparate to that of the disability movement, particularly in its emphasis on the retention of residential schools and social coexistence rather than inclusion (Corker 1998). Drawing from the intersection of disability studies with feminist and queer studies, I have suggested that the distinction between impairment and disability itself rests on a dichotomy between the individual and the social, with impairment being viewed primarily as an unexamined, commonly biological foundation for disability (Corker 1999b). There are, moreover, different ways in which both disability and the disabled individual can be understood from the perspective of a "social model" approach, which also tends to be marked by discrete boundaries.[3]

THE DISABILITY DISCRIMINATION ACT: JUSTIFYING ACTS OF INDIVIDUALISM

The complexity of disabled people's approaches to understanding disability and to articulating and effecting political action is important because these approaches represent how disabled people would wish to be treated under law. New disability discourses,[4] although they are becoming increasingly influential at the level of local policy and practice and in the academy, nevertheless remain minority discourses that coexist and are in competition with the dominant discourses of disability that drive U.K. government policy and its implementation (Corker 1998, Corker and French 1999). In spite of disabled people's intensive campaigns for disability rights, the failure of the U.K. social welfare and social security apparatus to deliver the goal of independent living for disabled people (Doyle 1999, 216), and concerted attempts since 1991 to move the Civil Rights (Disabled Persons) Bill modeled on the ADA 1990 (Doyle 1999, 217), Oliver's concept of disability "rights" has not reached the statute. What has been "achieved" is a legal instrument that has variously been described as "confusing, contorted and unsatisfactory" (Gooding 1996, 1), "a dissembling law not an enabling statute" (Doyle 1997, 78), and "one of the most ill-conceived pieces of legislation ever to reach the statute books" (Corker 1998, 115). This is the Disability Discrimination Act 1995 (DDA).

In both the DDA and the American ADA, disability is defined as "*either* a physical *or* a mental impairment" that has "a substantial and long-term adverse effect on his ability to carry out normal day-to-day activities" (DDA s.1) or "substantially limits one or more of the major life activities of such individual" (ADA s.3). The DDA "addresses the problem of discrimination against disabled persons in the employment field; in the provision of goods, facilities and services; in respect of the disposal and management of premises; and in a less direct and satisfactory fashion, the inaccessibility of education provision and transport" (Doyle 1999, 217–218). It is therefore limited in its scope and provisions when compared to the ADA.

Gooding (1996, 5) notes that "the conceptual framework of the DDA differs from both the British sex and race legislation and the American disability legislation," and in a comparative analysis of U.K. antidiscrimination law relating to disability, race and gender, I have emphasised the lack of correspondence between the statutes (Corker 1998, 117). For example, the Sex Discrimination Acts of 1975 and 1986 (SDA) and the Race Relations Act 1976 (RRA) cross-reference each other so that it is technically possible to make a claim under both acts if one is a black woman. The DDA, in its emphasis on "proof of disability" as it is defined under the act, renders uncertain the status of a black disabled woman making a claim of simultaneous discrimination for, as Shakespeare (1996, 109) notes: "disability is a very powerful identity, and one that has the power to transcend other identities." The definition of "race" in the RRA is neither as specified nor as exclusionary as the definition of disability though, significantly for the purposes of this essay, it does not include the community of Deaf sign language users who self-define as a linguistic minority. Similarly, while there is reference to "genuine occupational qualification" in both the SDA and the RRA, which makes provision for particular jobs to be advertised exclusively for women or people from ethnic minorities, the DDA (Section 64) contains reference only to occupations which are *not* covered by the Act.

As of June 1999, there had been 5,189 employment claims under the DDA, and it is estimated that 250 new claims are made every month (*The Disabled Century Debate,* BBC Television, June 10, 1999). It is more difficult, however, to judge the act's success in addressing disability discrimination on the basis of case law, since a high number of claims are settled out of court or under a confidentiality agreement. However, there is little doubt that the DDA represents a muddled combination of prohibition, justifiable discrimination and reasonable adjustment that can themselves act as a barrier to claimants who may be "isolated, possibly ill-informed, and under-resourced" (Gooding 1996, 6). Further, because the DDA legally justifies direct discrimination on the grounds of "disability" in what Gooding (1996, 6) describes as "dangerously vague" terms, and fails to incorporate a notion of the indirect discrimination experienced by disabled people, it seems an ineffective legal instrument for tackling the *institutionalized* oppression of disabled people. Unlike the ADA, the DDA is not at present supported within a constitutional Bill of Rights, though steps are currently being taken to introduce the European Convention on Human Rights into British law. (The Human Rights Act is due to come into force in October 2000.) This move has positive and negative dimensions, which, drawing on the U.S experience, I will explore further below. But from the legal perspective, and because disability and discrimination are defined in different ways in different legal instruments pertaining to education, community care and criminal law, for example, this introduction may prove to be a legislative nightmare.

The disabled people's movement's description of disability as being located at the systemic level clearly marks a significant departure from an individual model epitomized by dominant legal, medical, educational and scientific discourses of disability which reify disability as an individual "problem," "pathology," "deviance" or "dysfunction." However, concerns about an individual model as a model of formal justice are not confined to criticisms of its use within the DDA and the ADA. Many of the detailed critiques of antidiscrimination law *per se* focus on this issue. For example, Downing (1999) has recently argued that "First Amendment absolutists" who appear to urge the right to discriminatory language as free speech are imprisoned in the straitjacket formed by the priorities of legal discourse. These priorities ultimately require foundations to be laid that will rationalize and permit court decisions on individual cases at a particular moment in time. That is, they are framed primarily by the question: "Was or was not this particular individual damaged in some way in this place and time by this particular expression of discriminatory language?" Discriminatory language is seen as an individual act based on sociopsychological dynamics and with purely individual effects (Goldberg 1995). This focus exiles the societal and historical dimensions of discriminatory language along with its capacity to injure, as we will see below.

It could equally be said, however, that both the DDA and the ADA, as historically and culturally circumscribed texts, appear at first to be conceived from within similar sociocultural systems which tend to be individualist rather than collectivist.[5] Kim (1994) suggests that in some individualist societies, notably those that are described in terms of static individualism, emphasis is placed on the individual's "inalienable" rights and the institutions which uphold these. The welfare of disadvantaged, defenceless or powerless people is protected by law, as is the individual's right to autonomy and the freedom to pursue their own goals. However, because individuals tend to be unrelated to each other in static mode, they may not always act in responsible, moral, sane or humanitarian ways. The laws and regulations in such societies are therefore established and enforced so that people do not infringe the agreed group boundaries and no one enjoys special privileges, though individuals and groups can challenge these boundaries if they are regarded as a violation of their rights.

I would suggest that this description is characteristic of the current situation in the U.K. In other individualist societies, which are described in terms of aggregate individualism, individuals are expected to detach themselves from family, community and other ascribed relationships and are bound together by normative and ethical principles, rules and norms. Individuals base their interaction with others on these principles, which include an internalized concern for the welfare of others, a preparedness to take prosocial action, equality, competition, equity, noninterference and exchanges based on social contracts. Kim (1994) suggests that American culture is an example of aggregate individualism. In these circumstances, it may be important to examine Anita Silvers's (1999, 75) assertion that: "individuals with disabilities gain no greater recognition of their own equality if they seek a collective identity in disability itself. . . . To make identifying with the roles characteristic of disability the primary mark of their identity is to disregard, even to demean and devalue, how people with disabilities develop strong individualized approaches to living and functioning with their impairments." I will return to this in the final section. However, it may equally be said that a society is only individualist or collectivist to the extent that its members consent to or are coerced to support the individualist status quo and/or are able to engage in equitable social participation.

INTERROGATING "COMPETENCE" AND DISEMBODIMENT

Iris Marion Young (1990, 91) argues that "democracy is both an element and a condition of social justice" and therefore that "justice requires participation in public discussion and processes of democratic decision-making." She continues: "for a norm to be just, everyone who follows it must in principle have an effective voice in its consideration and be able to *agree* to it without *coercion*. For a social condition to be just, it must enable all to meet their needs and exercise their freedom; thus justice requires that all be able to express their needs" (1990, 34, emphasis added).

I now want to expand Young's thesis by interrogating both antidiscrimination law's dependency on a Cartesian mind-body dichotomy in its definition of disability, and its prescription and standardization of a particular authority on language. I will argue that, as an approach to formal justice, this actively works against democracy and social justice. Further, it does so in a way that has particular implications for people with language and communication impairments. To explain this, we must ask what it means to live in a postmodern "network society" (Castells 1996) founded on particularistic identities and information economies that increasingly "script" our lives (Cameron 1998), when discriminatory language is institutionalized and self-expression is disciplined through the imposition of barriers to language acquisition (language education, and particular approaches to mainstreaming and institutionalization, both educational and social) and use (language planning). When questioning is approached in this way, analysis becomes focused on the discursive construction of knowledge and a politics of resistance rather than being confined to subsidiary questions that ask, for example, what it means to be unable to hear in a society that discriminates through the privileging of oral performance, harbors a deep suspicion of relationships and communications that are not face to face, and places a very heavy emphasis on "direct talk, which is taken as the 'more honest' and 'more human' type of communication" (Lemert 1997, 45–46). However, this is not to diminish the significance of these latter questions, because they touch on the roots of institutionalized, systemic disability. They remind us that discriminatory language is endemic in society *even when we have no direct access to this language*, along with the corollary that our ignorance of it—or our silence in relation to it—does not mean that we lack complicity in its institutionalization. Thus we are also concerned with questions about responsibility and citizenship.

The "authority on language" adopted by antidiscrimination law is that exemplified by Jürgen Habermas's *Theory of Communicative Action* (1991a, 1991b).[6] He posits a model of language that depends upon the ability of "rational" interlocutors to reason and relies heavily on a paradigm of discursive argumentation while deemphasizing the metaphorical, rhetorical, playful, embodied aspects of speech and the affective dimension of expression that are an important aspect of its communicative effect (Young 1987) and are culturally embedded. Crossley (1997) suggests that Habermas's reduction of communicative action to rationalization amounts to cognitivism. He argues that when we communicate, we do not make only cognitive validity claims and our sole purpose is not always to have our claims understood and verified—at least this would be a very clumsy way of trying to describe some aspects of our interactions. However, the rationalist assumption that theorizing, in its ideal state, holds up a mirror to the world still dominates our thinking. The treatment of impairment as a regulatory ideal in dominant discourses of disability and its location in biological discourses occludes it and banishes it from its contingent and variable place in the social world. Thus Crossley also argues that in Habermas's critical theory, the body disappears and, in the absence of an alternative view of embodiment, human agency and communication are disembodied and confined to the expression of the symbolic:

> Communication for Habermas, is dependent upon the competence of concrete interlocutors. And linguistic competence, however much it is constituted and regulated by the conventions of the life-world, is nevertheless the acquired performative

skill of a concrete agent. This is important from the point of view of an analysis of embodiment because concrete communicative agents are necessarily embodied and theories of speech, therefore, presuppose a theory of the body. (Crossley 1997, 21)

Though Habermas indicates that a theory of communicative action must challenge the philosophy of consciousness that locates intentional egos as the ontological origins of social relations, and his theory of communicative action conceives individual identity not as an origin but as a product of linguistic and practical interaction, this emphasis on the competence of "concrete interlocutors" suggests a standpoint view of the communicator and of communication.

Habermas argues that language is a necessarily social and public act, which means that it is shared and, in order to be shared, it must be visible. For Crossley, this means it must be embodied, because a disembodied form of language would be invisible and inaudible and could not therefore function as a common or as a concrete reference point. Without embodiment, communication can be seen to occur by transmission, following a "conduit metaphor" that depicts speech as a three-step process. The speaker puts thoughts into word containers. These word-thought objects are then transferred from the speaker's mind through a conduit (the air) to the mind of the listener. Finally, the listener extracts the thoughts from the words. Communication is seen to work because speaker and listener are assumed to share a system of coding, or at least complementary systems for encoding and decoding.

Crossley's distinction could be interpreted in terms of the difference between *Deaf* and *deaf*. The *Deaf* way renders language visible through the bodily articulation of sign language, whereas *deaf* people are seen to be "silent," "invisible," and therefore to lack the "competence" of full expression because of a systemic distortion that privileges the "visual."[7] Further, as Alderson (1993), writing about children, suggests, "the most powerful way to justify coercion is to deny that children can reason, and to align reason with force; children's resistance is then seen as mindless 'self-destruction,' to be overridden by rational adults." Children "don't know what they don't know," so adults can choose what to tell them. Because one of the common stereotypes of disabled people is that they are "dependent," even childlike in their "need of care," such perspectives on children's competence are often extrapolated to apply to disabled people. Indeed, there are some instances where this is enshrined in U.K. law. For example, the 1991 Criminal Procedure (Insanity and Fitness to Plead) Act states that if a person is accused of even a minor offence and the judge deems that he or she does not understand the charge and is unfit to plead or "under disability,"[8] the only action the judge can take is to commit the defendant to a secure hospital (Chappell 1994). Case law demonstrates that some disabled people will be more vulnerable to this than others, notably those with cognitive and communication impairments.[9]

In Habermasian terms, then, the "visible" might be privileged, but the embodiment of communication does not remove the possibility for distortion, because it is only embodied discourses that are subject to distortion. Crossley continues:

> The systematic distortion of communication is that the possibility of open argument is negated through the influence of social-systemic factors: class, status, political power . . . these factors often enter into communication through the *mediation* of our embodiment e.g. accent, comportment, gesture, dress, bodily attitude. Or alternatively, the visible embodied signs (socially coded) of [*impairment, for example*]

may trigger a range of prejudicial interactive patterns [*direct discrimination*]. The way a person looks and acts comments upon what it is that they say and thus may detract from and distort it . . . bodily markers frame communicative encounters. (1997, 31, my additions in brackets)

It is here perhaps that we have the primary reason for the use of Habermasian perspectives on communication in legal discourse, because the capacity of embodiment for distortion means that the relationship between individuals, between the individual and society, and, therefore, the location of disability, is problematized through the act of multi-channelled, embodied communication. In the context of antidiscrimination law, this may mean, for example, that the provision of a TTY[10] or a sign language interpreter, though it may be regarded as "reasonable accommodation," may not *in practice* remove discrimination because of the capacity of these communication auxiliaries to emphasise distortion through what I have described as extra-embodiment (Corker 1999c). That is to say, these provisions externalize the act of communication, removing it from the embodied situation of the individual's lifeworld and instead placing it in the space between communicators in a conduit that is not neutral.[11]

Though embodied communication takes place at an "interval" or "between" and involves a rhythm or rather a synchronization of rhythms, an embodied conception of lifeworld must also include some understanding of the lived spatial and temporal organization of social life (Crossley 1996). To communicate is, at one level, to create and occupy (*qua* body-subject) a shared space and rhythm. Thus communication auxiliaries are more at the level of mediating our embodiment than embodying our communication. And, as Schutz's (1967) work on phenomenology shows, changes in time-space coordination have significant effects upon the possibility for communication. As embodied communicators, we must negotiate these time-space factors within the more general temporal and spatial factors of our lifeworld; but this is not within our control when communication is extra-embodied. The embodiment of communication may allow it to maximize its potential to be multilayered in a way that is essential to mutual understanding, but its mediation creates a high probability of systemic distortion because different layers can convey different and opposed messages that can be reduced or lost altogether in the act of mediation.

Following Williams's (1998) analysis of Leder's (1990) ideas about "the absent body," mediation also seems to dichotomize the hermeneutical and pragmatic dimensions of telic demand exerted by the interaction between disability and impairment in communication. However, because both these dimensions are ultimately important, it follows that the body in physical limbo and the body in communicative limbo, or the body apart and the body collective, for example, will produce different trajectories in relation to these dimensions which in turn create changes in "matter" which are "experienced" and "lived" differently and cannot be understood solely as the material creations and solutions of regulatory frameworks of "normality." Moreover, because all disabled people engage in some form of linguistic and social interaction, and much of this communicative action is regarded as "distorted" by a society engaged in normative practice, this can be extrapolated to the social category "disability."

Despite the possibilities of a communicative ethics, then, Habermas retains a commitment to the view that the reasoning subject abstracts from her or his own concrete contexts of need, desire and commitment, and regards others also from this general standpoint. Seyla Benhabib (1986, 348–351) suggests that, in that form, he retains a distinction between a public realm of rights and principles and a private realm of contextualized need.

And as Young (1990) further notes, his claim that participants in a dialogue implicitly aim at consensus echoes a strong strain of Kantian universalism that undermines any move to a radically pluralist participatory politics of need interpretation, and appears to hark back to the earlier discussion of individualism. Habermas's conception of dialogic reason finds valid only the expression of generalizable interests, a term whose meaning is *equivocal.* This creates further dichotomies between universal and particular, public and private, as needs and interests that may not be shareable, because they derive from a person's particular history and affiliations, are made liminal.

EMBODIED COMMUNICATION, "HATE SPEECH" AND UNIVERSALIST RIGHTS DISCOURSE

Earlier, I pointed out that the DDA contains no recognition of the concept of indirect discrimination, nor does its conceptualization of direct discrimination encompass an understanding of the role of communicative action in the transmission of discriminatory attitudes and stereotypes of disabled people. Habermas's project is certainly concerned with attempting to guarantee a communicative system in which political power and authority are dispersed and no one's speech disables or silences another's in a way that prevents them from using the performative. But as was noted above, arriving at such a guarantee relies heavily on speech acts being grounded in consensually established, univocal meaning: "the productivity of the process of understanding remains unproblematic only as long as all participants stick to the reference point of possibly achieving a mutual understanding in which the same utterances are assigned the same meaning" (Habermas 1987, 198). There are two problems with this "ideal unity of a civic public" (Young 1990). First, as Judith Butler (1997) suggests, there is a permanent diversity within the semantic field that constitutes an irreversible situation for political theorizing. Second, the drive for univocal meaning must involve a struggle for power of univocality, since diversity in the semantic field means that several meanings of disability coexist. Such a struggle, in Habermasian terms, would involve the production of "more speech" in order to resist universalist expressions of univocality that are seen to be oppressive, and the relegitimation and renegotiation of new disability discourse as it enters into the primary areas of social reproduction (Corker 1999a). This returns us to questions of "competence," "voice" and "access" in relation to censorship and silencing. In the U.K., as we have seen, this struggle takes place against the backdrop of legal discourse that justifies direct discrimination and emphasizes reactive justice. Indeed, I have suggested elsewhere (Corker 1998) that *inter alia,* U.K. law in relation to disability, in its confusion of liberty rights and welfare rights and in its propensity for dictating disabled people's prospects for self-determination in a way that reinforces the existing distribution of advantage and disadvantage, is more concerned with protecting the rights of the nondisabled majority.

Is there then a case for some form of universal approach to the question of civil or human rights, as is proposed? Much would depend on the model adopted and if and how it is enforced. But in searching for such a model, it may be important to address Wendy Brown's question: "What does it mean to write historically and culturally circumscribed experience into an ahistorical discourse, the universalist discourse of law? Is it possible to do this without rendering 'experience' as ontology, 'perspective' as Truth, and without unifying this ontology and this Truth in the Subject of Disability, and without encoding them in law as the basis of disabled people's rights?" Brown continues:

as a regulatory fiction of a particular identity is deployed to displace the hegemonic fiction of universal personhood, the discourse of rights converges insiduously with the discourse of disciplinarity to produce a spectactularly potent mode of juridicial regulatory domination . . . efforts at bringing subjugated discourses into the law merely constitute examples of what Foucault identified as the risk of recodification and recolonization of "disinterred knowledges" by those "unitary discourses," which first disqualified and then ignored them when they made their appearance. (1998, 319)

In other words, she suggests that the law *produces* the subjects it claims to protect or emancipate. Recent critiques of First Amendment absolutism in the U.S. (Downing 1999) and "hate speech" (Allen and Jensen 1995, Butler 1997) have highlighted the process of this production and have pointed to the drawbacks of universalist approaches. First Amendment absolutists argue that there is no reason for the U.S. Constitution to grant specific protection in relation to expressions of "hate speech" because such speech conflicts with the commitments to universal equality that are the fundamental tenets of the Constitution. However, Jensen and Arriola (1995) argue that the First Amendment offers illusory protections. The ideology that in the U.S. anyone can constitutionally say anything bypasses the social factors inhibiting the free and full expression of grievances and problems. "[T]he vast majority of survivors of sexual violence are ignored, blamed, pathologized, threatened, disbelieved, and otherwise revictimized when they protest the violation and try to hold their offenders accountable" (1995, 195–196). Thus women, ethnic minorities or disabled people with important stories to tell may not tell them because of a fear of what Jensen and Arriola describe as "oppressive silencing" (199–203). Moreover, the double bind is that those who are oppressed can comfortably be presumed by the public to have nothing of substance straitjacketing them because there is a talismanic First Amendment in existence (Downing 1999). In reality, then, the First Amendment does not protect their freedom to communicate or their right to freedom from hate-based communication or any other form of oppression that does straitjacket them in making "more speech."

Thus, following Butler (1997) and others, I would argue that, like reactive antidiscrimination legislation, universalist rights discourses, whilst perceived as being proactive, can be equally ineffective in dealing with institutionalized forms of linguistic oppression that have assumed the status of ritual. When combined with the mind-body dichotomy implicit in definitions of disability, Habermas's perspective on communicative action contrives a divorce between speech and action. Within this dichotomy, only discriminatory actions such as attacking individuals or direct discrimination against them are said to be appropriate for prohibitative legislation. As long as people restrain themselves to speech acts, no legal action can be taken against them. However, as Merleau-Ponty (1962, 178) notes: "speech, in the speaker, does not translate ready-made thought, but accomplishes it." Indeed, Downing (1999, 182) argues that the division between speakers and actors represents a "phantasmagorical social theory." He emphasises that discriminatory language seeks to create a climate within which hostilities are more and more likely to be perpetrated because they seem "excusable, even meritorious, even inevitable." Judith Butler (1997) elaborates on this perspective in a way that encompasses concepts of social agency and social injury.

Echoing Carey's (1989) distinction between transmission and ritual modes of communication, she says that language is injurious to the extent that it is given the form of a ritual repeated in time, and hence maintains a sphere of operation that is not restricted to the moment of the utterance itself. Further, the repetition of disabling performative acts produces over time "a set of corporeal styles that, in reified form, appear as the natural configuration of bodies" (Butler 1990, 140), into different impairments existing in a binary relation with one another.

Writing about race, Calvert (1997) suggests that the use of a ritual model would direct attention to indirect discrimination as the reinforcement of racism in society through the repetition of hate speech as a form of cultural ritual. This assumes importance in the light of the recommendations resulting from the findings of the Stephen Lawrence Enquiry in the U.K. (MacPherson 1999). These recommendations urge a much greater recognition of the role of racist speech in the incitement of institutionalized racial hatred and insist that steps be taken both to prohibit racist speech, even in the private domain, and to educate young people about its dangers through the school curriculum.[12] If a Bill of Rights is introduced into U.K. law, these recommendations must also apply to the institutionalized patterns of hate speech encountered by other disadvantaged groups, including disabled people. However, the report also recommends that those who experience "hate speech" and other forms of racial hatred must have the right to decide exactly what constitutes racist behavior and to explain why. Again we have the "more speech" dictum, with all the difficulties that presents.

CONCLUDING REMARKS

In this essay, I have interrogated antidiscrimination law's uncritical adoption of a Habermasian dialogical model of "equitable" social participation, arguing that it is one of the primary instruments through which the law produces the subjects it claims to protect and emancipate. In its disembodiment of communication, the conceptual separation of speech and action, and an emphasis on universalized, univocal expression, it is particularly deleterious to those whose lives are already characterized by systemic communication distortion. This happens because of its appropriation by legal discourse through the specification of "accommodations" that depend on the mediation of these lives, without addressing the displacement effected by culturally embedded, institutionalized and ritualized patterns of discriminatory language.

Additionally, I have suggested that there are problems with a legal framework that separates reactive, corrective justice from proactive, distributive social policy, a separation that renders both ineffective. It is for government and the legal profession to reconstruct the law, but it seems essential that such a reconstruction be effected through a dialogue with disabled people, through a public conversation with difference, through sameness—a conversation that is neither objectivist nor subjectivist. This stresses a different dialogic model based on the work of M. M. Bakhtin (1981). Like Habermas, Bakhtin is acutely aware of a strong potential in the postmetaphysical age for an expansion of participatory democracy and dialogue. However, his radical tolerance is not a form of tolerance that simply allows us to put up with the existence of pluralistic lifeworlds. Rather it aims at mutual recognition and co-understanding in a manner that opens up each lifeworld to a diversity of reciprocal influences and perspectives—a principle that must be central to the interrelationship of difference in the postmodern era of uncertainty because it emphasizes that "truth" itself is constituted dialogically: "The person who understands must not reject the possibility of changing or even abandoning his [*sic*] already prepared viewpoints and positions. In the act of understanding, a struggle occurs that results in mutual change and enrichment" (Bakhtin 1986, 142).

This is very different from Lyotard's (1984) construal of postmodern society as a collection of discrete and incommensurate forms of life. It means that, within law, people should have not only the right to be heard but also *the right to be understood.*

In this context, I remain concerned that in some sectors of the movement, disabled people's political resistance to systemic oppression and their insistence on visibility, ontological "purity" and the production of "more speech," has tended to reproduce Lyotard's vision, with very similar fragmentary outcomes. Based on my own work on the relationships between the Deaf community and the disability movement (Corker 1998), I tend to agree with Silvers's (1999, 98) assertion, following Helen Meekosha and Jan Pettman (1991), that: "the politics of collectivity is also categorically deleterious for people with disabilities. Not just specific political identities, but also the logic of transforming political identity into categorical group identity, result in performance norms that always will be oppressive and dismissive of (some) people with disabilities. This appears to be the case even when disability itself is made into a categorical group identity."

In part, it seems that this is because of the kind of collective we have constructed for ourselves and the fact that this collective exists in a world where we are coerced to consent to individualist ways of being and behaving. I do not think this means that we should abandon the collective, because it can be a tremendous source of strength to isolated individuals. Rather, it may be useful for the movement to look to the literature on collectivism and feminist notions of interdependency for examples of how we could address this problem. However, I think some of the movement's difficulties also happen because "the normative defects of interest-group politics are, first, that the privatized form of representation and decision-making it encourages *does not require these expressions of interests to appeal to justice,* and second, that inequality of resources, organization, and power allows some interests to dominate while others have little or no voice" (Young 1990, 92, emphasis added). This allows the most privileged and the most articulate members of a minority group to claim to "represent" their community (Meekosha and Pettman 1991; Corker 1998).

Letting go of assumptions about the cohesion of the grouping "disabled people" may open out a much richer range of explanatory possibilities, and this is not just a matter of adding inflections such as "Deaf," "lesbian," "black" or "woman" to the existing collectivity, but of entirely dismantling it. This means looking seriously at the diverse, discrete and interconnected moments of its construction through discourses and associated social practices as the basis for a truly proactive social policy.

NOTES

[1]The reader is referred to a number of wide-ranging British texts for this purpose (Morris 1991; Swain et al. 1993; Campbell and Oliver 1996; Barnes and Mercer 1997; Oliver 1996b; Shakespeare 1998; Barnes et al. 1999).

[2]The term "Deaf" refers to people with hearing impairments who use sign language.

[3]Priestley (1998), for example, presents a useful if ultimately simplified typology that depends upon such boundaries.

[4]It should be clear from this description that the term "disability" is used in both the social-model of disability and in dominant discourses. However, in the latter, the term refers to what social-model thinkers describe as impairment. In order to avoid confusion I will refer to social conceptualizations of disability as "new disability discourses" and to other conceptualizations as "dominant discourses on disability."

[5]Individualist societies are those which emphasize "I" consciousness, autonomy, emotional independence, individual initiative, the right to privacy, the need for specific friendship and universalism. Their stress on the I-versus-you distinction and on having an explicit and firm boundary between self and others takes an *independent* view of the self. Collective societies, in contrast, stress "we" consciousness, collective identity, emotional dependence, group solidarity, sharing, duties and obligations, a need for stable and predetermined friendship, group decision and particularism. They generally take an interdependent view of the self and are defined by specific and firm group boundaries which emphasis a we (the in-group)-versus-they (the out-group) distinction (see, for example, Kim et al. 1994; Rose and Kiger 1995; Corker 1996).

[6]In *Justice and the Politics of Difference* (1990), Young cites the title of Habermas's work as "The Theory of Communicative Competence," whereas in the most recent British translation of this work, it is called "The Theory of Communicative Action." It seems that there is a very subtle distinction between the terms "competence" and "action" which is particularly relevant for this essay, and though I refer to both, my analysis is focused on the concept of "communicative action."

[7]This distinction may also be of significance to the "politics of visibility" so often associated with identity politics and the practice of "passing" (see Seidman et al. 1999, in reference to sexuality).

[8]The criteria for defining "under disability" are: (i) the defendant must be able to understand the trial proceedings in order to make a proper defence; (ii) s/he must be able to understand the evidence; (iii) s/he must be able to instruct legal advisors; (iv) s/he is able to understand the charges and plead appropriately (Prins 1986: 19).

[9]See, for example, C. Williams 1995; Brennan and Brown 1997.

[10]A TTY or minicom is a telecommunications device which enables a deaf person to communicate through text with another party. Because the use of this device relies on written language, its effectiveness as a communication tool may depend, in Habermasian terms, on the "competence" of the deaf person to communicate in this way and on the ability of the receiver to decode the deaf person's English if he or she is not "competent."

[11]See Brennan and Brown (1997) and Metzger (1999) for further comments in relation to sign language interpreting.

[12]MacPherson marks a recognition that the "reactive" nature of legislation as framed by the 1976 Race Relations Act and its explication of direct discrimination (the projection of hostile attitudes or stereotypes), along with its definition of indirect discrimination (institutionalized discrimination), do not go far enough.

REFERENCES

Alderson, P. *Children's Consent to Surgery.* Buckingham, UK: Open University Press, 1993.

Allen, D. S. and Jensen, R., eds. *Freeing the First Amendment: Critical Perspectives on Freedom of Expression.* New York: New York University Press, 1995.

Bakhtin, M. M. *The Dialogic Imagination: Four Essays by M. M Bakhtin,* trans. C. Emerson and M. Holquist. Austin: University of Texas Press, 1981.

Bakhtin, M. M. *Speech Genres and Other Late Essays,* eds. C. Emerson and M. Holquist, trans. V. W. McGee. Austin: University of Texas Press, 1986.

Barnes, C. and Mercer, G. *Doing Disability Research.* Leeds, UK: The Disability Press, 1997.

Barnes, C., Mercer, G. and Shakespeare, T. *Exploring Disability: A Sociological Introduction.* Cambridge, UK: Polity, 1999.

Benhabib, S. *Critique, Norm and Utopia.* New York: Columbia University Press, 1986.

Brennan, M. and Brown, R. *Equality before the Law: Deaf People's Access to Justice.* 1997.

Brown, W. "Freedom's Silences," in R. C. Post, ed., *Censorship and Silencing: Practices of Cultural Regulation.* Los Angeles, CA: The Getty Research Institute, 1998.

Butler, J. *Gender Trouble: Feminism and the Subversion of Identity.* New York: Routledge, 1990.

Butler, J. *Excitable Speech.* New York: Routledge, 1997.

Calvert, C. "Hate Speech and Its Harms: A Communication Theory Perspective." *Journal of Communication* 47(l) (1997): 4–19.

Cameron, D. "Good to Talk?" Paper presented at the Sociolinguistics Symposium 12, University of London, March 1998.

Campbell, J. and Oliver, M. *Disability Politics: Understanding Our Past, Changing Our Future*. London: Routledge, 1996.

Carey, J. *Communication as Culture: Essays on Media and Society*. New York: Routledge, 1989.

Castells, M. *The Power of Identity*. Oxford: Blackwell, 1996.

Chappell, A. L. "Disability, Discrimination, and the Criminal Justice System." *Critical Social Policy*, 42 (Winter 1994/5): 19–33.

Corker, M. *Deaf Transitions*. London: Jessica Kingsley, 1996.

Corker, M. *Deaf and Disabled or Deafness Disabled?* Buckingham, UK: Open University Press, 1998.

Corker, M. "New Disability Discourse, the Principle of Optimization, and Social Change," in M. Corker and S. French, eds. *Disability Discourse*. Buckingham, UK: Open University Press, 1999a.

Corker, M. "Conflations, Foundations and Differences: The Limits to 'Accurate' Theoretical Representation of Disabled People's Experience?" *Disability and Society*, 14(5) (1999b): 627–642.

Corker, M. "A View from the Bridge: An Interdisciplinarian's Overview of the Social Relations of Disability Studies," *Disability Studies Quarterly* 19(4) (1999c): 305–317.

Corker, M. and French, S., eds. *Disability Discourse*. Buckingham, UK: Open University Press, 1999.

Crossley, N. *Intersubjectivity: The Fabric of Social Becoming*. London: Sage, 1996.

Crossley, N. "Corporeality and Communicative Action: Embodying the Renewal of Critical Theory." *Body and Society*, 3(1) (1997): 17–46.

Downing, J.D.H. "'Hate Speech' and 'First Amendment Absolutism' Discourses in the US." *Discourse and Society* 10(2) (1999): 175–189.

Doyle, B. "Enabling Legislation or Dissembling Law?—The Disability Discrimination Act 1995." *Modern Law Review* 64 (1997).

Doyle, B. "From Welfare to Rights? Disability and Legal Change in the United Kingdom in the Late 1990s," in M. Jones and L.A.B. Marks, eds. *Disability, Diversability and Legal Change*. The Hague: Martinus Nijhoff, 1999, 23.

Goldberg, D. T. "Afterword: Hate or Power?" in R. K. Whillock and D. Slayden, eds., *Hate Speech*. Thousand Oaks, CA: Sage, 1995.

Gooding, C. *Blackstone's Guide to the Disability Discrimination Act 1995*, London: Blackstone in association with RADAR, 1996.

Habermas, J. *The Philosophical Discourse of Modernity*, trans. Frederick Lawrence, Cambridge, MA: MIT Press, 1987.

Habermas, J. *The Theory of Communicative Action, Volume I—Reason and the Rationalization of Society*, trans. Thomas McCarthy. Cambridge, UK: Polity, 1991a.

Habermas, J. *The Theory of Communicative Action, Volume II—Lifeworld and System: A Critique of Functionalist Reason*, trans. Thomas McCarthy. Cambridge, UK: Polity, 1991b.

Hunt, P. "A Critical Condition," in P. Hunt, ed., *Stigma*. London: Geoffrey Chapman, 1996, reprinted in T. Shakespeare, ed., *The Disability Reader: Social Science Perspectives*. London: Cassell, 1998.

Jensen, R. and Arriola, E., "Feminism and Free Expression: Silence and Voice," in D. S. Allen and R. Jensen, eds. *Freeing the First Amendment: Critical Perspectives on Freedom of Expression*. New York: New York University Press, 1995.

Kim, U. "Individualism and Collectivism: Conceptual Clarification and Elaboration," in U. Kim, H. C. Triandis, C. Kagitcibasi, S-C Choi, G. Yoon, eds., *Individualism and Collectivism: Theory, Method and Applications*. Thousand Oaks, CA: Sage, 1994.

Leder, D. *The Absent Body*. Chicago: University of Chicago Press, 1990.

Lemert, C. *Postmodernism Is Not What You Think*. Oxford: Blackwell, 1997.

Linton, S. "Disability Studies: Not Disability Studies." *Disability and Society* 13(4) (1998a), 525–541.

Linton, S. *Reclaiming Disability: Knowledge and Identity*. New York: New York University Press, 1998b.

Lyotard, J-F. *The Postmodern Condition: A Report on Knowledge*. Minneapolis, MN: University of Minnesota Press, 1984.

MacPherson, Sir W. *The Stephen Lawrence Inquiry*. London: TSO, CM4262–1, 1999.

Meekosha, H. and Pettman, J. "Beyond Category Politics," *Hecate* 17(2) (1991): 75.

Merleau-Ponty, M. *Phenomenology of Perception*, trans. C. Smith. London: Routledge, 1962.

Metzger, M. *Sign Language Interpreting: Deconstructing the Myth of Neutrality*. Washington DC: Gallaudet University Press, 1999.

Morris, J. *Pride Against Prejudice*. London: The Women's Press, 1991.

Oliver, M. J. "Defining Impairment and Disability: Issues at Stake," in C. Barnes and G. Mercer, eds. *Exploring the Divide: Illness and Disability*. Leeds, UK: The Disability Press, 1996a.

Oliver, M. J. *Understanding Disability: From Theory to Practice*. Basingstoke, UK: MacMillan, 1996b.

Priestley, M. "Constructions and Creations: Idealism, Materialism, and Disability Theory." *Disability and Society* 13(1) (1998): 75–94.

Prins, H. *Dangerous Behaviour, the Law and Mental Disorder*. London: Tavistock, 1986.

Rose, P. and Kiger, G. "Intergroup Relations: Political Action and Identity in the Deaf Community." *Disability and Society* 10(4) (1995): 521–528.

Schutz, A. *The Phenomenology of the Social World*. Evanston, IL: Northwestern University Press, 1967.

Seidman, S., Meeks, C. and Traschen, F. "Beyond the Closet? The Changing Social Meaning of Homosexuality in the United States." *Sexualities* 2(1) (1999): 9–34, 24.

Shakespeare, T. "Disability, Identity and Difference," in C. Barnes and G. Mercer, eds. *Exploring the Divide: Illness and Disability*. Leeds, UK: The Disability Press, 1996.

Shakespeare, T., ed. *The Disability Reader: Social Science Perspectives*. London: Cassell, 1998.

Silvers, A. "Formal Justice," in A. Silvers, D. Wasserman, and M. B. Mahowald, eds. *Disability, Difference, Discrimination*. Lanham, MA: Rowman & Littlefield, 1998.

Silvers, A. "Double Consciousness, Triple Difference: Disability, Race, Gender and the Politics of Recognition," in M. Jones and L. A. B. Marks, eds. *Disability, Diversability and Legal Change*. The Hague: Martinus Nijhoff, 1999.

Swain, J, Finkelstein, V., French, S. and Oliver, M., eds. *Disabling Barriers Enabling Environments*. London: Sage in association with The Open University, 1993.

UPIAS. *The Fundamental Principles of Disability*. London: The Union of the Physically Impaired Against Segregation, 1976.

Williams, C. *Invisible Victims: Crime and Abuse against People with Learning Disabilities*. London: Jessica Kingsley, 1995.

Williams, S. J. "Bodily Dys-Order: Desire, Excess and the Transgression of Corporeal Boundaries," *Body and Society* 4(2) (1998): 59–82.

Young, I. M. "Impartiality and the Civic Public: Some Implications of Feminist Critiques of Moral and Political Theory." in S. Benhabib and D. Cornell, eds. *Feminism as Critique*. Minneapolis: University of Minnesota Press, 1987.

Young, I. M. *Justice and the Politics of Difference*. Princeton, NJ: Princeton University Press, 1990, 25.

A Bright New Era of Equality, Independence and Freedom
Casting an Australian Gaze on the ADA

MELINDA JONES AND LEE ANN BASSER MARKS

Gazing on the Americans with Disabilities Act from Australian shores offers a useful stand-point from which to assess a decade of experience of the ADA. An Australian view of the ADA brings with it the advantage of both distance and perspective. Because in many respects Australia is a new nation, struggling after two hundred years of white occupation to establish for itself an independent political identity, issues of rights and equality have a particular poignancy. The process of introspection has made Australians question the constructions of the political landscape and the values which ought to be considered fundamental. Issues of social justice are tied to the movement for an Australian republic, and there is mounting social pressure for (and opposition to) a Preamble to be added to the Australian Constitution which makes reference to the original occupants of the land and to fundamental freedoms. The rights of people with disabilities are among those rights which are under the microscope. As such, an analysis of how disability rights have evolved in the two countries should be illuminating for citizens of both nations.

This essay highlights differences and similarities between the Australian and the American experience of disability law and suggests that there are significant lessons to be gained in both directions. The particular matters with which we shall be concerned are first, the regulatory scheme in each jurisdiction. Second, we examine the very different definitional approaches to disability rights and the extent to which these reflect the cultural and social experience of each country. Third, the similarities and differences of individual complaints mechanisms are assessed. And finally, the Australian experiment with standards and action plans, which focus on the needs of people with disabilities as a group rather than responding to specific instances of discrimination, is investigated. We conclude that drawing on the groundbreaking U.S. legislation has provided the Australian disability movement with a model for legislative change and has given us the freedom to move beyond a complaints-based system. The U.S. experience of the law in action provides both recommendations and cautions.

Unlike the U.S., Australia has—the women's movement aside—no history of civil rights movements supporting the full inclusion of historically disadvantaged groups. Australia is just beginning to come to terms with the past mistreatment of our indigenous peoples. In this context, it is remarkable that there is a suite of legislation directed at the promotion of equality, and that this legislation prohibits discrimination not only on the grounds of sex and race, but also with respect to disability.[1] There is no doubt that the enactment of the federal Disability Discrimination Act (DDA) in 1992 was significantly influenced by the ADA. The "last civil rights movement" in the U.S.[2] has spawned not only U.S. domestic legislation but disability discrimination legislation around the common law world and beyond.

Superficially there are many similarities between the U.S. legal system and the Australian system. Both are constitutional democracies operating as a federation of states; both have a common-law heritage. However, the embodiment of a Bill of Rights in the U.S. Constitution creates fundamental differences between the two legal systems.

In Australia there is no comprehensive protection of rights in the Constitution, nor is there any provision which guarantees equality between members of the community. The rights and interests of people with disabilities are, however, addressed in a number of pieces of legislation at both a state and commonwealth level.[3] As in the U.S., even where legislation is not specifically directed at people with disabilities, all areas of law impact on the lives of people with disabilities. This is the case whether the law concerns education, health, local government, criminal justice, provision of basic services or civil and political rights. While in the U.S., to address legislative denial of rights and structural inequalities recourse can be had to the protections provided in the Constitution and the Bill of Rights, there is no generalized protection of rights in Australia and there is no mechanism, other than the DDA (and related state equal opportunity legislation), to address the structural inequalities and denial of rights that people with disabilities encounter in many areas of life.[4]

DISABILITY CIVIL RIGHTS MOVEMENTS IN AUSTRALIA AND THE U.S.

The geneses of the disability movements in Australia and the U.S. are very different. Even a cursory glance at the history of the disability rights movement in the U.S. reveals the impact of the success of the black civil right movements on the nascent disability rights movement in the early 1970s.[5] Disability groups run by people with disabilities for people with disabilities emerged actively lobbying for enabling, rights-based legislation and using the civil disobedience tactics of the civil rights movement. At the same time the interest in public-interest law was growing. Parents were lobbying for suitable education for their children with disabilities, and returning disabled Vietnam veterans were demanding to be included in mainstream American society. Against this background the Rehabilitation Act of 1973 was enacted. This act took a rights-based approach and contained radical anti-discrimination measures (Sections 501–504). It was tremendously important to the disability rights movement. As Scotch points out: "It would be going too far to say that Section 504 created the disability rights movement in the 1970s, but the existence of Section 504 did strengthen existing national and local organizations and contributed to the development of new ones. The social movement of disabled people became better organized and more broadly based as the result of federal civil rights activities."[6] From Australian shores it appears that it was this experience with the Rehabilitation Act which mobilized people with disabilities and ultimately led to the ADA.

By contrast, in Australia there has not been a cohesive, organized disability rights movement, and until the mid-1980s legislative provision for people with disabilities was premised on a "needs" model. Two distinctive features of the Australian political landscape bear on the nature of disability policy and law and on the nature of the disability movement. These are, on the one hand, the Australian welfare state being premised on wage security for the [male able-bodied] worker and, on the other hand, historically provided income support for people with disabilities based on "needs" as they "could not" work. Davis,[7] drawing on Castles,[8] notes that:

> the welfare state in Australia . . . developed along different lines from most other (especially European) welfare states . . . based on "wage security for the worker"

rather than "social security for the citizen." Paid work . . . has been the prime moral category of Australian social life. The focus of this "laborist" approach to welfare has been on shoring up wages and working conditions, as well as levels of employment. The problem for those who "couldn't work" was initially resolved by categorical exemptions for aged people and invalids. Over time, the range of categorical exemptions from the labour market was extended and the category of disability emerged as an elaboration of the invalidity category.

Davis documents the shift from a welfare/needs-based approach to rights-based reforms which have been embodied in more recent legislation.[9] Against a background of a long tradition of welfare support for all those outside the workforce (whatever the reason for this status), the Australian emphasis has not been on employment *per se*. This contrasts with the "rugged individualism" by which Americans are portrayed, where membership of the workforce appears to be paramount. Further, unlike in the U.S. the Australian impetus for the switch from a needs-based approach to one embedded in rights came from public policy rather than from public protest.

While there was disability activism at the time of the enactment of the DDA, the primary influence on both the scope and the detail of the DDA was exercised by lawyers with experience of the other civil rights acts and with experience of state antidiscrimination laws. This difference permeates much of the analysis of the law that is to follow.

THE DISABILITY DISCRIMINATION ACT

The DDA was introduced into Australia's Commonwealth Parliament, inspired by the idea of "a fairer Australia where people with disabilities are regarded as equals, with the same rights as all other citizens, with recourse to systems that redress any infringement of their rights . . . where difference is accepted, and where public instrumentalities, communities and individuals act to ensure that society accommodates difference."[10] In the absence of constitutional protections, it was believed that the legislation would "constitute the legal basis for the protection and promotion of the rights of people with disabilities and . . . help to overcome social and economic disadvantage by assisting people with disabilities to participate as equals in Australian society.[11] There is no doubt that the DDA has helped to put issues of disability rights onto the public agenda. The enactment of the legislation was in itself an important first step, recognizing as it does that people with disabilities are full members of Australian society.

The explicit purpose of the DDA is to ensure "that people with disabilities have the same rights to equality before the law as the rest of the community"[12] and "to promote recognition and acceptance within the community of the principle that persons with disabilities have the same fundamental rights as the rest of the community."[13] The objectives of the legislation are the elimination of discrimination on the ground of disability in the areas of work, accommodation, education, access to premises, clubs and sport and in the provision of goods, facilities, services and land.[14] There are many areas of life which are not covered by the DDA, and the act itself contains exclusions including superannuation and insurance, social security and immigration.[15] However, by comparison with the ADA, the Australian law is comprehensive.

In addition to the individual complaints mechanisms, the DDA contains four other mechanisms which have the potential to address structural inequalities affecting the lives of people with disabilities. These are action plans, standards, guidelines and investigations.[16] These features of the legislation are intended to address systemic discrimination and to have an impact on the lives of people with disabilities. The inclusion of these alternate mechanisms created great expectations among both people with disabilities and human rights activists. Their inclusion in what is otherwise a traditional civil rights statute was seen as both radical and empowering. The provision for alternate mechanisms to individual complaints clearly differentiates the Australian law from the ADA.

WHO CAN USE THE LEGISLATION: A QUESTION OF DEFINITION

The Australian DDA adopts a distinctive approach to the question of who is to count as a person with a disability and who is able to benefit from the legislation. Unlike the situation in almost any other jurisdiction including the U.S., the Australian legislation removes the necessity of surviving a threshold test of eligibility before the law comes into effect. This is achieved by the incorporation of a very broad definition of disability in Section 4 of the act.[17] Because of this broad definition, the focus of dispute is the act of discrimination rather than the status of the complainant.

For the purposes of the DDA, a disability includes the total or partial loss of the person's bodily or mental functions; the total or partial loss of a part of the body; the presence in the body of organisms causing disease or illness; the presence in the body of organisms capable of causing disease or illness; the malfunction, malformation or disfigurement of a part of the person's body; disorder or malfunction that results in the person learning differently from a person without the disorder or malfunction; and a disorder, illness or disease that affects a person's thought processes, perception of reality, emotions or judgment or that results in disturbed behavior. While there is no attempt in this definition to distinguish between impairment and disability, the definition is inclusive, embracing the full range of circumstances in which a person could be defined as disabled. There is no need to focus on the particular wording of the act or to establish that the disability alleged falls within a particular category of disability, for the legislation is concerned with the actions of the discriminator rather than the characteristics or worthiness of the complainant.

The coverage of the DDA is such that it moves well beyond people who would traditionally be seen as "people with disabilities." The act is unique in caring less about the categorization or the status of its beneficiaries than about discriminatory behavior of those coming into contact with people who are "different." This definition was specifically drafted as a result of the experience of state antidiscrimination law, where problems had arisen because of the interpretation of strict criteria of disability which focused on impairment and medical categorizations.[18] The effect of the breadth of the definition is that it is not necessary to show that a person is "deserving" of equal treatment or that the person was not implicated in the cause of the disability.[19] There is no requirement that the disability should be permanent, or even that the disability should affect the person continually and consistently. In fact the act potentially covers everyday illnesses and situations where the individual concerned has acted recklessly and could in some way be seen to have caused the disability. This has been a cause for criticism by many commentators with disabilities, for it is assumed that as a consequence the act is not operating to rectify historical disadvantage.

From the perspective of legal practitioners, the definition of disability removes the need to establish the client's "abnormality" as a threshold question and thereby both simplifies the process of bringing a claim and ensures that cases are not struck out on technical decisions about who is disabled. In the process the definition is empowering, because individuals do not need to prove their outsider status in order to use the act. This is quite different from the situation under the ADA.

Because the question of who is entitled to use the ADA involves a series of legal questions, there is a great deal of litigation about the applicability of the act to particular individuals. In the context of employment discrimination, Title 1 of the ADA requires individuals to pass another threshold test. The individual must be a "qualified individual with a disability" before an action can be commenced.

While the Australian law also recognizes that an employee must have the requisite skills to do the job and that justice to employers means that an employer must not be obliged to employ a person who is unable to perform the job, the issue of the "inherent requirements" of the job are neither personal to the applicant nor threshold questions. Once an applicant is able to demonstrate that she has been discriminated against by virtue of the disability, the focus shifts to the employer, who may be able to argue that the discrimination is not unlawful because the applicant is unable to perform the "inherent requirements" of the job.

It has been argued that the definition in the ADA is to be preferred to the broader, inclusionary approach of the Australian legislation because the definition of disability in Section 504 of the Rehabilitation Act and thus in the ADA: "establishes prejudice as the defining fact of disability and thus marks the break from the medical model to the social model for disability, by locating the 'handicap' in social perceptions and in the restrictions imposed by concrete living situations rather than listing medical conditions which come into the category of 'disabled.' "[20] From an Australian perspective, the opposite would seem to be the case. The ADA's definition is extremely narrow by comparison with that contained in the DDA.

From the Australian perspective, focus on the question of who should be entitled to be considered disabled creates unnecessary confusion and limits the effectiveness of the legislation. It also creates an anomaly that individuals who have been treated less favorably than "normal" members of the community because of an impairment are often unable to challenge their treatment or to be compensated for it. This situation could not arise in Australia, although an act of discrimination may not be unlawful in particular circumstances and hence no remedy may be available.

The advantage of the Australian approach is clear. It avoids emphasis on legal niceties and technicalities and at the same time affirms the individual's experience of impairment. In so doing, the Australian legislation does not automatically prioritize the rights and interests of people with disabilities, for it adopts other mechanisms by which to balance their interests with those of the community.

While there is no doubt that the definitions of disability in both the ADA and the DDA are informed by an understanding of the social causes of disability, the question of whether even the broad definition of disability in the DDA incorporates a social model of disability is a matter of dispute. The Australian definition operates in such a way as to redirect the focus of the inquiry from the individual and her "medical condition" to the question of the treatment of the person. Just as in the ADA, the DDA can be used not only by people who are currently disabled to challenge discriminatory behavior. It can also be used by those who are discriminated against as a result of a past disability or who are imputed to have a disability even if in fact they do not have one. Over and beyond this, a person who is discriminated against because of a future disabling condition can bring an action under the Australian legislation. An important feature of both the Australian and the U.S. law is that a nondisabled person can bring an action if he or she is discriminated against by virtue of his or her association with a person with a disability. In this situation the significance of not having to establish that the person with whom they are associate with is a "person with a disability" is substantial.

The simplicity of the Australian approach to the definition of disability can be seen as a direct result of the history of the disability civil rights movement in Australia. The definition as such does not empower particular historically disadvantaged groups. Nonetheless, in adopting a simple and broad definition of disability, the Australian legislation offers the potential of inculcating change at a fundamental level. By including minor or trivial disabilities within its scope, the legislation provides for a flexibility in treatment of all members of the community, which ultimately must be to the advantage of those whose difference is more acute. For people with disabilities to be accepted into society, there needs to be a great degree of flexibility and respect for individual difference. Responding to complaints of a minor nature can pave the way for the attitudinal change that is a prerequisite to social change. For example, where a university modifies the exam procedure to accommodate the needs of a student with a broken arm, it will be more open to providing exam modification for a person who has a permanent condition which affects the use of the arm. Further, the existence of flexibility granted to "normal" students normalizes the situation and makes it easier for a person with a disability to ask for support. Once accommodations are common and uncontroversial and not provided only for outsider groups, inclusion becomes a way of life and provides a backdrop for systemic change. As such, the flexible Australian approach to the question of disability appears to offer substantial advantages over its U.S. counterpart.

CONSTITUTING DISCRIMINATION

People with disabilities face a wide range of discrimination. They can be segregated from the rest of society. They can be excluded from or denied benefits, services or opportunities available to nondisabled people. They can face discrimination as a result of construction, transportation, architectural or communication barriers, or as the result of the adoption or application of standards, criteria, practices or procedures that are based on thoughtlessness or indifference.[21]

The extent to which these notions of discrimination are incorporated into legal constructions of disability varies. From an Australian perspective, the ADA seems to proscribe discrimination without exploring the nuances of the concept. Discrimination, in Australian law, means treating a person unequally because of a disability, whether that discrimination is directed at the person or simply impacts differently upon the person. As such, the distinction between intentional discrimination resulting from disparate treatment and the unintentional discrimination resulting from disparate impact, so important to U.S. antidiscrimination law, plays out somewhat differently in Australia.

The DDA prohibits four types of discrimination against people with disabilities. It is not only unlawful to discriminate directly against a person with a disability; it is equally unlawful to engage in indirect discrimination, to harass a person on the basis of disability and to ask discriminatory questions.[22] Direct discrimination, which is concerned with formal equality, occurs when a person with a disability is treated less favorably than another person because of her disability.[23] The test of direct discrimination is an objective test which focuses on the question of whether a person has been treated materially differently to a person without a disability. In other words, would the person have been discriminated against "but for" the disability? Indirect discrimination, on the other hand, is concerned with the principles of substantive equality. The test of indirect discrimination is whether a person is unfairly excluded from equal participation in society as a result of the imposition of a requirement or condition with which a disproportionate number of people with disabilities are unable to comply.

In Australian law a person can discriminate even if he or she is unaware that a person has a disability or if he or she is unaware that people with disabilities will be adversely affected by the requirement or condition. It does not matter whether there was an intention to discriminate or whether the discriminator believed that he or she was acting in the interests of the person with a disability.[24] Further, when determining whether there has been an act of discrimination, where there are multiple reasons for the act, the DDA specifies that if one of the reasons is the affected person's disability, this is sufficient to ground discrimination.[25] This is the case even if the person's disability is not the dominant or even a substantial reason for doing the act.

The High Court of Australia has held that motive and the intention to discriminate are irrelevant to the fact of discrimination.[26] The case of *Scott & Anor v. Telstra* (1995) EOC 92–717, a case of indirect discrimination, illustrates this point. Telstra had a blanket policy of providing a standard handset for telephones to all their customers. Telstra refused to provide any alternative telecommunications devices, which would make the telecommunications system accessible to people with hearing impairments.

Telstra argued that the service it provided was the telephone network. Telstra argued that it did not intend for there to be disparate treatment of people with disabilities. All it did was supply a standard handset in addition to the network service. HREOC, however, found that the service Telstra provided was communication over the network, and that the requirement that the network be accessed by standard handsets was clearly one with which a disproportionate number of people with profound hearing loss could not comply and which was patently unreasonable in the circumstances.

An important feature of the DDA is that there is no assumption that people with disabilities have rights which other members of the community do not have. As such, it is not necessary to employ a particular person because she or he has a disability. While reasonable adjustments must be put into place to make it possible for a person with a disability to succeed at the job, it is not expected that a person should be employed if she is unable to perform the "inherent requirements" of the job.[27]

The main question with respect to disability discrimination in employment is the extent to which the notion of "inherent requirement" can be seen to facilitate creative and lateral solutions to inclusion or is used to undermine real equality. The DDA attempts to find a balance between the needs of the employers and those of employees. The idea of "inherent requirements of the job" protects both the employer and the (potential) employee with a disability by ensuring that underlying prejudices are exposed while acknowledging that certain features of a job are essential.

At this point reference should be made to the case of *Commonwealth of Australia v. Human Rights and Equal Opportunity Commission & X* (1998) EOC 92–909, where the question of the lawfulness of the discharge from the Australian Defence Forces of a soldier who was HIV-positive was considered. Commissioner Carter took a narrow view of the inherent requirements of defence force personnel and accepted that the performance of noncombative duties would not be affected by HIV status. An appeal was made to the Full Federal Court, where this position was categorically rejected. The Full Court held that a broad approach to inherent requirements was not only legitimate but legally correct, and that on the facts of the particular case it would be dangerous to allow a person with HIV to serve as a soldier because of the inherent risk of injury and consequently of bleeding.

While there is good reason to be concerned by the judgment about bleeding, the interpretation of "inherent requirements" is extremely troubling. Justice Burchett in the Full Court commented that: "The inherent requirements of a particular employment are not to be limited to a mechanical performance of its tasks or skills. They will frequently involve an interaction with other employees, or with outsiders. In some occupations, for example, a psychological problem producing significant rudeness to others might be disabling. Although all assigned tasks might be performed, the employee might be unable to carry out the inherent requirement of maintaining a smooth working relationship with fellow workers or with the general public."[28] The case has gone on appeal to the High Court of Australia, which has currently reserved its judgment.

If allowed to stand, this interpretation of "inherent requirements" has the potential to minimize the utility of the DDA. The effect of the decision may leave it open for employers to argue that their clients would find employees with disabilities offensive; that the other staff members were unprepared to change their work practices to accommodate the needs of employees with disabilities; or that other organizations with which they had ongoing dealings were not prepared to deal with employees with disabilities. This would allow the position of people with disabilities to be treated in a manner which has been consistently rejected as unacceptable in the area of racial discrimination in Australia. It could allow inherently discriminatory environments to be maintained and legitimized as nondiscriminatory.

In the context of Australian law, this interpretation would place people with disabilities in a quite different position from people who are discriminated against on the basis of gender or race. While gazing on Australia from the U.S., this may not seem startling given the very different experience of discrimination law. However, casting an Australian eye on the U.S. situation, it seems anathema to the objectives of disability discrimination law to permit inherently discriminatory practices to continue.

LAWFUL DISCRIMINATION

The DDA has an extremely broad reach when compared to the ADA. Almost all aspects of life are covered by the terms and the operation of the DDA. While the act lists specific headings and provides specific detail with respect to the significant areas of employment and education, amongst others, these are not proffered as exceptions but as demonstrations of the principles involved. By comparison, to gain a full picture of the rights of people with disabilities in the U.S. it is necessary to consult a number of pieces of legislation. The rules relating to discrimination not only vary between pieces of legislation but also are different from title to title of the ADA. From the Australian perspective this creates enormous complexity and must present difficulty not only for lawyers but for people with disabilities attempting to know and assert their rights.

The DDA then, offers a comparatively straightforward and simple approach to the subject of disability discrimination. However, under the DDA not all discrimination is unlawful. Once discrimination is proven the burden of proof shifts to the respondent to show that, in the circumstances of the case, the discrimination was lawful. There are five situations in which discriminatory action are is provided for. These are: where the adjustments impose an unjustifiable hardship on the employer or service provider; where the action is not covered by the DDA or is explicitly exempted from it; where the action is covered by an exemption issued by HREOC; where the action is in "direct compliance" with legislation "prescribed" under the DDA; and where the action is in compliance with a disability standard.

Exemptions

The DDA specifically provides for exemptions in a number of areas. Some of the exemptions directly benefit people with disabilities. For example, special measures which promote the equal opportunity of people with disabilities and programs which target their special needs are exempt from the provisions of the DDA.[29] Similarly, charities may confer benefits on people with disabilities or on people with a particular disability.[30]

The other exemptions allow for discrimination against people with disabilities. These range from the exemption of domestic workers employed in the discriminator's home; to lawful discrimination in the areas of superannuation and insurance; certain pensions and allowances; or where people with disabilities have infectious diseases and the discrimination is reasonably necessary to protect public health.[31] Further, discriminatory provisions in certain statutes are specifically exempted from the operation of the DDA, such as the Migration Act 1958. Similarly, discrimination is allowed where combat duties and peacekeeping activities are concerned.[32]

In addition, the HREOC can grant further exemptions on the application by a concerned individual.[33] The commission has granted exemptions in a number of areas. For example, an exemption has been granted to the Public Transport Corporation in the State of Victoria with respect to certain trams and to the Minister for Transport in South Australia with respect to accessible buses. Other exemptions have been granted to a women's legal service and to the Lutheran Church. Exemptions are not "at large" and are granted for a limited time, usually to enable future compliance with the DDA.

Direct Compliance

Acts done by statutory authority are also exempt in certain circumstances.[34] These include acts done in direct compliance with a court order or a determination made by HREOC and those carried out in direct compliance with a prescribed law. The Commonwealth attorney general has the power to prescribe legislation under the DDA. In order to make use of the defense that the discriminatory action is taken in "direct compliance" with the prescribed legislation, the requirement that discriminatory action must be in direct compliance with the prescribed law is limited to situations where the person was compelled to act the way he did. This should to some extent allay the concerns of the disability community about the effect of prescribing particular legislation.

ALTERNATIVE STRATEGIES UNDER THE DDA

A distinctive feature of the Australian legislation is that it recognizes that the problems for people with disabilities operate at a deep level and that the structural inequalities which extend to so many areas of the lives of people with disabilities cannot possibly be addressed simply by complaints-handling mechanisms which are the traditional fare of antidiscrimination laws. While other Australian antidiscrimination laws, both at state level and federal laws dealing with sex and race, revolve around individual responses to particular instances of discrimination, the DDA provides a range of alternative mechanisms which have the potential to address systemic and structural disadvantage. These mechanisms function both at the level of guidance for voluntary organizational responses to rectifying social imbalance and at the level of legal demand to redesign specific aspects of social life to bring about social justice for people with disabilities.

Because the DDA is a late entry into the field of federal antidiscrimination law, it has been able to draw on the range of issues experienced in other jurisdictions. In the area of sex discrimination, it has been considered very important that affirmative-action programs go hand in hand with equal opportunity or antidiscrimination laws. Chris Ronalds, a barrister who played an important role in agitating for the DDA, writes:

> Affirmative action legislation places the onus on employers, rather than on a disadvantaged employee or prospective employee, to examine and if necessary to change organisational and institutional practices. It tackles the same issues as sex discrimination legislation but in a different way. Sex discrimination legislation is of value to the aggrieved individual and has a ripple effect which may cause a broader change to employment policy to ensure similar complaints do not arise. This is an indirect and ad hoc method of achieving the necessary structural changes required for equal employment opportunity. Affirmative action extends sex discrimination legislation by requiring employers to confront their practices directly and systematically."[35]

The DDA attempts to capture the benefits of affirmative action by introducing the strategies of inquiry, action plans, guidelines and standards. Disability standards and action plans are the main processes developed to address systemic discrimination; the other strategies, the adoption of guidelines and the use of HREOC's inquiry power have been so little used that it is impossible at this stage to comment on their significance. Nonetheless, together these are taken to be means by which people with disabilities could be empowered by the positive action of those they come into contact with. This is quite distinct from and additional to traditional complaints mechanisms that offer defensive antidiscrimination proceedings which are responsive to negative action.

Action Plans

Of all the strategies available, action plans have the greatest potential to bring about social change. Under Part 3 of the DDA, a service provider[36] may prepare and implement an action plan, which is really a document prepared by the service provider setting out its strategies to ensure elimination of disability discrimination. Action plans are, as such, individual organizational plans to be adopted in order for an organization to identify discriminatory practices and develop blueprints for bringing about change to those practices. Action plans place the onus on organizations rather than on disadvantaged individuals and suggest that it is within the power of the wider community to remove disabling barriers and to play an active part in the production of enabling environments.[37]

Action plans can be developed by any service provider relating to the services it provides, and may be lodged with the HREOC.[38] "Service providers" are widely defined to include anyone who provides services, offers goods or makes facilities available, whether free or at a cost.[39]

The aim of an action plan is to identify discriminatory behavior and set a timetable to overcome it. As action plans allow service providers to work on their own solutions to disability discrimination without the supervision of an outside agency,[40] service providers are able to become educated about disability discrimination in a safe environment. Further, by undertaking the process of developing an action plan, an organization will "own" the plan. This will potentially result in a commitment to bring about long-term change and a determination to make that change even if it involves a gradual approach to meeting principles of legislation.

The existence of an action plan registered with HREOC is not evidence in itself that measures will be taken to improve the position of people with disabilities. There is no requirement that people with disabilities be consulted in the formulation of action plans, nor does HREOC play any role in scrutinizing them to ensure they further the objects of the DDA. Furthermore, there is no mechanism to monitor compliance with action plans, so that even the best plan on paper may be ignored in practice.

The extent to which action plans have been developed is further evidence of their inability to make a real difference. As of July 23, 1999, of the thousands of organizations that could potentially utilize action plans, there were only 140 plans registered on the published Register of Action Plans. This is despite the fact that Commonwealth government departments and agencies were meant to have lodged action plans by the end of 1997. At this stage action plans have been lodged by 31 nongovernment and government business enterprises; 29 Commonwealth government departments and agencies; 12 state government departments and agencies; 50 local governments; and 20 educational institutions. At the time of writing, another 15 or so have been lodged with HREOC, but this amounts to a tiny percentage of those that could have been expected.

Disability Standards

The other major innovation of the DDA which is again distinctive and unique to the Australian context is the provision of disability standards, which are intended to respond to systemic and institutional discrimination against people with disabilities. Disability standards are included in the legislation as a mechanism to make rights and obligations under the DDA clearer, simpler and easier to comply with and enforce. The move away from a complaints-based approach to a standards-setting approach has been hailed as a radical means of addressing deeply embedded discrimination.[41] The Australian Law Reform Commission, in its review of the Sex Discrimination Act 1984 (SDA) commented:

> The standard setting function of the DDA has been described as an "innovation for Australian anti-discrimination law." The objective is to "specify requirements for equal opportunity and access for people with a disability in greater detail and with more certainty than is provided by the prohibition of discrimination by other provisions of the DDA." Standards require positive compliance with the legislation and should indicate the practices and policies that should be the rule rather than implying that these practices and policies are "special measures". . . . Standard setting would be a useful way to promote the objectives of the SDA, encourage compliance with its provisions and to indicate best practices under the Act. . . . Standard setting is a useful way to combat systemic discrimination.[42]

Under Section 31 of the DDA, the attorney general may formulate disability standards to specify rights and responsibilities regarding disability issues in specified areas. These are employment, education, accommodation, public transport and the administration of Commonwealth laws and programs. The Federal Government has recently announced its intention to amend the DDA to allow for standards in the area of access to premises.

The purposes of disability standards were described by the former Disability Discrimination Commissioner, Elizabeth Hastings, in a speech given in July 1997:

> There are two main reasons for the inclusion of this provision. The first is to provide clearer delineation of what actually must be done to ensure access and equity than is provided for in the Act itself, in which the requirements for equal access for people with disabilities are only broadly stated. This type of open-ended legislation has its advantages, but is limited in its capacity effectively and consistently to achieve equality for people with disabilities. The second reason for the standards-making

provision is to set time scales in place under the law for achieving equal access for people with disabilities in the areas covered by the DDA; plainly, it is not feasible to bring in far-reaching mandatory requirements and expect the world to change from that point on.[43]

The question as to what should be contained in standards, which is left open by the DDA, has been a source of confusion. In the process of trying to determine the content of standards, it has been suggested that there are a number of different types of standards which may be developed, and that the choice of standard type will affect decisions about the appropriate content of the standard. Standards have been characterized as principle-based, performance-based, prescriptive, process or product standards.[44] Principle-based standards are general statements of the objectives to be reached requiring interpretation according to the particular circumstances. Performance-based standards are those which specify the desired outcome in precise terms but which do not specify the method of achieving those outcomes. A prescriptive standard specifies what conduct is acceptable in particular circumstances, while product standards specify the design or performance of particular products such as textbooks or communication devices. Process standards are those which attempt to define the various roles, relationships and procedures in the particular area. In each case, the standard is intended to provide clarification of the application of legal principle to complex areas of life. However, it is doubtful whether any useful document could ever be drafted which would satisfy this objective, given the range of circumstances and the conflicting needs and interests of all the players.

The most significant issue relates to the content of standards. The DDA is very broad in its objectives and makes it clear that systemic solutions are required for systemic problems. However standards, once enacted, become part of the law. They take the form of regulations but differ in one significant element from ordinary regulations: because the standards become part of the legislation, they will be read down only in the light of the objectives of the legislation in the case of ambiguity.[45]

This means that if the disability standards actually water down the protection found in the DDA, it will not be possible to complain of discrimination if the discriminator has acted consistently with the standard. This will be the case even where the standard provides a lower standard than the rest of the DDA.

The process of drafting standards has given a key role to various stakeholders in the area. People with disabilities are considered to be only one player among many, and more often than not the interests of institutional groups have been given priority over people with disabilities. At present, the defence of unjustifiable hardship is available in only limited circumstances (in the area of education it is limited to enrollment). The draft standards, however, do not only offer minimum standards but also allow for an institution or organization to refuse to comply with the minimum standard on the basis of unjustifiable hardship.

Instead of using disability standards to spell out the scope of discriminatory conduct or embedded discrimination in practice, the standards process has been co-opted by stakeholders who wish to retain the status quo as far as possible—or even justify future discriminatory conduct. For this reason, there has been the suggestion that action plans should become mandatory and that standards should be avoided. If disability standards are to provide alternative mechanisms for overcoming discrimination, it is unsatisfactory if the only way in which they can be enforced is via the individual complaints-handling mechanism. Yet there are no provisions for ensuring compliance with the standards.

The availability of government funding or the provision of licences could be made dependent on compliance with standards. A monitoring agency could be established, not only with the power to investigate complaints but also with the power to initiate inquiries into compliance. Further, all those in the field should be obliged to comply with any requests of the monitoring agency and could, perhaps, be required to conduct regular audits of their practices which could be lodged with the agency. To be of real value, though, such an agency would need to have teeth. Reporting to Parliament and waiting for action is not sufficient.

The optimism which the drafters of the DDA felt and with which disability standards have been greeted by disability activists is beginning to wane. Instead of being statements of principle, bolstering the objectives of the DDA with subject-specific principles, standards, as currently in process, appear to be no different from traditional regulations which accompany almost every piece of legislation. In the U.S. context, regulations under disability legislation abound. Instead of clarifying the position for people with disabilities, these regulations appear to complicate and mystify the processes of the law. Standards, which cover very limited areas of life, are not intended to take this form.

USING THE LEGISLATION

The process of pursuing disability rights in the U.S. seems unnecessarily convoluted, to the point where it would seem likely to disenfranchise many potential complainants. The situation in Australia is much more straightforward. Complaints are lodged with HREOC, and this may be done either in writing or by telephone. Previously a complaint would be referred to the Disability Discrimination Commissioner, who had responsibility for investigating the complaint and for its conciliation. Decision-making in matters of disability-discrimination law now resides with the Federal Court. Recent changes have met with significant opposition from the disability community. These changes bring with them three issues which confront people with disabilities. These are the cost of bringing a matter in the Federal Court, the formality of the Federal Court and the lack of expertise in disability matters of the Federal Court. The issue of costs is of greatest concern. The issue of formality is also of concern. The Federal Court generally operates according to strict rules of evidence which may involve standards of proof with which victims of discrimination may be unable to comply. The final matter of concern relates to the decision-makers on the Federal Court bench. Many members of the Federal Court do in fact have experience in the area of discrimination law, but relatively few have the detailed experience of disability commissioners.

CONCLUSION

Casting an Australian gaze on the ADA 1990 allows us to see both advantages and problems of using a civil-rights statute to achieve justice for people with disabilities. The Australian experience is quite different from the U.S. experience because we have no history of a civil rights movement and no Bill of Rights from which to build the inclusion of outsider groups. Nonetheless, Australia has developed antidiscrimination mechanisms promoting rights on the basis of race, gender and disability. Australian law has followed the law of other jurisdictions and has taken both the ideals and the strategies from a range of sources while developing its own unique approach to the problem.

The assumption that with the ADA there would dawn "a bright new era of equality, independence and freedom" seems somewhat optimistic. There can be no doubt that the ADA has made very significant differences to the lives of people with disabilities in the U.S., and that as knowledge of it spreads, this will continue. In passing the ADA, the U.S. led the world in recognizing the rights of people with disabilities and their entitlement to inclusion in society. The ADA has provided a model law for many jurisdictions, including Australia.

Legislating for the rights of people with disabilities in both countries has made a significant difference to the visibility and acceptability of people with disabilities. Ensuring that all members of the community, whether they be people with or without disabilities, are treated with respect requires a deep commitment to justice and equality. Law can only take us so far. Both the DDA and the ADA provide important starting points which, with appropriate support from the community and sufficient commitment from the state, have the potential to bring about real change. Educating the community about the law and about the rights of people with disabilities is fundamental, and analysis and critique of the law are essential for this purpose. Only when people with disabilities achieve equality can the bright new era begin.

NOTES

[1] The suite of federal legislation includes: Racial Discrimination Act 1975; Sex Discrimination Act 1984; Affirmative Action (Equal Employment Opportunity for Women) Act 1986; Disability Discrimination Act 1992; and the Human Rights and Equal Opportunity Act 1986.

[2] D. Driedger. *The Last Civil Rights Movement: Disabled Peoples' International.* London: Hurst & Co, 1989.

[3] In addition to the federal legislation listed in note 1, see for example, state equal opportunity legislation: Anti-Discrimination Act 1977 (NSW); Anti-Discrimination Act 1991 (Qld); Equal Opportunity Act 1984 (SA); Equal Opportunity Act 1995 (Vic); Equal Opportunity Act 1984 (WA); Discrimination Act 1991 (ACT); Anti-Discrimination Act 1992 (NT) The power-sharing relationship in our federal system of government is such that where laws of the Commonwealth are within power and cover a field, the law of the Commonwealth will prevail: § 109 Commonwealth Constitution.

[4] For general discussion about the DDA, see J. Bourke "Mental Illness, Discrimination in Employment and the Disability Discrimination Act 1992," *J. L. & Med.* 3 (1996): 318; *Australian & New Zealand Equal Opportunity Law and Practice.* Sydney: CCH, 1999; Maeve McDonagh, "Disability Discrimination in Australia," in *Disability Discrimination in the United States, Australia and Canada,* G. Quinn, M. McDonagh and C. Kimber, eds. Oak Tree Press, 1993; Bonnie Tucker, "The Disability Discrimination Act; Ensuring Rights of Australians with Disabilities, Particularly Hearing Impairments," *Monash U. L. R.* 21 (1995): 15; M. C. Tyler, "The Disability Discrimination Act 1992: Genesis, Drafting and Prospects," *Melbourne U. L. R.* 19 (1993): 211.

[5] For a history of the disability law and the disability movement in the U.S., see Richard Scotch. *From Goodwill to Civil Rights: Transforming Federal Disability Policy.* Philadelphia: Temple University Press, 1984. See also Stephen Percy. *Disability, Civil Rights and Public Policy: The Politics of Implementation.* Tuscaloosa: University of Alabama Press, 1989. A brief summary of this history is found in Caroline Gooding. *Disabling Laws, Enabling Acts: Disability Rights in Britain and America.* London: Pluto Press, 1994, 19–26. Of course, the experience of disability groups in the U.S. dates from much earlier—for example, the work of the National Federation of the Blind, which was established in 1940. See Gooding, 20.

[6] Scotch 1984, 150.

[7] Lynne Davis, "Rights Replacing Needs: A New Resolution of the Distributive Dilemma for People with Disabilities in Australia?" in *Justice for People with Disabilities: Legal and Institutional Issues,* M. Hauritz, C. Sampford and S. Blencowe, eds. Sydney: The Federation Press, 1998, 17.

[8] F. Castles. "Welfare and Equality in Captialist Societies: How and Why Australia Was Different," in *Australian Welfare: Historical Sociology,* R. Kennedy, ed. New York: Macmillan, 1989, 69.

[9]In, for example, the Disability Services Act 1986. For an elaboration of Davis's thesis about citizenship and disability, see Davis 1998; and also Lynne Davis, "Riding with the Man on the Escalator: Citizenship and Disability" in Jones and Marks, eds., *Disability, Diversability and Legal Change*. The Hague: Martinus Nijhoff, 1999.

[10]The Hon. Brian Howe, Minister for Health Housing and Community Services, Second Reading Speech, *Parliamentary Debates* May 26, 1992, 2755.

[11]Ibid.

[12]DDA § 3(b).

[13]DDA § 3 (c).

[14]DDA § 3.

[15]DDA §§ 46, 51, and 52.

[16]DDA Part 3, §§ 31–34, 67(1)(k), and 67(1).

[17]It is interesting to note that the first draft of the ADA as introduced into the U.S. Senate contained a similarly broad definition of disability.

[18]For example, in the case of *Kitt v. Tourism Commissioner and Ors* (1987) EOC 92–196, it was found that the NSW Act did not cover epilepsy. Kitt had been employed as a temporary cave guide in the Jenolan Caves in the Blue Mountains outside Sydney. A medical examination was a precondition of permanent employment, and when it was discovered that Kitt had epilepsy, he was told he could not work in the caves and he was given a job selling tickets. A question of legal interpretation arose as to whether epilepsy constituted a physical impairment as defined by the NSW legislation. It was found that certain neurological disabilities (including epilepsy) and mental disorders were not covered by the legislation.

[19]Jerome Bickenbach demonstrates that these are significant limitations in both the Canadian and USA law. See J. Bickenbach, "Voluntary Disabilities and Everyday Illnesses" in *Disability Is Not Measles*, M. Rioux and M. Bach, eds. Toronto: Roeher Institute, 1994.

[20]Caroline Gooding. *Disabling Laws, Enabling Acts: Disability Rights in Britain and America*. London: Pluto Press, 1994, 59. See also Ruth Colker, who argues that the ADA is designed to promote the interests of an historically disadvantaged group: R. Colker, "Affirmative Action, Reasonable Accommodation and Capitalism: Irreconcilable Differences?" in M. Hauritz et al. 1998.

[21]Colker and Tucker 1998, 2.

[22]DDA §§ 6, 35–40, and 30.

[23]*Kinsella v. Queensland University of Technology* (unreported, August 10, 1997). Mr Kinsella, a wheelchair user, wished to participate in a university graduation ceremony on the same basis as his fellow graduates. However the venue chosen for the event could not be reasonably adapted to enable him to participate in all aspects of the ceremony. The Human Rights and Equal Opportunity Commission ordered the university to arrange a suitable alternative venue.

[24]DDA § 6.

[25]DDA § 10.

[26]See *Waters v. Public Transport Corporation* (1992) 103 ALR 513, 520 (HCA).

[27]DDA § 15(4)(a).

[28]1998, 78, 078.

[29]DDA § 45.

[30]DDA § 49.

[31]DDA §§ 15(3), 46, 51, and 48.

[32]DDA § 53 and also § 54 with respect to the peacekeeping role of the Australian Federal Police.

[33]DDA § 55.

[34]DDA § 47.

[35]Cited in R. Graycar and J. Morgan, *The Hidden Gender of Law*. Sydney: Federation Press, 1990, 109.

[36]For a definition of "service provider" for the purposes of the DDA, see § 59 outlined below.

[37]See Swain, J., Finkelstein, V., French, S. and Oliver, M. *Disabling Barriers—Enabling Environments*. London: Open University Press in association with Sage, 1993.

[38]DDA §§ 60 and 64.

[39]DDA § 59.

[40]However, HREOC has developed a number of very useful guides to help, *inter alia,* local government, nongovernment organizations, businesses and tertiary educational institutions to develop action plans.

[41]P. Tahmindjis, "The Law and Indirect Racial Discrimination: Of Square Pegs, Round Holes, Babies & Bathwater" in *Racial Discrimination Act 1975: Review.* Race Relations Commissioner, ed. Canberra: AGPS, 1995, 101 at 126.

[42]ALRC 1994 cited *Aboriginal Legal Issues* 2nd ed. H McRae, G. Nettheim and L Beacroft. Sydney: Federation Press, 1998, 94–95.

[43]"The Right to Belong—Disability Discrimination Law in Education," speech by Elizabeth Hastings, Disability Discrimination Commissioner, in Sydney, July 1997, "speeches," via Disability Rights Home Page, <http://wwwhreoc.gov.au/disability_rights/>.

[44]Disability Discrimination Act Standards Project. *Background Material for the Disability Sector on the MCEETYA Discussion Paper on DDA Standards in Education.* August 1997; see also Submission on Disability Standards in Education of the NSW Disability Discrimination Legal Centre.

[45]The general rule is that if a regulation goes beyond the scope of the legislation it will be *ultra vires* (that is, beyond power). However, because of the way in which the DDA is drafted with respect to standards, this rule does not apply, and the standard may therefore have the effect of limiting the operation of the law as it currently stands.

Appendix: Texts of Laws and Court Decisions

The following Internet sites contain full texts of laws and court decisions referred to in this book:

<http://www.law.cornell/edu/topics/disability.html>: Cornell University's Legal Information Institute's page on disability law. Syllabi of Supreme Court decisions and full texts of the Americans with Disabilities Act and other federal and state statutes can be found at this site.

<http://www.findlaw.com>: This is a comprehensive legal guide. Full texts of Supreme Court decisions can be found here.

<http://caselaw.findlaw.com/cgi-bin/getcase.pl?court=US&navby=year&year=1999>: For *Albertson's, Inc. v. Kirkingburg, Cleveland v. Policy Management Systems Corp., Murphy v. United Parcel Service, Inc., Olmstead v. LC.,* and *Sutton v. United Airlines, Inc.*

<http://caselaw.findlaw.com/cgi-bin/getcase.pl?court-US&navby=year&year=1998>: For *Bragdon v. Abbott.*

<http://caselaw.findlaw.com/cgi-bin/getcase.pl?court-US&navby=year&year=1985>: For *Alexander v. Choate,* and *Cleburne v. Cleburne Living Center, Inc.*

<http://caselaw.findlaw.com/scripts/getcase.pl?court=US&navby=year>: For all other Supreme Court cases.

Contributors

Ron Amundson is a philosopher of biology and disability activist who teaches at the University of Hawaii at Hilo. Amundson published one of the most often-cited philosophical contributions to disability studies, "Disability, Handicap, and the Environment,"in the *Journal of Social Philosophy* in 1992.

Lori B. Andrews is a professor at Chicago-Kent College of Law and the director of the Institute for Science, Law, and Technology at the Illinois Institute of Technology. She is the former chair of the federal Working Group on the Ethical, Legal, and Social Implications of the Human Genome Project. Andrews is the author of *The Clone Age: Adventures in the New World of Reproductive Technologies* and writes extensively about shifting legal understandings of disability, especially in relation to new reproductive technologies.

Richard J. Arneson is a professor of philosophy at the University of California, San Diego, where he was department chair from 1992 to 1996. He has held visiting appointments at California Institute of Technology, the University of California at Davis and Yale University, and has been a visiting fellow at Australian National University, Canberra. His research interests lie in political and moral philosophy, with a special emphasis on contemporary theories of justice. His recent writings work at formulating an egalitarian account of distributive justice that accommodates reasonable concerns about personal responsibility.

Andrew I. Batavia (J.D., M.S.) is an associate professor in the School of Policy and Management, College of Urban and Public Affairs of Florida International University. He has held several key disability policy positions in the federal government, including Executive Director of the National Council on Disability, Associate Director of the White House Domestic Policy Council, and Special Assistant to the Attorney General in the year the ADA regulations were promulgated. Batavia has authored two books and over fifty other publications on issues of disability policy. He is a founding associate editor of the *Journal of Disability Policy Studies* and a member of the state bars of Florida, California and the District of Columbia, and Georgetown University's Kennedy Institute of Ethics.

Lawrence C. Becker is William R. Kenan, Jr. Professor in the Humanities and Professor of Philosophy at the College of William and Mary. His most recent book is *A New Stoicism,* and previous books include *Property Rights: Philosophic Foundations* and *Reciprocity*. He is the editor, with Charlotte B. Becker, of the two-volume *Encyclopedia of Ethics*. Since 1985, he has been an associate editor of the journal *Ethics*.

Jerome E. Bickenbach is a professor in the Department of Philosophy, the Faculty of Law and School of Rehabilitation Therapy at Queen's University. His philosophical, legal and policy treatment of disability can be found in his book *Physical Disability and Social Policy*. Recently, he has been primarily engaged as a consultant for the World Health Organization in the areas of disability epidemiology and survey methodologies as applied to the development of disability classification and assessment tools and their policy applications.

Peter David Blanck is a professor of law, of psychology, and of preventive medicine at the University of Iowa. He received his Ph.D. in psychology from Harvard University and his J.D. from Stanford Law School, where he served as president of the *Stanford Law Review.* Blanck is the Director of the Law, Health Policy and Disability Center at the Iowa College of Law. He is a member of the President's Committee on the Employment of People with Disabilities. His books in the area include *The Americans with Disabilities Act and the Emerging Workforce* and the forthcoming *Employment, Disability, and the Americans with Disabilities Act.*

Dan W. Brock is Charles C. Tillinghast University Professor of Philosophy and Biomedical Ethics and director of the Center for Biomedical Ethics at Brown University. He writes and consults extensively on health care policy. He is the author of *Life and Death* and coauthor of *Deciding for Others* and the forthcoming *From Chance to Choice: Genetics and Justice.*

Ruth Colker holds the Heck-Faust Memorial Chair in Constitutional Law at the Ohio State University College of Law. She is the coauthor (with Bonnie P. Tucker) of the *Law of Disability Discrimination,* as well as the author of numerous books and articles on feminist theory, constitutional law and disability discrimination.

Mairian Corker is a senior research fellow in deaf and disability studies at the University of Central Lancashire, U.K. She is author and editor of numerous publications including *Deaf Transitions* (with Jessica Kingsley); *Deaf and Disabled or Deafness Disabled?; Disability Discourse* with Sally French (Open University Press); and *Disability and Postmodernity* with Tom Shakespeare (Cassell, forthcoming). She is also an executive editor of the international journal *Disability and Society.*

Mary Crossley is a professor of law at the University of California, Hastings College of the Law, where she teaches in the fields of health policy, bioethics and contracts. Her research focuses on the application of disability discrimination law to medical care and the health care financing system.

Norman Daniels is Goldthwaite Professor in the Department of Philosophy, Tufts University. His most recent books include *Benchmarks of Fairness for Health Care Reform* (with Don Light and Ron Caplan), *Justice and Justification* and *From Chance to Choice: Genetics and Justice* (with Allen Buchanan, Dan Brock and Dan Wikler, in press).

Lennard J. Davis is a professor of English at Binghamton University (SUNY). His works on disability include *Enforcing Normalcy: Disability, Deafness, and the Body,* which won the 1996 Gustavus Myers Center for the Study of Human Rights annual award for the best scholarship on the subject of intolerance in North America, and *The Disability Studies Reader.* His memoir *My Sense of Silence,* about growing up in a Deaf family, is forthcoming. Davis was a founding member of the Modern Language Association's Committee on Disability Issues in the Profession.

Matthew Diller is a professor of law at Fordham University. His areas of expertise include the ADA and disability benefits programs. He is currently chair of the Poverty Law Section of the American Association of Law Schools and Associate Director of the Stein Center on Ethics and Public Interest Law at Fordham Law School.

One of the most influential philosophers of law of our time, **Joel Feinberg** is emeritus professor of philosophy at the University of Arizona. Feinberg has published the four-volume

Moral Limits of the Criminal Law; Rights, Justice, and the Bounds of Liberty: Essays in Social Justice; Essays in Social Philosophy; Freedom and Fulfillment: Philosophical Essays; Doing and Deserving and many other books and papers. Feinberg is a former chair of the Board of Officers of the American Philosophical Association.

Leslie Francis is a professor of philosophy, a professor of law and an adjunct professor of internal medicine at the University of Utah. She received her Ph.D. in philosophy from the University of Michigan, and her J.D. from the University of Utah. She is the author of *Sexual Harassment as an Ethical Issue in Academic Life* and of many papers on affirmative action, justice in health care, and health care and the elderly. She is coeditor of *Genetics and Criminality* (American Psychological Association, 1999). She is a member of the American Bar Association's Commission on the Legal Problems of the Elderly, and past chair of the American Philosophical Association's Committee for the Defense of the Professional Rights of Philosophers.

Political scientist and disability theorist **Harlan Hahn** is one of the founding figures in disability studies. He is credited with formulating the minority model of disability and influencing the development of the political process which led to the Americans with Disabilities Act. Hahn now heads the Disability Forum. He is a professor of political science at the University of Southern California.

Michelle Hibbert is a graduate of Chicago-Kent College of Law. She has published on forensic DNA testing, prenatal screening and research on Native American remains. She practices law at Meyer, Hendricks, and Bivens in Phoenix.

Patricia Illingworth is an assistant professor of philosophy and religion at Northeastern University. She is also an attorney in Massachusetts. Professor Illingworth has published in the areas of professional ethics, AIDS and social policy, and health care policy.

Melinda Jones is the director of the Australian Human Rights Centre at the Faculty of Law, University of NSW, and Editor-in-Chief of the *Australian Journal of Human Rights*. With Lee Ann Basser Marks, Jones researches the area of law and the social construction of disability. Together they edited *Disability, Divers-ability and Legal Change*.

The late **Gregory S. Kavka** was a professor of philosophy and social sciences at the University of California, Irvine, where he taught moral and political philosophy. The author of *Hobbesian Moral and Political Theory* and *Moral Paradoxes of Nuclear Deterrence,* he also published many papers on the history of political philosophy, rational choice theory, moral theory and applied ethics. His "Disability and the Right to Work," reprinted here, is a classic study in the philosophy of disability.

Mark Kelman is the William Nelson Cromwell Professor of Law at Stanford University. He has written extensively about antidiscrimination law and tax policy/distributive ethics. He is the coauthor (with Gillian Lester) of *Jumping the Queue: An Inquiry into the Legal Treatment of Students with Learning Disabilities*.

Eva Feder Kittay is a professor of philosophy at SUNY, Stony Brook. She is mother of two children, one of whom is her disabled daughter Sesha, the subject of the essay included in this volume. She has written numerous articles on issues pertaining to women, ethics and social and political philosophy and is an expert on metaphor and the philosophy of language. Her most recent book is *Love's Labor: Essays on Women, Equality, and Dependency*.

The eminent moral philosopher **Alasdair MacIntyre**'s most recent book is *Dependent Rational Animals: Why Human Beings Need the Virtues,* which discusses the moral importance of the part people with disabilities play in the common life of communities. MacIntyre's other books include *A Short History of Ethics, After Virtue, Whose Justice? Which Rationality?* and *Three Rival Versions of Moral Enquiry.* He currently is Arts and Sciences Professor of Philosophy at Duke University.

Lee Ann Basser Marks is a senior lecturer in the School of Law and Legal Studies at Latrobe University, Latrobe, Australia. She researches and teaches family law and disability law. She is a coeditor of *Disability, Divers-ability and Legal Change,* an interdisciplinary, international collection of essays on law and disability.

Arlene Mayerson has been directing attorney of the Disability Rights Education and Defense Fund (DREDF) since 1981. One of the nation's leading experts in disability rights law, she has been a key advisor to both Congress and the disability community on the major legislation in this field. Mayerson has written and consulted in every disability rights case before the U.S. Supreme Court since the mid-1980s, either as counsel or as amicus. Mayerson serves by appointment of the Secretary of U.S. Department of Education on the Civil Rights Reviewing Authority.

David Orentlicher is Samuel R. Rosen Professor of Law and codirector of the Center for Law and Health at Indiana University School of Law-Indianapolis. A graduate of the Harvard Medical School and Harvard Law School, he is coauthor of *Health Care Law and Ethics* and has published widely on issues in bioethics and law. During the 1997–1998 academic year, he was the DeCamp Visiting Professor of Bioethics at Princeton University.

Wendy E. Parmet is a professor of law at Northeastern University School of Law in Boston, where she teaches disability law, health law and bioethics. Parmet has published articles on the ADA, HIV law and public health law and was cocounsel for the plaintiff, Sidney Abbott, in *Bragdon v. Abbott,* the Supreme Court's first case considering the ADA's definition of disability.

Thomas Pogge is an associate professor of philosophy at Columbia University. He has published extensively on theories and applications of Rawlsian approaches to justice. He is currently a member of the Princeton Institute for Advanced Study and is writing a book tentatively entitled *Real World Justice* for Oxford University Press.

Richard K. Scotch is an associate professor of sociology and political economy in the School of Social Sciences at the University of Texas at Dallas. His *From Good Will to Civil Rights: Transforming Federal Disability Policy* traces the development and implementation of Sections 503 and 504 of the Rehabilitation Act. Scotch has written extensively on American disability policy and social movements in the disability community, including two books and numerous articles and monographs.

Anita Silvers, professor of philosophy at San Francisco State University, is the coauthor of *Disability, Difference, Discrimination.* She is the coeditor of several books in bioethics, most recently *Physician Assisted Suicide: Expanding the Debate* and the forthcoming *Health Care and Distributive Justice.* She writes on ethics and bio-ethics, social philosophy, aesthetics, feminism, public policy and disability studies. Silvers received the California Faculty Association's Equal Rights Award for her advocacy of people with disabilities in higher education.

Michael Ashley Stein received a J.D. from Harvard Law School and a Ph.D. from Cambridge University. Among leading academics in the field of disability law, Stein is assistant professor at the College of William and Mary School of Law.

David Wasserman, (J.D., University of Michigan) is a research scholar at the Institute for Philosophy and Public Policy in the School of Public Affairs at the University of Maryland. He writes about the moral underpinnings of criminal law and legal practice, the concept of discrimination, and procedural and distributive justice, including ethical and policy issues in disability, reproduction, and genetic research and technology. In addition to numerous articles and book chapters, he has authored *A Sword For the Convicted: Representing Indigent Defendants on Appeal,* coauthored *Disability, Difference, Discrimination,* and coedited *Genetics and Criminal Behavior: Methods, Meanings, and Morals.*

Iris Marion Young is a professor of political science at the University of Chicago. She is the author of several books, including *Justice and the Politics of Difference, Intersecting Voices: Dilemmas of Gender, Political Philosophy and Policy,* and *Inclusion and Democracy* (forthcoming). Her influential work in social and political philosophy and in feminist philosophy has been systematically inclusive in examining issues important to people with disabilities. Young's writings are often cited in political theory scholarship in the field of disability studies.

Index